STRESS AND ADDICTION

Biological and Psychological Mechanisms

STRESS AND ADDICTION

Biological and Psychological Mechanisms

Edited by

MUSTAFA AL'ABSI, Ph.D.
University of Minnesota Medical School
Duluth, MN, USA

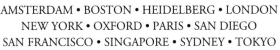

AMSTERDAM • BOSTON • HEIDELBERG • LONDON
NEW YORK • OXFORD • PARIS • SAN DIEGO
SAN FRANCISCO • SINGAPORE • SYDNEY • TOKYO
Academic Press is an imprint of Elsevier

Academic Press is an imprint of Elsevier
30 Corporate Drive, Suite 400, Burlington, MA 01803, USA
525 B Street, Suite 1900, San Diego, California 92101-4495, USA
84 Theobald's Road, London WC1X 8RR, UK

Library of Congress Cataloging-in-Publication Data
Application submitted

British Library Cataloguing-in-Publication Data
A catalogue record for this book is available from the British Library.

ISBN 13: 978-0-12-370632-4
ISBN 10: 0-12-370632-7

For information on all Academic Press publications
visit our Web site at www.books.elsevier.com

Printed in the United States of America
06   07   08   09   10   9   8   7   6   5   4   3   2   1

Contents

Contributors

Numbers in parentheses indicate the chapter(s) contributed by the authors.

Mustafa al'Absi (13, 18) University of Minnesota Medical School, Department of Behavioral Sciences, 1035 University Avenue, Duluth, MN 55812

Kristin G. Anderson (12) University of California, San Diego, Department of Psychology, McGill Hall, 9500 Gilman Drive, La Jolla, CA 92093-0109

Jean C. Beckham (16) Duke University Medical Center, Durham Veterans Affairs Medical Center, 508 Fulton St., Durham, NC, 27705

Sandra A. Brown (12) University of California, San Diego, Department of Psychology, McGill Hall, 9500 Gilman Drive, MC 0109, La Jolla, CA 92093-0109

Rachel Y. Chong (4) The Johns Hopkins University School of Medicine, Senior Clinical and Research Fellow, 720 Rutland Ave., Ross Building, Baltimore, MD 21205

Gary L. Davis (13) University of Minnesota Medical School, Department of Behavioral Sciences, 1035 University Drive, Duluth, MN 55812

Christopher B. Donahue (9, 15) University of Minnesota, Department of Psychiatry, Fairview-Riverside Hospital, F282/2A West 2450 Riverside Ave., Minneapolis, MN 55454

Michael Ellery (14) Department of Psychology, Dalhousie University, Life Sciences Centre, 1355 Oxford St., Halifax, NS B3H 4J1, Canada

Mary-Anne Enoch (6) National Institute on Alcohol Abuse and Alcoholism, NIH, Laboratory of Neurogenetics, 5625 Fishers Lane, Bethesda, MD 20892-8110

Suzanne Erb (7) University of Toronto, Associate Professor, Department of Life Science, 1265 Military Trail, Scarborough, Ontario M1C 1A4, Canada

Daniel P. Evatt (8) University of Illinois at Chicago, Department of Psychology, 1007 W. Harrison St., Behavioral Sciences Building, Chicago, IL 60607-7137

Nicholas E. Goeders (2) Louisiana State University Health Sciences Center, Department of Pharmacology, Toxicology & Neuroscience, 1501 Kings Highway, Shreveport, LA 71130-3932

Jon E. Grant (9) Butler Hospital, Director, Impulse Control Disorders Clinic, 345 Blackstone Blvd., Providence, RI 02906

Justin E. Greenstein (8) University of Illinois at Chicago, Department of Psychology, 1007 W. Harrison St., Behavioral Sciences Building, Chicago, IL 60607-7137

Mark Hamer (10) University College London, Department of Epidemiology & Public Health, 1–19 Torrington Place, London WC1E 6BT, United Kingdom

Jane Hovland (13) University of Minnesota Medical School, Department of Behavioral Sciences, 1035 University Avenue, Duluth, MN 55812

Jon D. Kassel (8) University of Illinois at Chicago, Department of Psychology, 1007 W. Harrison St., Behavioral Sciences Building, Chicago, IL, 60607-7137

Priscilla Kehoe (5) University of California at Irvine, School of Biological Sciences, Irvine, CA 92697-1450

Clemens Kirschbaum (1) Dresden University of Technology, Department of Psychology, Zellescher Weg 17, A220, D-01062, Dresden, Germany

Therese A. Kosten (5) Yale University School of Medicine, VA-CT Hospital System, Division of Substance Abuse, 950 Campbell Ave., West Haven, CT 06516

Brigitte M. Kudielka (1) University of Trier, Department of Theoretical and Clinical Psychobiology, Johanniterufer 15, 54290 Trier, Germany

Matt G. Kushner (15) University of Minnesota, Department of Psychiatry, Fairview-Riverside Hospital, F282/2A West 2450 Riverside Ave., Minneapolis, MN 55454

William R. Lovallo (11) VA Medical Center, Director, Behavioral Sciences Labs, 921 NE 13th St., Oklahoma City, OK 73104

Michela Marinelli (3) Rosalind Franklin University of Medicine & Science, The Chicago Medical School, Department Cellular & Molecular Pharmacology, 3333 Green Bay Rd., North Chicago, IL 60064

Scott D. Moore (16) Duke University Medical Center, Durham Veterans Affairs Medical Center, 508 Fulton St., Durham, NC 27705

Bonnie J. Nagel (12) University of California, San Diego, Department of Psychology, McGill Hall, 9500 Gilman Drive, La Jolla, CA 92093-0109

Charles B. Nemeroff (17) Emory University School of Medicine, Department of Psychiatry & Behavioral Sciences, Woodruff Memorial Research Building, 101 Woodruff Circle, Atlanta, GA 30322

Katherine A. Patterson (12) University of California, San Diego, Department of Psychology, McGill Hall, 9500 Gilman Drive, La Jolla, CA 92093-0109

Miguel E. Roberts (16) Duke University Medical Center, Durham Veterans Affairs Medical Center, 508 Fulton St., Durham, NC 27705

Linda L. Roesch (8) University of Illinois at Chicago, Department of Psychology, 1007 W. Harrison St., Behavioral Sciences Building, Chicago, IL 60607-7137

Daniel Saal (17) Emory University School of Medicine, Department of Psychiatry & Behavioral Sciences, Suite 4000, Woodruff Memorial Research Building, 101 Woodruff Circle, Atlanta, GA 30322

Andrew Steptoe (10) University College London, Department of Epidemiology & Public Health, 1-19 Torrington Place, London WC1E 6BT, United Kingdom

Sherry H. Stewart (14) Dalhousie University, Professor, Department of Psychology, Halifax, Nova Scotia, B3H 4J1, Canada

Susan R. Tate (12) University of California, San Diego, Department of Psychology, McGill Hall, 9500 Gilman Drive, La Jolla, CA, 92093-0109

Magdalena Uhart (4) The Johns Hopkins University School of Medicine, Research Fellow, 720 Rutland Ave., Ross Building, Room 863, Baltimore, MD 21205

Jennifer C. Veilleux (8) University of Illinois at Chicago, Department of Psychology, 1007 W. Harrison St., Behavioral Sciences Building, Room 1009 (MC 285), Chicago, IL 60607-7137

Gary S. Wand (4) The Johns Hopkins University School of Medicine, Professor of Medicine & Psychiatry, 720 Rutland Ave., Ross Building, Room 863, Baltimore, MD 21205

Margaret C. Wardle (8) University of Illinois at Chicago, Department of Psychology, 1007 W. Harrison St., Behavioral Sciences Building, Room 1009 (MC 285), Chicago, IL 60607-7137

Marisa C. Yates (8) University of Illinois at Chicago, Department of Psychology, 1007 W. Harrison St., Behavioral Sciences Building, Room 1009 (MC 285), Chicago, IL 60607-7137

Foreword

Stress has been defined as the nonspecific response to any common demand upon the body (Hans Selye, *Nature* 1936) or any alteration in psychological homeostatic processes (Susan Burchfield, *Psychosomatic Medicine* 1979). Paralleling these conceptual advances in our understanding of stress has been major advances in our understanding not only of the control of hormonal responses to stressors (definition 1), but also major advances in the neurobiological stress mechanisms independent of a direct action of the classic hormonal systems (definition 2). The evolution of our understanding of the body's stress response has also been accompanied by a major evolution in our understanding of the neurobiology of addiction. Addiction has been conceptualized as a chronic relapsing disorder with roots both in impulsivity and compulsivity and neurobiological mechanisms that change as the subject moves from one domain to the other. The convergence of the two major fields of stress and addiction has led to inevitable convergence of these two fields allowing advances and insights from both fields to inform the other.

The present treatise is an outstanding compendium that broaches the subject of the neurobiology of stress and addiction from two major trajectories (or themes) that meet and interact but provide an excellent framework for future study. One trajectory is the developmental trajectory that contains chapters defining and diagnosing stress and stress disorders and provides key information about psychometric measures necessary. The developmental trajectory also explores the evolution of the interaction of stress and addiction from adolescent vulnerability to actual psychopathology such as posttraumatic stress and other anxiety disorders. The second major trajectory or theme is how environmental factors and genetics provide a vulnerability to stress and addiction. Psychosocial factors, early life stressors, genetic factors in multiple sources of reinforcement, genetic factors in individuals with a family history of addiction, negative affect and impulsivity.

Intertwined in the influence of environment and genetics upon the developmental trajectory is the key element of the neurobiological mechanisms involved which provides the glue holding these themes together to understand such a complex interaction. Emphasis is placed in several chapters on the key role of the hormonal stress response systems to interact with the mesolimbic dopamine system in the initiation of the addictive process. However, equally exciting are the chapters exploring the role of hormonal and brain stress systems in modulating negative affect and relapse components of the drug addiction cycle. One particularly excitf ing theme from the book is how understanding the brain and hormonal stress components of addiction can lead to novel treatments for drug addiction.

Historically, a major cause of relapse in drug addiction long after the dissipation of acute early withdrawal has been the presence of either a stressor or a state oprotracted abstinence associated with a state of stress. A number of chapters in this book address the key role for stress systems in various components of relapse, from glucocorticoid responses predicting the actions of opioid antagonists in preventing relapse, to excessive drinking, to the compelling animal data suggesting that extrahypothalamic corticotropin-releasing factor has an important role in blocking stress-induced reinstatement as demonstrated by administration of selective CRF antagonists. Perhaps equally important are data showing that the *state of stress* produced by acute and protracted abstinence to alcohol and other drugs of abuse as measured in animal models of anxiety is blocked by CRF antagonists. These observations provide a key role for brain stress systems, largely, but not exclusively, coordinated by brain CRF systems in various aspects of the trajectories outlined in the book. CRF certainly controls the hypothalamic-pituitary adrenal response to stressors which contributes impulsivity associated with adolescent drug taking and the vulnerability to addiction. CRF has an important role in controlling autonomic and behavioral responses to stressors, both independent of the pituitary adrenal responses to stressors, which can contribute to dysregulated homeostatic functions associated with the negative emotional state associated with acute withdrawal. CRF clearly has a role in stress-induced reinstatement associated with animal models of relapse. One can envision a stress response system that begins with acute excessive drug intake and an activation of the hypothalamic pituitary adrenal response to stressors, followed by activation of the extrahypothalamic CRF system having a critical role in the compulsivity associated with the loss of control over drug seeking behavior. One might speculate that such an activation drives not only its own dysregulation but also the extrahypothalamic stress systems producing an out of control stress response that can only be temporarily and immediately suppressed by . . . . taking more drug!

Such wild speculation aside, the present treatise provides a broad and in depth perspective of the many domains by which stress and addiction may intersect. Compiled by leaders of the field and representing a translational approach, the book provides a much needed resource for research already completed and a resource that will stimulate new research in the field. Given the burgeoning interest in novel treatments for drug addiction, the information in the present work also provides new conceptualizations and novel frameworks for the aspects of the addiction process clearly driven by a dysregulated stress system.

George F. Koob, Ph.D.
Professor, Molecular and
Integrative Neurosciences Department
The Scripps Research Institute
La Jolla, California

Preface

The idea for this book was conceived after fruitless search for a text covering the scientific evidence of the effects of stress on addiction. Available books either focused on providing advice for recovering drug users on how to deal with stress or reviewed scientific work on addiction or stress alone. Therefore, in the absence of an appropriate textbook, many scientists, practitioners, or instructors resort to using multiple books and/or several selected readings from published articles in order to provide comprehensive didactic training on the topic.

This book was developed to address the need for a comprehensive sourcebook that integrates the basic scientific information with corresponding applied strategies dealing with the topic of stress and addiction. It provides highly focused coverage of the available knowledge on the role of stress in addiction. The breadth and diversity of the materials covered will make it of great interest to researchers, practitioners, and students in the field of addiction and stress-related disorders. Chapters include reviews of state-of-the-art research that set the stage for advanced translational research.

Stress is one of the most common risk factors for drug use and is considered a primary trigger of relapse to drug abuse. In the past two decades, a number of significant advances have been achieved in research focusing on the neurobiological aspects of stress and addiction. With this knowledge came the recognition of the importance of understanding the interaction of stress and addiction and how this interaction may influence risk for initiation and maintenance of addictive behaviors. The results have influenced the way we think about addiction and its etiology and have introduced promising possibilities for developing effective prevention and treatment strategies.

This is a timely book in light of the need to synthesize and summarize the growing knowledge about the biological and psychosocial effects of stress on addiction and relapse. In these stressful times, people who are vulnerable to addiction or who are trying to overcome an addiction may face substantial difficulties. In trying to remedy the lack of integrated materials, I was fortunate to assemble leading transdisciplinary scientists in the area of addiction and stress research to contribute chapters that set the agenda for advancement of research and clinical knowledge to help this vulnerable population afflicted with addiction and stress-related disorders.

The book is divided into three sections. The first includes discussions of the basic physiology and anatomy of addiction and stress. It also includes up-to-date reviews of the biological bases of rewards and vulnerability to addiction and relapse. The second section addresses issues related to psychosocial processes that contribute to stress sensitivity and vulnerability to addiction. The final section deals with the clinical implications of the interactions between stress and addiction with a specific focus on assessment methods, co-morbid conditions, and treatment-related challenges.

Mustafa al'Absi
Duluth, MN
2006

Acknowledgments

I would like to thank my many colleagues and staff at the University of Minnesota Medical School for providing help and support during the development of this book. I am grateful to colleagues who provided valuable inputs on the need for this book. I also owe gratitude to many colleagues and scientists who have influenced my ideas and my approach to this project, especially William R. Lovallo, Larry Wittmers, Gary Davis, Dorothy Hatsukami, Jane Hovland, Stephan Bongard, and Natalie Ceballos. The assistance of Carol Peterman, Angie Harju, Steven Carr, Deanna Ellestad, Barbara Gay, and Tracy Kemp in editing and facilitating timely completion of the manuscripts is highly appreciated.

I would like to thank all the authors for their outstanding manuscripts and for their cooperation and timeliness throughout the preparation of this book. I also would like to acknowledge the support of my research program by the National Institute for Drug Abuse and the National Cancer Institute. Thanks go to the Elsevier publishing team who worked with me on this project: Sara Purdy for management of the initial phase of development, Kirsten Funk for her dedication and efficiency in preparing the book for production, Jeff Freeland for his work on production, and Johannes Menzel for guiding the overall development of the book.

My wife Maha and our daughters Sarah, Susan, and Hana continue to cope well with interruptions to our regular family life whenever I take on additional writing and academic responsibilities. They have done that with love, support, and understanding that have been critical in achieving the successful completion of my work.

Mustafa al'Absi
Duluth, MN
2006

NEUROBIOLOGY OF STRESS AND ADDICTION

1

Biological Bases of the Stress Response

BRIGITTE M. KUDIELKA AND CLEMENS KIRSCHBAUM

In this introductory chapter, we give an overview on the biological bases of the stress response. The major components of the stress response system are the corticotropin-releasing hormone and the locus coeruleus-noradrenaline/autonomic system with their peripheral effectors, the pituitary-adrenal (HPA) axis and the autonomic system.

This chapter is organized in five sections. After a brief introductory section, the second part gives an overview on physiological stress research encompassing the origin of stress research, definitions of stress, stress research, and McEwen's concept of allostatic load. In the third section, the major components of the biological stress response system are characterized in more detail, namely the CRH and LC-noradrenaline/autonomic system. In the body, the stress system interacts with several other important physiological systems. Therefore, other stress-responsive classical endocrine axes like the hypothalamus-pituitary-gonadal (HPG) axis, the hypothalamus-pituitary-growth hormone (HPGH) axis, the hypothalamus-pituitary-prolactinergic (HPP) system, and the hypothalamus-pituitary-thyroid (HPT) axis are introduced in the fourth section. In section five, two further important stress-responsive systems, the immune system and the blood coagulation system, are addressed. First, immune system responses and immune system responses to stress are described. Second, regulation of coagulation and fibrinolysis and functioning of the blood coagulation system under stress are briefly summarized.

I. INTRODUCTION

Stress is a common condition of life and is significantly involved in the maintenance of health or the development of disease. In response to stress, different regulatory systems of the body are activated to improve the ability of the organism to adapt to internal or external challenges. Adaptive responses can be specific to the stressor or can be generalized and nonspecific (see Chrousos and Gold, 1992). The major physiological components of the stress response system are the corticotropin-releasing hormone (CRH) and the locus coeruleus (LC)-noradrenaline/autonomic system with their peripheral effectors, the pituitary-adrenal axis, and the autonomic system. They trigger the release of glucocorticoids (e.g., cortisol in humans) from the adrenal cortex and catecholamines (adrenaline and noradrenaline) from the sympathetic nerves and adrenal medulla, respectively (see Axelrod and Reisine, 1984; Chrousos and Gold, 1992). There are numerous interactions among the components of the hypothalamus-pituitary-adrenal (HPA) axis and the LC-noradrenaline/autonomic (sympathetic) system and other brain elements involved in the regulation of emotion, cognitive function, and behavior (see Axelrod and Reisine, 1984; Chrousos and Gold, 1992). The stress system also interacts with other important physiological systems like the immune system and other classical endocrine axes, which are responsible for reproduction, growth, or thyroid function (see below). In this chapter, we first provide the reader with a brief account of the origins of stress research and trends in physiological stress research, including a description of the model of allostatic load as introduced by McEwen and co-workers (see McEwen, 1998b). Thereafter, we give an overview of the main components of the stress regulating system. Furthermore, other stress-responsive hormone axes are briefly described (e.g., the hypothalamus-pituitary-gonadal axis, the hypothalamus-pituitary-growth-hormone axis, the hypothalamus-pituitary-thyroid axis, etc.). Finally, basic functioning of the immune system and stress-related immunological changes are summarized as well as stress-related changes in other systems, like the blood coagulation system.

II. PHYSIOLOGICAL STRESS RESEARCH

A. The Origin of Stress Research

The term *stress* is most closely associated with the physician Hans Selye, who for the first time defined *stress* as a nonspecific response of the body to any demand characterized by the secretion of glucocorticoids. Selye developed the concept of the *general adaptation syndrome (GAS)*, which encompasses an alarm reaction, a stage of resistance, and finally a stage of exhaustion. The physiological responses to massive or ongoing stress were summarized in the *stress triad*, including the enlargement and hyperactivity of the adrenal cortex; the shrinking or atrophy of the thymus, spleen, lymph nodes, and the lymphatic system; and the appearance of gastrointestinal and bowel ulceration (Selye, 1936, 1937). Regarding health consequences, Selye argued that stress plays a role in the development of every disease and that there is always a particularly weak organ or system (due to heredity or external conditions) that is thus likely to break down under stress. Hence, he concluded that individuals can develop different types of diseases under the influence of the same kind of stressor. In his concept of four basic variations of stress, Selye (1983) pointed out that stress can be based on overstress ("hyperstress"), understress ("hypostress"), damaging stress ("distress"), or good stress ("eustress").

However, Selye's idea of an unspecific stress response to all kinds of stimuli was challenged by Mason (1968a, 1968b, 1971), who underlined the importance of specific emotional reactions that determine a specific endocrine stress response. Mason could show that specific situational characteristics, such as novelty, uncontrollability, unpredictability, ambiguity, anticipation of negative consequences, and high ego-involvement, lead to specific hormonal stress responses.

B. Definition of Stress

Diverse stress definitions have been proposed in the past without final agreement. In their contribution "What is stress?" Levine and Ursin (1991) offered a comprehensive definition of stress, distinguishing between input or stress stimuli, individual processing, and outcome which encompasses physiological (e.g., HPA axis, sympathetic nervous system, immune system responses), behavioral (e.g., attention, arousal, and vigilance), and subjective/

verbal stress reactions (e.g., interpretations, cognitions, and emotions). In this concept, stimuli that require processing are defined as loads. The appraisal process principally determines whether a load becomes a stressor. Individual differences in processing might be based on genetic, ontogenetic, early life and lifelong experiences as well as social factors. A related idea was introduced earlier in the cognitive-transactional model by Lazarus and Folkman (1984). However, several (physiological) stimulus inputs elicit automatic stress responses without prior evaluation, like hemorrhaging. Therefore, others categorize stressors upon their character (systemic versus neurogenic/processive, physical versus psychological), chronicity (acute versus chronic), intermittency, and intensity. According to Levine and Ursin (1991), stress responses to physical and psychological stimuli are primarily determined by the individual interpretation, the individual's ability to effectively "cope" with the stressor, but also by the social context, the social status, genetic factors, gender, developmental stage, and individual lifelong experiences (see also Biondi and Picardi, 1999). Finally, this concept contrasts an unspecific stress response (general alarm) and a specific individual stress reaction. With this idea, their approach offers an integrational view of Selye's and Mason's first approaches to a definition of stress.

C. Stress Research

Two decades after Mason's seminal work, Henry (1992) posited that the HPA axis is activated when a sense of uncontrollability and helplessness emerges while the sympathetic-adrenal-medulla (SAM) axis system (see below) is predominantly activated when an individual is confronted with a challenging situation which can be mastered actively by effort. Studies by Frankenhäuser and co-workers yielded some empirical support for an endocrine stress response model contrasting "effort with distress" (HPA axis) versus "effort without distress" (SAM axis) in humans (Frankenhaeuser et al., 1980; Lundberg, 1983). However, evidence whether cortisol is released specifically in response to uncontrollable situations in humans remains inconclusive (Buchanan et al., 1999; Peters et al., 1998) while more support can be found in animal literature (for more details on this debate see Dickerson and Kemeny, 2004).

In 1999, Biondi and Picardi (1999) provided a review of experimental studies in humans summarizing the effects of different stressors on neuroendocrine stress-responsive axes. The authors emphasized that little is still known about the generalizability of laboratory results and that such data cannot easily be extrapolated to real-life stress conditions. Since there is a marked variability in individual responses to different stressors, they assumed that the subjective perception of the situation might be a main determinant of the psychoendocrine response pattern. In line with a constructivistic perspective, Biondi and Picardi (1999) stated that every given stressor has a strictly personal and idiosyncratic meaning and might lose its "objective" characteristics (see also above). Also Pacak and McCarty (2000) concluded that each stressor produces a specific neurochemical "signature" involving quantitatively, if not qualitatively, distinct central and peripheral mechanisms.

Based on the observation that several studies using different types of negative situations have failed to induce significant cortisol changes, Dickerson and Kemeny (2004) recently conducted a meta-analysis of 208 laboratory studies of acute psychological stressors in order to delineate the essential situational elements capable of eliciting HPA axis responses. Their results showed that motivated performance tasks elicit cortisol responses if they are uncontrollable, creating a context of forced failure, in which a subject is unable to avoid negative consequences or cannot succeed despite best effort, or are characterized by a social component called social-evaluative threat, where task performance could be negatively judged by others. Tasks containing both components (uncontrollability and social-evaluative threat) were associated with the largest HPA axis stress responses and the longest recovery times. The meta-analytical findings fit the theoretical reasoning based on the social self-preservation theory that "uncontrollable threats to the goal of maintaining the 'social self' would trigger reliable and substantial cortisol changes." Dickerson and Kemeny (2004) concluded that the Trier Social Stress Test (TSST) is one of the few available laboratory stress protocols that satisfies the criteria of a motivated performance task that combines elements of uncontrollability and high levels of social-evaluative threat (Kirschbaum et al., 1993; Kudielka et al., In press-a, In press-b).

Besides controlled stress experiments in a laboratory setting, stress researchers are often interested in stress responses to real-life situations or momentary assessment of daily stress. One major advantage of the assessment of cortisol (or other stress parameters) in saliva is that samples can be obtained in the field, i.e., in the natural (social) environment of a subject/patient or in a special setting (ambulatory assessment). Saliva samples can easily be obtained even independently of the researcher. Recently, we could show that electronic monitoring devices can be employed to monitor and improve subjects' adherence to saliva sampling protocols outside the laboratory (Broderick et al., 2004; Kudielka et al., 2003).

D. The Concept of Allostatic Load

1. Introduction to the Model of Allostatic Load

Physiological changes after stress help the organism to adapt to increased demands and maintain homeostasis after challenge and can protect the body in the short run. In contrast, they can cause

damage in the long run and can finally promote development of several stress-related diseases. Following a model introduced by McEwen and Stellar (1993), the biological "costs" of short-term adaptation to stress are described as *allostatic load*. Homeostatic regulation reflects stability within a narrow range (homeostatic systems like body temperature, blood volume and composition, blood oxygen, blood pH, glucose levels must be maintained within a narrow range) while allostatic regulation means stability through change. That means that deviations in a homeostatic system trigger a restorative response to correct the changes. In contrast, the regulation of allostatic (adaptive) systems can operate in a relatively broad range of regulation. Following Sterling and Eyer (1988), allostasis is the regulation of the internal milieu through dynamic change in hormonal and physical parameters. Allostasis is defined as the ability of the body to increase or decrease vital functions to a new steady state.

McEwen and Stellar (1993) concluded that the concept of homeostasis is not helpful in explaining the hidden costs of chronic stress on the organism. Therefore, they extended the concept of allostasis over the dimension of time and introduced the idea of allostatic load. Allostatic load is defined as the cost of chronic exposure to elevated or fluctuating endocrine or neural responses resulting from chronic or repeated challenges that the individual experiences as stressful linking subjective perceptions of stress to the development of diseases (McEwen and Seeman, 1999). Following the model, primary mediators (e.g., cortisol, catecholamines, DHEA-S) lead to primary effects and then to secondary outcomes (e.g., blood pressure, waist-hip ratio, HDL cholesterol, cholesterol/HDL ratio, glycosylated hemoglobin), which lead, finally, to tertiary outcomes that represent actual disease. In the long run, a high allostatic load might result in a number of negative health outcomes, such as diabetes, hypertension, cancer, and cardiovascular disease (McEwen, 1998a,

1998b; McEwen and Seeman, 1999; McEwen and Stellar, 1993).

2. Types of Allostatic Load

According to the model of McEwen (McEwen, 1998a, 1998b), four different scenarios can cause allostatic load: (1) frequent exposure to stress, (2) inability to habituate to repeated challenges, or (3) inability to terminate a stress response. In these three types, allostatic load is promoted by an organism's increased exposure to stress hormones and other allostatic mediators. Finally, (4) an inadequate allostatic response in one allostatic system could be related to an increased activation or inadequate (compensatory) response of another. The model emphasizes that allostatic load not only reflects the impact of lifelong experiences ("wear and tear"), but also covers early life experiences, genetic predispositions, environmental factors, as well as psychological and behavioral parameters. The cascading relationships between these factors could explain individual differences in the susceptibility to stress and, in some cases, disease. For example, early life experiences can calibrate the lifelong pattern of physiological stress responses (Liu et al., 2000; Meaney et al., 1991). Neonatal handling resulted in reduced HPA and SAM axes stress responsiveness for the entire life span. With respect to genetic factors, Wüst and co-workers observed increasing heritability estimates for markers of stimulated HPA axis reactivity with repeated psychosocial stress exposure and reported on a medium-sized, yet distinct genetic influence on the cortisol awakening rise (Federenko et al., 2004; Wüst et al., 2000, 2005). A detailed discussion of the role of genes in the regulation of stress systems can also be found in Koch and Stratakis (2000). Psychological factors, such as anticipating negative consequences, pessimism, anxiety, or worry, also contribute to allostatic load. While the origin of allostatic load can be based on an individual psychological appraisal process, psychological factors can prolong, intensify,

expand, or aggravate the amount of existing allostatic load. Finally, there seems to be a bidirectional influence of stress and lifestyle factors. A further summary of stress and health research and the concept of allostatic load can be found in Kudielka and Kirschbaum (2001).

III. MAJOR COMPONENTS OF THE BIOLOGICAL STRESS RESPONSE SYSTEM

The major physiological stress response systems in the organism are the hypothalamus-pituitary-adrenal (HPA) axis and the LC-noradrenaline/sympathetic system, which trigger the release of glucocorticoids and catecholamines, respectively.

A. The Hypothalamus-Pituitary-Adrenal (HPA) Axis

The HPA axis is a central control and regulatory system of the organism. This hierarchical hormone system encompasses the hypothalamus, the pituitary gland, and the adrenal cortex with their respective hormonal secretagogues (Kupfermann, 1991). Besides its role in stress regulation, the HPA axis is vital for supporting normal physiological functioning.

In face of an internal or external challenge, nerval stimulation of the paraventricular nucleus of the hypothalamus (PVN) initiates the secretion of corticotropin-releasing hormone (CRH). Important afferent stimulation or inhibition of the PVN originates from brain areas like the brain stem, in particular the locus coeruleus and the nucleus tractus solitarius, the amygdala, and hippocampus. In the pituitary, CRH leads to cleavage of proopiomelanocortin (POMC) into adrenocorticotropin (ACTH), beta-endorphin, and other peptides and with subsequent release of these peptides. CRH is the most potent but not the only trigger of ACTH release. Other ACTH secretagogues, like vasopressin, oxytocin, adrenaline, and noradrenaline, significantly modulate the effects of CRH. After release, ACTH is transported via the bloodstream to the adrenal cortex and triggers the secretion of glucocorticoids (predominantly cortisol in humans and corticosterone in rats).

The largest proportion of cortisol is bound to transport proteins in blood (90–95%), only 5–10% of total plasma cortisol circulates as biologically active, "free" cortisol (Mendel, 1989). In contrast to CRH (McClennen et al., 1998) and cortisol (Hiramatsu and Nisula, 1987), ACTH does not bind to transport molecules and therefore is subject to significantly faster enzymatic degradation. Overall functioning of the HPA axis is controlled by several negative feedback loops (Darlington and Dallman, 1995), regulated by mineralocorticoid and glucocorticoid receptors (de Kloet et al., 1998).

Cortisol exerts its effects via genomic as well as nongenomic pathways (McEwen, 1991, 1994). It has a wide range of physiological effects since virtually every nucleated cell in the body has cortisol receptors and significant amounts of glucocorticoids penetrate the blood-brain barrier (de Kloet et al., 1998, 2005). Under stress, cortisol redirects energy utilization among various organs. It simultaneously amplifies energy mobilizing mechanisms and inhibits less relevant organ functions (e.g., promotion of gluconeogenesis and glycogenolysis, reduction of glucose consumption in tissues, lipolysis, mobilization of free fatty acids from fat depots, etc.; Chrousos and Gold, 1992; McEwen, 2003). This helps to overcome the increased metabolic demand presented by a host of challenges. Cortisol also impacts on other important physiological systems. It enhances functioning of the cardiovascular system (in part by increasing the sensitivity for catecholamines), impacts on the immune system (e.g., anti-inflammatory and anti-allergic effects, enhancement of initial trafficking of activated immune cells to sites of infection), regulates fluid volume and response to hemorrhage, exerts significant effects on affective and cognitive processes

(for a meta-analytic review of cortisol effects on memory, see Het et al., 2005), and suppresses stress-induced increases in central neural levels of noradrenaline. CRH, ACTH, and cortisol exhibit pronounced circadian rhythms with maximal cortisol levels shortly after awakening (cortisol awakening rise, CAR) and continuously decreasing levels thereafter (Born et al., 1999; Weitzman et al., 1971; for a review, see Clow et al., 2004).

The HPA axis can be activated by physical activity, psychological stress, or the application of pharmacological substances (Heuser et al., 1994; Mason, 1968a; Rose, 1984). The intensity of a respective endocrine response appears to be dependent of the circadian activity (Windle et al., 1998; but compare Kudielka et al., 2004b). Applying the Trier Social Stress Test, ACTH and cortisol levels rise two- to threefold in about 70–80% of all tested subjects with peak levels around 1–20 minutes after cessation of the task (Kirschbaum et al., 1993; Kudielka et al., 2007a, 2007b).

Since alterations in HPA axis stress responses appear to be a close correlate of different diseases or disease progression, the characterization of an individual's HPA axis response pattern to psychosocial stress is of major interest. In 1992, Chrousos and Gold concluded "that the theoretical framework for testing the hypothesis that a dysregulation in the stress system can lead to human disease has been set in place with the potential for improved understanding, diagnosis, and treatment of such disorders." A dysfunctional HPA axis is associated with manifestations of psychosomatic and psychiatric disorders (for reviews, see Chrousos and Gold, 1992; Heim et al., 2000; Holsboer, 1989; Raison and Miller, 2003; Stratakis and Chrousos, 1995; Tsigos and Chrousos, 1994; Tsigos and Chrousos, 2002). For example, HPA axis hyperactivity is often found in major depression and also seems to be associated with susceptibility to infectious diseases and cardiovascular problems. A hyperactive CRH system, respectively hyperactive HPA axis under stress, may also be associated with chronic active alcoholism, alcohol and narcotic withdrawal, as well as an increased vulnerability to narcotic self-administration and predisposition to develop amphetamine addiction (see Chrousos and Gold, 1992). Hyporeactivity of the HPA axis system is associated with autoimmune processes such as lupus erythematosis, multiple sclerosis, neurodermatitis or fibromyalgia, chronic fatigue syndrome, and rheumatoid arthritis. Is has been argued that sex differences in HPA axis stress responses might be causally linked, at least in part, to sex differences in stress-related diseases (for overview, see Kudielka et al., 2000; Kudielka and Kirschbaum, 2005). It is generally accepted that exposure to stress can cause and/or intensify numerous existing diseases.

B. The Locus Coeruleus-Noradrenaline/ Autonomic System

The central regulatory components of the locus coeruleus (LC)-noradrenaline/ autonomic system are the hypothalamus and the locus coeruleus (LC). These structures build the conjunction to the classical endocrine system. Activation of the LC-noradrenaline/autonomic (sympathetic) nervous system, located in the brain stem, leads to the discharge of the neurotransmitter noradrenaline from a dense network of neurons throughout the brain, resulting in enhanced arousal, vigilance, and increased anxiety (Chrousos and Gold, 1992). As outlined by Chrousos and Gold, major brain systems like the amygdala/hippocampus complex and the mesocortical and meso-limbic dopamine systems (which innervate the prefrontal cortex) are activated by the stress system and in turn influence its activity. In contrast to other classical endocrine axes, the sympathetic-adrenal-medulla (SAM) axis is not characterized by a hierarchical organization with integrated feedback loops. Sympathetic nerve fibers project to single chromaffin mark cells

in the adrenal medulla with cholinergic synapses. Interestingly, the endocrine cells in the adrenal medulla can be regarded as modified sympathetic postganglionic cells. The sympathetic nerves, innervated by the CNS, stimulate the adrenal medulla, which in turn secretes adrenaline (~80%) and noradrenaline (~20%). In the medulla, the conversion of noradrenaline to adrenalin is mediated by cortisol. In sum, adrenaline (and to a lesser extent noradrenaline) is released peripherally from the adrenal medulla, while noradrenaline is released from sympathetic nerve terminals throughout the remainder of the sympathethic nervous system. Under resting conditions, the adrenal medulla releases only low levels of catecholamines into the blood. During stress, significant amounts may be secreted from the adrenal medulla (up to approximately 35% of the total circulating noradrenaline), while the remaining is released from sympathetic nerve endings and may enter the bloodstream from the site of release. Catecholamines are then transported throughout the body and impact on organ systems (except parts of the CNS with intact blood-brain barrier).

Adrenaline and noradrenaline secreted from the adrenal medulla can have the same target organs as the neurotransmitter of postganglionic sympathetic neurons. However, noradrenaline released from sympathetic nerve endings acts mainly locally with only a small proportion of released noradrenaline reaching the bloodstream. In order to interpret plasma noradrenaline levels in response to stress, one must therefore consider the indirect and distant relationship between plasma noradrenaline levels and sympathetic nerve activity. Although adrenaline has several equivalent effects on the body as direct sympathetic stimulation, the effects last considerably longer and can, via the bloodstream, also reach organs without direct sympathetic innervations (for reviews, see Goldstein, 2000; Hjemdahl, 2000; Kvetnansky and McCarty, 2000; Pollard, 2000). The effects of catecholamines are exerted via membrane alpha and beta adrenoreceptors. In general, adrenaline and noradrenaline show only gradually different effects; however, due to differential affinity for alpha and beta adrenergic receptors, different physiological effects can emerge. In the bloodstream, catecholamines are mostly bound to sulfate and show a short half-life (1–2 minutes). The effect of a sympathetic nerve impulse is even shorter. Inactivation takes place due to a rapid reuptake in postganglionic neurons and fast enzymatic degradation by catechol-O-methyltransferase (COMT) or monoamine oxidase (MAO), respectively (Hoeldtke et al., 1983). In general, the adrenal medulla may function in concert with the sympathetic nervous system, or it may function somewhat independently in meeting homeostatic demands (Kvetnansky and McCarty, 2000).

Besides extreme heat or cold, pain, blood loss, and lack of oxygen supply, etc., physical effort (e.g., physical labor, exercising like bicycle ergometry and treadmill running) and psychological stress (e.g., parachute jumps, exams, free speeches, cognitive conflict tasks, the Trier Social Stress Test) activate catecholamine release (Axelrod and Reisine, 1984; Mason, 1968b; Schommer et al., 2003). Interestingly, under repeated psychosocial stress, the reactivity of the HPA axis and the SAM system dissociates. Although HPA axis responses quickly habituate, the SAM system shows rather uniform activation patterns with repeated exposure to psychosocial challenge (Schommer et al., 2003). The fundamental role of catecholamine secretion is the rapid mobilization of stored energy depots (e.g., supply of free fatty acids and glucose, glucogenolysis, lipolysis) and to downregulate less important organ functions (e.g., the gastrointestinal tract, reproduction; see also below). In respect to cardiovascular functioning during stress, catecholamines mediate the so-called defense reaction with increases in heart rate, cardiac output, and blood pressure

(for reviews, see Hjemdahl, 2000; Pollard, 2000). Catecholamines also facilitate the oxygen supply via dilatation of the bronchial tubes; enhance platelet aggregation and reduce clotting time (see below); and impact on the vascular smooth muscles causing the shunting of blood away from the skin, mucosa, and kidney to the coronary arteries, skeletal muscle, and the brain. Furthermore, central noradrenergic neurons terminate in the PVN and synapse on CRH neurons directly activating CRH neurons (see above). Some of these stress-related adaptational processes were identified as the "fight-and-flight" response by Cannon as early as at the beginning of the last century (Cannon, 1929).

IV. OTHER STRESS-RESPONSIVE HORMONE AXES

Besides the HPA and SAM axes, several other endocrine systems contribute to a reestablishment of homeostasis under stress. Some of these systems that show significant alterations during periods of acute stress are briefly presented in the following section. These systems act directly by changes in the release or the biological effects of endocrine stress mediators, or act more indirectly by changing levels of monitored parameters which then in turn provoke homeostatic adjustment.

A. The Hypothalamus-Pituitary-Gonadal (HPG) Axis

Under stress, there is a temporary decrease in reproductive function to shift energy to other more important organ systems, which are vital for immediate survival. The inhibition of reproduction under stressful conditions probably serves the purpose to delay reproduction to a more auspicious time (McEwen and Seeman, 1999). Under chronic stress conditions, all levels of HPG axis functioning (hypothalamus, anterior pituitary, and gonads) seem to be decreased resulting in lowered GnRH (gonadotropin-releasing hormone), LH (luteinizing hormone), and FSH (follicle-stimulating hormone), as well as reduced sex hormone levels, an effect which can mainly be ascribed to stress-induced increases in HPA axis activity (for reviews, see Berga and Loucks, 2005; Biondi and Picardi, 1999; Pacak and McCarty, 2000; Rivier and Rivest, 1991).

However, evidence from human and animal studies also suggested that acute stress exposure can lead to slightly increased plasma androgen levels and LH (and sometimes FSH) concentrations which are mostly temporary. Altered androgen levels in humans appear not to reflect increased androgen secretion but decreased metabolic clearance and transient alterations in plasma volume. It was speculated that LH levels might increase due to an ACTH-dependent GnRH stimulation in the hypothalamus, though other pathways are possible. Furthermore, the stress-induced LH increase seems to depend on estrogen availability, and it has been speculated whether estrogens might provide some protection against adverse and inhibitory effects of acute stress on HPG axis regulation. Furthermore, noradrenaline, serotonin, and interleukin-1 probably exert inhibitory effects upon HPG axis functioning during acute stress (Knol, 1991; Pacak and McCarty, 2000). In respect to addiction, alterations in HPG axis regulation could be observed in chronic alcoholics during withdrawal (Heinz et al., 1995).

B. The Hypothalamus-Pituitary-Growth Hormone (HPGH) Axis

Growth hormone (GH) shows a strong circardian rhythm and is released from the anterior pituitary triggered by a hypothalamic GHRH (growth hormone-releasing hormone) signal. GH-binding to receptors leads to hepatic secretion of insulin-like growth factor-1 (IGF-1) that mediates many GH effects (Merimee and Grant, 1995). Stress-related activation or inhibition of GH secretion appears to depend

significantly on the type of stressor and the duration of stress (for reviews, see Biondi and Picardi, 1999; Delitala et al., 1987; Pacak and McCarty, 2000). Acute induction or exposure to physical exercise, pain, surgery, hemorrhage, or hypoglycemia, and sometimes confrontation with psychological stress tasks like mental arithmetic, public speaking, exams, or parachute jumps led to a release of growth hormone (GH). In contrast, stressors like cold, hypertonic saline, electric shock, or handling (in animals) resulted in decreased plasma GH concentrations. While acute administration of glucocorticoids stimulates GH secretion, chronically elevated glucocorticoid levels inhibit the release of GH exerting significant effects on actions of the IGF-1 system in the periphery. There is also evidence suggesting that GH responses correlate with changes in catecholamine content in several hypothalamic nuclei. To date, the neural mechanisms regulating stress-induced activation or inhibition of growth hormone secretion are poorly understood (see Pacak and McCarty, 2000).

C. The Hypothalamus-Pituitary-Prolactinergic (HPP) System

Prolactin is also synthesized by the anterior pituitary. Its secretion is mainly regulated by an inhibiting factor of the hypothalamus called prolactin-release-inhibiting hormone (PIH) which is identical to dopamine. In humans and animals, prolactin concentrations predominantly increase during surgery, but may also increase under hypoglycemia, hemorrhage, acute blood withdrawal, pain stress, and physical exercise. By contrast, prolactin responses to psychological stress have not been consistently reported. Some studies found increases in prolactin in response to psychological stress like parachute jumps, exams, or work stress (Anderzen and Arnetz, 1999; Arnetz, 1996; Lokk and Arnetz, 1997; Theorell, 1992). However, other studies yielded contradictory results.

The regulatory mechanisms identifying how prolactin secretion is signaled under stress and what the physiological consequences of stress-related prolactin secretion are remain unclear (for reviews, see Biondi and Picardi, 1999; Delitala et al., 1987; Pacak and McCarty, 2000).

D. The Hypothalamus-Pituitary-Thyroid (HPT) Axis

Secretion of TRH (thyrotropin-releasing hormone) from the hypothalamus triggers the release of thyroid-stimulating hormone (TSH=thyrotropin) by the anterior pituitary which regulates the release of T4 (tetraiodothyronine=thyroxine) and T3 (triiodothyronine) from the thyroid gland. Effects of the thyroid hormones are multifaceted. For instance, in response to cold, the body responds with a marked activation of the HPT axis in order to generate significant amounts of energy to maintain body temperature. Thyroid hormones increase core body temperature since they promote heat production. The catecholamines seem to play an important role in HPT axis thermogenesis. In animals, also forced swimming and noise led to an activation of the HPT axis (Pacak and McCarty, 2000). Pronounced stress-related HPA axis activation is related to a reduction of HPT axis functioning with lowered secretion of TRH and TSH, and a reduced conversion from the relatively inactive T4 to the more biologically active T3. As for HPG axis regulation, it has been speculated that a reduction of HPT axis functioning during (severe) stress is a beneficial defense mechanism that helps to conserve energy resources for other more important organ systems which are vital for immediate survival and restoration of homeostasis. CRH, somatostatin, and cyctokines (e.g., interleukin-1, interleukin-6) are potential inhibitors of HPT axis functioning under acute stress (for reviews, see Chrousos and Gold, 1992; Helmreich et al., 2005; Visser and Fliers,

2000). With respect to addiction, results by Baumgartner et al. (1994) showed numerous abnormalities in HPT axis regulation in chronic alcoholics during withdrawal and after abstinence.

V. OTHER STRESS-RESPONSIVE SYSTEMS

A. The Immune System

1. Immune System Responses

The immune system consists of organs (e.g., bone marrow, spleen, thymus, lymph nodes), cells (leucocytes such as T/B lymphocytes, natural killer cells, monocytes/macrophages, and granulocytes), and messenger molecules (cytokines, chemokines, prostaglandins, etc.). Dhabhar (2000a) classified the functions of the immune system into six major categories, namely (a) surveillance of the body in preparation for potential immunological challenges, detection and elimination of (b) infectious agents like bacteria, viruses, fungi etc., (c) noninfectious foreign matter, as well as (d) tumors and neoplastic tissues, (e) wound repair and healing, and finally (f) clearance of debris from apoptosis processes. Metaphorically, Dhabhar (2000a) circumscribed the immune system as the body's "army" with "soldiers" (immune cells) moving from their "barracks" (bone marrow, lymph nodes, spleen, thymus) through "highways" (blood vessels and lymphatic ducts) and patrolling almost all organs within the body, especially organs that may serve as potential "battle stations," should the body's defenses be breached. Communication between immune cells and between immune cells and the rest of the body is regulated by messenger molecules such as cytokines and chemokines.

The innate (natural) or unspecific immunity is characterized by immediate activation, nonspecifity, and no memory formation. In contrast the adaptive or specific immunity is characterized by the formation of an immunological memory. As outlined by Segerstrom and Miller (2004), cells involved in natural immunity do not provide defense against any particular pathogen; rather, they are all-purpose cells that can attack a number of different pathogens and do so in a relatively short time frame when challenged. Therefore, the innate immune response is also called the "first defense line," which is mainly regulated by plasma complement proteins and phagocytic cells. Phagocytic cells consist of monocytes (=precursors of macrophages), macrophages, and neutrophils (which belong to the group of granulocytes). All these cells belong to the family of leukocytes (white blood cells). The recognition system of phagocytic cells is nonspecific and rather primitive, but allows for an immediate response. Their main aim is the elimination of pathogens as by capture and digestion of microbes. Activated cells secrete so-called pro-inflammatory cytokines such as TNF-alpha (tumor necrosis factor-alpha), IL-1, and IL-6 (interleukin-1 and -6) in a cascade-like fashion. These cytokines stimulate the secretion of acute phase proteins in the liver, amplify the local immune response by recruiting more phagocytic cells to the infection site, and communicate the infection to the CNS.

If necessary, monocytes and macrophages (besides other cells) present antigen fragments to cells of the adaptive immune system, starting a three-phasic process encompassing an induction, activation, and effector phase (McEwen et al., 1997). Different types of lymphocytes, T and B lymphocytes (T and B cells) mediate the adaptive immune response. T cells can be further divided into cytotoxic T cells (which destroy infected cells) and T helper cells (which help other lymphocytes to intervene). Subgroups of T cells can be distinguished from each other by specific cell surface molecules; for example, cytotoxic T cells are called CD8 positive cells because they express a glycoprotein known as CD8 (see Dantzer, 2000). Binding of an antigen-presenting cell activates a respective T helper cell and triggers

the release of IL-2 and expression of a high affinity IL-2 receptor. IL-2 in turn activates the proliferation and differentiation of naïve (CD4) T cells to mature T effector cells. Activated T helper cells then initiate either a cell-mediated immune response (through phagocytes and cytotoxic T cells) or a humoral-mediated immune response (antibody production of B lymphocytes). T cells that support primarily cellular immunity are so-called TH1 or inflammatory T cells, while those supporting humoral immunity are called TH2 cells (Mosmann et al., 1986; Mosmann and Sad, 1996). The most effective inducer of TH1/TH2 differentiation is the cytokine environment present during the development of the precursor cells (e.g., the pro-inflammatory cytokines TNF-alpha and IL-12 support differentiation into TH1 cells, while the anti-inflammatory cytokines IL-4 and IL-10 support differentiation into TH2 cells (Fearon and Locksley, 1996; Rincon and Flavell, 1997). TH1 cells secrete interferon-gamma (INF-gamma), TNF-beta, and IL-2 (so-called type 1 cytokines), mediate phagocyte activation, and stimulate macrophages to produce TNF-alpha, IL-1, and IL-6. These cytokines attract further inflammatory cells to the site of infection. TH2 cells produce IL-4, IL-5, IL-10, and IL-13 (so-called type 2 cytokines) that primarily act as growth and differentiation factors for B cells, and thereby evoke strong antibody responses. Antibodies are soluble proteins (so-called immunoglobulins, Ig) that neutralize extracellular infectious agents, which are then destroyed by macrophages, neutrophils, or complement proteins. A TH1 immune response is essential for the fight against intracellular bacteria, while the TH2 response is required to combat extracellular infections. Though, overactivation of TH1 or TH2 immune responses appears to be related to different diseases (Elenkov and Chrousos, 1999; Romagnani, 1996). Despite these classifications, an immune response is often a combination of innate (specific) and adaptive (acquired) immune reactions. A concise overview can also be found in the recent excellent review by Segerstrom and Miller (2004).

2. Stress and Immune System Responses

The immune system is an important component of acute stress responses, and numerous changes in immune functioning can be observed under different kinds of stress including psychological stimuli (for reviews, see Glaser, 2005; Kiecolt-Glaser et al., 2002; Kiecolt-Glaser and Glaser, 1995). For example, stress influences leukocyte trafficking (away from the blood), natural killer cell activity (NK cells are identified by surface molecules such as CD16 and CD56), lymphocyte proliferation, antibody production, effector cell function, and cell-mediated immune reactions (Dhabhar, 2000b). A stress-related increase of pro-inflammatory cytokines helps to maintain immunologic homeostasis during stressful situations and in turn participates in HPA axis regulation. As shown in animal research, the inflammatory cytokines TNF-alpha, IL-1, and IL-6 (through activation of CRH neurons in the PVN) are potent stimulators of hypothalamic CRH (Bernardini et al., 1990; Naitoh et al., 1988; Sapolsky et al., 1987). Also, immune activation itself can induce a stress response similar to psychological or other physiological stimuli (Besedovsky et al., 1991).

Stress-induced elevated glucocorticoids are known to suppress inflammation and the acute phase response to infections mainly by altered leukocyte functioning/redistribution or by decreased production of cytokines/mediators of inflammation (e.g., type 1 cytokines). Immunosuppressive effects of glucocorticoids are essential to keep stress-related immune responses under control to minimize damage that the immune system might inflict in case of overactivation (Munck et al., 1984). In line with this, Lewis rats characterized by an innate hyporesponsive HPA axis show an increased susceptibility to inflammatory diseases upon exposure to stressful stimuli (Sternberg et al., 1989a, 1989b). At the same time, glucocorticoids

enhance initial mobilization of immune cells to sites of infection and shape the nature of the immune response, favoring for example humoral over cellular immunity, or under some conditions enhance cytokine function and proliferative responses and phagocytosis (Dhabhar, 2000b; McEwen, 2003).

Recently, Dhabhar and McEwen (1999) reported that stress has bidirectional effects on immune function such that acute stress is merely immunoenhancing, while chronic stress is rather immunosuppressive. This is in line with findings that CRH, catecholamines, and sympathetic activation can have both stimulating and inhibitory effects upon diverse components of the immune system (Chrousos, 1995; Dhabhar, 2000b; Reichlin, 1993; Sapolsky et al., 2000). In their recent review and meta-analysis of over 300 empirical stress studies, Segerstrom and Miller (2004) concluded that acute (laboratory) stressors were predominantly associated with adaptive upregulation of some parameters of natural immunity and downregulation of some functions of specific immunity, while naturalistic stressors (like academic exams) tended to suppress cellular immunity but preserved humoral immunity. Chronic stress was accompanied by suppression of both cellular and humoral parameters, respectively.

B. The Blood Coagulation System

1. Regulation of Coagulation and Fibrinolysis

Fibrin is the main component of a blood clot (thrombus). In the human blood, a small amount of fibrin is permanently formed and dissolved. Via a cascade-like activation of different coagulation factors, prothrombin is converted into thrombin, which in turn converts fibrinogen into fibrin. The action of thrombin is inhibited by binding to antithrombin III and the formation of a thrombin/antithrombin III-complex (TAT) in order to prevent overactivity of the coagulation process. In the fibrinolytic process, fibrin is dissolved by activation of plasmin.

In this process, fibrin degradation products are generated (e.g., D-dimer). Heightened levels of TAT and D-dimer indicate increased formation of thrombin and fibrin, respectively, and are thought to be potential indices of a hypercoagulable state or activity of the coagulation cascade (for a more detailed overview, see von Känel, 2003).

2. Stress and the Blood Coagulation System

Although acute stress simultaneously activates procoagulant molecules (e.g., fibrinogen, von Willebrand Factor or vWF) as well as fibrinolytic molecules (e.g., tissue plasminogen activator, t-PA), the physiological equilibrium between coagulation and fibrinolysis might be altered under stress favoring a hypercoagulable state (von Känel et al., 2001a, 2001b, 2004, 2005). A chronic hypercoagulable state, e.g., due to chronic stress conditions, may increase cardiovascular risk (von Känel et al., 2001a, 2001b, 2004, 2005). Changes in blood coagulation and fibrinolysis with stress are largely mediated by the sympathetic nervous system via catecholamine and adrenergic receptor activity. Stress might also affect coagulation activity via an influence on the regulation of genes coding for coagulation and fibrinolysis molecules (von Känel, 2003; von Känel and Dimsdale, 2000).

VI. FINAL REMARKS

More than 10 years of research with a standardized stress protocol in our as well as in other laboratories worldwide confirmed that acute psychosocial stress in a laboratory setting elicits a concert of physiological changes in the human body (see Kudielka et al., 2007a, 2007b). For example, exposure to the Trier Social Stress Test (TSST) elicits significant activation of HPA axis hormones and catecholamines; increases in heart rate, blood pressure, growth hormone, prolactin and testosterone levels, alpha-amylase concentrations, several immune parameters (e.g., neutrophils, eosinophils, basophils, lym-

phocytes, IL-6, TNF-alpha); and measures of hemoconcentration (hematocrit, hemoglobin, plasma volume) (Buske-Kirschbaum et al., 2002; Kirschbaum et al., 1993; Kudielka et al., 2004a; Kudielka and Kirschbaum, 2005; Nater et al., 2005, 2006, Rohleder et al., 2004; Schommer et al., 2003; von Känel et al., 2006; Zgraggen et al., 2005).

REFERENCES

Anderzen, I., and Arnetz, B. B. (1999). Psychophysiological reactions to international adjustment. Results from a controlled, longitudinal study. *Psychother Psychosom, 68*, 67–75.

Arnetz, B. B. (1996). Techno-stress: A prospective psychophysiological study of the impact of a controlled stress-reduction program in advanced telecommunication systems design work. *J Occup Environ Med, 38*, 53–65.

Axelrod, J., and Reisine, T. D. (1984). Stress hormones: Their interaction and regulation. *Science, 224*, 452–459.

Baumgartner, A., Rommelspacher, H., Otto, M., Schmidt, L. G., Kurten, I., Graf, K. J., Campos-Barros, A., and Platz, W. (1994). Hypothalamic-pituitary-thyroid (HPT) axis in chronic alcoholism. I. HPT axis in chronic alcoholics during withdrawal and after 3 weeks of abstinence. *Alcohol Clin Exp Res, 18*, 284–294.

Berga, S. L., and Loucks, T. L. (2005). The diagnosis and treatment of stress-induced anovulation. *Minerva Ginecol, 57*, 45–54.

Bernardini, R., Kamilaris, T. C., Calogero, A. E., Johnson, E. O., Gomez, M. T., Gold, P. W., and Chrousos, G. P. (1990). Interactions between tumor necrosis factor-alpha, hypothalamic corticotropin-releasing hormone, and adrenocorticotropin secretion in the rat. *Endocrinology, 126*, 2876–2881.

Besedovsky, H. O., del Rey, A., Klusman, I., Furukawa, H., Monge Arditi, G., and Kabiersch, A. (1991). Cytokines as modulators of the hypothalamus-pituitary-adrenal axis. *J Steroid Biochem Mol Biol, 40*, 613–618.

Biondi, M., and Picardi, A. (1999). Psychological stress and neuroendocrine function in humans: The last two decades of research. *Psychother Psychosom, 68*, 114–150.

Born, J., Hansen, K., Marshall, L., Molle, M., and Fehm, H. L. (1999). Timing the end of nocturnal sleep. *Nature, 397*, 29–30.

Broderick, J. E., Arnold, D., Kudielka, B. M., and Kirschbaum, C. (2004). Salivary cortisol sampling compliance: Comparison of patients and healthy volunteers. *Psychoneuroendocrinology, 29*, 636–650.

Buchanan, T. W., al'Absi, M., and Lovallo, W. R. (1999). Cortisol fluctuates with increases and decreases in negative affect. *Psychoneuroendocrinology, 24,* 227–241.

Buske-Kirschbaum, A., Gierens, A., Hollig, H., and Hellhammer, D. H. (2002). Stress-induced immuno-modulation is altered in patients with atopic dermatitis. *J Neuroimmunol, 129,* 161–167.

Cannon, W. B. (1929). Organization of physiological homeostasis. *Physiol Rev, 9,* 399–431.

Chrousos, G. P. (1995). The hypothalamic-pituitary-adrenal axis and immune-mediated inflammation. *N Engl J Med, 332,* 1351–1362.

Chrousos, G. P., and Gold, P. W. (1992). The concepts of stress and stress system disorders. Overview of physical and behavioral homeostasis. *JAMA, 267,* 1244–1252.

Clow, A., Thorn, L., Evans, P., and Hucklebridge, F. (2004). The awakening cortisol response: Methodological issues and significance. *Stress, 7,* 29–37.

Dantzer, R. (2000). Psychoneuroimmunology. In G. Fink, Ed., *Encyclopedia of stress* (Vol. 2, pp. 294–298). San Diego: Academic Press.

Darlington, D. N., and Dallman, M. F. (1995). Feedback control in endocrine systems. In K. L. Becker, Ed., *Endocrinology and metabolism* (chap 4). Philadelphia: J. B. Lippincott Company.

de Kloet, E. R., Joels, M., and Holsboer, F. (2005). Stress and the brain: From adaptation to disease. *Nat Rev Neurosci, 6,* 463–475.

de Kloet, E. R., Vreugdenhil, E., Oitzl, M. S., and Joels, M. (1998). Brain corticosteroid receptor balance in health and disease. *Endocr Rev, 19,* 269–301.

Delitala, G., Tomasi, P., and Virdis, R. (1987). Prolactin, growth hormone and thyrotropin-thyroid hormone secretion during stress states in man. *Baillieres Clin Endocrinol Metab, 1,* 391–414.

Dhabhar, F. S. (2000a). Immune cell distribution, Effects of. In G. Fink, Ed., *Encyclopedia of stress* (Vol. 2, pp. 507–514). San Diego: Academic Press.

Dhabhar, F. S. (2000b). Immune function, stress-induced enhancement of. In G. Fink, Ed., *Encyclopedia of stress* (Vol. 2, pp. 515–523). San Diego: Academic Press.

Dhabhar, F. S., and McEwen, B. S. (1999). Enhancing versus suppressive effects of stress hormones on skin immune function. *Proc Natl Acad Sci U S A, 96,* 1059–1064.

Dickerson, S. S., and Kemeny, M. E. (2004). Acute stressors and cortisol responses: A theoretical integration and synthesis of laboratory research. *Psychol Bull, 130,* 355–391.

Elenkov, I. J., and Chrousos, G. P. (1999). Stress hormones, Th1/Th2 patterns, pro/anti-inflammatory cytokines and susceptibility to disease. *Trends Endocrinol Metab, 10,* 359–368.

Fearon, D. T., and Locksley, R. M. (1996). The instructive role of innate immunity in the acquired immune response. *Science, 272,* 50–53.

Federenko, I. S., Nagamine, M., Hellhammer, D. H., Wadhwa, P. D., and Wüst, S. (2004). The heritability of hypothalamus pituitary adrenal axis responses to psychosocial stress is context dependent. *J Clin Endocrinol Metab, 89,* 6244–6250.

Frankenhaeuser, M., Lundberg, U., and Forsman, L. (1980). Dissociation between sympathetic-adrenal and pituitary-adrenal responses to an achievement situation characterized by high controllability: Comparison between type A and type B males and females. *Biol Psychol, 10,* 79–91.

Glaser, R. (2005). Stress-associated immune dysregulation and its importance for human health: A personal history of psychoneuroimmunology. *Brain Behav Immun, 19,* 3–11.

Goldstein, D. S. (2000). Sympathetic nervous system. In G. Fink, Ed., *Encyclopedia of stress* (Vol. 3, pp. 558–565). San Diego: Academic Press.

Heim, C., Ehlert, U., and Hellhammer, D. H. (2000). The potential role of hypocortisolism in the pathophysiology of stress-related bodily disorders. *Psychoneuroendocrinology, 25,* 1–35.

Heinz, A., Rommelspacher, H., Graf, K. J., Kurten, I., Otto, M., and Baumgartner, A. (1995). Hypothalamic-pituitary-gonadal axis, prolactin, and cortisol in alcoholics during withdrawal and after three weeks of abstinence: Comparison with healthy control subjects. *Psychiatry Res, 56,* 81–95.

Helmreich, D. L., Parfitt, D. B., Lu, X. Y., Akil, H., and Watson, S. J. (2005). Relation between the hypothalamic-pituitary-thyroid (HPT) axis and the hypothalamic-pituitary-adrenal (HPA) axis during repeated stress. *Neuroendocrinology, 81,* 183–192.

Henry, J. P. (1992). Biological basis of the stress response. *Integr Physiol Behav Sci, 27,* 66–83.

Het, S., Ramlow, G., and Wolf, O. T. (2005). A meta-analytic review of the effects of acute cortisol administration on human memory. *Psychoneuroendocrinology, 30,* 771–784.

Heuser, I., Yassouridis, A., and Holsboer, F. (1994). The combined dexamethasone/CRH test: A refined laboratory test for psychiatric disorders. *J Psychiatr Res, 28,* 341–356.

Hiramatsu, R., and Nisula, B. C. (1987). Erythrocyte-associated cortisol: *Measurement, kinetics of dissociation, and potential physiological significance. J Clin Endocrinol Metab, 64,* 1224–1232.

Hjemdahl, P. (2000). Cardiovascular system and stress. In G. Fink, Ed., *Encyclopedia of stress* (Vol. 1, pp. 389–403). San Diego: Academic Press.

Hoeldtke, R. D., Cilmi, K. M., Reichard, G. A., Jr., Boden, G., and Owen, O. E. (1983). Assessment of norepinephrine secretion and production. *J Lab Clin Med, 101,* 772–782.

Holsboer, F. (1989). Psychiatric implications of altered limbic-hypothalamic-pituitary-adrenocortical activity. *Eur Arch Psychiatry Neurol Sci, 238,* 302–322.

Kiecolt-Glaser, J. K., and Glaser, R. (1995). Psychoneuro-immunology and health consequences: Data and shared mechanisms. *Psychosom Med, 57,* 269–274.

Kiecolt-Glaser, J. K., McGuire, L., Robles, T. F., and Glaser, R. (2002). Psychoneuroimmunology: Psychological influences on immune function and health. *J Consult Clin Psychol, 70,* 537–547.

Kirschbaum, C., Pirke, K. M., and Hellhammer, D. H. (1993). The 'Trier Social Stress Test'—A tool for investigating psychobiological stress responses in a laboratory setting. *Neuropsychobiology, 28,* 76–81.

Knol, B. W. (1991). Stress and the endocrine hypothalamus-pituitary-testis system: A review. *Vet Q, 13,* 104–114.

Koch, C. A., and Stratakis, C. A. (2000). Genetic factors and stress. In G. Fink, Ed., *Encyclopedia of stress* (Vol. 2, pp. 205–212). San Diego: Academic Press.

Kudielka, B. M., Broderick, J. E., and Kirschbaum, C. (2003). Compliance with saliva sampling protocols: Electronic monitoring reveals invalid cortisol daytime profiles in noncompliant subjects. *Psychosom Med, 65,* 313–319.

Kudielka, B. M., Buske-Kirschbaum, A., Hellhammer, D. H., and Kirschbaum, C. (2007a). Differential heart rate reactivity and recovery after psychosocial stress (TSST) in healthy children, younger adults, and elderly adults: The impact of age and gender. *Int J Behav Med, 11,* 116–121.

Kudielka, B. M., Hellhammer, D. H., and Kirschbaum, C. (2000). Sex differences in human stress response. In G. Fink, Ed., *Encyclopedia of stress* (Vol. 3, pp. 424–429). San Diego: Academic Press.

Kudielka, B. M., Hellhammer, D. H., and Kirschbaum, C. (2007a). Ten years of research with the Trier Social Stress Test (TSST)—revisited. In E. Harmon-Jones and P. Winkielman, Eds., Fundamentals in *Social neuroscience.* New York: Guilford Press.

Kudielka, B. M., and Kirschbaum, C. (2001). Stress and health research. In N. J. Smelser and P. B. Baltes, Eds., *The international encyclopedia of the social and behavioral sciences* (Vol. 22, pp. 15170–15175). Oxford, England: Elsevier.

Kudielka, B. M., and Kirschbaum, C. (2005). Sex differences in HPA axis responses to stress: A review. *Biol Psychol, 69,* 113–132.

Kudielka, B. M., Schommer, N. C., Hellhammer, D. H., and Kirschbaum, C. (2004b). Acute HPA axis responses, heart rate, and mood changes to psychosocial stress (TSST) in humans at different times of day. *Psychoneuroendocrinology, 29,* 983–992.

Kudielka, B. M., Wüst, S., Kirschbaum, C., and Hellhammer, D. H. (2007b). The Trier Social Stress Test (TSST). In G. Fink, Ed., *Encyclopedia of stress* (2nd ed.). San Diego: Academic Press.

Kupfermann, I. (1991). Hypothalamus and limbic system: Peptidergic neurons, homeostasis, and emotional behaviour. In E. R. Kandel, J. H. Schwartz, and T. M. Jessell, Eds., *Principles of neural science* (pp. 735–749). Norwalk, Connecticut: Appleton & Lange.

Kvetnansky, R., and McCarty, R. (2000). Adrenal medulla. In G. Fink, Ed., *Encyclopedia of stress* (Vol. 1, pp. 63–70). San Diego: Academic Press.

Lazarus, R. S., and Folkman, S. (1984). *Stress, appraisal, and coping.* New York: Springer.

Levine, S., and Ursin, H. (1991). What is stress? In M. R. Brown, G. F. Koob, and C. Rivier, Eds., *Stress—Neurobiology and neuroendocinology* (pp. 3–21). New York: Marcel Dekker.

Liu, D., Caldji, C., Sharma, S., Plotsky, P. M., and Meaney, M. J. (2000). Influence of neonatal rearing conditions on stress-induced adrenocorticotropin responses and norepinepherine release in the hypothalamic paraventricular nucleus. *J Neuroendocrinol, 12,* 5–12.

Lokk, J., and Arnetz, B. (1997). Psychophysiological concomitants of organizational change in health care personnel: Effects of a controlled intervention study. *Psychother Psychosom, 66,* 74–77.

Lundberg, U. (1983). Sex differences in behaviour pattern and catecholamine and cortisol excretion in 3–6 year old day-care children. *Biol Psychol, 16,* 109–117.

Mason, J. W. (1968a). A review of psychoendocrine research on the pituitary-adrenal cortical system. *Psychosom Med, 30,* (Suppl), 576–607.

Mason, J. W. (1968b). A review of psychoendocrine research on the sympathetic-adrenal medullary system. *Psychosom Med, 30,* (Suppl), 631–653.

Mason, J. W. (1971). A re-evaluation of the concept of 'non-specificity' in stress theory. *J Psychiatr Res, 8,* 323–333.

McClennen, S. J., Cortright, D. N., and Seasholtz, A. F. (1998). Regulation of pituitary corticotropin-releasing hormone-binding protein messenger ribonucleic acid levels by restraint stress and adrenalectomy. *Endocrinology, 139,* 4435–4441.

McEwen, B. S. (1991). Non-genomic and genomic effects of steroids on neural activity. *Trends Pharmacol Sci, 12,* 141–147.

McEwen, B. S. (1994). Steroid hormone actions on the brain: When is the genome involved? *Horm Behav, 28,* 396–405.

McEwen, B. S. (1998a). Protective and damaging effects of stress mediators. *N Engl J Med, 338,* 171–179.

McEwen, B. S. (1998b). Stress, adaptation, and disease. Allostasis and allostatic load. *Ann N Y Acad Sci, 840,* 33–44.

McEwen, B. S. (2003). Interacting mediators of allostasis and allostatic load: Towards an understanding of resilience in aging. *Metabolism, 52,* 10–16.

McEwen, B. S., Biron, C. A., Brunson, K. W., Bulloch, K., Chambers, W. H., Dhabhar, F. S., Goldfarb, R. H., Kitson, R. P., Miller, A. H., Spencer, R. L., and Weiss, J. M. (1997). The role of adrenocorticoids as modulators of immune function in health and disease: Neural, endocrine and immune interactions. *Brain Res Brain Res Rev, 23,* 79–133.

McEwen, B. S., and Seeman, T. (1999). Protective and damaging effects of mediators of stress. Elaborating and testing the concepts of allostasis and allostatic load. *Ann N Y Acad Sci, 896,* 30–47.

McEwen, B. S., and Stellar, E. (1993). Stress and the individual. Mechanisms leading to disease. *Arch Intern Med, 153,* 2093–2101.

Meaney, M. J., Viau, V., Bhatnagar, S., Betito, K., Iny, L. J., O'Donnell, D., and Mitchell, J. B. (1991). Cellular mechanisms underlying the development and expression of individual differences in the hypothalamic-pituitary-adrenal stress response. *J Steroid Biochem Mol Biol, 39,* 265–274.

Mendel, C. M. (1989). The free hormone hypothesis: A physiologically based mathematical model. *Endocr Rev, 10,* 232–274.

Merimee, T. J., and Grant, M. B. (1995). Growth hormone and its disorders. In K. L. Becker, Ed., *Principles and practice of endocrinology and metabolism* (pp. 129–140). Philadelphia: Lippincott Company.

Mosmann, T. R., Cherwinski, H., Bond, M. W., Giedlin, M. A., and Coffman, R. L. (1986). Two types of murine helper T cell clone. I. Definition according to profiles of lymphokine activities and secreted proteins. *J Immunol, 136,* 2348–2357.

Mosmann, T. R., and Sad, S. (1996). The expanding universe of T-cell subsets: Th1, Th2 and more. *Immunol Today, 17,* 138–146.

Munck, A., Guyre, P. M., and Holbrook, N. J. (1984). Physiological functions of glucocorticoids in stress and their relation to pharmacological actions. *Endocr Rev, 5,* 25–44.

Naitoh, Y., Fukata, J., Tominaga, T., Nakai, Y., Tamai, S., Mori, K., and Imura, H. (1988). Interleukin-6 stimulates the secretion of adrenocorticotropic hormone in conscious, freely-moving rats. *Biochem Biophys Res Commun, 155,* 1459–1463.

Nater, U. M., La Marca, R., Florin, L., Moses, A., Langhans, W., Koller, M. M., and Ehlert, U. (2006). Stress-induced changes in human salivary alpha-amylase activity-associations with adrenergic activity. *Psychoneuroendocrinology, 31,* 49–58.

Nater, U. M., Rohleder, N., Gaab, J., Berger, S., Jud, A., Kirschbaum, C., and Ehlert, U. (2005). Human salivary alpha-amylase reactivity in a psychosocial stress paradigm. *Int J Psychophysiol, 55,* 333–342.

Pacak, K., and McCarty, R. (2000). Acute stress response: Experimental. In G. Fink, Ed., *Encyclopedia of stress* (Vol. 1, pp. 8–17). San Diego: Academic Press.

Peters, M. L., Godaert, G. L., Ballieux, R. E., van Vliet, M., Willemsen, J. J., Sweep, F. C., and Heijnen, C. J. (1998). Cardiovascular and endocrine responses to experimental stress: Effects of mental effort and controllability. *Psychoneuroendocrinology, 23,* 1–17.

Pollard, T. M. (2000). Adrenaline. In G. Fink, Ed., *Encyclopedia of stress* (Vol. 1, pp. 52–58). San Diego: Academic Press.

Raison, C. L., and Miller, A. H. (2003). When not enough is too much: The role of insufficient glucocorticoid signaling in the pathophysiology of stress-related disorders. *Am J Psychiatry, 160,* 1554–1565.

Reichlin, S. (1993). Neuroendocrine-immune interactions. *N Engl J Med, 329,* 1246–1253.

Rincon, M., and Flavell, R. A. (1997). T-cell subsets: Transcriptional control in the Th1/Th2 decision. *Curr Biol, 7,* R729–732.

Rivier, C., and Rivest, S. (1991). Effect of stress on the activity of the hypothalamic-pituitary-gonadal axis: Peripheral and central mechanisms. *Biol Reprod, 45,* 523–532.

Rohleder, N., Nater, U. M., Wolf, J. M., Ehlert, U., and Kirschbaum, C. (2004). Psychosocial stress-induced activation of salivary alpha-amylase: An indicator of sympathetic activity? *Ann N Y Acad Sci, 1032,* 258–263.

Romagnani, S. (1996). Th1 and Th2 in human diseases. *Clin Immunol Immunopathol, 80,* 225–235.

Rose, R. M. (1984). Overview of endocrinology of stress. In G. M. Brown, S. H. Koslow, and S. Reichlin, Eds., *Neuroendocrinology and psychiatric disorder* (pp. 95–122). New York: Raven Press.

Sapolsky, R., Rivier, C., Yamamoto, G., Plotsky, P., and Vale, W. (1987). Interleukin-1 stimulates the secretion of hypothalamic corticotropin-releasing factor. *Science, 238,* 522–524.

Sapolsky, R. M., Romero, L. M., and Munck, A. U. (2000). How do glucocorticoids influence stress responses? Integrating permissive, suppressive, stimulatory, and preparative actions. *Endocr Rev, 21,* 55–89.

Schommer, N. C., Hellhammer, D. H., and Kirschbaum, C. (2003). Dissociation between reactivity of the hypothalamus-pituitary-adrenal axis and the sympathetic-adrenal-medullary system to repeated psychosocial stress. *Psychosom Med, 65,* 450–460.

Segerstrom, S. C., and Miller, G. E. (2004). Psychological stress and the human immune system: A meta-analytic study of 30 years of inquiry. *Psychol Bull, 130,* 601–630.

Selye, H. (1936). A syndrome produced by diverse noxious agents. *Nature, 32.*

Selye, H. (1937). Studies on adaptation. *Endocrinology, 21,* 169–188.

Selye, H. (1983). The stress concept: Past, present, and future. In C. L. Cooper, Ed., *Stress research* (pp. 1–20). New York: McGraw Hill.

Sterling, P., and Eyer, J. (1988). Allostasis: A new paradigm to explain arousal pathology. In S. Fisher and H. S. Reason, Eds., *Handbook of life stress, cognition and health* (pp. 629–649). New York: Wiley.

Sternberg, E. M., Hill, J. M., Chrousos, G. P., Kamilaris, T., Listwak, S. J., Gold, P. W., and Wilder, R. L. (1989a). Inflammatory mediator-induced hypothalamic-pituitary-adrenal axis activation is defective in streptococcal cell wall arthritis-susceptible Lewis rats. *Proc Natl Acad Sci U S A, 86,* 2374–2378.

Sternberg, E. M., Young, W. S., 3rd, Bernardini, R., Calogero, A. E., Chrousos, G. P., Gold, P. W., and Wilder, R. L. (1989b). A central nervous system defect in biosynthesis of corticotropin-releasing hormone is associated with susceptibility to streptococcal cell wall-induced arthritis in Lewis rats. *Proc Natl Acad Sci U S A, 86,* 4771–4775.

Stratakis, C. A., and Chrousos, G. P. (1995). Neuroendocrinology and pathophysiology of the stress system. Annals of the New York academy of sciences. In G. P. Chrousos, R. McCarty, K. Pacâk, G. Cizza, E. Sternberg, P. W. Gold, and R. Kvetnanský, Eds., *Stress: Basic mechanisms and clinical implications* (Vol. 771, pp. 1–18). New York: The New York Academy of Sciences.

Theorell, T. (1992). Prolactin—A hormone that mirrors passiveness in crisis situations. *Integr Physiol Behav Sci, 27,* 32–38.

Tsigos, C., and Chrousos, G. P. (1994). Physiology of the hypothalamic-pituitary-adrenal axis in health and dysregulation in psychiatric and autoimmune disorders. *Endocrinol Metab Clin North Am, 23,* 451–466.

Tsigos, C., and Chrousos, G. P. (2002). Hypothalamic-pituitary-adrenal axis, neuroendocrine factors and stress. *J Psychosom Res, 53,* 865–871.

Visser, T. J., and Fliers, E. (2000). Hypothalamo-pituitary-adrenal axis. In G. Fink, Ed., *Encyclopedia of stress* (Vol. 3, pp. 605–612). San Diego: Academic Press.

von Känel, R. (2003). Changes in blood coagulation in stress and depression—From evolution to gene regulation. *Ther Umsch, 60,* 682–688.

von Känel, R., and Dimsdale, J. E. (2000). Effects of sympathetic activation by adrenergic infusions on hemostasis in vivo. *Eur J Haematol, 65,* 357–369.

von Känel, R., Dimsdale, J. E., Ziegler, M. G., Mills, P. J., Patterson, T. L., Lee, S. K., and Grant, I. (2001a). Effect of acute psychological stress on the hypercoagulable state in subjects (spousal caregivers of patients with Alzheimer's disease) with coronary or cerebrovascular disease and/or systemic hypertension. *Am J Cardiol, 87,* 1405–1408.

von Känel, R., Kudielka, B. M., Hanebuth, D., Preckel, D., and Fischer, J. E. (2005). Different contribution of interleukin-6 and cortisol activity to total plasma fibrin concentration and to acute mental stress-induced fibrin formation. *Clin Sci (Lond), 109,* 61–67.

von Känel, R., Kudielka, B. M., Preckel, D., Hanebuth, D., and Fischer, J. E. (2006). Delayed response and lack of habituation in plasma interleukin-6 to acute mental stress in men. *Brain Behav Immun, 20,* 40–48.

von Känel, R., Mills, P. J., Fainman, C., and Dimsdale, J. E. (2001b). Effects of psychological stress and psychiatric disorders on blood coagulation and fibrinolysis: A biobehavioral pathway to coronary artery disease? *Psychosom Med, 63,* 531–544.

von Känel, R., Preckel, D., Zgraggen, L., Mischler, K., Kudielka, B. M., Haeberli, A., and Fischer, J. E. (2004). The effect of natural habituation on coagulation responses to acute mental stress and recovery in men. *Thromb Haemost, 92,* 1327–1335.

Weitzman, E. D., Fukushima, D., Nogeire, C., Roffwarg, H., Gallagher, T. F., and Hellman, L. (1971). Twenty-four hour pattern of the episodic secretion of cortisol in normal subjects. *J Clin Endocrinol Metab, 33,* 14–22.

Windle, R. J., Wood, S. A., Shanks, N., Lightman, S. L., and Ingram, C. D. (1998). Ultradian rhythm of basal corticosterone release in the female rat: Dynamic interaction with the response to acute stress. *Endocrinology, 139,* 443–450.

Wüst, S., Federenko, I., Hellhammer, D. H., and Kirschbaum, C. (2000). Genetic factors, perceived chronic stress, and the free cortisol response to awakening. *Psychoneuroendocrinology, 25,* 707–720.

Wüst, S., Federenko, I. S., van Rossum, E. F., Koper, J. W., and Hellhammer, D. H. (2005). Habituation of cortisol responses to repeated psychosocial stress—further characterization and impact of genetic factors. *Psychoneuroendocrinology, 30,* 199–211.

Zgraggen, L., Fischer, J. E., Mischler, K., Preckel, D., Kudielka, B. M., and von Känel, R. (2005). Relationship between hemoconcentration and blood coagulation responses to acute mental stress. *Thromb Res, 115,* 175–183.

2

The Hypothalamic-Pituitary-Adrenal Axis and Addiction

NICHOLAS E. GOEDERS

Anecdotal and scientific evidence suggests a link between substance abuse and stress. One explanation for the high concordance between stress-related disorders and drug addiction is the self-medication hypothesis, which suggests that a dually-diagnosed person often uses the abused substance to cope with tension associated with life stressors or to relieve symptoms of anxiety and depression resulting from a traumatic event. However, another characteristic of self-administration is that drug delivery and its subsequent effects on the HPA axis are under the direct control of the individual. This controlled activation of the HPA axis may result in the production of an internal state of arousal or stimulation that is actually sought by the individual (i.e., the sensation-seeking hypothesis). During abstinence, exposure to stressors or drug-associated cues can stimulate the HPA axis to remind the individual about the effects of the abused substance, thus producing craving and promoting relapse. These cues trigger the HPA axis unpredictably and without warning so that the addict feels a loss of control, and the relapse to drug use helps the individual regain control over his

or her HPA axis activation. These data suggest that stress reduction in combination with pharmacotherapies targeting the HPA axis may prove beneficial in reducing cravings and promoting abstinence in individuals seeking treatment for addiction.

I. INTRODUCTION

It is not that surprising that scientists have uncovered a link between drug addiction and the hypothalamo-pituitary-adrenal (HPA) axis. How many times have you heard an alcoholic rationalize his or her addiction by asserting that "I drink to forget" or "I drink for courage" or "I drink to cope"? Or have you heard relapsing cigarette smokers claim that their cravings for cigarettes became too much to bear following exposure to one stressor or another? Cocaine addicts often claim that they use cocaine because it produces feelings of power or control and clarity of thought. Obviously, drug addiction is a much more complex physical and psychological phenomenon than the simplistic statements above indicate, but at the same time increasing evidence suggests

Stress and Addiction: Biological and Psychological Mechanisms
Edited by **Mustafa al'Absi, Ph.D.**

that an addict's belief that his or her drug of choice provides relief from stress or control over life's stressors, which is an important component of addiction, has a biological basis. In general, addictive drugs tend to alter HPA axis activity. Cocaine and other psychomotor stimulants increase HPA axis activity (Goeders, 2002b), as does cigarette smoking (Mendelson et al., 2005; Steptoe and Ussher, 2005) and alcohol intoxication and withdrawal (Adinoff et al., 1998; Adinoff et al., 2003). Conversely, heroin users typically exhibit a hyporesponsive HPA axis and decreased plasma cortisol (Facchinetti et al., 1985; Kreek et al., 2005). This chapter will review the evidence for a physiological basis underlying the role for the HPA axis in drug addiction. Since the majority of the work we have conducted over the last 20 years has primarily involved cocaine, this chapter will focus on the HPA axis and cocaine addiction.

II. STRESS AND THE HPA AXIS

If you were to ask 10 different people for their definitions of stress, you would likely get 10 different answers that would all generally focus on the negative ramifications associated with exposure to stress. Some people might describe stress on the job, stress from dealing with family or friends, or stress related to a traumatic event, and in each case they would likely relate the negative impact the stressor produced, which could include problems sleeping, increased anxiety, ulcers, heart disease, depression and other more serious psychiatric disorders. This is a common misconception since in reality stress is not necessarily exclusively associated with negative events. The modern definition of stress and its implication for disease were developed by the pioneering neuroendocrinologist Hans Selye, who defined stress as the nonspecific response of the body to any demand placed upon it to adapt, whether that demand produces

pleasure or pain (Selye, 1975). Therefore, positive events can be just as "stressful" to the body as negative events. Accordingly, stress can result from the loss of a loved one or from a marriage or birth of a child, a job promotion or the loss of a job, moving into a new house or losing one's home, or any number of events that impact upon an individual's daily life.

Exposure to stress results in the activation of at least two functionally related biological systems, the sympathetic nervous system and the hypothalamo-pituitary-adrenal (HPA) axis (Stratakis and Chrousos, 1995). The activation of these systems makes it possible for an individual to cope with (adapt to) an environmental event through the production of a stress response or the "stress cascade." The sympathetic nervous system is part of the autonomic nervous system, which by definition suggests that the functions of the sympathetic nervous system occur below the level of consciousness (i.e., automatically). The activation of the sympathetic nervous system results in an increase in heart rate, a rise in blood pressure, a shift in blood flow to skeletal muscles, an increase in blood glucose, a dilatation of the pupils, and an increase in respiration. This automatic response, also called the "fight or flight" response, makes it possible for the individual to face the stressor or attempt to escape from it. In reality, however, people cannot run away from (or fight) many of life's stressors but instead must learn to adapt to the environmental (and internal physiological) changes. During positive events (e.g., a marriage ceremony) an individual may perceive his or her increased heart rate as excitement, while an increased heart rate resulting from a negative event (e.g., narrowly avoiding an auto accident) may be perceived as anger or fear. Many abused substances also produce changes in the activity of the sympathetic nervous system (Sinha et al., 2003), and these effects are felt differently by different individuals. One person may relish the increased heart rate (or rush) produced by cocaine, while the same autonomic response may cause another individual to panic.

The HPA axis consists of a complex, well-regulated interaction between the brain, the anterior pituitary gland, and the adrenal cortex (Goeders, 2002a). The initial step in the activation of the HPA axis is the neuronal-regulated secretion of the peptide corticotropin-releasing hormone (CRH). Although CRH is distributed in a number of brain regions (the importance of which will be revealed later in this chapter), it is those CRH-containing neurons localized in the parvocellular division of the paraventricular nucleus (PVN) of the hypothalamus projecting to the external zone of the median eminence that initiate HPA axis activity. These neurons release the peptide into the adenohypophyseal portal circulation in a circadian manner or in response to neuronal stimulation. The interaction of CRH with receptors located on anterior pituitary corticotrophs results in the synthesis of proopiomelanocortin (POMC), a large precursor protein which is proteolytically cleaved to produce several smaller biologically active peptides, including β-endorphin and adrenocorticotropin hormone (ACTH). POMC-derived ACTH diffuses through the general circulation until it reaches the adrenal glands. There it stimulates the biosynthesis of adrenocorticosteroids, most notably the glucocorticoids, cortisol (in humans), and corticosterone (in rats), which results in their secretion from the adrenal cortex. Two types of adrenocorticosteroid receptors have been identified, both of which bind corticosterone (Joëls and de Kloet, 1994). The type I mineralocorticoid receptor has a higher affinity for corticosterone and is usually fully occupied at basal concentrations of the hormone. This receptor also displays a high affinity for the mineralocorticoid, aldosterone. In contrast, the type II glucocorticoid receptor has a lower affinity for corticosterone and is more likely to be occupied when plasma corticosterone is elevated (e.g., during "stress"). This receptor also has a high affinity for the synthetic glucocorticoid, dexamethasone. As mentioned above, psychomotor stimulants (Goeders, 2002b), nicotine-containing cigarettes (Mendelson et al., 2005; Steptoe and Ussher, 2005), and ethanol (Adinoff et al., 1998; Adinoff et al., 2003) increase HPA axis activity, while opioids suppress the HPA axis (Facchinetti et al., 1985; Kreek et al., 2005). The following sections will review the interactions between addiction, stress, and the subsequent activation of the HPA axis.

III. STRESS, THE HPA AXIS, AND THE ACQUISITION OF DRUG TAKING

During the acquisition of drug-taking behavior (e.g., intravenous drug self-administration), an animal comes into contact with a drug and its potentially rewarding effects for the first time (Goeders, 2002a). This is also when the animal learns to make the response that leads to drug delivery, thereby producing reinforcement. Environmental events (e.g., stressors) that decrease the lowest dose of a drug that is recognized by the animal as a reinforcer are considered to be events that increase vulnerability or the propensity for an animal to acquire self-administration. Acquisition can also be facilitated by events that decrease the time required to reach a specified behavioral criterion indicative of self-administration.

The ability of various stressors to alter the acquisition of drug taking in rats has received considerable attention (Goeders, 2002a; Piazza and Le Moal, 1998). The acquisition of amphetamine and cocaine self-administration is enhanced in rats exposed to social isolation (Schenk et al., 1987) or tail pinch (Piazza et al., 1990), in rats witnessing other rats being subjected to electric foot shock (Ramsey and Van Ree, 1993) and in rats born of female rats exposed to restraint during pregnancy (Deminière et al., 1992). Housing with female rats also increases psychomotor stimulant self-administration by male rats (Lemaire et al., 1994), as do other forms of "social stress" including female rats exposed to an attack by a lactating female rat (Haney et al., 1995) or male rats exposed to an attack by an aggressive male (Haney et al., 1995), exposed to the threat of attack following several defeats (Tidey and Miczek, 1997) or exposed to only the threat of attack (Miczek and Mutschler, 1996).

In a classic experiment, we investigated the effects of exposure to response-contingent ("controllable stress") and noncontingent ("uncontrollable stress") electric foot shock on the acquisition of intravenous cocaine self-administration in rats (Goeders and Guerin, 1994). In these experiments, one rat from a group of three randomly received an electric foot shock when it pressed a response lever that also resulted in the presentation of food (response-contingent shock). Although this resulted in a conflict between obtaining food reinforcement and avoiding foot shock, these animals were in some control over whether or not and when shock was delivered. Shock presentation for the second rat in each triad was yoked to the first rat, so that the second rat received foot shock regardless of whether or not it had pressed its food response lever at all (noncontingent shock). Therefore, these rats had no control over the delivery of the stressor. The third rat in each triad responded under the same schedule of food reinforcement as the other two rats but was never shocked. When responding under this food reinforcement/electric foot-shock schedule stabilized for all three rats, testing for the acquisition of cocaine self-administration commenced. These rats were initially tested with an extremely low dose of cocaine (i.e., 0.031 mg/kg/infusion) for 1 week, and this concentration was subsequently doubled weekly through 0.5 mg/kg/infusion, a dose that is readily self-administered by rats. Doses were tested in an ascending order in all of our acquisition experiments since exposure to higher doses of psychomotor stimulants can sensitize

rats to lower doses (Schenk and Partridge, 1997), resulting in the acquisition of self-administration at doses of these drugs that would not otherwise maintain responding. Rats exposed to uncontrollable stress were more sensitive to low doses of cocaine than rats exposed to controllable stress or that were not shocked at all, which emphasizes the importance of controllability over stressor presentation on the effects of that stressor on drug reward (Goeders, 2002b).

Since uncontrollable stress made animals more vulnerable to cocaine, we hypothesized that this process may be mediated through corticosterone (cortisol in humans), which is secreted as the final step of HPA axis activation. Therefore, we next studied the effects of daily injections of corticosterone on the acquisition of cocaine taking (Mantsch et al., 1998). Daily pretreatment with corticosterone produced an increase in sensitivity to cocaine that was almost identical to what we saw with uncontrollable stress. In a related experiment, the adrenal glands were surgically removed (i.e., by adrenalectomy) prior to acquisition testing to effectively eliminate the final step in HPA axis activation. These adrenalectomized rats did not self-administer cocaine at any dose tested even though they quickly learned to respond on another lever for food pellets, indicating that the rats could still learn and perform the necessary lever-pressing response but that cocaine was no longer rewarding (Goeders and Guerin, 1996). In another series of experiments, the synthesis of corticosterone was blocked with daily injections of ketoconazole, a corticosterone synthesis inhibitor, and this reduced both the rate of acquisition of cocaine self-administration and the number of rats reaching the criterion for acquisition under conditions of food restriction (Campbell and Carroll, 2001). Taken together, these preclinical data suggest an important role for stress and the subsequent activation of the HPA axis in the vulnerability for drug taking.

How does exposure to a stressor increase the vulnerability for drug taking? This biological phenomenon likely occurs via a process analogous to sensitization, whereby repeated but intermittent injections of cocaine increase the behavioral and neurochemical responses to subsequent exposure to the drug (Piazza and Le Moal, 1998). Interestingly, exposure to stressors or injections of corticosterone can also result in sensitization to the behavioral and neurochemical responses to cocaine, and these effects are attenuated in rats with their adrenal glands removed or when corticosterone synthesis is inhibited. Although exposure to the stressor itself may be aversive in many cases, the net result is reflected as an increased sensitivity to the drug. This suggests that if certain individuals are more sensitive to stress and/or if they find themselves in an environment where they do not feel that they have adequate control over this stress, then these individuals may be more likely to engage in substance abuse.

IV. STRESS AND VULNERABILITY TO ADDICTION IN HUMANS

There is a growing clinical literature describing the link between stress and addiction (Brady and Sonne, 1999; Brady and Sinha, 2005; Kreek et al., 2005). One group of individuals who appear to be at greater risk for substance abuse are combat veterans, especially those suffering from post-traumatic stress disorder (PTSD), and a number of studies have identified individuals with the dual diagnosis of combat-related PTSD and substance abuse (Keane and Kaloupek, 1997; Kulka et al., 1988). Veterans with PTSD typically report a higher lifetime use of nicotine, alcohol, cocaine, and heroin than veterans screening negative for PTSD (Keane and Kaloupek, 1997; Zaslav, 1994). However, people exposed to stressors other than combat, such as an unhappy marriage, dissatisfac-

tion with employment, or harassment, also report increased rates of addiction (Breslau et al., 1991; Breslau et al., 2003; Gianoulakis, 1998; Kessler et al., 1995). Sexual abuse, trauma, and sexual harassment are also more likely to produce symptoms of PTSD and alcoholism and/or other addictions in women than in men (Newton-Taylor et al., 1998). Adolescents are especially susceptible to social stressors and traumatic life events, and exposure to these stressors can significantly impact their substance use (Arnsten and Shansky, 2004; Baker et al., 2004; McFarlane et al., 2005; Zweben et al., 1994). Examples of such events range from childhood sexual abuse or other childhood trauma to the inability to effectively cope with the demands produced by everyday family or social stressors.

This raises the question of which came first? Do stressors, sexual trauma, and/or PTSD actually lead to subsequent substance use, or does substance use contribute to the occurrence of the traumatic events and/or the development of PTSD in the first place? Obviously, not everyone who experiences trauma and PTSD is a substance abuser, and not every drug addict can trace the etiology of his or her addiction to some specific stressor or traumatic event. Nevertheless, prevalence estimates suggest that rates of substance abuse among individuals with PTSD may be as high as 60–80%, while the rates of PTSD among substance abusers is between 40–60% (Brady and Sinha, 2005; Donovan et al., 2001), indicating that there is a clear relationship between PTSD and increased substance use. One explanation for the high concordance between PTSD (and related disorders) and drug addiction (i.e., dual diagnosis) is the self-medication hypothesis. According to this hypothesis, a dually diagnosed person often uses the abused substance to cope with tension associated with life stressors or to relieve or suppress symptoms of anxiety, irritability, and depression resulting from a traumatic event (Khantzian, 1985), just as highlighted in the introduction to this chapter. Others may also engage in substance abuse to manage symptoms of anxiety and/or depression that may be unrelated to a specific life event.

V. THE HPA AXIS AND THE MAINTENANCE OF DRUG TAKING

In our earliest work in this area, we reported that pretreatment with the benzodiazepine chlordiazepoxide significantly decreased intravenous cocaine self-administration in rats (Goeders et al., 1989). This effect was attenuated when the unit dose of cocaine was increased, suggesting that chlordiazepoxide decreased cocaine reinforcement. In pilot experiments, diazepam also attenuated intravenous cocaine self-administration maintained under a progressive-ratio schedule of reinforcement in rats (Dworkin et al., 1989). However, since these decreases in drug-intake may have resulted from a nonspecific disruption of the ability of the rats to respond, an additional study was conducted. Alprazolam was tested in rats responding under a multiple schedule of intravenous cocaine presentation and food reinforcement, with cocaine available during 1 hour of the session and food presentations available during the other (Goeders et al., 1993). Food reinforcement was used to generate a control performance to evaluate whether or not the effects of alprazolam were specific for cocaine-maintained responding. Initially, responding maintained by both food and cocaine was reduced following exposure to alprazolam. However, tolerance quickly developed to the sedative effects of alprazolam on food-maintained responding during subsequent testing. On the other hand, no tolerance was observed on the ability of alprazolam to reduce cocaine self-administration. The results of these experiments demonstrate that upon repeated administration, alprazolam decreased cocaine self-administration without affecting food-maintained respond-

ing. This outcome suggests that these effects may result from specific actions on cocaine reinforcement rather than nonspecific effects on the ability of the rats to respond. In a more recent experiment, it was shown that alprazolam also reduces cocaine self-administration in baboons without affecting food-maintained responding (Weerts et al., 2005). Benzodiazepines also reduce the subjective effects of d-amphetamine in humans (Rush et al., 2004), and $GABA_A$ receptor agonists (including benzodiazepines) were recently reported to decrease the discriminative stimulus effects of cocaine in rats (Barrett et al., 2005) and rhesus monkeys (Negus et al., 2000) and to reduce cocaine self-administration in rats without affecting food-maintained responding (Barrett et al., 2005). These data indicate that benzodiazepines and other agonists at $GABA_A$ receptors (Sofuoglu and Kosten, 2005) may be useful in the treatment of addiction to psychomotor stimulants.

Benzodiazepines may decrease cocaine self-administration and the subjective effects of the drug because of the effects of these compounds on corticosterone and other "stress" hormones and peptides. Benzodiazepines decrease plasma corticosterone (Keim and Sigg, 1977), cortisol, and ACTH (Meador-Woodruff and Greden, 1988; Torpy et al., 1993) and attenuate cocaine-induced increases in plasma corticosterone (Yang et al., 1992), suggesting that this may be one mechanism by which these drugs decrease cocaine reinforcement. Thus, decreasing plasma corticosterone itself may also reduce cocaine reward. The following experiments were therefore designed to investigate the effects of corticosterone synthesis inhibitors on the maintenance of cocaine self-administration using metyrapone (Goeders and Guerin, 1996) and ketoconazole (Goeders et al., 1998).

Metyrapone blocks the 11β-hydroxylation reaction in the production of corticosterone, thereby resulting in decreases in plasma concentrations of the hormone (Haleem et al., 1988; Haynes, 1990). Pretreatment with metyrapone resulted in significant dose-related decreases in plasma corticosterone and ongoing cocaine self-administration, suggesting that corticosterone is involved in the maintenance as well as the acquisition of cocaine self-administration (Goeders and Guerin, 1996). However, it was not clear whether these effects were specific for cocaine reinforcement or were the result of nonspecific effects on the ability of the rats to respond. An additional experiment was designed to address this problem through the use of a multiple, alternating schedule of food presentation and cocaine self-administration.

Ketoconazole is an oral antimycotic agent with a broad spectrum of activity and low toxicity that is used in the treatment of fungal disease (Sonino, 1987; Thienpont et al., 1979). This drug also inhibits the 11β-hydroxylation and 18-hydroxylation steps in the synthesis of adrenocorticosteroids (Engelhardt et al., 1985) and may also function as a glucocorticoid receptor antagonist (Loose et al., 1983). Furthermore, clinical studies have shown that ketoconazole is effective in the treatment of hypercortisolemic depression that is resistant to standard antidepressant therapy (Ghadirian et al., 1995; Murphy et al., 1991; Wolkowitz et al., 1993). Since depression and anxiety are often manifested during cocaine withdrawal in humans (Gawin and Ellinwood, 1989) and since corticosterone has been implicated in cocaine reinforcement (Goeders, 1997), the following experiments were therefore designed to investigate the effects of the corticosterone synthesis inhibitor ketoconazole on intravenous cocaine self-administration in rats (Goeders et al., 1998).

In these experiments, rats were allowed alternating 15-minute periods of access to food reinforcement and cocaine self-administration during daily 2-hour sessions. Pretreatment with ketoconazole reduced low dose (i.e., 0.125–0.25 mg/kg/infusion) cocaine self-administration without affecting food-reinforced responding. In fact, pretreatment with ketoconazole resulted in rates

and patterns of self-administration at these doses of cocaine that were indistinguishable from those observed during cocaine extinction, when responding only resulted in infusions of saline. However, these effects were surmounted when the highest dose of cocaine tested was self-administered (i.e., 0.5 mg/kg/infusion). Although basal levels were not altered, ketoconazole also reduced plasma corticosterone in rats trained with the lower doses of cocaine but did not significantly affect the hormone when the highest dose was self-administered. These data suggest that ketoconazole may have reduced drug-intake, at least in part, through its effects on corticosterone.

In our earlier experiments, exposure to uncontrollable electric foot shock shifted the ascending limb of the cocaine acquisition dose-response curve upwards and to the left without affecting the descending limb (Goeders and Guerin, 1994). In other words, electric foot-shock–induced elevations in plasma corticosterone increased low dose cocaine self-administration, but had little or no effect on responding maintained by higher doses of the drug (Goeders and Guerin, 1994). Likewise, exogenous injections of corticosterone also shifted the ascending limb of the acquisition curve for cocaine self-administration to the left without affecting the descending limb (Mantsch et al., 1998). This is a critical distinction since the ascending limb of the cocaine dose-response curve is believed to be more involved with the reinforcing effects of the drug, while the descending limb is also affected by the rate-decreasing effects resulting from higher doses of the drug (Woods et al., 1987). Interestingly, ketoconazole reduced only low dose cocaine self-administration, indicating that the ascending limb of the dose-response curve was specifically affected. These data suggest a potential role for corticosterone in the maintenance of cocaine reinforcement. These data further suggest that the anxiety and depression associated with chronic cocaine use and withdrawal in humans may be related to changes in HPA axis responsiveness resulting from the prolonged and repeated stimulation of ACTH and cortisol secretion.

While the experiments described above suggested an important role for corticosterone in cocaine self-administration, cocaine-induced increases in plasma corticosterone ultimately result from the effects of the drug on CRH secretion from the hypothalamus (Rivier and Vale, 1987; Sarnyai et al., 1992). Therefore, the following experiment was designed to determine the effects of pretreatment with CP-154,526, a centrally active, small molecule CRH1 receptor antagonist, on intravenous cocaine self-administration in rats (Goeders and Guerin, 2000). Rats were trained to respond under the same multiple, alternating schedule of food reinforcement and cocaine self-administration described above. Pretreatment with CP-154,546 did not affect food-maintained responding. However, cocaine self-administration was significantly attenuated, and in some cases completely eliminated, following pretreatment with CP-154,526. Drug intake was decreased across all doses of cocaine tested, with the dose-response curve for cocaine self-administration effectively shifted downward and flattened, suggesting that CP-154,526 decreased cocaine reinforcement. Furthermore, responding on the cocaine lever following CP-154,526 pretreatment was significantly suppressed even during the first 15 minutes of the session, a time when rats typically sample the cocaine lever during extinction (Goeders et al., 1998), suggesting that CRH may be involved in the conditioned effects of cocaine as well (DeVries and Pert, 1998). These data underscore a potential role for CRH in cocaine reinforcement and further suggest a role for the HPA axis in cocaine addiction and withdrawal.

VI. RELAPSE TO ADDICTION

Exposure to external cues previously associated with drug use can trigger relapse in recovering addicts (Ehrman et al., 1992;

Kilgus and Pumariega, 1994), suggesting that pharmacotherapies designed to help these individuals cope with those cues that promote relapse need to be developed. Thus, the development of more effective and efficient strategies for the treatment of addiction depends on an understanding of how these cues contribute to the precipitation of relapse. Accordingly, the development of animal models that reflect many of the salient features of relapse in humans has recently received considerable attention (Markou et al., 1993). One well-studied animal model of relapse involves a reinstatement procedure (Gerber and Stretch, 1975; Stewart and de Wit, 1987). Using this model, rats are trained to self-administer a given drug. Once stable self-administration is observed, the rats are subjected to repeated extinction whereby responding is no longer reinforced by the delivery of the drug or to a period of abstinence from drug availability. Once extinction has been successful or the period of abstinence has been reached, the rats are exposed to various events in an attempt to reinstate drug-seeking behavior.

In humans and nonhumans, the acute re-exposure to the addictive drug itself is a potent event for provoking relapse to drug seeking (de Wit, 1996; Stewart and de Wit, 1987). This drug-induced reinstatement has been observed for both stimulant (de Wit and Stewart, 1981; Gerber and Stretch, 1975; Slikker et al., 1984) and opiate (Davis and Smith, 1976; de Wit and Stewart, 1983) self-administration. Exposure to stress (Wills and Shiffman, 1985), or simply the presentation of stress-related imagery (Li et al., 2005; Sinha et al., 1999, 2000, 2003), is another event that induces craving and relapse in humans. In rats, exposure to stress in the form of intermittent electric foot shock has been reported to reinstate heroin- (Shaham and Stewart, 1995) and cocaine-seeking behavior (Ahmed and Koob, 1997; Erb et al., 1996) in rats without affecting food-seeking behavior (Ahmed and Koob, 1997). We have conducted similar experiments, and in our hands electric foot shock significantly increased responding on the cocaine-paired lever compared to that observed during the previous extinction sessions (Mantsch and Goeders, 1999a). Pretreatment with the corticosterone synthesis inhibitor ketoconazole blocked stress-induced reinstatement. Although plasma corticosterone was still slightly elevated above basal levels in these rats, ketoconazole pretreatment significantly decreased the plasma corticosterone response to electric foot shock, suggesting an important role for corticosterone in the ability of this stressor to reinstate cocaine-seeking behavior in rats. These data also imply that adrenocorticosteroids may be involved in stress-induced cocaine craving in humans as well.

We have also investigated the ability of a cue previously paired with cocaine self-administration to reinstate extinguished cocaine-seeking behavior (Goeders and Clampitt, 2002; Goeders et al., 2000; Meil and See, 1996; See, 2005). In these experiments, responding during reinstatement testing resulted in the contingent presentation of a tone and house light cue that had been paired with cocaine delivery during self-administration training, and this compound stimulus reliably reinstated extinguished cocaine-seeking behavior. Conditioned increases in plasma corticosterone were evident during cocaine extinction as well as during reinstatement (Goeders and Clampitt, 2002). However, while plasma corticosterone returned to basal levels by the end of the session during extinction, it remained elevated through the end of the session during reinstatement, suggesting a potential relationship between HPA axis activation and cue-induced cocaine seeking. In humans, exposure to drug-related cues also increases plasma cortisol and ACTH and activates the sympathetic nervous system (Sinha et al., 2003), suggesting an important involvement of the HPA axis and sympathetic nervous system during drug cue-induced cocaine craving. In our animal studies, pretreatment with ketoconazole reversed the conditioned cue-induced reinstatement of extinguished cocaine-seeking behavior and also attenuated the conditioned increases in plasma corticosterone observed during reinstatement (Goeders and Clampitt, 2002; Goeders et al., 2000), which further underscores a role for the HPA axis in this behavior. In other studies (Clampitt et al., 2001), we demonstrated that pretreatment with oxazepam or alprazolam also prevented the cue-induced reinstatement of extinguished cocaine seeking, suggesting that benzodiazepine therapy may be useful in combating craving induced by conditioned cues associated with cocaine use.

As reported above, CRH1 receptor antagonists are effective in reducing cocaine self-administration (Goeders and Guerin, 2000). However, these compounds also decrease the stress- (Erb et al., 1998; Erb et al., 2001; Shaham et al., 1998) and cocaine- (Erb et al., 1998) induced reinstatement of extinguished cocaine-seeking behavior in rats. We have reported that pretreatment with the CRH receptor antagonist CP-154,526 also reduces the ability of conditioned cues to reinstate extinguished cocaine seeking (Goeders and Clampitt, 2002). We also conducted another series of related experiments based on the observation that animals will respond for days on the lever previously associated with cocaine, even if only saline is delivered (i.e., during extinction), when presented with cues that had been associated with cocaine in the past. It has been hypothesized that such responding is another model of cue-induced cocaine seeking (Weiss et al., 2000). We used this model to test the involvement of CRH1 receptors in cue-induced cocaine seeking by using the selective CRH1 receptor antagonist CP-154,526 (Gurkovskaya and Goeders, 2001). Rats were trained to self-administer cocaine, and when responding stabilized, saline was substituted for cocaine and the animals were tested for extinction for the first time. Other rats were allowed to self-administer cocaine for an additional 30 days, and extinction was tested once again. CP-154,526-treated animals responded significantly less than vehicle-treated animals during extinction on the first day of testing and also after 30 days of self-administration. Interestingly, CP-154,526 did not suppress plasma corticosterone, suggesting that the effects of this compound were acting, in part, independently of the HPA axis and were likely mediated at sites located outside the hypothalamus. However, these data further underscore an important role for CRH in the ability of environmental cues to stimulate cocaine-seeking behavior in rats.

VII. INCONSISTENCIES

Several laboratories have published reports inconsistent with our results with ketoconazole. We reported that pretreatment with ketoconazole at doses that suppress low dose cocaine self-administration (Goeders et al., 1998) and block the stress- (Mantsch and Goeders, 1999a) and cue- (Goeders and Clampitt, 2002) induced reinstatement of extinguished cocaine seeking did not affect the subjective effects of cocaine using a drug discrimination task in rats (Mantsch and Goeders, 1999b). Other laboratories have also demonstrated that ketoconazole fails to alter the subjective effects of cocaine in rats (Filip et al., 2000) and humans (Ward et al., 1998). Thus it appears evident that blocking the synthesis of corticosterone (or cortisol) does not affect the subjective effects of cocaine, suggesting that if a cocaine addict uses cocaine while on ketoconazole treatment, he or she will still likely experience the desired effects of the drug. To this end, we conducted an open-label clinical trial on the effects of chronic ketoconazole on cocaine craving in five cocaine addicts (unpublished results). While all of the subjects reported decreases in cocaine cravings as measured using the Addiction Severity Index and two of the five subjects were completely drug free at the end of the 6 week study, the subjects reported that they could still "get high" if they chose to use cocaine. Other laboratories have reported that ketoconazole does not block the self-administration of cocaine maintained under a fixed-ratio 30 time-out 10-minute schedule of cocaine self-administration in rhesus monkeys (Broadbear et al., 1999), although the lack of effects in this case may have been influenced by nature of the schedule of reinforcement, the behavioral history of the animals or other factors. The results of a 12-week, double-blind clinical trial indicated that chronic ketoconazole treatment increased rather than decreased both heroin and cocaine use in methadone-maintained patients with a history of cocaine abuse or dependence (Kosten et al., 2002). However, it must also be highlighted that these patients also received cortisol to prevent the possibility of ketoconazole-induced adrenal insufficiency, and morning cortisol levels were no different than in patients receiving placebo. All patients were also maintained on methadone. Any of these factors may have mitigated the effects of ketoconazole on cocaine craving. Taken together, however, these data demonstrate that the subjective effects of cocaine are unrelated to changes in plasma corticosterone (or cortisol).

Nevertheless, cocaine has been reported to stimulate HPA axis activity in a manner analogous to various other stressors, which indicates that this system has the potential to influence many of the neurochemical and behavioral effects of the drug. For example, the acute administration of cocaine dose-dependently increases plasma concentrations of corticosterone, ACTH, and β-endorphin in rats (Borowsky and Kuhn, 1991; Moldow and Fischman, 1987; Rivier and Vale, 1987). Cocaine also stimulates the release of ACTH and cortisol in humans (Baumann et al., 1995; Mendelson et al., 1989) and nonhuman primates (Sarnyai et al., 1996) by increasing the peak amplitude of secretory pulses of these hormones without altering pulse frequency, suggesting that these increases are driven by hypothalamic CRH (Mendelson et al., 1989; Sarnyai et al., 1996; Teoh et al., 1994). However, while the HPA axis is important for addiction, especially with respect to the effects of conditioned environmental cues on craving and relapse, we have also recently collected data that suggest that many of the effects we have observed are mediated through sites outside the hypothalamus. For example, as stated above, pretreatment with the CRH receptor antagonist does not produce reliable, reproducible effects on plasma corticosterone (Gurkovskaya and Goeders, 2001). We have seen similar effects (or the lack of effect) in other investigations of this compound (e.g., Goeders and Guerin, 2000), which suggests that the effects of CP-154,526 may be mediated through brain regions outside the hypothalamus.

We have collected additional data suggesting that the medial prefrontal cortex may function as an interface between the HPA axis and the central nervous system. One series of experiments involved the effects of cocaine on benzodiazepine receptor binding. Chronic, daily injections of cocaine for 15 days resulted in differential effects on central benzodiazepine receptor binding in various regions of the rat brain (Goeders et al., 1990a; Goeders, 1991). In general, cocaine decreased binding in terminal fields for the mesocorticolimbic dopaminergic system, while increasing labeling in terminal fields for the nigrostriatal system. Statistically significant decreases in binding in the medial prefrontal cortex and increases in the ventral tegmental area (VTA) were still observed for up to 2 weeks following the final injection of cocaine, suggesting that benzodiazepine receptors in these brain regions may be especially sensitive to the effects of the drug. These cocaine-induced changes in binding appeared to be mediated, at least in part, through the effects of the drug on dopaminergic neuronal activity since intraventricular injections of 6-hydroxydopamine (6-OHDA) attenuated or reversed these effects (Goeders, 1991). Continuous exposure to cocaine has also been reported to alter benzodiazepine receptor binding in various structures of the rat brain (Lipton et al., 1995; Ziegler et al., 1991).

Some of the major symptoms associated with cocaine withdrawal often include severe anxiety, restlessness, and agitation (Crowley, 1987; Gawin and Ellinwood, 1989; Tarr and Macklin, 1987), suggesting that benzodiazepines may be useful for alleviating these negative symptoms during the early stages of withdrawal. These drugs are also useful in the emergency room for the treatment of some of the medical complications associated with cocaine intoxication since convulsions are often apparent following an acute overdose. These seizures can be treated with intravenous diazepam (Gay, 1981; Tarr and Macklin, 1987). Interestingly, the number of benzodiazepine receptors in platelets from chronic cocaine users has been reported to be augmented when compared to those obtained from alcoholics or normal controls (Chesley et al., 1990). In addition, peripheral benzodiazepine receptors labeled with [3H]PK11195 were decreased in neutrophil membranes from the blood of male inpatients following 3 weeks of cocaine abstinence (Javaid et al., 1994). These data indicate that benzodiazepine receptors may mediate some of the biological effects of cocaine in humans. We and others have shown (reviewed above) that benzodiazepines are effective in reducing cocaine self-administration (Barrett et al., 2005; Dworkin et al., 1989; Goeders et al., 1989; Goeders et al., 1993; Weerts et al., 2005) and the cue-induced reinstatement of extinguished cocaine seeking (Clampitt et al., 2001), which suggests that benzodiazepines may be useful in the treatment of cocaine addiction.

In rats, cocaine-induced increases in ACTH and corticosterone can be blocked by pretreatment with the CRH antagonist α-helical CRF9-41 (Sarnyai et al., 1992), by immunoneutralization of CRH with an anti-CRH antibody (Rivier and Vale, 1987; Sarnyai et al., 1993), or by bilateral electrolytic lesions of the PVN (Rivier and Lee, 1994), indicating that these increases are also mediated by the cocaine-induced release of CRH from parvocellular neurons in the PVN. It has been reported that cocaine administration also results in increases in hypothalamic CRH mRNA (Rivier and Lee, 1994; Zhou et al., 1996) and alters CRH receptor binding measured autoradiographically in various regions of the rat brain (Goeders et al., 1990b). These data suggest that the complex relationship between cocaine reinforcement and corticosterone secretion we have previously reported may ultimately result from actions on extra-hypothalamic CRH.

Accordingly, we have also confirmed that ketoconazole-induced changes in cocaine self-administration and reinstatement do not always correspond with decreases in plasma corticosterone, which suggests that other mechanisms must be underlying the behavioral effects that we observe. We recently investigated the effects of acute, repeated, and chronic ketoconazole administration on CRH content in hypothalamic and extrahypothalamic brain sites in rats following the same dosing regimen that we have used in our behavioral studies (Smagin and Goeders, 2004). We found a significant increase in CRH content in the median eminence after the acute administration of ketoconazole that just failed to reach statistical significance following repeated or chronic administration. However, acute, repeated, and chronic treatment with ketoconazole each significantly increased CRH content in the medial prefrontal cortex, but did not consistently affect the peptide in any other brain region studied (Smagin and Goeders, 2004). Since the medial prefrontal cortex and CRH have been implicated in the neurobiology of cocaine (Goeders, 1997; Goeders and Smith, 1983), CRH-induced alterations in dopaminergic neurotransmission may play an important role in this peptide's effects on cocaine responsiveness. Taken together, these data suggest that ketoconazole, as well as CRH receptor antagonists, may affect cocaine reward, at least in part, through interactions with dopamine and CRH within the medial prefrontal cortex.

To this end, we have conducted several neurochemical experiments that support this hypothesis. We investigated the effects of CP-154,526 on cocaine-induced dopamine overflow in the nucleus accumbens and medial prefrontal cortex measured using *in vivo* microdialysis (Gurkovskaya et al., 2005). Rather than decreasing dopamine content as we hypothesized, CP-154,526 actually enhanced the cocaine-induced increases in dopamine in the medial prefrontal cortex and the rostral part of the nucleus accumbens, but did not alter these increases in dopamine in the rest of the nucleus accumbens. In a separate study, we demonstrated that ketoconazole produced a similar augmentation of cocaine-induced increases in dopamine overflow in the medial prefrontal cortex (Smagin and Goeders, 2000). These data implicate prefrontal cortex dopamine in the ability of CRH-receptor antagonists and the corticosterone synthesis inhibitor ketoconazole to attenuate cocaine seeking in rats.

Finally, we recently conducted a study designed to determine differences in the neurochemical and neuroendocrine responses to cocaine during response-contingent and response-independent cocaine administration in rats (Goeders et al., 2004). Male rats were divided into triads of three rats each: One rat was selected as the self-administration rat, while the other two rats were designated as the yoked-cocaine and yoked-saline rats, respectively. Self-administration rats were trained to self-administer cocaine, and each infusion was accompanied by an identical simultaneous cocaine infusion to the yoked-cocaine rat and saline to the yoked-saline rat. Twenty minute microdialysis samples were collected 2 hours prior to, during, and after the self-administration session, and dialysates were analyzed for corticosterone by radioimmunoassay. Baseline corticosterone in the medial prefrontal cortex was low and stable in all groups prior to the start of the self-administration session and remained stable throughout the entire experiment in the yoked-saline rats, suggesting that the procedure itself was not stressful. Medial prefrontal cortex corticosterone was significantly elevated in the microdialysates from the self-administration rats during cocaine self-administration (269% increase), while corticosterone was increased 553% above baseline in the medial prefrontal cortex of the yoked-cocaine rats (Goeders et al., 2004). Medial prefrontal cortex corticosterone was significantly higher in the yoked-cocaine rats compared to the self-administration rats. We conducted similar experiments in the amygdala and the nucleus accumbens, but we did not observe any consistent, reproducible changes in corticosterone in these brain regions. These data suggest that corticosterone in the medial prefrontal cortex may mediate the differences between cocaine reward (in the self-administration rats) and the more aversive aspects of cocaine (in the yoked-cocaine rats; Dworkin et al., 1995), further highlighting the role for this brain region in addiction and suggesting that the medial prefrontal cortex may also serve as an interface between the central nervous system and the HPA axis.

In humans, exposure to cues associated with cocaine induces craving and results in changes in blood flow and metabolic activity in the orbitofrontal cortex and the dorsolateral and anterior cingulate cortices, which loosely correspond to the prefrontal cortex in rats. Increases in glucose metabolism using ^{18}F fluorodeoxyglucose were observed in the dorsolateral cortex and medial orbitofrontal cortex after the presentation of cues associated with cocaine when compared to neutral cues (Grant et al., 1996). In a more recent study by the same group that was designed to extend these initial findings, increases in glucose metabolism were found in the right superior frontal gyrus in the dorsolateral prefrontal cortex and the left lateral orbitofrontal cortex (Bonson et al., 2002). In contrast, glucose metabolism in the left medial prefrontal cortex and the ventromedial frontal pole decreased after the presentation of cocaine-associated cues. Wang et al.

(1999) demonstrated that an interview with the subjects about cocaine use produced increases in metabolism in the orbitofrontal gyrus, but not in the frontal cortex or cingulate gyrus. Both the anterior cingulate cortex and the dorsolateral prefrontal cortex were activated after the subjects watched a cocaine-related video as measured by blood oxygenation using functional magnetic resonance imaging (fMRI; Maas et al., 1998). In a more extensive study, the activation of the left dorsolateral cortex as well as the left anterior cingulate cortex and the left posterior cingulate cortex were also identified using fMRI (Garavan et al., 2000). Finally, cerebral blood flow, measured using ^{15}O-labeled water, increased in the anterior cingulate cortex (Childress et al., 1999; Kilts et al., 2001), but not in the orbitofrontal cortex, in research subjects after internally generated craving (Kilts et al., 2001) or following the presentation of a cocaine-related video (Childress et al., 1999). Taken together, these data highlight the importance of the frontal cortex in cocaine craving in humans, and taken with the preclinical data reviewed above, these data further suggest that the prefrontal cortex may mediate the induction of craving resulting from the cue-induced activation of the HPA axis.

VIII. CONCLUSIONS AND IMPLICATIONS FOR THE TREATMENT OF ADDICTION

There is a clear link between stress and the subsequent activation of the HPA axis and vulnerability for drug addiction. A growing clinical literature highlights this link, with an especially high concordance between PTSD (and related disorders) and drug addiction (i.e., dual diagnosis). One explanation for this phenomenon is the self-medication hypothesis (Khantzian, 1985) whereby a dually diagnosed person often uses the abused substance to cope with tension associated with life stressors. On the surface, however, this may appear somewhat counterintuitive. Many abused substances (especially psychomotor stimulants such as cocaine) can induce anxiety and panic in humans and anxiogenic-like responses in animals through direct effects on CRH release (Goeders, 1997; Goeders, 2002a). Accordingly, one might expect that drug-induced increases in HPA axis activity would enhance the aversive effects of the drug and reduce the motivation for it. During acquisition, however, exposure to aversive, stressful stimuli may actually sensitize individuals, making them more sensitive to drug reward. Once self-administration has been acquired, the positive aspects of drug reward likely mitigate the drug's potential anxiogenic effects (Goeders, 2002b).

However, another characteristic of self-administration is that drug delivery and its subsequent effects on the HPA axis are under the direct control of the individual. This is an important consideration since the controllability and predictability of a stressor significantly decrease its aversive effects (Levine, 2000). The individual controls when the drug is administered and, therefore, when the activation of the HPA axis occurs. This controlled activation of the HPA axis may result in the production of an internal state of arousal or stimulation that is actually sought by the individual (Goeders, 2002b). This internal state may be analogous to novelty or sensation seeking that has been reported in humans (e.g., thrill seekers or sensation seekers) and suggested to be involved in drug reward (Wagner, 2001). Drug taking by this subgroup of substance abusers may represent an attempt to seek out specific sensations, with the internal state produced being very similar to that perceived by individuals who engage in risky, thrill-seeking behavior. These sensation seekers have been reported to be at greater risk for abusing a variety of substances including cocaine, opioids, alcohol, cannabis, and nicotine.

The role for the HPA axis during ongoing drug use is less clear. Inhibiting the synthesis of corticosterone (cortisol) reduces cocaine self-administration (Goeders et al., 1998), but only when low doses of cocaine are available; increasing the unit dose of cocaine overcomes the effects of corticosterone synthesis inhibitors. In addition, corticosterone does not appear to be involved in the subjective effects of cocaine. These data suggest that corticosterone is not an important component of cocaine reward. Rather, corticosterone appears to be more involved with the conditioned effects of cocaine and other drugs. The drug-induced activation of the HPA axis during self-administration becomes associated with specific aspects of the addict's environment, and these environmental cues take on the properties of a conditioned stimulus following repeated pairings. Thus, once drug use has terminated during abstinence, exposure to drug-associated cues (or stressors) stimulates the sympathetic nervous system and activates the HPA axis to remind the individual about the effects of the abused substance, thus producing craving and promoting relapse (Goeders, 2002b). These cues trigger the HPA axis unpredictably and without warning so that the addict feels a loss of control, and the relapse to drug use helps the individual regain control of his or her HPA axis activation. This drug-induced pharmacological activation of the HPA axis overcomes the cue-induced activation of the HPA axis, thereby returning control to the drug user.

What are the implications for the HPA axis in the development of novel pharmacotherapies for the treatment of cocaine and other addictions? Although corticosterone (cortisol) synthesis inhibitors will dampen the ability of environmental cues to activate the HPA axis and stimulate craving during abstinence, these compounds will not alter cocaine reward. Preclinical data suggest that CRH receptor antagonists would be effective in treating ongoing cocaine use as well as dampening the ability of various stimuli (e.g., the drug itself, stressors, and drug-associated cues) to elicit craving and relapse. Unfortunately, as of the date this chapter is being written, there are no CRH receptor antagonists that are FDA approved for use in humans. A growing body of behavioral and biological data suggest that benzodiazepines are capable of reducing cocaine reward, blocking the subjective effects of cocaine and other psychomotor stimulants and reversing the cue-induced reinstatement of extinguished cocaine seeking. However, clinicians are reluctant to prescribe benzodiazepines for the treatment of addictions since there is also an inherent abuse liability associated with these drugs (Tarr and Macklin, 1987).

We have recently collected preliminary data on a novel combination pharmacotherapy with potential for the treatment of cocaine abuse. Using this model, two (or more) drugs with divergent mechanisms of action, but that ultimately produce similar effects on the body's responses to stressors, are administered together at doses that are ineffective when administered alone. In these experiments, we tested doses of a benzodiazepine (e.g., oxazepam) and a corticosterone synthesis inhibitor (e.g., metyrapone) that did not affect cocaine self-administration when administered alone. However, when rats were pretreated with both compounds together, we observed a dramatic and significant decrease in self-administration across several doses of cocaine with no effects on food-maintained responding. We have observed similar effects on the cue-induced reinstatement of extinguished cocaine seeking. While these effects may be partly due to changes in pharmacokinetics, they may also result from the combined, synergistic effects of the two compounds to reduce HPA axis activity. These data suggest a new direction for medications development. By using lower doses, the potential abuse liability of benzodiazepines and the potential hepatotoxic and other side effects of corticosterone synthesis inhibitors can be minimized. Continued investigations into how stress and the subsequent activation of the HPA axis impact addiction will result in the identification of more effective and efficient treatment for substance abuse in humans. Stress reduction and coping strategies, in combination with pharmacotherapies targeting the HPA axis as described above, may prove beneficial in reducing cravings and promoting abstinence in individuals seeking treatment for addiction.

ACKNOWLEDGMENTS

This work was supported by USPHS grants DA06013 and DA13463 from the National Institute on Drug Abuse.

REFERENCES

Adinoff, B., Iranmanesh, A., Veldhuis, J., and Fisher, L. (1998). Disturbances of the stress response: The role of the HPA axis during alcohol withdrawal and abstinence. *Alcohol Health Res. World, 22*, 67–72.

Adinoff, B., Ruether, K., Krebaum, S., Iranmanesh, A., and Williams, M. J. (2003). Increased salivary cortisol concentrations during chronic alcohol intoxication in a naturalistic clinical sample of men. *Alcohol. Clin. Exp. Res., 27*, 1420–1427.

Ahmed, S. H., and Koob, G. F. (1997). Cocaine- but not food-seeking behavior is reinstated by stress after extinction. *Psychopharmacology, 132*, 289–295.

Arnsten, A. F., and Shansky, R. M. (2004). Adolescence: Vulnerable period for stress-induced prefrontal cortical function? Introduction to part IV. *Ann. N. Y. Acad. Sci., 1021*, 143–147.

Baker, T. B., Brandon, T. H., and Chassin, L. (2004). Motivational influences on cigarette smoking. *Annu. Rev. Psychol., 55*, 463–491.

Barrett, A. C., Negus, S. S., Mello, N. K., and Caine, S. B. (2005). Effect of GABA agonists and GABA-A receptor modulators on cocaine- and food-maintained responding and cocaine discrimination in rats. *J. Pharmacol. Exp. Ther., 315*, 858–871.

Baumann, M. H., Gendron, T. M., Becketts, K. M., Henningfield, J. E., Gorelick, D. A., and Rothman, R. B. (1995). Effects of intravenous cocaine on plasma cortisol and prolactin in human cocaine abusers. *Biol. Psychiatry, 38*, 751–755.

Bonson, K. R., Grant, S. J., Contoreggi, C. S., Links, J. M., Metcalfe, J., Weyl, H. L., Kurian, V., Ernst, M., and London, E. D. (2002). Neural systems and cue-induced cocaine craving. *Neuropsychopharmacology, 26*, 376–386.

Borowsky, B., and Kuhn, C. M. (1991). Monoamine mediation of cocaine-induced hypothalamo-pituitary-adrenal activation. *J. Pharmacol. Exp. Ther., 256*, 204–210.

Brady, K. T., and Sinha, R. (2005). Co-occurring mental and substance use disorders: The neurobiological effects of chronic stress. *Am. J. Psychiatry, 162*, 1483–1493.

Brady, K. T., and Sonne, S. C. (1999). The role of stress in alcohol use, alcoholism treatment, and relapse. *Alcohol Res. Health, 23*, 263–271.

Breslau, N., Davis, G. C., Andreski, P., and Peterson, E. (1991). Traumatic events and posttraumatic stress disorder in an urban population of young adults. *Arch. Gen. Psychiatry, 48*, 216–222.

Breslau, N., Davis, G. C., and Schultz, L. R. (2003). Posttraumatic stress disorder and the incidence of nicotine, alcohol, and other drug disorders in persons who have experienced trauma. *Arch. Gen. Psychiatry, 60*, 289–294.

Broadbear, J. H., Winger, G., and Woods, J. H. (1999). Cocaine-reinforced responding in rhesus monkeys: Pharmacological attenuation of the hypothalamic-pituitary-adrenal axis response. *J. Pharmacol. Exp. Ther., 290*, 1347–1355.

Campbell, U. C., and Carroll, M. E. (2001). Effects of ketoconazole on the acquisition of intravenous cocaine self-administration under different feeding conditions in rats. *Psychopharmacology, 154*, 311–318.

Chesley, S. F., Scharzki, A. D., DeUrrutia, J., Greenblatt, D. J., Shader, R. I., and Miller, L. G. (1990). Cocaine augments peripheral benzodiazepine binding in humans. *J. Clin. Psychiatry, 51*, 404–406.

Childress, A. R., Mozley, P. D., McElgin, W., Fitzgerald, J., Reivich, M., and O'Brien, C. P. (1999). Limbic activation during cue-induced cocaine craving. *Am. J. Psychiatry, 156*, 11–18.

Clampitt, D. M., Peltier, R. L., and Goeders, N. E. (2001). The effects of alprazolam on the ability of conditioned cues to reinstate extinguished cocaine-seeking behavior in rats. *Drug Alcohol Depend., 63*, (Suppl. 1) S28.

Crowley, T. J. (1987). Clinical issues in cocaine abuse. In S. Fisher, A. Raskin, and E. H. Uhlenhuth, (Eds.), *Cocaine: Clinical and biobehavioral aspects* (pp. 193–211). New York: Oxford University Press.

Davis, W. M., and Smith, S. G. (1976). Role of conditioned reinforcers in the initiation, maintenance and extinction of drug-seeking behavior. *Pavolv. J. Bio. Sci., 11*, 222–236.

Deminière, J. M., Piazza, P. V., Guegan, G., Abrous, N., Maccari, S., Le Moal, M., and Simon, H. (1992). Increased locomotor response to novelty and propensity to intravenous amphetamine self-administration in adult offspring of stressed mothers. *Brain Res., 586*, 135–139.

DeVries, A. C., and Pert, A. (1998). Conditioned increases in anxiogenic-like behavior following exposure to contextual stimuli associated with cocaine are mediated by corticotropin-releasing factor. *Psychopharmacology, 137*, 333–340.

de Wit, H. (1996). Priming effects with drugs and other reinforcers. *Exp. Clin. Psychopharmacol., 4*, 5–10.

de Wit, H., and Stewart, J. (1981). Reinstatement of cocaine-reinforced responding in the rat. *Psychopharmacology, 75*, 134–143.

de Wit, H., and Stewart, J. (1983). Drug reinstatement of heroin-reinforced responding in the rat. *Psychopharmacology, 79*, 29–31.

Donovan, B., Padin-Rivera, E., and Kowaliw, S. (2001). "Transcend": Initial outcomes from a posttraumatic stress disorder/substance abuse treatment program. *J. Trauma Stress, 14*, 757–772.

Dworkin, S. I., D'Costa, A., Goeders, N. E., and Hoffman, E. (1989). A progressive-ratio schedule for cocaine administration: Effects of cocaine dose and diazepam. *Neurosci. Abstr., 15*, 802.

Dworkin, S. I., Mirkis, S., and Smith, J. E. (1995). Response-dependent versus response-independent presentation of cocaine: Differences in the lethal effects of the drug. *Psychopharmacology, 117*, 262–266.

Ehrman, R. N., Robbins, S. J., Childress, A. R., and O'Brien, C. P. (1992). Conditioned responses to cocaine-related stimuli in cocaine abuse patients. *Psychopharmacology, 107*, 523–529.

Engelhardt, D., Dörr, G., Jaspers, C., and Knorr, D. (1985). Ketoconazole blocks cortisol secretion in man by inhibition of adrenal 11β-hydroxylase. *Klin. Wochenschr., 63*, 607–612.

Erb, S., Salmaso, N., Rodaros, D., and Stewart, J. (2001). A role for the CRF-containing pathway from central nucleus of the amygdala to bed nucleus of the stria terminalis in the stress-induced reinstatement of cocaine seeking in rats. *Psychopharmacology, 158*, 360–365.

Erb, S., Shaham, Y., and Stewart, J. (1996). Stress reinstates cocaine-seeking behavior after prolonged extinction and a drug-free period. *Psychopharmacology, 128*, 408–412.

Erb, S., Shaham, Y., and Stewart J. (1998). The role of corticotropin-releasing factor and corticosterone in stress- and cocaine-induced relapse to cocaine seeking in rats. *J. Neurosci., 18*, 5529–5536.

Facchinetti, F., Volpe, A., Farci, G., Petraglia, F., Porro, C. A., Barbieri, G., Cioni, A., Balestrieri, A., and Genazzani, A. R. (1985). Hypothalamus-pituitary-adrenal axis of heroin addicts. *Drug Alcohol Depend., 15*, 361–366.

Filip, M., Nowak, E., Siwanowicz, J., and Przegalinski, E. (2000). Effects of corticosterone and its synthesis blockade on the cocaine-induced discriminative stimulus effects in rats. *Pol. J. Pharmacol., 52*, 411–421.

Garavan, H., Pankiewicz, J., Bloom, A., Cho, J. K., Sperry, L., Ross, T. J., Salmeron, B. J., Risinger, R., Kelley, D., and Stein, E. A. (2000). Cue-induced cocaine craving: Neuroanatomical specificity for drug users and drug stimuli. *Am. J. Psychiatry, 157*, 1789–1798.

Gawin, F. H., and Ellinwood, E. H. (1989). Cocaine dependence. *Annu. Rev. Med., 40,* 149–161.

Gay, G. R. (1981). You've come a long way baby! Coke time for the new American Lady of the eighties. *J. Psychoactive Drugs, 13,* 297–318.

Gerber, G. J., and Stretch, R. (1975). Drug-induced reinstatement of extinguished self-administration behavior in monkeys. *Pharmacol. Biochem. Behav., 3,* 1055–1061.

Ghadirian, A. M., Engelsmann, F., Dhar, V., Filipini, D., Keller, R., Chouinard, G., and Murphy, B. E. P. (1995). The psychotropic effects of inhibitors of steroid biosynthesis in depressed patients refractory to treatment. *Biol. Psychiatry, 37,* 369–375.

Gianoulakis, C. (1998). Alcohol-seeking behavior: The roles of the hypothalamic-pituitary-adrenal axis and the endogenous opioid system. *Alcohol Health Res. World, 22,* 202–210.

Goeders, N. E. (1991). Cocaine differentially affects benzodiazepine receptors in discrete regions of the rat brain: Persistence and potential mechanisms mediating these effects. *J. Pharmacol. Exp. Ther., 259,* 574–581.

Goeders, N. E. (1997). A neuroendocrine role in cocaine reinforcement. *Psychoneuroendocrinology, 22,* 237–259.

Goeders, N. E. (2002a). The HPA axis and cocaine reinforcement. *Psychoneuroendocrinology, 27,* 13–33.

Goeders, N. E. (2002b). Stress and cocaine addiction. *J. Pharmacol. Exp. Ther., 301,* 785–789.

Goeders, N., Bell, V., Guidroz, A., and McNulty, M. (1990b). Dopaminergic involvement in the cocaine-induced up-regulation of benzodiazepine receptors in the rat striatum. *Brain Res., 515,* 1–8.

Goeders, N. E., Bienvenu, O. J., and De Souza, E. B. (1990a). Chronic cocaine administration alters corticotropin-releasing-factor receptors in the rat brain. *Brain Res., 531,* 322–328.

Goeders, N. E., Clampitt, D., Peltier, R. L., and Guerin, G. F. (2000). Reinstatement of cocaine-seeking behavior using a conditioned reinforcer: Role for the hypothalamo-pituitary-adrenal (HPA) axis. NIDA Research Monograph, Problems of Drug Dependence, 1999, L. S. Harris (Ed.) NIH publication number 00–4737, p. 92.

Goeders, N. E., and Clampitt, D. M. (2002). Potential role for the HPA axis in the conditioned reinforcer-induced reinstatement of extinguished cocaine seeking in rats. *Psychopharmacology, 161,* 222–232.

Goeders, N. E., and Guerin, G. F. (1994). Noncontingent electric footshock facilitates the acquisition of intravenous cocaine self-administration in rats. *Psychopharmacology, 114,* 63–70.

Goeders, N. E., and Guerin, G. F. (1996). Effects of surgical and pharmacological adrenalectomy on the initiation and maintenance of intravenous cocaine self-administration in rats. *Brain Res., 722,* 145–152.

Goeders, N. E., and Guerin, G. F. (2000). Effects of the CRH receptor antagonist CP-154,526 on intravenous cocaine self-administration in rats. *Neuropsychopharmacology, 23,* 577–586.

Goeders, N. E., McNulty, M. A., Mirkis, S., and McAllister, K. H. (1989). Chlordiazepoxide alters intravenous cocaine self-administration in rats. *Pharmacol. Biochem. Behav., 33,* 859–866.

Goeders, N. E., McNulty, M. A., and Guerin, G. F. (1993). Effects of alprazolam on intravenous cocaine self-administration in rats. *Pharmacol. Biochem. Behav., 44,* 471–474.

Goeders, N. E., Peltier, R. L., and Guerin, G. F. (1998). Ketoconazole reduces low dose cocaine self-administration in rats. *Drug Alcohol Depend., 53,* 67–77.

Goeders, N. E., Smagin, G. N., and Palamarchouk, V. S. (2004). Effects of self-administered and passive cocaine infusions on medial prefrontal cortex (MPC) and nucleus accumbens (NA) corticosterone and activity of the hypothalamo-pituitary-adrenal (HPA) axis. Program No. 916.4. 2004 Abstract Viewer/Itinerary Planner. Washington, DC: Society for Neuroscience, 2004. Online.

Goeders, N. E., and Smith, J. E. (1983). Cortical dopaminergic involvement in cocaine reinforcement. *Science, 221,* 773–775.

Grant, S., London, E. D., Newlin, D. B., Villemagne, V. L., Liu, X., Contoreggi, C., Phillips, R. L., Kimes, A. S., and Margolin, A. (1996). Activation of memory circuits during cue-elicited cocaine craving. *Proc. Natl. Acad. Sci. U. S. A., 93,* 12040–12045.

Gurkovskaya, O., and Goeders, N. E. (2001). Effects of CP-154,526 on responding during extinction from cocaine self-administration. *Eur. J. Pharmacol., 432,* 53–56.

Gurkovskaya, O. V., Palamarchouk, V., Smagin, G., and Goeders, N. E. (2005). Effects of corticotropin-releasing hormone receptor antagonists on cocaine-induced dopamine overflow in the medial prefrontal cortex and nucleus accumbens of rats. *Synapse, 57,* 202–212.

Haleem, D. J., Kennet, G., and Curzon, G. (1988). Adaptation of female rats to stress: Shift to male pattern by inhibition of corticosterone synthesis. *Brain Res., 458,* 339–347.

Haney, M., Maccari, S., Le Moal, M., Simon, H., and Piazza, P. V. (1995). Social stress increases the acquisition of cocaine self-administration in male and female rats. *Brain Res., 698,* 46–52.

Haynes, R. C. Jr. (1990). Adrenocorticotropic hormone; adrenocortical steroids and their synthetic analogs; inhibitors of the synthesis and actions of adrenocortical hormones. In A. G. Gilman, T. W. Rall, A. S. Nies, P. Taylor (Eds.), *The pharmacological basis of therapeutics* (8th edition, pp. 1431–1462). New York: Pergamon Press.

Javaid, J. I., Notorangelo, M. P., Pandey, S. C., Reddy, P. L., Pandey, G. N., and Davis, J. M. (1994). Peripheral benzodiazepine receptors are decreased during cocaine withdrawal in humans. *Biol. Psychiatry, 36,* 44–50.

Joëls, M., and de Kloet, E. R. (1994). Mineralocorticoid and glucocorticoid receptors in the brain. Implications for ion permeability and transmitter systems. *Prog. Neurobiol., 43*, 1–36.

Keane, T. M., and Kaloupek, D. G. (1997). Comorbid psychiatric disorders in PTSD. Implications for research. *Ann. N. Y. Acad. Sci., 821*, 24–34.

Keim, K. L., and Sigg, E. B. (1977). Plasma corticosterone and brain catecholamines in stress: Effect of psychotropic drugs. *Pharmacol. Biochem. Behav., 6*, 79–85.

Kessler, R. C., Sonnega, A., Bromet, E., Hughes, M., and Nelson, C. B. (1995). Posttraumatic stress disorder in the National Comorbidity Survey. *Arch. Gen. Psychiatry, 52*, 1048–1060.

Khantzian, E. J. (1985). The self-medication hypothesis of addictive disorders: Focus on heroin and cocaine dependence. *Am. J. Psychiatry, 142*, 1259–1264.

Kilgus, M. D., and Pumariega, A. J. (1994). Experimental manipulation of cocaine craving by videotaped environmental cues. *South Med. J., 87*, 1138–1140.

Kilts, C. D., Schweitzer, J. B., Quinn, C. K., Gross, R. E., Faber, T. L., Muhammad, F., Ely, T. D., Hoffman, J. M., and Drexler, K. P. (2001). Neural activity related to drug craving in cocaine addiction. *Arch. Gen. Psychiatry, 58*, 334–341.

Kosten, T. R., Oliveto, A., Sevarino, K. A., Gonsai, K., and Feingold. A. (2002). Ketoconazole increases cocaine and opioid use in methadone maintained patients. *Drug Alcohol Depend., 66*, 173–180.

Kreek, M. J., Nielsen, D. A., Butelman, E. R., and LaForge, K. S. (2005). Genetic influences on impulsivity, risk taking, stress responsivity and vulnerability to drug abuse and addiction. *Nat. Neurosci., 8*, 1450–1457.

Kulka, R. A., Schlenger, W. E., Fairbank, J. A., Hough, R. L., Jordan, B. K., Marmar, C. R., and Weiss, D. S. (1988). *National Vietnam Veterans Readjustment Study (NVVRS): Description, current status, and initial PTSD prevalence estimates.* Washington, DC: Veterans Administration.

Lemaire, V., Deminière, J. M., and Mormède, P. (1994). Chronic social stress conditions differentially modify vulnerability to amphetamine self-administration. *Brain Res., 649*, 348–352.

Levine, S. (2000). Influence of psychological variables on the activity of the hypothalamic-pituitary-adrenal axis. *Eur. J. Pharmacol., 405*, 149–160.

Li, C. S., Kemp, K., Milivojevic, V., and Sinha, R. (2005). Neuroimaging study of sex differences in the neuropathology of cocaine abuse. *Gend. Med., 2*, 174–182.

Lipton, J. W., Olsen, R. W., and Ellison, G. D. (1995). Length of continuous cocaine exposure determines the persistence of muscarinic and benzodiazepine receptor alterations. *Brain Res., 676*, 378–385.

Loose, D. S., Stover, E. P., and Feldman, D. (1983). Ketoconazole binds to glucocorticoid receptors and exhibits glucocorticoid antagonist activity in cultured cells. *J. Clin. Invest., 72*, 404–408.

Maas, L. C., Lukas, S. E., Kaufman, M. J., Weiss, R. D., Daniels, S. L., Rogers, V. W., Kukes, T. J., and Renshaw, P. F. (1998). Functional magnetic resonance imaging of human brain activation during cue-induced cocaine craving. *Am. J. Psychiatry, 155*, 124–126.

Mantsch, J. R., and Goeders, N. E. (1999a). Ketoconazole blocks the stressor-induced reinstatement of cocaine-seeking behavior in rats: Relationship to the discriminative stimulus effects of cocaine. *Psychopharmacology, 142*, 399–407.

Mantsch, J. R., and Goeders, N. E. (1999b). Ketoconazole does not block cocaine discrimination or the cocaine-induced reinstatement of cocaine-seeking behavior. *Pharmacol. Biochem. Behav., 64*, 65–73.

Mantsch, J. R., Saphier, D., and Goeders, N. E. (1998). Corticosterone facilitates the acquisition of cocaine self-administration in rats: Opposite effects of the glucocorticoid receptor agonist, dexamethasone. *J. Pharmacol. Exp. Ther., 287*, 72–80.

Markou, A., Weiss, F., Gold, L. H., Caine, B., Schulteis, G., and Koob, G. F. (1993). Animal models of drug craving. *Psychopharmacology, 112*, 163–182.

McFarlane, A., Clark, C. R., Bryant, R. A., Williams, L. M., Niaura, R., Paul, R. H., Hitsman, B. L., Stroud, L., Alexander, D. M., and Gordon, E. (2005). The impact of early life stress on psychophysiological, personality and behavioral measures in 740 nonclinical subjects. *J. Integr. Neurosci., 4*, 27–40.

Meador-Woodruff, J. H., and Greden, J. F. (1988). Effects of psychotropic medications on hypothalamic-pituitary-adrenal regulation. *Endocrinol. Metab. Clin. North Am., 17*, 225–234.

Meil, W. M., and See, R. E. (1996). Conditioned cued recovery of responding following prolonged withdrawal from self-administered cocaine in rats: An animal model of relapse. *Behav. Pharmacol., 7*, 754–763.

Mendelson, J. H., Mello, N. K., Teoh, S. K., Ellingboe, J., and Cochin, J. (1989). Cocaine effects on pulsatile secretion of anterior pituitary, gonadal, and adrenal hormones. *J. Clin. Endocrinol. Metab., 69*, 1256–1260.

Mendelson, J. H., Sholar, M. B., Goletiani, N., Siegel, A. J., and Mello, N. K. (2005). Effects of low- and high-nicotine cigarette smoking on mood states and the HPA axis in men. *Neuropsychopharmacology, 30*, 1751–1763.

Miczek, K. A., and Mutschler, N. A. (1996). Activational effects of social stress on IV cocaine self-administration in rats. *Psychopharmacology, 128*, 256–264.

Moldow, R. L., and Fischman, A. J. (1987). Cocaine induced secretion of ACTH, beta-endorphin, and corticosterone. *Peptides, 8*, 819–822.

Murphy, B. E. P., Dhar, V., Ghadirian, A. M., Chouinard, G., and Keller, R. (1991). Response to steroid suppression in major depression resistant to antidepressant therapy. *J. Clin. Psychopharmacol., 11*, 121–126.

Negus, S. S., Mello, N. K., and Fivel, P. A. (2000). Effects of GABA agonists and GABA-A receptor modulators on cocaine discrimination in rhesus monkeys. *Psychopharmacology, 152,* 398–407.

Newton-Taylor, B., DeWit, D., and Gliksman, L. (1998). Prevalence and factors associated with physical and sexual assault of female university students in Ontario. *Health Care Women Int., 19,* 155–164.

Piazza, P. V., Deminière, J. M., Le Moal, M., and Simon, H. (1990). Stress- and pharmacologically-induced behavioral sensitization increases vulnerability to acquisition of amphetamine self-administration. *Brain Res., 514,* 22–26.

Piazza, P. V., and Le Moal, M. (1998). The role of stress in drug self-administration. *Trends Pharmacol. Sci., 19,* 67–74.

Ramsey, N. F., and Van Ree, J. M. (1993). Emotional but not physical stress enhances intravenous cocaine self-administration in drug-naive rats. *Brain Res., 608,* 216–222.

Rivier, C., and Lee, S. (1994). Stimulatory effects of cocaine on ACTH secretion: Role of the hypothalamus. *Mol. Cell. Neurosci., 5,* 189–195.

Rivier, C., and Vale, W. (1987). Cocaine stimulates adrenocorticotropin (ACTH) secretion through a corticotropin-releasing factor (CRF)-mediated mechanism. *Brain Res., 422,* 403–406.

Rush, C. R., Stoops, W. W., Wagner, F. P., Hays, L. R., and Glaser, P. E. (2004). Alprazolam attenuates the behavioral effects of d-amphetamine in humans. *J. Clin. Psychopharmacol., 24,* 410–420.

Sarnyai, Z., Bíró, É., Gardi, J., Vecsernyés, M., Julesz, J., and Telegdy, G. (1993). Alterations of corticotropin-releasing factor-like immunoreactivity in different brain regions after acute cocaine administration in rats. *Brain Res., 616,* 315–319.

Sarnyai, Z., Bíró, É., Penke, B., and Telegdy, G. (1992). The cocaine-induced elevation of plasma corticosterone is mediated by endogenous corticotropin-releasing factor (CRF) in rats. *Brain Res., 589,* 154–156.

Sarnyai, Z., Mello, N. K., Mendelson, J. H., Eros-Sarnyai, M., and Mercer, G. (1996). Effects of cocaine on pulsatile activity of the hypothalamic-pituitary-adrenal axis in male rhesus monkeys: Neuroendocrine and behavioral correlates. *J. Pharmacol. Exp. Ther., 277,* 225–234.

Schenk, S., Lacelle, G., Gorman, K., and Amit, Z. (1987). Cocaine self-administration in rats influenced by environmental conditions: Implications for the etiology of drug abuse. *Neurosci. Lett., 81,* 227–231.

Schenk, S., and Partridge, B. (1997). Sensitization and tolerance in psychostimulant self-administration. *Pharmacol. Biochem. Behav., 57,* 543–550.

See, R. E. (2005). Neural substrates of cocaine-cue associations that trigger relapse. *Eur. J. Pharmacol., 526,* 140–146.

Selye, H. (1975). Confusion and controversy in the stress field. *J. Hum. Stress, 1,* 37–44.

Shaham, Y., Erb, S., Leung, S., Buczek, Y., and Stewart, J. (1998). CP-154,526, a selective, non-peptide antagonist of the corticotropin-releasing factor-1 receptor attenuates stress-induced relapse to drug seeking in cocaine- and heroin-trained rats. *Psychopharmacology (Berl), 137,* 184–189.

Shaham, Y., and Stewart, J. (1995). Stress reinstates heroin self-administration behavior in drug-free animals: An effect mimicking heroin, not withdrawal. *Psychopharmacology, 119,* 334–341.

Sinha, R., Catapano, D., and O'Malley, S. (1999). Stress-induced craving and stress response in cocaine dependent individuals. *Psychopharmacology, 142,* 343–351.

Sinha, R., Fuse, T., Aubin, L. R., and O'Malley, S. S. (2000). Psychological stress, drug-related cues and cocaine craving. *Psychopharmacology, 152,* 140–148.

Sinha, R., Talih, M., Malison, R., Cooney, N., Anderson, G. M., and Kreek, M. J. (2003). Hypothalamic-pituitary-adrenal axis and sympatho-adreno-medullary responses during stress-induced and drug cue-induced cocaine craving states. *Psychopharmacology, 170,* 62–72.

Slikker, W., Brocco, M. J., and Killam, K. F. (1984). Reinstatement of responding maintained by cocaine or thiamylal. *J. Pharmacol. Exp. Ther., 228,* 43–52.

Smagin, G. M., and Goeders, N. E. (2000). Ketoconazole enhances cocaine-induced dopamine release in the medial prefrontal cortex (Mpfc) in rats. *Neurosci. Abstr., 26,* 1822.

Smagin, G. N., and Goeders, N. E. (2004). Effects of acute and chronic ketoconazole administration on hypothalamo-pituitary-adrenal axis activity and brain corticotropin-releasing hormone. *Psychoneuroendocrinology, 29,* 1223–1228.

Sofuoglu, M., and Kosten, T. R. (2005). Novel approaches to the treatment of cocaine addiction. *CNS Drugs, 19,* 13–25.

Sonino, N. (1987). The use of ketoconazole as an inhibitor of steroid production. *N. Engl. J. Med., 317,* 812–818.

Steptoe, A., and Ussher, M. (2005, December 5). Smoking, cortisol and nicotine. *Int. J. Psychophysiol.* [Epub ahead of print].

Stewart, J., and de Wit, H. (1987). Reinstatement of drug-taking behavior as a method of assessing incentive motivational properties of drugs. In M. A. Bozarth, (Ed.), *Methods of assessing the reinforcing properties of abused drugs* (pp. 21–227). New York: Springer.

Stratakis, C. A., and Chrousos, G. P. (1995). Neuroendocrinology and pathophysiology of the stress system. *Annu. N. Y. Acad. Sci., 771,* 1–18.

Tarr, J. E., and Macklin, M. (1987). Cocaine. *Pediatr. Clin. North Am., 34,* 319–331.

Teoh, S. K., Sarnyai, Z., Mendelson, J. H., Mello, N. K., Springer, S. A., Sholar, J. W., Wapler, M., Kuehnle, J. C., and Gelles, H. (1994). Cocaine effects on pulsatile secretion of ACTH in men. *J. Pharmacol. Exp. Ther., 270,* 1134–1138.

Thienpont, D., Van Cutsem, J., Van Gerven, F., Heeres, J., and Janssen, P. A. J. (1979). Ketoconazole—a new broad spectrum orally active antimycotic. *Experientia, 35*, 606–607.

Tidey, J. W., and Miczek, K. A. (1997). Acquisition of cocaine self-administration after social stress: Role of accumbens dopamine. *Psychopharmacology, 130*, 203–212.

Torpy, D. J., Grice, J. E., Hockings, G. I., Walters, M. M., Crosbie, G. V., and Jackson, R. V. (1993). Alprazolam blocks the naloxone-stimulated hypothalamo-pituitary-adrenal axis in man. *J. Clin. Endocrinol. Metab., 76*, 388–391.

Wagner, M. K. (2001). Behavioral characteristics related to substance abuse and risk-taking, sensation-seeking, anxiety sensitivity, and self-reinforcement. *Addict. Behav., 26*, 115–120.

Wang, G. J., Volkow, N. D., Fowler, J. S., Cervany, P., Hitzemann, R. J., Pappas, N. R., Wong, C. T., and Felder, C. (1999). Regional brain metabolic activation during craving elicited by recall of previous drug experiences. *Life Sci., 64*, 775–784.

Ward, A. S., Collins, E. D., Haney, M., Foltin, R. W., and Fischman, M. W. (1998). Ketoconazole attenuates the cortisol response but not the subjective effects of smoked cocaine in humans. *Behav. Pharmacol., 9*, 577–586.

Weerts, E. M., Froestl, W., and Griffiths, R. R. (2005). Effects of GABAergic modulators on food and cocaine self-administration in baboons. *Drug Alcohol Depend., 80*, 369–376.

Weiss, F., Maldonado-Vlaar, C. S., Parsons, L. H., Kerr, T. M., Smith, D. L., and Ben-Shahar, O. (2000). Control of cocaine-seeking behavior by drug-associated stimuli in rats: Effects on recovery of extinguished operant-responding and extracellular dopamine levels in amygdala and nucleus accumbens. *Proc. Natl. Acad. Sci. U. S. A., 97*, 4321–4326.

Wills, T. A., and Shiffman, S. (1985). Coping and substance use: A conceptual framework. In S. Shiffman T. A. Wills (Eds.) *Coping and substance abuse* (pp. 3–24). New York: Academic Press.

Wolkowitz, O. M., Reus, V. I., Manfredi, F., Ingbar, J., Brizendine, L., and Weingartner, H. (1993). Ketoconazole administration in hypercortisolemic depression. *Am. J. Psychiatry, 150*, 810–812.

Woods, J. H., Winger, G. D., and France, C. P. (1987). Reinforcing and discriminative stimulus effects of cocaine: Analysis of pharmacological mechanisms. In S. Fisher, A. Raskin, E. H. Uhlenhuth (Eds.), *Cocaine: Clinical and biobehavioral aspects* (pp. 21–65). New York: Oxford University Press.

Yang, X. M., Gorman, A. L., Dunn, A. J., and Goeders, N. E. (1992). Anxiogenic effects of acute and chronic cocaine administration: Neurochemical and behavioral studies. *Pharmacol. Biochem. Behav., 41*, 643–650.

Zaslav, M. R. (1994). Psychology of comorbid posttraumatic stress disorder and substance abuse: Lessons from combat veterans. *J. Psychoactive Drugs, 26*, 393–400.

Zhou, Y., Spangler, R., LaForge, K. S., Maggos, C. E., Ho, A., and Kreek, M. J. (1996). Corticotropin-releasing factor and type 1 corticotropin-releasing factor receptor messenger RNAs in rat brain and pituitary during "binge"-pattern cocaine administration and chronic withdrawal. *J. Pharmacol. Exp. Ther., 279*, 351–358.

Ziegler, S. D., Lipton, J. W., Toga, A. W., and Ellison, G. D. (1991). Continuous cocaine administration produces persisting changes in brain neurochemistry and behavior. *Brain Res., 552*, 27–35.

Zweben, J. E., Clark, H. W., and Smith, D. E. (1994). Traumatic experiences and substance abuse: Mapping the territory. *J. Psychoactive Drugs, 26*, 327–344.

3

Dopaminergic Reward Pathways and Effects of Stress

MICHELA MARINELLI

The aim of this chapter is to review literature on the dopamine reward system, how it is affected by stress, and its relevance to addiction. The first two sections will provide a brief definition of stress and an introduction on the dopamine system, including methods used to evaluate its activity. The third section will describe the role of the dopamine system in drug addiction. It will also examine the effects of addictive drugs on different aspects of dopaminergic transmission, such as dopamine overflow and action potential output. The fourth section will focus on the effects of stress on dopaminergic transmission. It will highlight how stress has an inverted-U-shaped effect: Mild/moderate stressors increase dopaminergic transmission, whereas intense unpredictable stressors can decrease it. Possible mechanisms underlying the effects of stress on the dopamine system, including the important role of glucocorticoid stress hormones, will also be discussed. The review will conclude by examining how an interaction between stress and dopamine could play an important role in the development of addiction-associated behaviors; it will also provide

different views that try to reconcile findings showing that increased dopamine transmission is seen after both rewarding and stressful stimuli.

I. DEFINING STRESS

Stress is a complex term that requires a brief description at the onset of this chapter. Biologically, stressful events cause a rise in blood levels of glucocorticoids, which are considered as major stress hormones (for review, see Axelrod and Reisine, 1984; Bohus, 1975; Dallman et al., 1989; de Kloet, 2000; Munck and Guyre, 1986). Psychologically, stress generally bears a negative value as it is commonly believed that individuals will avoid stressful stimuli; however, this is not always the case. In humans, some individuals show preference for situations that enhance stress levels (e.g., "sensation-seekers"; Zuckerman, 1990); similar traits exist in animals as well (Dellu et al., 1996). Rats with enhanced hormonal reactivity to stress also choose to spend more time in stressful situations (Kabbaj et al., 2000). In other words, some individuals seek "stressful" situations that promote the release of stress hormones. On a similar line, rats voluntarily self-administer corticosterone, the major glucocorticoid hormone in the rat (Deroche et al., 1993b; Piazza et al., 1993).

In addition to recognizing that stress is not necessarily an avoided condition, it is important to distinguish different degrees of stress. Stressors could have diverse effects according to their intensity, duration, and predictability. Mild stressors such as changes in the social setting, mild foot shock, brief tail pinch, short-term food deprivation, and mild food restriction can increase arousal and produce a state of activation. On the other hand, intense, unpredictable, and prolonged stressors such as those performed during a "chronic mild stress" procedure, which is not that "mild" after all (Cabib, 1997), produce learned helplessness and depressive-like symptoms in animals (Cabib, 1997; Cabib and Puglisi-Allegra, 1996b; Willner, 1997). Somewhat similar findings are seen in humans; repeated administration of low doses of corticosteroids can produce euphoria in some humans (Klein, 1992; Plihal et al., 1996), but chronic stress or chronically elevated levels of glucocorticoids are associated with major depression (for review, see Andrews, 2005; Holsboer, 2001; Muller et al., 2004; Steckler et al., 1999).

Thus, stress has an inverted U-shaped curve, in which low to moderate stressors may be excitatory and higher levels are inhibitory. This has been documented using a variety of paradigms and has been particularly investigated in the learning and memory field (Conrad et al., 1999; Luine, 1994, 1997; Sandi, 1998). For example, low levels of the stress hormone corticosterone facilitate the acquisition and retention of hippocampal-dependent memory tasks (Akirav et al., 2004; Luine, 1997; Sandi et al., 1997; Sandi, 1998), whereas high levels of the hormones or extensive exposure to psychological stress impair performance in both animals and humans (Dachir et al.,

1993; Diamond et al., 1996; Luine et al., 1993; Lupien et al., 1997; Newcomer et al., 1994). On a similar line, administration of low levels of stress hormones increases hippocampal synaptic plasticity, whereas repeated exposure to high levels of the hormone decreases it (Diamond and Rose, 1994; Diamond et al., 1992, 1994).

Overall these data emphasize the notion that stress exhibits an inverted U-shaped curve, in which low to moderate stressors have activating effects, whereas intense or prolonged stressors have inhibitory effects. This is also true for behavioral responses to psychostimulant drugs; thus, cocaine-seeking behavior is not modified by the administration of low doses of the stress hormone corticosterone; it is increased by high doses of the hormone and reduced again by very high (nonphysiological) levels of the hormone (Deroche et al., 1997). In addition, this inverted U-shaped function is particularly notable on the dopamine system and will be discussed in more detail in the following sections.

II. THE MESENCEPHALIC DOPAMINE SYSTEM

A. Dopamine Neurons

Dopamine was recognized as a neurotransmitter in the 1950s (Benes, 2001; Carlsson, 1959), and its localization in the rat brain was initially characterized by Dahlström and Fuxe (Dahlstrom, 1971; Dahlstrom and Fuxe, 1964). In the midbrain, dopamine neurons comprise about 75% of all of the dopamine cells of the brain. They are located in three main areas: the retrorubral field, which projects to the dorsal striatum (A8 pathway); the substantia nigra pars compacta, also mostly projecting to the dorsal striatum (A9 pathway); and the ventral tegmental area, mostly projecting to the ventral striatum (nucleus accumbens), amygdala, olfactory tubercule, and limbic cortex (A10 pathway; for review, see Anden et al., 1965; Dahlstrom, 1971; German et al., 1983; Oades and Halliday, 1987). Direct or indirect excitatory glutamatergic inputs to midbrain dopamine neurons originate from structures such as the prefrontal cortex, the bed nucleus of the stria terminalis, the subthalamic nucleus, the pedunculo pontine nucleus, the laterodorsal tegmental nucleus, and the superior colliculus (for review, see Adell and Artigas, 2004; Haber and Fudge, 1997; Kalivas, 1993; Mathon et al., 2003). Inhibitory GABAergic inputs arise mostly from the striatal complex, which includes inputs from the nucleus accumbens, caudate nucleus, globus pallidus, and ventral pallidum (for review, see Groenewegen et al., 1993; Smith and Bolam, 1990; Somogyi et al., 1981; Von Krosigk et al., 1992; White, 1996). Another important GABAergic input arises from local neurons in the midbrain (Bayer and Pickel, 1991; Hajos and Greenfield, 1994; Kosaka et al., 1987).

B. Evaluating the Activity of the Dopaminergic Pathway

1. Extracellular Concentrations of Dopamine

Extracellular concentrations of dopamine can be measured with different techniques that offer different disadvantages/advantages with respect to their temporal resolution and their selectivity for the detected compounds. Commonly used techniques will be described below and have also been described in other thorough reviews (Marsden et al., 1988; Di Chiara, 1990a, 1990b; Robinson et al., 2003; Phillips and Wightman, 2003; Phillips et al., 2003a).

a. Microdialysis and Postmortem Tissue Analysis Extracellular concentrations of dopamine can be measured with microdialysis techniques, both in anesthetized animals and in freely moving ones (Arbuthnott et al., 1990; Church et al., 1987b; Hamilton et al., 1992; Hurd et al., 1988; Osborne et al., 1990; Sharp et al., 1987; Zetterstrom et al.,

1988). A concentric probe composed of an inner and outer tube is lowered in the region of interest (Santiago and Westerink, 1990). A perfusate whose composition should mimic that of cerebrospinal fluid (Moghaddam and Bunney, 1989; Osborne et al., 1991b) is slowly pumped through the inner probe via the inlet and collected at the outlet from the outer tube. The probe is composed of a semipermeable membrane (1–2 mm in length, 0.2–0.5 mm in diameter), so it allows diffusion of small molecules between the extracellular fluid and the perfusion fluid. This exchange of molecules occurs in both directions, and the direction of flow is governed by the concentration gradient. The collected dialysate is separated by high performance/pressure liquid chromatography, and dopamine can be measured with different techniques such as ultraviolet detection, oxidative-reductive electrochemical detection, and photoluminescence following electron-transfer detection, all of which offer a high degree of chemical selectivity (Carter, 1994; Church et al., 1987b; Hurd et al., 1988; Jung et al., 2006; Plotsky et al., 1977; Refshauge et al., 1974; Wightman et al., 1977).

The above-mentioned detection techniques can also be used to analyze dopamine levels in brain tissue *postmortem*. In *postmortem* studies, the brain tissue of interest is removed and homogenized; dopamine is extracted with an organic solvent and subsequently analyzed. Subtle changes in dopamine levels are seldom detected, especially because these studies allow only for a snapshot of dopamine at a single timepoint for each animal; time-related changes in dopamine levels could be missed easily. Generally, *postmortem* studies provide a gross quantification of extracellular concentration of dopamine, as well as of dopamine metabolites. Ratios of metabolites to dopamine can provide an indication of dopamine turnover.

The concentration of collected dopamine in the dialysate, or of any other compound, depends on the size of the probe, the difference in concentration between the perfusate and the extracellular fluid, as well as on the diffusion coefficient of the compound through the extracellular fluid. The flow rate of the perfusate is also important; it is usually around 0.5–2 µL/min for dopamine, which represents a compromise between diffusion rate, collected volume, and adequate sampling timescales. Given these considerations, dialysate samples with detectable dopamine concentrations are usually collected over several minutes (15–20 minutes). In some conditions, when microbore/small-bore chromatography columns are used, dopamine can be detected in shorter (1–5 minutes) timescales, and its detection limit is improved about 50 times with respect to conventional bore columns (Carter, 1994; Church et al., 1987b; Moghaddam et al., 1990; Parsons et al., 1998). It should be noted that once the microdialysis probe is lowered in the brain, a minimum period of about 1 hour of stabilization is required prior to sample collection (due to tissue damage), and it is not until 2–3 days after probe insertion that dopamine concentrations are most stable. Dopamine concentrations decrease again on day 4 after the insertion of the probe, probably because of development of gliotic tissue around the microdialysis probe (Osborne et al., 1991a). After their collection, dialysate samples should be analyzed immediately, as dopamine oxidizes rapidly; adding antioxidants such as ascorbic acid in the perfusate only partly obviates this problem (Parry et al., 1990; Thorre et al., 1997)

It is essential to recognize that dopamine assayed with microdialysis studies simply reflects the extracellular concentrations of the neurotransmitter, which are the common product of neurotransmitter release, reuptake, diffusion, and degradation. So data obtained with microdialysis should not be misinterpreted to reflect neurotransmitter release, even though this might be the case under certain conditions. The fact that microdialysis can reflect changes in dopamine release is shown by findings showing increases in dopamine after treatments that increase neurotransmitter release (e.g., potassium, veratrine, ouabain, and amphetamine), and reductions in dopamine by treatments that lower transmitter release (e.g., low concentrations of calcium) or those that block impulse flow (e.g., tetrodotoxin) (Arbuthnott et al., 1990; Cosford et al., 1994; Fairbrother et al., 1990a, 1990b; Hurd and Ungerstedt, 1989a; Moghaddam and Bunney, 1989; Moghaddam et al., 1990; Osborne et al., 1991b; Zetterstrom et al., 1988). However, rises in extracellular dopamine after pharmacological treatments can also reflect changes in neurotransmitter reuptake, even when neurotransmitter release is actually decreased, such as after the administration of nomifensine, GBR 12909, and bupropion (Benwell et al., 1993; Church et al., 1987a; Hurd and Ungerstedt, 1989b; Nomikos et al., 1990). Thus, because of its unclear origin, dopamine detected with the microdialysis technique should be referred to as dopamine "overflow," "levels," or simply "extracellular concentrations," but never as "dopamine release."

Given all of these considerations, it is clear that the microdialysis technique is very valuable for studies that require monitoring extracellular concentrations of dopamine for extended periods of time (hours to days). Using this technique, it was shown that extracellular concentrations of dopamine in baseline (rest) conditions are in the range of 1–20 nM in the striatal complex. As Figure 3-1 shows, concentrations are highest in the dorsal striatum with respect to the nucleus accumbens, where levels are higher in the shell with respect to the core (Barrot et al., 1999; Justice, Jr., 1993, although see Abercrombie et al., 1989). These differences between core and shell were also found using *postmortem* analysis of core and shell tissue (Deutch and Cameron, 1992).

Concerning the microdialysis technique, the 1–20 minute sampling rate is ideal for studies detecting changes in dopamine overflow that occur over minutes/hours (e.g., after the administration of drugs of abuse

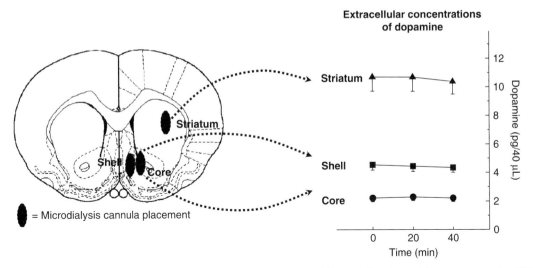

FIGURE 3-1 Basal extracellular concentrations of dopamine in different subregions of the striatal complex. Values were obtained with *in vivo* microdialysis in the freely moving rat, and probe placements are indicated on the coronal section. Dopamine levels are highest in the dorsolateral striatum (Striatum), then in the nucleus accumbens shell (Shell), followed by the nucleus accumbens core (Core). Modified with permission, from Barrot et al., 1999.

or certain stressful stimuli, as shown in the next sections). However, microdialysis is insensitive to dopamine transients, such as those occurring in behaving animals or produced by transient/phasic changes in dopamine neuron activity (Borland et al., 2005; Budygin et al., 2000; Floresco et al., 2003; Lu et al., 1998; Peters and Michael, 1998). Such changes in extracellular concentrations of dopamine produced by phasic changes in neuronal activity can be seen with microdialysis, but generally only if dopamine reuptake is blocked pharmacologically (Floresco et al., 2003; Lu et al., 1998). Otherwise, techniques with a better temporal resolution are required (see below).

b. Voltammetry and Amperometry Dopamine transients are best detected with techniques with good spatial and temporal resolution (Robinson et al., 2003), such as differential normal pulse voltammetry (minute timescale), high-speed chronoamperometry (1–5 second timescale), fast-scan cyclic voltammetry (~100 msec), and constant potential amperometry (msec timescale).

In constant potential amperometry, a potential is constantly applied to the electrode, which is sufficient to produce a redox reaction in the molecule of interest. Electrode responses are extremely rapid, giving the best temporal resolution among such techniques. However, selectivity is poor, so it is difficult to differentiate between molecules requiring similar redox potentials. Because of its poor selectivity, this technique should be used only to study the kinetics of electrically evoked dopamine transients in the tissue slice or in anesthetized rats. It is inappropriate for transients observed in behaving animals, as there is too little confidence on the nature of the measured compound (Dugast et al., 1994; Robinson et al., 2003).

Fast-scan cyclic voltammetry is perhaps one of the best techniques to study transient changes in extracellular concentrations of dopamine, especially in behaving animals. This technique provides excellent temporal and spatial resolution, while maintaining a good selectivity (Ewing et al., 1982; Kuhr and Wightman, 1986; Rice and Nicholson, 1989; Wiedemann et al., 1991; Wightman et al., 1988). In addition, the sampling electrode is extremely small (25–400 μm long, ~10 μm in diameter), which causes minimal tissue damage (Bungay et al., 2003), and allows for sampling in precise brain areas, without overflowing in adjacent structures. During fast-scan cyclic voltammetry, a triangular voltage waveform is applied repeatedly to a carbon electrode (Cahill et al., 1996; Ewing et al., 1982; Rice and Nicholson, 1989). The parameters of the triangle waveform have changed over the years, and they have been optimized to improve sensitivity and stability. This cycling through alternating positive and negative voltages produces a background current of the electrode (a cyclic voltammogram), attributable to movement of charged species around the electrode. During these cycles, dopamine molecules around the electrode are also oxidized (when positive voltage is applied) and reduced (with negative voltage). This transfer of current produced by oxidation and reduction of dopamine adds to the background current of the electrode. Given that the background current of the electrode is stable over several seconds, the background can be digitally subtracted, to reveal current changes produced by redox reactions of dopamine. The magnitude of the current changes is directly proportional to changes in dopamine concentration. Although background current is stable over seconds, it can drift over minutes, so while this technique is ideal for measuring transient changes in dopamine, it is not suitable for studies on the long-term changes in neurotransmitter levels (Robinson et al., 2003). It is also noteworthy to mention that changes in the pH of the microenvironment do not change the efficiency of the detection, but they do interfere by producing a competitive signal. Fast-scan cyclic voltammetry is able to distinguish between changes in pH and changes in analyte levels, whereas other techniques are not always able to make this distinction (Phillips and Wightman, 2003; Venton et al., 2003a).

Using fast-scan cyclic voltammetry, it was shown that baseline concentrations of dopamine in the striatal complex are in the range of 5–10 nM in resting and anesthetized conditions (Kawagoe et al., 1992; Kuhr and Wightman, 1986; Wightman et al., 1988) and that they can transiently (over ~2 s) increase to 50–200 nM in behaving animals (Rebec et al., 1997a, 1997b; Robinson and Wightman, 2004; Stuber et al., 2005). Although fast-scan cyclic voltammetry technically measures extracellular concentrations of dopamine, its fast temporal resolution allows to record changes in dopamine clearance as well as in dopamine release, such as the release produced by the electrical stimulation of dopamine neurons (Chergui et al., 1994; Garris et al., 2003; Gonon, 1988; Kuhr and Wightman, 1986; Suaud-Chagny et al., 1992), especially in conditions that mimic the release produced by natural burst-firing activity (Phillips and Wightman, 2004; Venton et al., 2003b).

High-speed chronoamperometry is also an excellent technique to measure rapid changes in extracellular concentrations of dopamine (Brazell et al., 1987; Gerhardt et al., 1999; Gratton et al., 1989). It is not as rapid as fast-scan cyclic voltammetry, but still offers second-to-second resolution and has satisfactory selectivity for dopamine. During chronoamperometry, a fused silica-based single carbon fiber electrode is lowered in the brain region of interest, and a reference electrode is implanted in the cortex. The small dimension of the recording probe (30–33 μm in diameter) causes little tissue damage and its short length (100–200 μm) provides structure selectivity. Repetitive 100 ms square-wave pulses are applied to the electrode, and dopamine surrounding the electrode undergoes a redox reaction; the resulting oxidation current (measured during rising phase of the step) and reduction current (measured during descending phase) are then digitally integrated. This technique shows stable results over at least 5 consecutive days and can therefore provide information on rapid transients over prolonged periods of time (Gerhardt et al., 1999). In addition, the probe can be adapted to include a microejection system; this allows combining the local application of neurotransmitters and other chemicals with the electrochemical recordings. Using these techniques the clearance kinetics of dopamine were assessed in different brain structures, and it was found that dopamine is cleared more rapidly in the nucleus accumbens with respect to the dorsal striatum (Cass et al., 1993). Finally, this technique is well adapted to freely moving animals; initial studies showed periodic interference by artifacts produced by rat movement, but simple mathematical approaches can now be applied to eliminate random noise effects (Sabeti et al., 2002a). Its stability over time makes this technique particularly suitable for long-term studies.

2. Dopamine Neuron Activity

Electrophysiological studies have been used to evaluate the action potential output of midbrain dopamine neurons. *In vivo* recordings (performed in anesthetized or awake animals) are performed with extracellular electrodes that record the voltage change produced by neuronal firing. The tip of these electrodes is very small (1–10 μm in diameter), causing minimal tissue damage. This setting provides information on the firing rate and pattern of these neurons, in the context of normal circuitry. *In vitro* recordings are generally performed in the tissue slice with a variety of recording techniques: extracellular, patch clamp (voltage or current clamp mode), or intracellular (current clamp mode with sharp electrodes). Therefore, these studies are more reductionistic, but they provide valuable information on the mechanisms that regulate neuronal activity.

During *in vivo* extracellular recordings, electrical signals are fed from the electrode into a high-impedance amplifier; they are then filtered through well-defined low- and high-pass bands that significantly influence the shape of the signal (Marinelli et al., 2006). Neurons are defined as dopaminergic if they fulfill specific electrophysiological

requirements, including a typical dopamine "signature" with a triphasic waveform (+/−/+) of long duration (Grace and Bunney, 1983; Marinelli et al., 2006; Ungless et al., 2004). Using this technique, it was shown that dopamine neuron activity is relatively similar in awake and anesthetized animals (Fa et al., 2003; Freeman et al., 1985; Hyland et al., 2002; Kiyatkin and Rebec, 1998); however, recordings are technically demanding in awake animals, as the recorded cell is easily lost with slight movements of the animal. Therefore, this technique is most commonly used in anesthetized preparations.

In both anesthetized and awake animals, dopamine neurons *in vivo* can be silent, or spontaneously active. Among spontaneously active neurons, the action potential output can show slow regular, slow irregular, or fast-bursting activity. Bursts are characterized by spikes that are clustered in high-frequency events that generally show spike-frequency adaptation and accommodation (Bunney et al., 1973; Grace and Bunney, 1983, 1984a; Guyenet and Aghajanian, 1978). Bursting can exist to different degrees. Few cells show no bursting activity at all, but most neurons show moderate levels of bursting (5–50% of bursting spikes). Some neurons show elevated bursting (>80% of bursting spikes); cells with high levels of bursting are characterized by numerous burst events and/or numerous spikes within each burst event. It is important to note that spontaneous bursting is generally unique to the *in vivo* situation, and it is seldom observed *in vitro* (Grace and Bunney, 1984b; Kita et al., 1986; Sanghera et al., 1984; Shepard and Bunney, 1988), most likely because many of the excitatory synaptic inputs responsible for bursting have been severed in the tissue slice. *In vitro*, firing activity is extremely regular (pacemaker-like). The different firing patterns seen *in vivo*, and the regular firing observed *in vitro* are illustrated in Figure 3-2.

As mentioned above, bursting activity *in vivo* has been shown to produce an increase in terminal dopamine release (Gonon, 1988;

Firing patterns of dopamine neurons

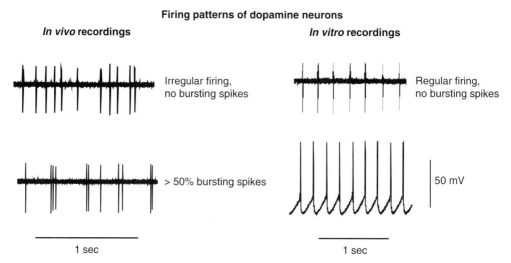

FIGURE 3-2   Firing patterns of dopamine neurons recorded in the ventral tegmental area of rodents. Left traces represent *in vivo* extracellular recordings in anesthetized animals, whereas right traces are *in vitro* recordings in the tissue slice using cell-attached or current clamp recordings. *In vivo*, dopamine neurons show irregular firing, with different degrees of bursting activity. Bursts are characterized by clusters of spikes (see text). *In vitro*, neurons do not burst spontaneously, and they show regular spiking activity. Data obtained by M. Marinelli for the purpose of this book chapter.

Phillips et al., 2003a; Suaud-Chagny et al., 1992; Venton et al., 2003b). However, because neurotransmitter reuptake by the dopamine transporters is rapid, such phasic increases in peri-synaptic dopamine are only detectable using techniques with good temporal resolution, such as fast-scan cyclic voltammetry or chronoamperometry (Dugast et al., 1994; Garris et al., 1997; Phillips and Wightman, 2004). They can be detected with microdialysis only if dopamine reuptake is experimentally blocked, such as after the administration of the reuptake blocker nomifensine (Floresco et al., 2003).

III. DOPAMINE AND ADDICTION

A. Role of Dopamine in Addiction

The dopamine system is one of the major players mediating the rewarding effects of addictive drugs. It is not the scope of this chapter to provide a comprehensive review of literature on the importance of dopa-

mine in addiction; please refer to excellent reviews on this subject (Adinoff, 2004; Di Chiara et al., 2004; Everitt and Wolf, 2002; Franken et al., 2005; Kiyatkin, 2002; Koob et al., 1994; Robinson and Berridge, 2000; White and Kalivas, 1998; Wise, 1998, 2005). I will only summarize the most relevant studies for the purpose of this chapter.

Indirect evidence for a role of increased dopaminergic activity in addiction is shown by the positive relationship between drug self-administration behavior and the level of activation of the dopamine system. Compared with animals showing low activity of the dopaminergic system, animals showing heightened dopaminergic transmission (high levels of dopamine in the nucleus accumbens and high action potential output of dopamine neurons) are more likely to acquire psychostimulant and opiate self-administration behavior (Glick et al., 1992; Hooks et al., 1991; Hooks et al., 1992; Marinelli and White, 2000; Rouge-Pont et al., 1993). On a similar line, recordings in freely moving animals have shown that dopamine neuron activity peaks right before animals engage in heroin self-admin-istration behavior (Kiyatkin and Rebec, 1997, 2001). Similarly, dopamine release, measured with fast-scan cyclic voltamme-try, increases immediately prior to respond-ing for cocaine (about 1 second prior to lever pressing for the drug), as well as after presentation of a drug-related cue and the drug itself (Phillips et al., 2003a; Stuber et al., 2005). In addition, evoking dopamine release on such a short timescale, by elec-trical stimulation, promotes drug seeking (Phillips et al., 2003b). Microdialysis stud-ies do not have this time resolution, as the sampling timescale is multiple minutes; nevertheless, they are consistent with the notion that dopamine increases in response to conditioned drug-related stimuli, dis-criminative stimuli, and drug responding (Bradberry, 2000; Ito et al., 2002; Weiss et al., 2000). Overall this suggests that an increase in dopamine transmission facilitates drug-associated behaviors.

Pharmacological studies also corrobo-rate the idea that dopamine is important in addiction-related behaviors. Drugs that decrease dopaminergic transmission gen-erally produce a decrease in drug reward. Thus, the systemic administration of the GABA$_B$ receptor agonist baclofen, at doses that inhibit dopamine neuron activity and release, has been shown to reduce self-administration of psychostimulants and opiates under different schedules of rein-forcement (Brebner et al., 2000, 2002; Di Ciano and Everitt, 2003; Roberts et al., 1996; Shoaib et al., 1998; Xi and Stein, 1999; Xi and Stein, 2000). Similar findings were reported after direct infusion of baclofen into the ventral tegmental area (Blokhina et al., 2005; Hyytia et al., 1999; Ranaldi et al., 1996; Schenk et al., 1993), or by administration of the ionotropic glutamate receptor blockers into this structure (Kalivas and McFarland, 2003; Shaham et al., 2003), indicating that the effects are probably specific to decreases in dopamine neuron activity.

In addition to being important for self-administration behavior, dopamine also has an important role in drug-seeking behavior, which represents a valid model of drug relapse in humans. Pharmacological inacti-vation of the ventral tegmental area (Stewart, 1984; Vorel et al., 2001), or the administra-tion of drugs that putatively decrease dopa-mine neuron activity (Bossert et al., 2004; Di Ciano and Everitt, 2003, 2004; Marinelli et al., 2003b; McFarland and Kalivas, 2001), reduces drug-seeking behavior in animals that were previously trained on self-admin-istration tasks. On the other hand, treat-ments that are known to enhance dopamine neuron activity, such as stimulation of affer-ent structures or the local infusions of glu-tamate or morphine, intensify responding in drug-seeking paradigms (Stewart, 1984; Vorel et al., 2001). It should be noted, how-ever, that direct stimulation of the medial forebrain bundle with brief burst events (3-spike/burst) does not produce an increase in drug-seeking behavior (Vorel et al., 2001); this suggests that a physiological increase in bursting, such as that obtained with synaptic stimulation (i.e., several spikes/bursts fol-lowed by long pauses) might be important for seeking behavior. Supporting this, stud-ies mentioned above show that stimulation of dopamine fibers, using protocols that are known to increase dopamine transients (24 spikes/bursts) will promote drug-seeking behavior (Phillips et al., 2003b).

Despite the relationship between experi-mentally induced increases/decreases in dopamine neuron activity and seeking behavior, there is no relationship between the enhanced dopamine neuron activity observed at short withdrawal times from psychostimulant self-administration and drug-seeking behavior. In fact, seeking behavior increases over time, and it is usually lowest at short withdrawal times from drug intake (Grimm et al., 2001; Tran-Nguyen et al., 1998) when, instead, neuronal activity is highest (Marinelli et al., 2003b). It is possible that, at early withdrawal times, the observed upregulation of dopamine transporter levels and increased dopamine clearance via these transporters prevents increases in dopamine neuron activity to translate into accumulation of dopamine (Cass et al., 1992; Mash et al., 2002; Meiergerd et al., 1997; Pierce and Kalivas, 1997; Sabeti et al., 2002b).

While the above studies mostly point to a role of increased dopaminergic tone as a facilitator of addiction, there is also ample evidence for decreases in dopamine to be related with addiction (Melis et al., 2005). As noted in the next section, withdrawal from long-term use of addictive drugs can lead to a hypo-dopaminergic state. It has been argued that this state could decrease an individual's interest in stimuli that are not related to drugs. At the same time, though, it would promote the search for drug, so as to counteract the decrease in dopaminergic tone (Imperato et al., 1992b; Melis et al., 2005; Volkow et al., 2002). These views are not incompatible; it has thus been proposed that drug craving and relapse in the addicted individual could be the result of two separate phenomena. "Chronic craving" would be the result of a reduced dopaminergic tone; in this case, the individual would take drugs to alleviate this hypo-dopaminergic state (Melis et al., 2005; Volkow et al., 2002). "Instant craving," instead, would be caused by a temporary increase in dopaminergic transmission, which would act like a trigger to precipitate relapse (Leyton et al., 2002; Oswald et al., 2005). For more discussion on the "dual" role for dopamine in addiction and craving, see Pilla et al. (1999); Childress and O'Brien (2000); Franken et al. (2005).

B. Effects of Addictive Drugs on Dopaminergic Transmission

1. Effects of Addictive Drugs on Extracellular Concentrations of Dopamine

Additional evidence for a role of dopamine in addiction comes from studies showing that addictive drugs have the common property of producing an increase in extracellular levels of dopamine in the striatal complex (Carboni et al., 1989;

Di Chiara et al., 1993). This action is the consequence of different mechanisms of action (Hurd et al., 1998; Klitenick et al., 1992; Leone et al., 1991), such as increase in dopamine neuron firing rate (opiates and ethanol), reversal of the dopamine transporter, and release from synaptic vesicles (amphetamine) or blockade of dopamine reuptake (e.g., cocaine and amphetamine). Recent data suggest that cocaine can also increase extracellular concentrations of dopamine by mobilizing a reserve pool of the neurotransmitter from synaptic vesicles (Venton et al., 2006).

In early studies, there was an apparent debate on whether psychostimulant drugs equally increase dopamine levels in the dorsal striatum (caudate) and ventral striatum (nucleus accumbens). A set of reports indicated a preferential increase in the ventral striatum, whereas another set showed that psychostimulant-induced dopamine levels were highest in the dorsal striatum (Carboni et al., 1989; Cass et al., 1993; Paulson and Robinson, 1995; Robinson and Camp, 1990). This apparent contradiction was resolved by examining the way the data were analyzed (Robinson and Camp, 1990). In fact, percent increases in extracellular concentrations of dopamine are inversely correlated with baseline values (Weiss et al., 1992b); they are greater when baseline values are low, because any small variation is translated into a large percent change. Given that baseline levels of dopamine are low in the nucleus accumbens (about 3–5 times lower than in the dorsal striatum), the percent change in dopamine efflux produced by psychostimulant drugs appears greatest in this structure. Instead, changes in the striatum appear smaller, even though drug-induced absolute values are actually higher in this structure.

Recently, the effects of addictive drugs on accumbens dopamine have been further examined by subdividing the nucleus accumbens into the shell and core, which are functionally and anatomically distinct subsets of this nucleus (Zahm and Brog, 1992). These data show that, regardless of the way data are presented, drug-induced increases in dopamine are highest in the shell of the accumbens with respect to the core. Then, according to the way data are presented, levels are higher in the striatum or the core (Barrot et al., 1999; Ferraro et al., 2000; Hedou et al., 1999; Pontieri et al., 1995). Figure 3-3 shows cocaine-induced increases in extracellular concentrations of dopamine in the core, shell and dorsal striatum.

It is important to note that while the acute or repeated administration of addictive drugs increases dopamine levels, withdrawal from their repeated administration generally, but not always, produces a decrease in dopamine in the striatal complex (Crippens et al., 1993; Crippens et al., 1994; Parsons et al., 1991; Pothos et al., 1991; Robertson et al., 1991; Robinson et al., 1994; Rossetti 1992a, 1992b; and Weiss et al., 1992a).

2. Effects of Addictive Drugs on Dopamine Neuron Activity

Although addictive drugs all increase dopamine levels, their action on dopamine neuron activity varies. Acute administration of psychostimulant drugs such as amphetamine (Rebec and Segal, 1978; Wang, 1981), cocaine (Bunney et al., 2001; Einhorn et al., 1988; Lacey et al., 1990), methylphenidate (Brandon et al., 2003; Federici et al., 2005; Rebec and Segal, 1978) or caffeine (Stoner et al., 1988) produces a decrease in dopamine neuron activity. This is due to the augmentation in extracellular concentrations of dopamine produced by these drugs in the somatodendritic region of dopamine neurons (Bradberry and Roth, 1989). Such an elevation in somatodendritic dopamine activates somatodendritic impulse-regulating autoreceptors, which inhibits neuronal activity (Aghajanian and Bunney, 1977; Einhorn et al., 1988; Gariano et al., 1989). Amphetamine may also modify neuronal firing indirectly, via feedback from the activation of forebrain structures (Bunney and Aghajanian, 1977; Paladini and Williams, 2004; Paladini et al., 2001).

It is important to note that psychostimulant drugs decrease dopamine neuron activity while the drugs are onboard; however, withdrawal from their repeated administration produces the opposite effect—that is, a transient increase in dopamine neuron firing. This is seen after repeated experimenter-administered drugs as well as after voluntary drug self-administration (Marinelli et al., 2003b; White and Kalivas, 1998). Given its transient nature, the increase in dopamine cell activity seen after psychostimulant withdrawal does not appear to influence the expression of addictive behaviors (which persist long after dopamine cell activity has recovered). However, it appears to be critical for their development (Vezina, 2004; Wolf et al., 1994). Thus, such a short-lived increase

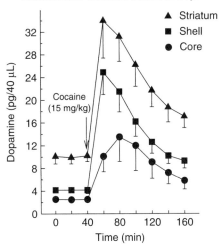

Extracellular concentrations of dopamine

FIGURE 3-3 Effects of cocaine on extracellular concentrations of dopamine in different subregions of the striatal complex. Data were obtained using *in vivo* microdialysis in freely moving rats (see Figure 3-1 for probe location). The administration of cocaine (15 mg/kg, IP) produces an increase in extracellular concentrations of dopamine in all regions. However, this increase is proportionally greater in the nucleus accumbens shell (Shell) with respect to the nucleus accumbens core (Core) or the dorsolateral striatum (Striatum). Modified with permission, from Barrot et al., 1999.

in dopamine cell activity is thought to be a "driving force" for transferring information to the forebrain, where drug-induced neuroadaptations are persistent.

Exposure to other addictive drugs, such as ethanol, opiates, or cannabinoids, has effects that are opposite to those produced by psychostimulant drugs. Thus, the acute administration of these drugs produces an increase in dopamine cell activity (Brodie et al., 1999; Gessa et al., 1998; Gysling and Wang, 1983; Mereu et al., 1984). The mechanism by which ethanol increases dopamine neuron activity is not fully understood, but appears to involve direct excitation of dopamine neurons, via inhibition of delayed rectifying potassium channels (Appel et al., 2003). Cannabinoids increase dopamine cell activity by acting on cannabinoid 1 receptors (Cheer et al., 2003; Melis et al., 2004), possibly by decreasing inhibitory GABAergic input to dopamine neurons (Szabo et al., 2002). The increase in dopamine neuron activity produced by the acute administration of opiate drugs is the consequence of μ opioid receptor activation; this inhibits local GABA neurons, which removes tonic GABA inhibition of these cells (Gysling and Wang, 1983; Johnson and North, 1992). On this line, animals that lack μ opioid receptors show enhanced GABAergic input onto dopamine neurons measured by increased frequency of spontaneous inhibitory postsynaptic currents (Mathon et al., 2005a); they also show blunted activity of dopamine cell firing (Mathon et al., 2005b). Again, withdrawal from their repeated administration produces an effect that is opposite to that seen when the drug is onboard; thus neuronal activity decreases transiently during withdrawal from repeated administration of these drugs (Bailey et al., 2001; Diana et al., 1993, 1995, 1998).

Overall, these data indicate that dopamine neurons respond to addictive drugs with either excitation or inhibition, according to the mechanism of action of the drugs. The effects observed while the drug is onboard are usually opposite to those produced when the drug treatment is withdrawn. It is conceivable that such neuroadaptations represent a compensatory response whereby withdrawal from a drug produces a rebound effect on neuronal activity.

IV. DOPAMINE AND STRESS

A. Dopaminergic Activity Is Higher in Animals with Greater Reactivity to Stress

The activity of the dopamine system differs across individuals, and a first indirect link between stress and dopamine comes from studies showing that individuals with higher reactivity to mild stress (High Responders, HRs) show greater dopaminergic activity compared with individuals with a lower reactivity to stress (Low Responders, LRs). Higher reactivity to stress is measured by a greater (Kabbaj et al., 2000) or longer (Piazza et al., 1991a) corticosterone secretion in response to a stressful situation, such as the exposure to a novel setting or to restraint stress. It is also characterized by greater or longer locomotor response to a novel environment (for review, see Marinelli, 2005b). Thus, animals with enhanced reactivity to stress (HRs) show higher baseline firing and bursting activity of dopamine neurons compared with animals with low reactivity to stress (LRs; Marinelli and White, 2000). Greater neuronal activity is paralleled by enhanced extracellular levels of dopamine in the nucleus accumbens, both in basal conditions and in response to stress or psychostimulant drugs (Bradberry et al., 1991; Hooks et al., 1991; Piazza et al., 1991b; Rouge-Pont et al., 1998). Interestingly, these animals with heightened stress and dopaminergic activity also show greater susceptibility to acquire psychostimulant self-administration behavior (Grimm and See, 1997; Marinelli and White, 2000; Piazza et al., 1990; Suto et al., 2001). This suggests that an interaction between stress and dopamine neurons could be a mechanism by which stress favors the development of addiction (Marinelli and Piazza, 2002; Piazza and Le Moal, 1996).

B. Effects of Stress on Dopaminergic Transmission

1. *Effects of Stress on Extracellular Concentrations of Dopamine*

The effects of stress have been examined on extracellular concentrations of dopamine, measured using *in vivo* microdialysis, voltammetry, or chronoamperometry techniques. Data show that stress exhibits an inverted U-shaped curve, in which mild to moderate stressors have activating effects (they increase dopaminergic transmission), whereas intense, chronic, and unpredictable stressors have inhibitory effects (they decrease dopaminergic transmission).

a. Effects of Mild Stress on Extracellular Concentrations of Dopamine Perhaps one of the first studies examining the effects of stress on dopaminergic transmission was published 30 years ago. Using *postmortem* analysis of tissue dopamine and its metabolites, it was found that a brief (3 minute) foot-shock stress increases dopamine turnover (the ratio between the deamination product of dopamine and dopamine) in the frontal cortex of rodents (Thierry et al., 1976). These *postmortem* findings were reproduced and expanded, using similar or slightly different stressors such as different foot-shock paradigms (Blanc et al., 1980; Carlson et al., 1991; Deutch et al., 1985; Fadda and Liguori, 1981; Fadda et al., 1978; Herman et al., 1982; Lavielle et al., 1979), exposure to a mate undergoing foot shock or exposure to the environment previously associated with the shock (Deutch et al., 1985; Herman et al., 1982; Kaneyuki et al., 1991), restraint (Carlson et al., 1991; Morrow et al., 1993), exposure to cold (Dunn and File, 1983), brief (24-hour) food deprivation (Carlson et al., 1987). Most of these studies show similar results: Mild stress produces

large increases in dopamine turnover in the frontal cortex (~80% increase), small and sometimes insignificant increases in the nucleus accumbens (~35% increases), and very small, but mostly no changes at all, in the striatum. Stress-induced increases in dopamine turnover are preferentially seen in the ventral tegmental area, which projects to the prefrontal cortex and the nucleus accumbens, as opposed to the substantia nigra, which projects to the striatum (Deutch et al., 1985), in line with preferential increase in the cortex and accumbens compared with the striatum. Studies using stressors of different intensities confirm these results; very low-level stressors activate dopamine turnover only in the prefrontal cortex, whereas mild-moderate stressors produce a more generalized increase in dopamine utilization (Carlson et al., 1991; Deutch and Roth, 1990; Inoue et al., 1994; Lavielle et al., 1979; Roth et al., 1988). This suggests that meso-prefrontal dopamine neurons are particularly sensitive to the effects of stress, perhaps because of differences in dopamine reuptake and afferent excitatory input to these neurons with respect to meso-striatal ones (for review, see Finlay and Zigmond, 1997). Increased reactivity of meso-prefrontal dopamine neurons to stress is also strengthened by findings showing that restraint stress selectively activates (as measured by expression of c-Fos protein) dopamine neurons projecting to the prefrontal cortex (Deutch et al., 1991); this effect is paralleled by a preferential increase of dopamine levels (measured *postmortem*) in the prefrontal cortex, as opposed to the nucleus accumbens.

Further studies have been performed using microdialysis techniques, which can detect more subtle changes in extracellular dopamine and can capture time-dependent changes that could go unnoticed using *postmortem* studies. Studies comparing dopamine levels across structures confirm the heterogeneous response to stress, although differences in prefrontal cortex and accumbens are not always as robust.

Different stressors such as intermittent tail shock, exposure to cold, handling or mild tail pinch produce increases in dopamine efflux that tend to be greater in the prefrontal cortex (~50–95% increase) as opposed to the nucleus accumbens (~40–50% increase) or the striatum (~25% increase). Dopamine levels peak approximately 15 minutes after termination of the stressor in the nucleus accumbens and striatum, and they often follow a more rapid time-course in the prefrontal cortex (Abercrombie et al., 1989; Cenci et al., 1992; Gresch et al., 1994; Imperato et al., 1991; Kalivas and Duffy, 1989).

Other, single-structure, microdialysis studies have also reported increases in prefrontal cortex dopamine following stress. Thus, brief exposure to foot shock, to the foot-shock environment, as well as restraint stress, social defeat, tail pinch or brief handling, increase dopamine levels in the prefrontal cortex of rats (Enrico et al., 1998; Finlay et al., 1995; Imperato et al., 1991; Jedema and Moghaddam, 1994; Sorg and Kalivas, 1993; Tidey and Miczek, 1996; Wedzony et al., 1996). On the same line, stressors similar to those described above have been shown to increase dopamine overflow in the nucleus accumbens (Imperato et al., 1991; Imperato et al., 1992a; Puglisi-Allegra et al., 1991; Sorg and Kalivas, 1991). Importantly, not only does stress increase dopamine levels, but it also increases dopaminergic reactivity to addictive drugs. Thus, as will be discussed in the last section, stressed animals show greater drug-induced increases in accumbens dopamine than nonstressed individuals (Balakrishna et al., 1995; Sorg, 1992).

While stress has been shown to increase accumbens dopamine, it is important to recognize that such increases are not homogeneous across individuals and strains. Thus some individual rats, or rat strains, react to stress more than others (Bertolucci-D'Angio et al., 1990b; Giorgi et al., 1997; Leggio et al., 2003; Rouge-Pont et al., 1993, 1998); similarly, different strains of mice can be more or less sensitive to the dopaminergic effects of stress (Herve et al., 1979; Puglisi-Allegra et al., 1990; Shanks et al., 1990). In addition, reactivity to stress can differ within the different subregions of nucleus accumbens (the core and the shell). This probably explains why earlier studies, which did not distinguish between core and shell, observed only modest or sometimes inconsistent effects of stress on accumbens dopamine. When the core/shell distinction is made, *postmortem* studies indicate that immediately following the exposure to restraint stress, animals have greater dopamine utilization in the shell versus the core of the nucleus accumbens (Deutch and Cameron, 1992). Microdialysis studies provide more detail on the time-course of the effects of stress. They show that another stressor (20-minute exposure to mild foot shock) produces a marked elevation of dopamine in the nucleus accumbens shell; this increase is evident approximately 10–20 minutes after the end of the stressor. Whereas stress increases dopamine levels in the shell, it has no effects in the core (Kalivas and Duffy, 1995). Additional microdialysis studies using a weaker stressor confirm the above findings. Thus, the intraperitoneal injection of saline produces an increase in dopamine overflow in the shell of the nucleus accumbens, which occurs within 20 minutes from the end of the stressor; this same stress does not alter dopamine levels in the core. In fact, the core is similar to the dorsal striatum in its inability to be activated by mild stressors (Barrot et al., 1999). These structure-related differences in reactivity to stress are illustrated in Figure 3-4; interestingly, they are similar to those seen in response to addictive drugs (Barrot et al., 1999 and Figure 3.3).

Studies using voltammetry also show that stress enhances extracellular concentrations of dopamine or its metabolites. However, brain areas showing greatest effects vary across studies. For example, it was shown that a brief (1 minute) electric shock to the animal's tail or a 20–30 minute exposure to a shallow ice-cold water bath increases dopamine levels in the striatum (Keller, Jr.

Extracellular concentrations of dopamine

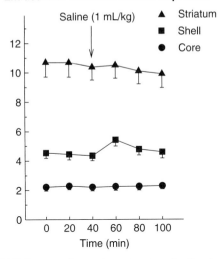

FIGURE 3-4 Effects of an injection of saline (a minor stressor) on extracellular concentrations of dopamine in different subregions of the striatal complex. Data were obtained using *in vivo* microdialysis in freely moving rats (see Figure 3-1 for probe location). The administration of saline does not modify extracellular concentrations of dopamine in the dorsolateral striatum (Striatum) or the nucleus accumbens core (Core). However, the saline injection increases dopamine by about 25% in the nucleus accumbens shell (Shell). Thus, the nucleus accumbens shell shows reactivity to a mild stressor, whereas the other two subregions do not. Modified from Barrot et al., 1999.

et al., 1983). The increase is transient and peaks only 4–7 minutes after the stressor, which is probably why it is detected with this technique only with greater temporal resolution and sensitivity. In a different study, tail pinch, immobilization stress, and forced locomotion produced a greater increase in dopamine metabolites in the nucleus accumbens with respect to the prefrontal cortex; no changes in the striatum were observed (Bertolucci-D'Angio et al., 1990a). Similar results indicating a preferential increase of dopamine metabolism in the accumbens over the prefrontal cortex were obtained with a pharmacological anxiogenic stressor (Bertolucci-D'Angio et al., 1990a). Other studies monitoring dopamine levels show that foot-shock stress increases dopamine clearance in the prefrontal cortex

(Meiergerd et al., 1997) or that a brief (2 minute) tail pinch increases overflow in the prefrontal cortex, an effect that lasts longer in the left versus the right prefrontal cortex (Sullivan and Gratton, 1998).

Finally, though brief and mild stressors can increase dopamine levels, if the stressor is prolonged (e.g., prolonged restraint or foot shock), it will eventually produce a decrease in dopamine (Puglisi-Allegra et al., 1991). Similarly, if the stress is intensified or becomes unpredictable, it will switch from increasing dopamine to decreasing it (Carlson et al., 1993). This is consistent with the notion that stress has an inverted U-shaped function on dopaminergic transmission and that strong stressors depress dopaminergic transmission. This will be discussed further in the next section.

b. Effects of Intense Stress on Extracellular Concentrations of Dopamine Chronic food restriction (about 20–30% of body weight loss), which can be considered an intense stressor, produces a marked decrease in baseline levels of nucleus accumbens dopamine, as measured with microdialysis techniques (Pothos et al., 1995a, 1995b). Another strong stress, such as a 7-day exposure to inescapable electric shock, also produces a net decrease in basal levels of dopamine in the nucleus accumbens shell; a longer (3-week) exposure to this stressor also lowers basal levels of accumbens dopamine, and dopamine levels remain low for at least 2 weeks after termination of the stress (Mangiavacchi et al., 2001). The exposure to a variety of stressors, administered repeatedly (such as electric shock, physical restraint, and exposure to an environment previously associated with electric shock), also produces a net decrease in baseline levels of accumbens dopamine (Gambarana et al., 1999). Not only is baseline dopamine decreased, but drug-induced accumulation of dopamine is also lessened. Thus, chronic stress reduces cocaine and amphetamine-induced increase in accumbens dopamine (Gambarana et al., 1999; Mangiavacchi et al.,

2001). Similar results on baseline and drug-stimulated dopamine are also observed in the prefrontal cortex. Interestingly, however, 2 weeks after the exposure to chronic stress, baseline dopamine is back to normal levels in the prefrontal cortex, and cocaine-induced accumulation of dopamine is actually increased, suggesting a rebound increase in dopaminergic transmission after its suppression (Mangiavacchi et al., 2001).

Other experiments have been performed using other classically used chronic mild stress procedures (Moreau et al., 1995; Willner, 1997). In these experiments, animals were subjected for 4 weeks to daily unpredictable mild stressors that included reversal of the light-dark cycle, brief withdrawal of food or water, exposure to a soiled or a small cage, and so on. Using this procedure, Di Chiara and colleagues (1999) did not observe a significant decrease in basal levels of accumbens or prefrontal cortex dopamine; yet, similar to the above studies, they observed a blunted dopaminergic response to the presentation of a rewarding stimulus such as palatable food (Di Chiara and Tanda, 1997; Di Chiara et al., 1999). Interestingly, though chronic stress decreased the dopaminergic response to a positive stimulus, it produced an opposite effect in response to an aversive stimulus (a 10-minute tail pinch). In these experiments a 10-minute tail pinch produced a slight depression of accumbens dopamine in control animals but a marked increase in dopamine overflow in chronically stressed rats. In the prefrontal cortex, tail pinch elevated dopamine levels in all animals, but more so in chronically stressed rats (Di Chiara et al., 1999). This indicates that, in these conditions, chronic mild stress did not modify the tonic modality of dopaminergic transmission (basal levels), but only the phasic one (in response to rewarding or stressful/aversive stimuli). It should be noted, however, that in the latter studies, the chronic mild stress procedure did not impair the animal's *behavioral* ability to approach the rewarding stimulus; it only blunted the *dopaminergic*

reactivity to that stimulus. This indicates that the stress procedure did not necessarily cause pronounced *behavioral* inhibition and anhedonia, as is sometimes seen with prolonged stress protocols; a *behavioral* hallmark of anhedonia is inhibition of behavioral responses, such as consumption and preference for palatable sweet solutions (Muscat and Willner, 1992; Papp et al., 1991). In studies in which chronic stress has been shown to produce overt signs of behavioral inhibition, basal levels of dopamine were also reduced (Gambarana et al., 1999). It is therefore possible that tonic dopaminergic transmission is decreased only when the chronic stressor is strong enough to produce marked *behavioral* inhibition, which further corroborates the notion that stress has an inverted U-shaped effect on dopaminergic transmission.

2. Effects of Stress on Dopamine Neuron Activity

Although most studies focused on the effects of stress on dopamine levels using neurochemical methods, a few have analyzed the effects of stress on dopamine neuron activity, measured by evaluating the firing rate and pattern of these cells. Some of these studies have yielded contradictory results, as they have shown that "stress" has no effects, produces a transient decrease, or produces a long-lasting increase in dopamine neuron activity.

a. Effects of Mild Stress on Dopamine Neuron Activity Indirect evidence that stress affects the activity of dopamine neurons came from a study in which stress-induced increases in dopamine content of the nucleus accumbens were prevented by blocking action potentials in the medial forebrain bundle with tetrodotoxin (Keefe et al., 1993).

Direct evidence for the effects of stress on dopamine neuron activity is provided by electrophysiological studies. Different stressful conditions that increase glucocorticoids levels, such as a reduction in food availability, restraint stress, and cold swim stress (Dallman et al., 2004; Deroche et al., 1993a, 1995; Huber et al., 2001; Shalev et al., 2003), have all been shown to increase dopamine neuron activity. A 12–20 day food restriction (10% in body weight reduction produced by reduction in daily ration of food) or a single day of complete food deprivation produces an increase in the firing and bursting activity of ventral tegmental area dopamine neurons of anesthetized rats (Figure 3-5). Similarly, a 5-minute exposure to cold swim also increases action potential output. This effect is seen within 2 hours after exposure to the stressor and persists for about 24 hours after the end of the stressor; baseline firing is reestablished 48–72 hours thereafter (Figure 3-5). Chronic exposure to a cold room reduces the number of active dopamine neurons, but it also produces an increase in the proportion of neurons with high levels of bursting activity (Moore et al., 2001), suggesting that this stress might facilitate the switch from regular firing to burst-firing activity. In awake rats, a 30-minute restraint stress also increases the firing

activity of dopamine neurons. This stress also augments bursting activity in 80% of the neurons, and it does so preferentially in those neurons with high burst rates under resting conditions (Anstrom and Woodward, 2005). In awake-behaving cats, the exposure to the stress of a conditioned emotional reaction, which is known to increase stress hormones, also increases dopamine neuron activity (Trulson and Preussler, 1984). Finally, the administration of glucocorticoid hormones, in the range between low and high peaks of the circadian cycle, has been shown to increase glutamate-induced bursting activity of dopamine neurons (Overton et al., 1996).

b. Effects of Brief Aversive Stimuli on Dopamine Neuron Activity

Whereas exposure to moderate stressors has been shown to increase dopamine neuron activity, brief exposure to mildly aversive situations has been shown to increase neuronal activity, has no effect, or more generally produces a transient decrease in neuronal firing rate.

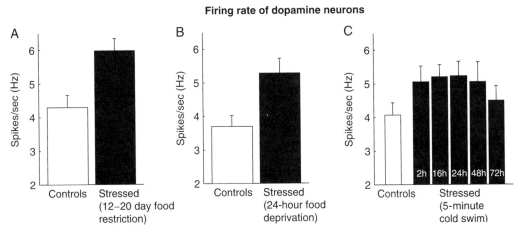

FIGURE 3-5 Effects of mild stress on dopamine neuron activity, recorded with *in vivo* extracellular recordings in anesthetized rats. The activity of dopamine neurons (number of spikes/sec) is increased by (A) repeated (12–20 days) food restriction (approximately 8–10% body weight loss), (B) acute, 24 hours of food deprivation (approximately 7–8% body weight loss), and (C) a brief (5-minute) exposure to cold swim. For this stressor, neuronal activity is increased 2 hours after the end of the stress; firing rate remains elevated until 48 hours after the end of the stress. Values return to baseline levels 72 hours after the end of the stress. Modified from Marinelli et al., 2006 (a and b) or preliminary observations obtained by M. Marinelli and C. N. Rudick (C).

In awake cats, the brief presentation of aversive stimuli, such as a tail pinch, the immersion of the paws in cold water, exposure to white noise or to inaccessible food, does not cause significant changes in dopamine neuronal firing (Strecker and Jacobs, 1985). In rats, pinching the paw while the animal is anesthetized has been shown to slow down neuronal firing in about 85% of identified dopamine neurons (Ungless et al., 2004). Similar findings were shown in earlier studies; different brief aversive (but not necessarily painful) stimuli, such as tail pressure, light flashes, and air puffs to the snout, produce a mild depression of neuronal activity in cells with typical electrophysiological parameters indicating their dopaminergic nature; instead, these same stimuli increase activity in neurons with waveforms of shorter duration (Chiodo et al., 1980), which were unlikely dopaminergic cells (Grace and Bunney, 1983; Marinelli et al., 2006; Ungless et al., 2004). In a different study, tail pinching was shown to depress firing activity in 25% of putative dopamine neurons projecting to cortical regions, but to increase it in 65% of this mesocortical population, and to have no effect on the remainder of the neurons (Mantz et al., 1989). Similarly, the effects of a noxious radiant heat have been shown to have heterogeneous effects on dopamine neurons of the midbrain (Barasi, 1979). It is possible that differences in nature of the cells (projection sites of these cells, or possibly dopamine versus nondopamine identity) might account for this discrepancy in rodent studies. Heterogeneous results are somewhat seen in primate studies too. In monkeys, a pinching stimulus has been shown to decrease action potential output in 50% of the dopamine cell population, but to increase it in 25% of the cells and to have no effect in the remainder of the population (Schultz and Romo, 1987). A decrease in dopamine neuron activity was also seen when monkeys experienced an aversive stimulus: Primates that were trained to expect a juice reward upon responding were not offered such a reward (Schultz et al., 1997;

Schultz, 2002). A milder aversive stimulus (non-noxious air puffs) has not been shown to produce significant changes in dopamine cell activity (Mirenowicz and Schultz, 1996), suggesting that aversive stimuli should be of greater intensity to produce an effect or that dopamine neurons do not respond to certain types of aversive stimuli.

3. Differences between Aversive and Stressful Stimuli, and between Dopamine Levels and Dopamine Neuron Activity

Overall, data described above indicate that acute and brief (<1 minute) presentation of aversive stimuli generally decrease dopamine neuron activity. Instead, exposure to longer and possibly more stressful stimuli increases neuronal activity. The nature of this discrepancy between brief aversive stimuli and longer stressful stimuli is unclear. It is possible that "aversive" and "stressful" stimuli could be different in nature—one causing depression, the other excitation. In fact, exposure to quinine, an aversive stimulus, has been shown to produce a transient decrease in accumbens dopamine levels measured with fast-scan cyclic voltammetry consistent with the notion of aversion leading to suppression of dopaminergic transmission (Roitman et al., 2005). Such a depression is not seen using techniques such as microdialysis (Levita et al., 2002; Wilkinson et al., 1998), probably because rapid phasic changes are seldom detected with this technique (see II.B., "Evaluating the Activity of the Dopaminergic Pathway," above). Instead, increases in dopamine produced by prolonged stressful events are detected by microdialysis, because such increases are produced over prolonged periods of time, long enough for dopamine to accumulate in the extracellular space.

Alternatively, if one views aversive stimuli as being, to some degree, "stressful," it is possible that their brevity and low intensity might not make them "stressful enough" to activate dopaminergic transmission. Such stimuli might need to be presented repeatedly, or they might require long periods of time in order to become "stressful enough" to increase dopaminergic transmission. On this line, it has been suggested that increases in dopaminergic transmission are manifested only when environmental events produce prolonged increases in stress hormone levels (Marinelli and Piazza, 2002). Consistent with the notion that increases in stress hormones are necessary to produce increases in dopamine neuron activity are studies showing that stress produces an increase in dopamine neuron excitability, and this effect is prevented by the administration of a glucocorticoid receptor antagonist (Saal et al., 2003); more information on the role of glucocorticoids in the effects of stress will be provided in the following sections.

Perhaps a complementary explanation to reconcile why brief aversive stimuli depress dopamine neuron activity, whereas prolonged exposure to mild stressors increase it, could be that increased cell activity represents a "rebound" effect from initial depression. This rebound is seen only after prolonged exposure to the stimulus, which is why it is observed only after repeated or prolonged mild stress, but not after brief aversive stimuli. This could be analogous to what happens with psychostimulant drugs; administration of these drugs causes an initial decrease in neuronal activity and a rebound increase during their withdrawal. Such a hypothesis has not been tested directly, and further electrophysiological studies are required to determine the nature of stress- and aversive stimulus-induced changes in dopamine neuron action potential output.

4. Role of Stress Hormones

Stress activates the hypothalamo-pituitary-adrenal axis and elevates levels of corticotropin-releasing hormone and glucocorticoids; as suggested above, such increases in hormone levels could mediate, at least in part, the effects produced by stressful events on dopaminergic transmission. The interaction between glucocorticoids and dopamine has been revised extensively (de Jong and de Kloet, 2004; Marinelli and Piazza, 2002, 2003; Piazza and Le Moal, 1996; Piazza et al., 1996b); here I will focus mostly on stress-induced glucocorticoids secretion. For a more detailed review on the role of basal glucocorticoids secretion, please refer to the above reviews.

a. Effects of Stress Hormones on Dopaminergic Transmission As seen above, stress increases excitatory synaptic inputs onto dopamine neurons. These effects appear to be mediated by glucocorticoids because stress-induced increases in synaptic transmission are blocked by the administration of a glucocorticoid receptor antagonist (Saal et al., 2003). Stress-induced increases in corticotropin-releasing hormone are also a likely factor contributing to increases in synaptic transmission because the administration of corticotropin-releasing hormone potentiates NMDA receptor-mediated synaptic transmission in dopamine neurons (Ungless et al., 2003).

Further evidence for an involvement of glucocorticoids on dopamine transmission comes from studies showing that suppression of glucocorticoids by adrenalectomy reduces basal extracellular concentrations of dopamine in the nucleus accumbens, measured with *in vivo* microdialysis (Barrot et al., 2000; Piazza et al., 1996a). These effects depend on corticosterone because they are reversed by administration of the hormone. It is interesting to note that glucocorticoids have a specificity of action in the nucleus accumbens. Suppressing glucocorticoid hormones by adrenalectomy selectively decreases baseline dopamine levels in the shell of the accumbens, without modifying them in the core (Barrot et al., 2000). A similar effect is seen for stress-induced dopamine increases; thus adrenalectomy prevents the increase in dopamine produced by a mildly stressful situation (an intraperitoneal injection of saline). Similarly, blockade of stress-induced corticosterone secretion prevents the increase in accumbens dopamine induced by a 10-minute tail pinch stressor (Rouge-Pont et al., 1998). These effects are mediated by glucocorticoid receptors but not mineralocorticoid receptors because the administration of a mineralocorticoid antagonist does not modify extracellular levels of dopamine in the accumbens shell, whereas the administration of glucocorticoid receptor antagonist decreases dopamine levels in a dose-dependent manner (Marinelli et al., 1998). It should be noted, however, that other studies reported that adrenalectomy does not prevent changes in dopamine produced by restraint stress (Imperato et al., 1989; Imperato et al., 1991). Given the specificity of action of glucocorticoids, it is possible that differences in the location of the microdialysis probe (core versus shell) could explain these discrepancies.

Studies on dopamine levels following the administration of the stress hormone corticosterone are somewhat controversial. Using *in vivo* microdialysis, it was found that administration of corticosterone produces a modest increase in accumbens dopamine, but these effects are obtained only with concentrations of corticosterone that are well above the physiological range (Imperato et al., 1989, 1991). Instead, voltammetry studies found that dopamine levels are increased following administration of stress-like levels of corticosterone (Mittleman et al., 1992). This could be explained by possible state-dependent effects of glucocorticoid hormones. In fact, it has been shown that corticosterone increases accumbens dopamine if it is administered during the dark phase, when animals are active, but not during the light phase, when animals are inactive (Piazza et al., 1996c). Similarly, the effects of corticosterone are greater if it is administered when the animals are about to engage in eating behavior (Piazza et al., 1996c). In addition, corticosterone produces greater increases in accumbens dopamine in animals that already show a higher base-line dopaminergic tone (Rouge-Pont et al., 1998). In other words, the glucocorticoid corticosterone increases accumbens dopamine only if it is administered when the dopamine system is in an activated state, such as during the dark phase (Paulson and Robinson, 1994), during food intake (Hoebel et al., 1989; Taber and Fibiger, 1997), or in animals with an increased baseline dopaminergic tone (Rouge-Pont et al., 1993).

b. Possible Mechanisms of Stress Hormone Action The mechanisms by which glucocorticoid stress hormones modify dopaminergic transmission are not well characterized. They could modify dopamine neuron activity and release, as well as neurotransmitter synthesis, metabolism, and/or clearance of the neurotransmitter from the synaptic region. With respect to dopamine cell activity, it has been shown that glucocorticoids have a facilitatory role on glutamate-induced activity (Cho and Little, 1999; Overton et al., 1996). They also seem to impact basal neuronal activity, as mice lacking brain glucocorticoid receptors show low baseline firing of dopamine neurons compared to their wild-type littermates (Marinelli et al., 2003a; Turiault et al., 2005). Although glucocorticoid receptors are located in the midbrain (Harfstrand et al., 1986), they do not seem to be present on dopamine neurons (Czyrak and Chocyk, 2001). This suggests an indirect action of these hormones on dopamine cells. Such an indirect action is supported by preliminary showing that mice lacking glucocorticoid receptors in dopamine D1-expressing neurons show reduced firing rate of midbrain dopamine neurons, similar to that observed in mice lacking the receptors in the entire brain (Marinelli et al., 2003a; Turiault et al., 2005).

Concerning dopamine synthesis, glucocorticoids have been shown to have a facilitatory action on tyrosine hydroxylase (TH), the rate-limiting enzyme in dopamine synthesis (Dunn et al., 1978;

Iuvone et al., 1977; Ortiz et al., 1995); however, see Lindley et al. (1999). With respect to dopamine-metabolism, glucocorticoid hormones have been shown to decrease the activity of dopamine-metabolizing enzymes, such as monoamine oxidases; however, they have no effects on catechol-O-methyltransferase (Caesar et al., 1970; Ho-Van-Hap et al., 1967; Parvez and Parvez, 1973; Veals et al., 1977). Finally, it has been shown that these hormones could modify dopaminergic transmission by acting at the level of dopamine transporter sites. Thus, suppression of glucocorticoids decreases the number of dopamine-binding sites in the nucleus accumbens, and replacement of the hormone reverses this effect (Sarnyai et al., 1998). The effects are specific to the nucleus accumbens shell, where the authors observed a positive correlation between corticosterone and dopamine transporter levels. This is in line with findings showing that stress (repeated restraint) increases dopamine transporter function; however, this can also be seen as a compensatory change for increased dopamine levels, not necessarily as its cause, and not necessarily dependent on secretion of glucocorticoids (Copeland et al., 2005).

5. Other Factors Mediating the Effects of Stress on Dopaminergic Transmission

In addition to modifying dopamine synthesis, degradation and/or reuptake, stress and/or stress hormones could act on dopaminergic transmission by modifying other intrinsic or synaptic properties of dopamine cells. Dopaminergic transmission is regulated by numerous intrinsic and synaptic factors, which have been reviewed extensively in many reviews (Kitai et al., 1999; Marinelli et al., 2006; Mathon et al., 2003; Overton and Clark, 1997; White, 1996). I will give a brief overview of some factors that could be implicated in mediating the effects of stress or stress hormones on dopaminergic transmission.

a. Dopamine Autoreceptors Impulse-regulating autoreceptors play an important role in providing an efficient auto-inhibition onto dopamine neurons. These receptors are of the D2-class dopamine receptor family and are located in the somatodendritic region of midbrain dopamine neurons (Bunney et al., 1987; Clark and Chiodo, 1988; Mercuri et al., 1992). Somatodendritically released dopamine (Beart et al., 1979; Cheramy et al., 1981; Kalivas and Duffy, 1991) binds to these autoreceptors; this causes dissociation of the coupled Gi/o protein into the βγ dimer which activates G-protein–coupled inward-rectifying potassium channels (Davila et al., 2003; Innis and Aghajanian, 1987; Lacey et al., 1987; Mercuri et al., 1992; Williams and Lacey, 1988). Potassium outflow hyperpolarizes the cells, causing its inhibition. The functional state of these somatodendritic dopamine autoreceptors thus plays an important role in determining the level of activity of dopamine neurons (Marinelli et al., 2006).

Binding and *in situ* hybridization studies indicate that stress decreases expression of dopamine D2 receptors in the midbrain (Cabib et al., 1998; Dziedzicka-Wasylewska et al., 1997). Preliminary electrophysiological studies support these results and show that stress reduces the functional output of these receptors. Thus, mild food restriction reduces the ability of dopamine neuron to inhibit their activity after the administration of an autoreceptor agonist (Figure 3-6). Although such studies require further electrophysiological, molecular, and biochemical validation, it is tempting to speculate that a decrease in the expression of these receptors, or in their coupling to the Gi/o protein could be responsible for stress-induced increased dopamine neuron activity. Changes in the expression of G-protein-coupled inward-rectifying potassium channels could also mediate the effects of stress on dopamine neuron activity. Although data are absent

Firing rate of dopamine neurons: inhibition by auto-receptor activation

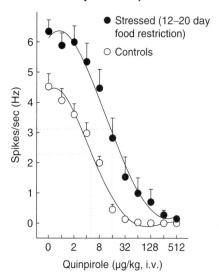

FIGURE 3-6 Reactivity of dopamine neurons to autoreceptor activation (administration of the autoreceptor agonist quinpirole, administered IV through the tail vein) in baseline conditions (Controls) or after repeated exposure to food restriction stress (Stressed). Data were obtained with *in vivo* extracellular recordings in anesthetized rats. Quinpirole dose-dependently inhibits dopamine cell activity in all animals; however, its ability to inhibit neuronal firing is decreased in stressed animals. Thus, stressed animals require higher doses of quinpirole to produce 50% of neuronal inhibition. Modified from Marinelli et al., 2002.

for the midbrain, it has been shown that administration of stress hormones can modify protein expression for these channels in the hippocampus (Muma and Beck, 1999).

b. Excitatory Synaptic Input Dopamine neuron activity is greatly influenced by the degree of excitatory glutamatergic input to these cells. Application of glutamate onto the cell body of dopamine neurons increases firing rate and bursting activity of these cells (Meltzer et al., 1997; Overton and Clark, 1991, 1992). Such effects are largely mediated by activation of AMPA and NMDA glutamate receptors, which mediate the majority of excitatory input to dopamine neurons (Mathon et al., 2003;

Overton and Clark, 1997; Wang and French, 1993a, 1993b). One way to evaluate the status of glutamatergic excitatory synaptic inputs onto dopamine neurons can be to quantify the ratio of AMPA to NMDA receptor-mediated synaptic currents (the "AMPA/NMDA ratio") after synaptic stimulation. Such AMPA/NMDA ratio can be a useful assay for changes in synaptic strength; higher ratios reflect greater synaptic potentiation (Saal et al., 2003; Ungless et al., 2001). Using this approach, it was shown that stress can enhance excitatory synaptic input onto dopamine cells. A brief, 5-minute exposure to cold swim stress enhances the ratio of AMPA to NMDA currents recorded in dopamine neurons after synaptic stimulation (Saal et al., 2003). Interestingly, a similar increase in AMPA/NMDA ratio is also seen after exposure to addictive drugs (Borgland et al., 2004; Faleiro et al., 2003; Saal et al., 2003; Thomas et al., 2000; Ungless et al., 2001) indicating that drugs and stress produce a common neuronal adaptation in the reward system; they share the common property of enhancing dopamine neuron reactivity to excitatory synaptic input. This is a very important finding because changes in synaptic strength have been implicated in learning and memory formation; so such strengthening of synaptic transmission in the reward circuit (Bonci et al., 2003; Jones and Bonci, 2005; Kauer, 2004) could facilitate the development of addiction (Kelley, 2004; Lovinger et al., 2003; Wolf et al., 2004).

While dopamine autoreceptors and excitatory inputs are possible substrates for stress action, it cannot be excluded that stress and/or stress hormones modify dopaminergic transmission via other direct or indirect mechanisms. Stress could, for example, influence countless other brain systems (opioids, GABA, serotonin, norepinephrine, etc.) which, in turn are susceptible of modulating the activity of midbrain dopamine cells. Given space limitation, many of these other potential mechanisms have not been examined.

V. CONCLUSIONS

A. Possible Relevance of Stress- and Drug-Induced Increases in Dopaminergic Transmission

Data presented above show that both stress and drugs of abuse can independently increase dopaminergic transmission; in fact, many scientists have studied this parallel between the effects of stress and drugs of abuse (Antelman et al., 1980; Bland et al., 2004a; Kalivas and Duffy, 1989; Meiergerd et al., 1997; Miczek et al., 1999; Prasad et al., 1995; Sorg, 1992; Sorg and Kalivas, 1991). So, it is somewhat puzzling that apparently opposite phenomena, such as mild stress and addictive drugs, actually have a similar effect on dopaminergic transmission. Several reviews have been published precisely to discuss this quandary.

Increases in dopamine are thought to be involved in aspects of sensorimotor functions that are important for both appetitive and aversive stimuli; thus stress- or drug-induced increases in dopamine could facilitate sensorimotor integration of the environment and surrounding stimuli, and would indirectly influence execution of complex behaviors (Salamone, 1992; Salamone, 1994). In this scenario, dopamine acts as an enabler to overcome response costs or difficulties; this improves behavioral reactivity and facilitates the execution of behaviors that increase probability of survival (Salamone, 1996; Salamone and Correa, 2002; Salamone et al., 1997).

It has also been suggested that elevations of dopamine in response to salient and arousing conditions, regardless of their valence, could mediate the effects of arousal on several behavioral functions, which could facilitate successful execution of goal-directed behaviors (Horvitz, 2000). In an analogous manner, it was proposed that dopamine

released during certain salient situations (whether positive or negative) could allow paying attention to stimuli that would otherwise go unnoticed; in this context dopamine would play a role in attributing attention toward otherwise familiar stimuli (Joseph et al., 2003). The fact that dopamine cells of stressed animals show stronger responsiveness to excitatory synaptic inputs (Saal et al., 2003) also suggests that stress increases reactivity to environmental stimuli; this could serve as a survival mechanism allowing animals to increase their attention toward behaviorally relevant stimuli.

The concept of dopamine being important for attention has been given much consideration by other authors as well. Phasic increases in dopamine neuron activity could help orient attention and behavior toward subsequent salient stimuli (Redgrave et al., 1999). This could facilitate associative learning (Bundesen et al., 2005) and serve as a preparatory stimulus for the appropriate reaction to a significant event (Redgrave et al., 1999). On a similar line, a large body of work has shown that dopaminergic transmission, especially to cortical areas, plays an important role in arousal (for example, see Coull, 1998; Feenstra et al., 2002; Nieoullon, 2002; Robbins et al., 1998). It is therefore possible that stress-induced enhancement of dopaminergic transmission increases the state of arousal, which would facilitate the individual's ability to perceive or react to environmental stimulations.

By viewing the behavioral responses to both positive and negative stimuli as "approach to safety," it has also been suggested that increases in dopaminergic transmission (seen during both positive and negative stimuli) could invigorate such approach responses. In positive contexts, dopamine increases approach toward the stimuli of survival values. In negative contexts, dopamine increases approach toward safety. In addition, increases in dopamine during the presentation of salient stimuli could enable the environment to acquire incentive properties. This view reconciles the role for dopamine in the context for the learning of associations with both positive and negative stimuli. Dopamine would be involved in such a learning process so that animals have an appropriate "approach to safety" response when they subsequently encounter a similar environment (Ikemoto and Panksepp, 1999).

Finally, it was proposed that stress-induced increases in dopaminergic transmission could represent an adaptive response that helps the individual cope with the stressful situation. Stress-induced increase in dopamine levels could reduce the aversive effects of stress and possibly make it "reinforcing"; this would increase the individual's ability to cope with the stressful situation, rather than to flee or become learned helpless (Marinelli and Piazza, 2002; Marinelli et al., 2006). Another interesting speculation can be made by examining the relationship between dopamine neuron activity and risk-taking behavior. Sustained increase in dopamine neuron activity has been suggested to reinforce risk-taking behavior (Fiorillo et al., 2003). Thus, the increase in dopamine neuron activity produced by stressors could facilitate risk-taking behavior, thereby broadening the animal's capacity to respond to the stressor.

B. Interaction between Stress, Dopamine, and Addiction

Regardless of its evolutionary relevance, could stress-induced increases in dopamine have any consequences on addiction-associated behaviors? In fact, increases in dopamine favor addiction-associated behaviors, and stressful events powerfully increase addiction-associated behaviors (for review, see Goeders, 2002; Marinelli and Piazza, 2002, 2003; Piazza and Le Moal, 1996, 1998; Shaham et al., 2000; Shalev et al., 2000; Stewart, 2000). So it is possible that stress-induced increases in dopaminergic transmission could represent a mechanism by which stressful events could lead to changes in an individual's reactivity to

drugs and enhance drug-associated behaviors. This will be examined below for behaviors such as drug-induced locomotion, drug self-administration, and drug seeking.

A first link between stress, dopamine, and drug responding comes from studies showing a concomitant increase in dopamine overflow and drug-self administration behavior in stressed animals. Exposure to social threat increases dopamine levels in the nucleus accumbens. This increase is greater in rats that have previously experienced social defeat. Such previously defeated rats, exhibiting high levels of accumbens dopamine, acquire cocaine self-administration about twice as quickly as nondefeated rats, which show lower dopamine levels (Tidey and Miczek, 1996, 1997). These data suggest that stress-induced increases in dopaminergic transmission may increase the individual's susceptibility to acquire stimulant self-administration. A somewhat similar pattern also exists in humans. Thus, there is a positive relationship between secretion of stress hormones, dopaminergic activity, and the subjective response to amphetamine (Oswald et al., 2005).

Studies on other drug-associated behaviors support the idea that an interaction between stress and dopamine exacerbates drug responding. Blockade of dopamine D1 receptors with a selective antagonist reverses the increase in the rewarding and locomotor-activating effects of amphetamine produced by food restriction stress (Carr et al., 2001). In another study, stress-induced increase in amphetamine place-preference was reversed by either D1 or D2 dopamine receptor antagonists (az-Otanez et al., 1997; Capriles and Cancela, 1999), suggesting that stress-induced increases in dopamine levels were probably responsible for the observed effects. However, changes in dopamine levels are not necessarily the only change in dopaminergic transmission underlying stress-induced increases in reward-related behaviors. In fact, it was shown that food restriction increases the sensitivity to a dopamine D1 receptor agonist during brain-stimulation reward (Carr et al., 2001). This indicates that food restriction-induced augmentation of reward can also bypass the dopamine terminal, and acts postsynaptically by increasing dopamine D1 receptor-mediated effects.

The above findings suggest that stress facilitates the development of reward and drug-related behaviors by enhancing the activity of the dopaminergic system. It is also likely that stress modifies the way in which the dopamine system reacts to addictive drugs, in a manner that could favor the development of addiction. This can be tested by evaluating dopaminergic responses to addictive drugs in stressed versus control animals. Indirect evidence for differential dopaminergic reactivity to drugs in stressed versus control animals comes from studies investigating the behavioral response to centrally injected psychostimulants or opiates. The motor response induced by the injection of psychostimulants in the nucleus accumbens is dopamine-dependent (Delfs et al., 1990; Vezina and Stewart, 1984), as is the one induced by administration of opiates in the ventral tegmental area (Joyce and Iversen, 1979; Kalivas and Duffy, 1989). It was shown that stress (food restriction) enhances this behavioral response, and this can be prevented by inhibiting the hormonal response to stress (Deroche et al., 1995). Work that directly examines dopamine overflow with microdialysis confirms that stress exacerbates the dopaminergic response to drugs of abuse. As briefly discussed previously, the repeated exposure to foot-shock stress enhances cocaine-induced increase in accumbens extracellular dopamine levels (Balakrishna et al., 1995; Kalivas and Duffy, 1989; Sorg and Kalivas, 1991; Sorg and Steketee, 1992). Similar results are obtained for tail shock in response to morphine (Bland et al., 2003, 2004a, 2004b) and for restraint stress and reactivity to amphetamine (Pacchioni et al., 2002). Food restriction stress is another stressor that also heightens cocaine-induced dopamine overflow; in addition, as shown in Figure 3-7,

these effects are prevented by inhibiting stress-induced secretion of stress hormones (Rouge-Pont et al., 1995). These same studies show that blocking stress-induced increases in dopamine levels also blocks stress-induced increases in the locomotor response to drugs (Rouge-Pont et al., 1995), which further suggests that stress-induced potentiation of the dopaminergic response to drugs is responsible for stress-induced potentiation of the behavioral effects of drugs.

The converse is also true in most cases: Not only do stressed animals show greater dopaminergic reactivity to drugs, but animals exposed to drugs show greater dopaminergic reactivity to stress. Numerous studies have shown that stress can produce a greater

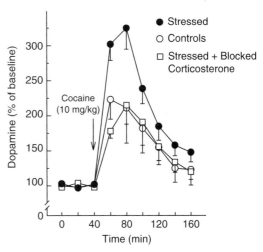

Extracellular concentrations of dopamine

FIGURE 3-7 Effects of cocaine on extracellular concentrations of dopamine in the nucleus accumbens of control rats (Controls), stressed rats (Stressed: 8 days of food restriction, 10% body weight loss), and stressed rats whose stress-induced corticosterone secretion was blocked by metyrapone, a corticosterone synthesis inhibitor (Stressed + Blocked Corticosterone). Cocaine produces an increase in extracellular levels of accumbens dopamine in all groups. However, this increase is greater in stressed animals. This effect of stress is prevented by blocking stress-induced corticosterone secretion, indicating that increases in stress hormones are required to produce the stress-induced exacerbation of the dopaminergic reactivity to cocaine. Modified with permission from Rougé-Pont et al., 1995.

activation of the dopamine system in animals that have been previously exposed to different addictive drugs such as cocaine and amphetamine. This has been documented by monitoring dopamine neuron activity with electrophysiological techniques (Marinelli, 2005a), as well by measuring dopamine levels in the nucleus accumbens and prefrontal cortex using microdialysis or *postmortem* techniques (Hamamura and Fibiger, 1993; Kalivas and Duffy, 1989; Robinson et al., 1987, 1988). However, such an increased reactivity to stress in drug-pretreated animals has not been reported in other studies using microdialysis (Sorg, 1992; Sorg and Kalivas, 1991, 1993), perhaps because of differences in probe location, intensity of the stress (foot shock), or the drug pretreatment and/or withdrawal regimen.

It is therefore likely that drug-experienced individuals exhibit greater dopaminergic reactivity to stressful events, which could be responsible for the well-documented increases in drug responding and relapse produced by stress. In fact, it has been shown that stress produces a parallel increase in accumbens dopamine and in drug-seeking behavior. This effect is reversed by the administration of dopamine receptor antagonists, indicating, once again, that the effects of stress are likely mediated by increased dopaminergic transmission (Shaham and Stewart, 1995, 1996).

Interestingly, an inverted U-shaped curve also exists for the interaction between stress, dopamine, and addictive drugs. Thus while mild/moderate stressors enhance dopaminergic and behavioral response to drugs (see above), intense stressors do not have this effect. As mentioned previously, the repeated presentation of intense stressors dampens dopaminergic reactivity to cocaine and amphetamine, and this effect is paralleled by decreased behavioral reactivity to these drugs (Gambarana et al., 1999). Interestingly, a relatively long (60-minute) restraint stress increases dopamine levels in drug-naïve animals but decreases it in amphetamine-exposed ones (Weiss et

al., 1997). If stress increases dopaminergic activity with an inverted U-shaped function, it is possible that this moderate-to-strong stressor is on the peak of the inverted U-shaped curve for control animals. However, if drug pre-exposure increases its effect, it could push it over to the descending limb of the curve. This is only seen with relative strong stressors (which are at the peak of the inverted U-shaped curve) but not with mild ones (which are on the bottom part of the ascending limb of the curve). In this case, an increase in stress effects would produce further enhancement of dopaminergic transmission.

Together, these findings indicate a positive relationship between stress, drug-induced dopamine overflow, and behavioral response to drugs. Mild stress, by interacting with the dopamine system, could facilitate the behavioral effects of addictive drugs. However, when stress becomes excessive, dopaminergic activity decreases, which offsets the individual's homeostatic state and could lead to decreased dopaminergic activity, depressive-like states, and decreased reactivity to drugs (Birman, 2005; Cabib, 1997; Cabib and Puglisi-Allegra, 1996a; Imperato et al., 1993; Willner, 1997).

C. Summary

Midbrain dopamine neurons originate in the ventral tegmental area and substantia nigra pars compacta, and project to forebrain structures such as the nucleus accumbens, the dorsal striatum, and the prefrontal cortex. The activity of the dopamine system can be measured using different techniques; they include microdialysis, which measures extracellular concentrations of dopamine, and fast-scan cyclic voltammetry and chronoamperometry, which measure extracellular concentrations of dopamine and can provide information on dopamine release and clearance. Electrophysiological studies are used to determine the action potential output of dopamine neurons.

The dopamine system plays an important role in addiction-associated behaviors. Its activity correlates positively with drug self-administration behavior in rodent models. In addition, addictive drugs have the common property of increasing extracellular concentrations of dopamine in the nucleus accumbens. Stressful events also modify dopaminergic transmission; they do so in an inverted U-shaped manner, according to the intensity and duration of the stressor. Mild stressors increase the activity of the dopamine system (extracellular concentrations of dopamine and neuronal firing), whereas intense prolonged and unpredictable stressors decrease dopaminergic transmission.

Though both stressors and addictive drugs can independently increase dopaminergic transmission, they can also interact. Mild stressors can enhance the dopaminergic effects of addictive substances. Stressed individuals show exacerbated dopaminergic responses to drugs such as cocaine, amphetamine, and morphine. This stress-induced increase in dopaminergic activity can exacerbate addiction-associated behaviors, such as locomotor activity in response to drugs, drug self-administration, and drug seeking.

In conclusion, stress, by increasing dopaminergic transmission and its reactivity to drugs, could facilitate the development of addiction-associated disorders and precipitate relapse to drug-seeking behaviors. Uncovering the cellular and molecular mechanisms that mediate the effects of stress on dopaminergic activity could help to better understand the interaction between stress and addiction, and to develop new therapeutic strategies for the treatment of this pathology.

ACKNOWLEDGMENTS

I would like to express my thanks to Drs. Satoshi Ikemoto and Mitchell Roitman for very helpful comments on several sections of this chapter. I thank Dr. Marco Diana for useful discussions on the role of hypodopaminergia in addiction, and Dr. Mark Ungless for very useful comments on several sections of this chapter, and for his input and ideas on the rebound effect of stress on dopamine neuron activity.

REFERENCES

Abercrombie, E. D., Keefe, K. A., DiFrischia, D. S., and Zigmond, M. J. (1989). Differential effect of stress on in vivo dopamine release in striatum, nucleus accumbens, and medial frontal cortex. *J. Neurochem.*, 52, 1655–1658.

Adell, A., and Artigas, F. (2004). The somatodendritic release of dopamine in the ventral tegmental area and its regulation by afferent transmitter systems. *Neurosci. Biobehav. Rev.*, 28, 415–431.

Adinoff, B. (2004). Neurobiologic processes in drug reward and addiction. *Harv. Rev. Psychiatry*, 12, 305–320.

Aghajanian, G. K., and Bunney, B. S. (1977). Dopamine "autoreceptors": Pharmacological characterization by microiontophoretic single cell recording studies. *Naunyn Schmiedebergs Arch. Pharmacol.*, 297, 1–7.

Akirav, I., Kozenicky, M., Tal, D., Sandi, C., Venero, C., and Richter-Levin, G. (2004). A facilitative role for corticosterone in the acquisition of a spatial task under moderate stress. *Learn. Mem.*, 11, 188–195.

Anden, N. E., Dahlstrom, A., Fuxe, K., and Larsson, K. (1965). Mapping out of catecholamine and 5-hydroxytryptamine neurons innervating the telencephalon and diencephalon. *Life Sci.*, 4, 1275–1279.

Andrews, J. S. (2005). Glucocorticoid antagonists and depression. In: *Handbook on stress and the brain; Part 2: Integrative and clinical aspects* (T. Steckler, N. H. Kalin, and J. M. H. M. Reul, Eds.) (Vol. 15, pp. 437–450.) Amsterdam: Elsevier Science.

Anstrom, K. K., and Woodward, D. J. (2005). Restraint increases dopaminergic burst firing in awake rats. *Neuropsychopharmacology*.

Antelman, S. M., Eichler, A. J., Black, C. A., and Kocan, D. (1980). Interchangeability of stress and amphetamine in sensitization. *Science*, 207, 329–331.

Appel, S. B., Liu, Z., McElvain, M. A., and Brodie, M. S. (2003). Ethanol excitation of dopaminergic ventral tegmental area neurons is blocked by quinidine. *J. Pharmacol. Exp. Ther.*, 306, 437–446.

Arbuthnott, G. W., Fairbrother, I. S., and Butcher, S. P. (1990). Dopamine release and metabolism in the rat striatum: An analysis by 'in vivo' brain microdialysis. *Pharmacol. Ther.*, 48, 281–293.

Axelrod, J., and Reisine, T. D. (1984). Stress hormones: Their interaction and regulation. *Science*, 224, 452–459.

az-Otanez, C. S., Capriles, N. R., and Cancela, L. M. (1997). D1 and D2 dopamine and opiate receptors are involved in the restraint stress-induced sensitization to the psychostimulant effects of amphetamine. *Pharmacol. Biochem. Behav., 58*, 9–14.

Bailey, C. P., O'Callaghan, M. J., Croft, A. P., Manley, S. J., and Little, H. J. (2001). Alterations in mesolimbic dopamine function during the abstinence period following chronic ethanol consumption. *Neuropharmacology, 41*, 989–999.

Balakrishna, M., Prasad, B. M., Sorg, B. A., Ulibarri, C., and Kalivas, P. W. (1995). Sensitization to stress and psychostimulants. *Involvement of dopamine transmission versus the HPA axis.* 617–625.

Barasi, S. (1979). Responses of substantia nigra neurones to noxious stimulation. *Brain Res., 171*, 121–130.

Barrot, M., Marinelli, M., Abrous, D. N., Rouge-Pont, F., Le Moal, M., and Piazza, P. V. (1999). Functional heterogeneity in dopamine release and in the expression of Fos-like proteins within the rat striatal complex. *Eur. J. Neurosci., 11*, 1155–1166.

Barrot, M., Marinelli, M., Abrous, D. N., Rouge-Pont, F., Le Moal, M., and Piazza, P. V. (2000). The dopaminergic hyper-responsiveness of the shell of the nucleus accumbens is hormone-dependent. *Eur. J. Neurosci., 12*, 973–979.

Bayer, V. E., and Pickel, V. M. (1991). GABA-labeled terminals form proportionally more synapses with dopaminergic neurons containing low densities of tyrosine hydroxylase-immunoreactivity in rat ventral tegmental area. *Brain Res., 559*, 44–55.

Beart, P. M., McDonald, D., and Gundlach, A. L. (1979). Mesolimbic dopaminergic neurones and somato-dendritic mechanisms. *Neurosci. Lett., 15*, 165–170.

Benes, F. M. (2001). Carlsson and the discovery of dopamine. *Trends Pharmacol. Sci., 22*, 46–47.

Benwell, M. E., Balfour, D. J., and Lucchi, H. M. (1993). Influence of tetrodotoxin and calcium on changes in extracellular dopamine levels evoked by systemic nicotine. *Psychopharmacology (Berl), 112*, 467–474.

Bertolucci-D'Angio, M., Serrano, A., and Scatton, B. (1990a). Differential effects of forced locomotion, tail-pinch, immobilization, and methyl-beta-carboline carboxylate on extracellular 3,4-dihydroxyphenyl-acetic acid levels in the rat striatum, nucleus accumbens, and prefrontal cortex: An in vivo voltammetric study. *J. Neurochem., 55*, 1208–1215.

Bertolucci-D'Angio, M., Serrano, A., and Scatton, B. (1990b). Mesocorticolimbic dopaminergic systems and emotional states. *J. Neurosci. Methods, 34*, 135–142.

Birman, S. (2005). Arousal mechanisms: Speedy flies don't sleep at night. *Curr. Biol., 15*, R511–R513.

Blanc, G., Herve, D., Simon, H., Lisoprawski, A., Glowinski, J., and Tassin, J. P. (1980). Response to stress of mesocortico-frontal dopaminergic neurones in rats after long-term isolation. *Nature, 284*, 265–267.

Bland, S. T., Hargrave, D., Pepin, J. L., Amat, J., Watkins, L. R., and Maier, S. F. (2003). Stressor controllability modulates stress-induced dopamine and serotonin

efflux and morphine-induced serotonin efflux in the medial prefrontal cortex. *Neuropsychopharmacology, 28*, 1589–1596.

Bland, S. T., Schmid, M. J., Watkins, L. R., and Maier, S. F. (2004a). Prefrontal cortex serotonin, stress, and morphine-induced nucleus accumbens dopamine. *Neuroreport, 15*, 2637–2641.

Bland, S. T., Twining, C., Schmid, M. J., Der-Avakian, A., Watkins, L. R., and Maier, S. F. (2004b). Stress potentiation of morphine-induced dopamine efflux in the nucleus accumbens shell is dependent upon stressor uncontrollability and is mediated by the dorsal raphe nucleus. *Neuroscience, 126*, 705–715.

Blokhina, E. A., Kashkin, V. A., Zvartau, E. E., Danysz, W., and Bespalov, A. Y. (2005). Effects of nicotinic and NMDA receptor channel blockers on intravenous cocaine and nicotine self-administration in mice. *Eur. Neuropsychopharmacol., 15*, 219–225.

Bohus, B. (1975). Environmental influences on pituitary-adrenal system function. *Probl. Actuels. Endocrinol. Nutr., 19*, 55–62.

Bonci, A., Bernardi, G., Grillner, P., and Mercuri, N. B. (2003). The dopamine-containing neuron: Maestro or simple musician in the orchestra of addiction? *Trends Pharmacol. Sci., 24*, 172–177.

Borgland, S. L., Malenka, R. C., and Bonci, A. (2004). Acute and chronic cocaine-induced potentiation of synaptic strength in the ventral tegmental area: Electrophysiological and behavioral correlates in individual rats. *J. Neurosci., 24*, 7482–7490.

Borland, L. M., Shi, G., Yang, H., and Michael, A. C. (2005). Voltammetric study of extracellular dopamine near microdialysis probes acutely implanted in the striatum of the anesthetized rat. *J. Neurosci. Methods, 146*, 149–158.

Bossert, J. M., Liu, S. Y., Lu, L., and Shaham, Y. (2004). A role of ventral tegmental area glutamate in contextual cue-induced relapse to heroin seeking. *J. Neurosci., 24*, 10726–10730.

Bradberry, C. W. (2000). Acute and chronic dopamine dynamics in a nonhuman primate model of recreational cocaine use. *J. Neurosci., 20*, 7109–7115.

Bradberry, C. W., Gruen, R. J., Berridge, C. W., and Roth, R. H. (1991). Individual differences in behavioral measures: Correlations with nucleus accumbens dopamine measured by microdialysis. *Pharmacol. Biochem. Behav., 39*, 877–882.

Bradberry, C. W., and Roth, R. H. (1989). Cocaine increases extracellular dopamine in rat nucleus accumbens and ventral tegmental area as shown by in vivo microdialysis. *Neurosci. Lett., 103*, 97–102.

Brandon, C. L., Marinelli, M., and White, F. J. (2003). Adolescent exposure to methylphenidate alters the activity of rat midbrain dopamine neurons. *Biol. Psychiatry, 54*, 1338–1344.

Brazell, M. P., Kasser, R. J., Renner, K. J., Feng, J., Moghaddam, B., and Adams, R. N. (1987).

Electrocoating carbon fiber microelectrodes with Nafion improves selectivity for electroactive neurotransmitters. *J. Neurosci. Methods*, 22, 167–172.

Brebner, K., Childress, A. R., and Roberts, D. C. (2002). A potential role for GABA(B) agonists in the treatment of psychostimulant addiction. *Alcohol Alcohol*, 37, 478–484.

Brebner, K., Phelan, R., and Roberts, D. C. (2000). Effect of baclofen on cocaine self-administration in rats reinforced under fixed-ratio 1 and progressive-ratio schedules. *Psychopharmacology (Berl)*, 148, 314–321.

Brodie, M. S., Pesold, C., and Appel, S. B. (1999). Ethanol directly excites dopaminergic ventral tegmental area reward neurons. *Alcohol Clin. Exp. Res.*, 23, 1848–1852.

Budygin, E. A., Kilpatrick, M. R., Gainetdinov, R. R., and Wightman, R. M. (2000). Correlation between behavior and extracellular dopamine levels in rat striatum: Comparison of microdialysis and fast-scan cyclic voltammetry. *Neurosci. Lett.*, 281, 9–12.

Bundesen, C., Habekost, T., and Kyllingsbaek, S. (2005). A neural theory of visual attention: Bridging cognition and neurophysiology. *Psychol. Rev.*, 112, 291–328.

Bungay, P. M., Newton-Vinson, P., Isele, W., Garris, P. A., and Justice, J. B. (2003). Microdialysis of dopamine interpreted with quantitative model incorporating probe implantation trauma. *J. Neurochem.*, 86, 932–946.

Bunney, E. B., Appel, S. B., and Brodie, M. S. (2001). Electrophysiological effects of cocaethylene, cocaine, and ethanol on dopaminergic neurons of the ventral tegmental area. *J. Pharmacol. Exp. Ther.*, 297, 696–703.

Bunney, B. S., and Aghajanian, G. K. (1977). D-amphetamine–induced inhibition of central dopaminergic neurons: Direct effect or mediated by a striatonigral feedback pathway? *Adv. Biochem. Psychopharmacol.*, 16, 577–582.

Bunney, B. S., Sesack, S. R., and Silva, N. L. (1987). Midbrain dopaminergic systems: Neurophysiology and electrophysiological pharmacology. In: *Psychopharmacology: The third generation of progress* (H. Y. Meltzer, Ed.) (pp. 113–126.) New York: Raven Press.

Bunney, B. S., Walters, J. R., Roth, R. H., and Aghajanian, G. K. (1973). Dopaminergic neurons: Effect of antipsychotic drugs and amphetamine on single cell activity. *J. Pharmacol. Exp. Ther.*, 185, 560–571.

Cabib, S. (1997). What is mild in mild stress? *Psychopharmacology (Berl)*, 134, 344–346.

Cabib, S., Giardino, L., Calza, L., Zanni, M., Mele, A., and Puglisi-Allegra, S. (1998). Stress promotes major changes in dopamine receptor densities within the mesoaccumbens and nigrostriatal systems. *Neuroscience*, 84, 193–200.

Cabib, S., and Puglisi-Allegra, S. (1996a). Different effects of repeated stressful experiences on meso-cortical and mesolimbic dopamine metabolism. *Neuroscience*, 73, 375–380.

Cabib, S., and Puglisi-Allegra, S. (1996b). Stress, depression and the mesolimbic dopamine system. *Psychopharmacology (Berl)*, 128, 331–342.

Caesar, P. M., Collins, G. G., and Sandler, M. (1970). Catecholamine metabolism and monoamine oxidase activity in adrenalectomized rats. *Biochem. Pharmacol.*, 19, 921–926.

Cahill, P. S., Walker, Q. D., Finnegan, J. M., Mickelson, G. E., Travis, E. R., and Wightman, R. M. (1996). Microelectrodes for the measurement of catecholamines in biological systems. *Anal. Chem.*, 68, 3180–3186.

Capriles, N., and Cancela, L. M. (1999). Effect of acute and chronic stress restraint on amphetamine-associated place preference: Involvement of dopamine D(1) and D(2) receptors. *Eur. J. Pharmacol.*, 386, 127–134.

Carboni, E., Imperato, A., Perezzani, L., and Di Chiara, G. (1989). Amphetamine, cocaine, phencyclidine and nomifensine increase extracellular dopamine concentrations preferentially in the nucleus accumbens of freely moving rats. *Neuroscience*, 28, 653–661.

Carlsson, A. (1959). The occurrence, distribution and physiological role of catecholamines in the nervous system. 490–493.

Carlson, J. N., Herrick, K. F., Baird, J. L., and Glick, S. D. (1987). Selective enhancement of dopamine utilization in the rat prefrontal cortex by food deprivation. *Brain Res.*, 400, 200–203.

Carlson, J. N., Fitzgerald, L. W., Keller, R. W., Jr., and Glick, S. D. (1991). Side and region dependent changes in dopamine activation with various durations of restraint stress. *Brain Res.*, 550, 313–318.

Carlson, J. N., Fitzgerald, L. W., Keller, R. W., Jr., and Glick, S. D. (1993). Lateralized changes in prefrontal cortical dopamine activity induced by controllable and uncontrollable stress in the rat. *Brain Res.*, 630, 178–187.

Carr, K. D., Kim, G. Y., and Cabeza, D. V. (2001). Rewarding and locomotor-activating effects of direct dopamine receptor agonists are augmented by chronic food restriction in rats. *Psychopharmacology (Berl)*, 154, 420–428.

Carter, A. J. (1994). Microbore high-performance liquid chromatographic method for the measurement of dopamine and its metabolites: Recommendations for optimal sample collection and storage. *J. Chromatogr. B Biomed. Appl.*, 660, 158–163.

Cass, W. A., Gerhardt, G. A., Mayfield, R. D., Curella, P., and Zahniser, N. R. (1992). Differences in dopamine clearance and diffusion in rat striatum and nucleus accumbens following systemic cocaine administration. *J. Neurochem.*, 59, 259–266.

Cass, W. A., Zahniser, N. R., Flach, K. A., and Gerhardt, G. A. (1993). Clearance of exogenous dopamine in rat dorsal striatum and nucleus accumbens: Role of metabolism and effects of locally applied uptake inhibitors. *J. Neurochem.*, *61*, 2269–2278.

Cenci, M. A., Kalen, P., Mandel, R. J., and Bjorklund, A. (1992). Regional differences in the regulation of dopamine and noradrenaline release in medial frontal cortex, nucleus accumbens and caudate-putamen: A microdialysis study in the rat. *Brain Res.*, *581*, 217–228.

Cheer, J. F., Kendall, D. A., Mason, R., and Marsden, C. A. (2003). Differential cannabinoid-induced electrophysiological effects in rat ventral tegmentum. *Neuropharmacology*, *44*, 633–641.

Cheramy, A., Leviel, V., and Glowinski, J. (1981). Dendritic release of dopamine in the substantia nigra. *Nature*, *289*, 537–542.

Chergui, K., Suaud-Chagny, M. F., and Gonon, F. (1994). Nonlinear relationship between impulse flow, dopamine release and dopamine elimination in the rat brain in vivo. *Neuroscience*, *62*, 641–645.

Childress, A. R., and O'Brien, C. P. (2000). Dopamine receptor partial agonists could address the duality of cocaine craving. *Trends Pharmacol. Sci.*, *21*, 6–9.

Chiodo, L. A., Antelman, S. M., Caggiula, A. R., and Lineberry, C. G. (1980). Sensory stimuli alter the discharge rate of dopamine (DA) neurons: Evidence for two functional types of DA cells in the substantia nigra. *Brain Res.*, *189*, 544–549.

Cho, K., and Little, H. J. (1999). Effects of corticosterone on excitatory amino acid responses in dopamine-sensitive neurons in the ventral tegmental area. *Neuroscience*, *88*, 837–845.

Church, W. H., Justice, J. B., Jr., and Byrd, L. D. (1987a). Extracellular dopamine in rat striatum following uptake inhibition by cocaine, nomifensine and benztropine. *Eur. J. Pharmacol.*, *139*, 345–348.

Church, W. H., Justice, J. B., Jr., and Neill, D. B. (1987b). Detecting behaviorally relevant changes in extracellular dopamine with microdialysis. *Brain Res.*, *412*, 397–399.

Clark, D., and Chiodo, L. A. (1988). Electrophysiological and pharmacological characterization of identified nigrostriatal and mesoaccumbens dopamine neurons in the rat. *Synapse*, *2*, 474–485.

Conrad, C. D., Lupien, S. J., and McEwen, B. S. (1999). Support for a bimodal role for type II adrenal steroid receptors in spatial memory. *Neurobiol. Learn. Mem.*, *72*, 39–46.

Copeland, B. J., Neff, N. H., and Hadjiconstantinou, M. (2005). Enhanced dopamine uptake in the striatum following repeated restraint stress. *Synapse*, *57*, 167–174.

Cosford, R. J., Parsons, L. H., and Justice, J. B., Jr. (1994). Effect of tetrodotoxin and potassium infusion on microdialysis extraction fraction and extracellular dopamine in the nucleus accumbens. *Neurosci. Lett.*, *178*, 175–178.

Coull, J. T. (1998). Neural correlates of attention and arousal: Insights from electrophysiology, functional neuroimaging and psychopharmacology. *Prog. Neurobiol.*, *55*, 343–361.

Crippens, D., Camp, D. M., and Robinson, T. E. (1993). Basal extracellular dopamine in the nucleus accumbens during amphetamine withdrawal: A 'no net flux' microdialysis study. *Neurosci. Lett.*, *164*, 145–148.

Crippens, D., and Robinson, T. E. (1994). Withdrawal from morphine or amphetamine: Different effects on dopamine in the ventral-medial striatum studied with microdialysis. *Brain Res.*, *650*, 56–62.

Czyrak, A., and Chocyk, A. (2001). Search for the presence of glucocorticoid receptors in dopaminergic neurons of rat ventral tegmental area and substantia nigra. *Pol. J. Pharmacol.*, *53*, 681–684.

Dachir, S., Kadar, T., Robinzon, B., and Levy, A. (1993). Cognitive deficits induced in young rats by long-term corticosterone administration. *Behav. Neural Biol.*, *60*, 103–109.

Dahlstrom, A. (1971). Regional distribution of brain catecholamines and serotonin. *Neurosci. Res. Program Bull.*, *9*, 197–205.

Dahlstrom, A., and Fuxe, K. (1964). Evidence for the existence of monoamine-containing neurones in the central nervous system. I. Demonstration of monoamines in the cell bodies of brain stem neurones. 1–55.

Dallman, M. F., Akana, S. F., Strack, A. M., Scribner, K. S., Pecoraro, N., La Fleur, S. E., Houshyar, H., and Gomez, F. (2004). Chronic stress-induced effects of corticosterone on brain: Direct and indirect. *Ann. N. Y. Acad. Sci.*, *1018*, 141–150.

Dallman, M. F., Darlington, D. N., Suemaru, S., Cascio, C. S., and Levin, N. (1989). Corticosteroids in homeostasis. *Acta Physiol. Scand. Suppl.*, *583*, 27–34.

Davila, V., Yan, Z., Craciun, L. C., Logothetis, D., and Sulzer, D. (2003). D3 dopamine autoreceptors do not activate G-protein–gated inwardly rectifying potassium channel currents in substantia nigra dopamine neurons. *J. Neurosci.*, *23*, 5693–5697.

de Jong, I. E., and de Kloet, E. R. (2004). Glucocorticoids and vulnerability to psychostimulant drugs: Toward substrate and mechanism. *Ann. N. Y. Acad. Sci.*, *1018*, 192–198.

de Kloet, E. R. (2000). Stress in the brain. *Eur. J. Pharmacol.*, *405*, 187–198.

Delfs, J. M., Schreiber, L., and Kelley, A. E. (1990). Microinjection of cocaine into the nucleus accumbens elicits locomotor activation in the rat. *J. Neurosci.*, *10*, 303–310.

Dellu, F., Piazza, P. V., Mayo, W., Le Moal, M., and Simon, H. (1996). Novelty-seeking in rats—biobehavioral characteristics and possible relationship with the sensation-seeking trait in man. *Neuropsychobiology*, *34*, 136–145.

Deroche, V., Marinelli, M., Le Moal, M., and Piazza, P. V. (1997). Glucocorticoids and behavioral effects of psychostimulants. II: Cocaine intravenous self-administration and reinstatement depend on glucocorticoid levels. *J. Pharmacol. Exp. Ther., 281,* 1401–1407.

Deroche, V., Marinelli, M., Maccari, S., Le Moal, M., Simon, H., and Piazza, P. V. (1995). Stress-induced sensitization and glucocorticoids. I. Sensitization of dopamine-dependent locomotor effects of amphetamine and morphine depends on stress-induced corticosterone secretion. *J. Neurosci., 15,* 7181–7188.

Deroche, V., Piazza, P. V., Casolini, P., Le Moal, M., and Simon, H. (1993a). Sensitization to the psychomotor effects of amphetamine and morphine induced by food restriction depends on corticosterone secretion. *Brain Res., 611,* 352–356.

Deroche, V., Piazza, P. V., Deminiere, J. M., Le Moal, M., and Simon, H. (1993b). Rats orally self-administer corticosterone. *Brain Res., 622,* 315–320.

Deutch, A. Y., and Cameron, D. S. (1992). Pharmacological characterization of dopamine systems in the nucleus accumbens core and shell. *Neuroscience, 46,* 49–56.

Deutch, A. Y., Lee, M. C., Gillham, M. H., Cameron, D. A., Goldstein, M., and Iadarola, M. J. (1991). Stress selectively increases Fos protein in dopamine neurons innervating the prefrontal cortex. *Cereb. Cortex, 1,* 273–292.

Deutch, A. Y., and Roth, R. H. (1990). The determinants of stress-induced activation of the prefrontal cortical dopamine system. *Prog. Brain Res., 85,* 367–402.

Deutch, A. Y., Tam, S. Y., and Roth, R. H. (1985). Footshock and conditioned stress increase 3,4-dihydroxyphenylacetic acid (DOPAC) in the ventral tegmental area but not substantia nigra. *Brain Res., 333,* 143–146.

Di Chiara, G. (1990a). Brain dialysis of neurotransmitters: A commentary. *J. Neurosci. Methods, 34,* 29–34.

Di Chiara, G. (1990b). In-vivo brain dialysis of neurotransmitters. *Trends Pharmacol. Sci., 11,* 116–121.

Di Chiara, G., Bassareo, V., Fenu, S., De Luca, M. A., Spina, L., Cadoni, C., Acquas, E., Carboni, E., Valentini, V., and Lecca, D. (2004). Dopamine and drug addiction: The nucleus accumbens shell connection. *Neuropharmacology, 47* (Suppl 1), 227–241.

Di Chiara, G., Loddo, P., and Tanda, G. (1999). Reciprocal changes in prefrontal and limbic dopamine responsiveness to aversive and rewarding stimuli after chronic mild stress: Implications for the psychobiology of depression. *Biol. Psychiatry, 46,* 1624–1633.

Di Chiara, G., and Tanda, G. (1997). Blunting of reactivity of dopamine transmission to palatable food: A biochemical marker of anhedonia in the CMS model? *Psychopharmacology (Berl), 134,* 351–353.

Di Chiara, G., Tanda, G., Frau, R., and Carboni, E. (1993). On the preferential release of dopamine in the nucleus accumbens by amphetamine: Further evidence obtained by vertically implanted concentric dialysis probes. *Psychopharmacology (Berl), 112,* 398–402.

Diamond, D. M., Bennett, M. C., Fleshner, M., and Rose, G. M. (1992). Inverted-U relationship between the level of peripheral corticosterone and the magnitude of hippocampal primed burst potentiation. *Hippocampus, 2,* 421–430.

Diamond, D. M., Fleshner, M., Ingersoll, N., and Rose, G. M. (1996). Psychological stress impairs spatial working memory: Relevance to electrophysiological studies of hippocampal function. *Behav. Neurosci., 110,* 661–672.

Diamond, D. M., Fleshner, M., and Rose, G. M. (1994). Psychological stress repeatedly blocks hippocampal primed burst potentiation in behaving rats. *Behav. Brain Res., 62,* 1–9.

Diamond, D. M., and Rose, G. M. (1994). Stress impairs LTP and hippocampal-dependent memory. *Ann. N. Y. Acad. Sci., 746,* 411–414.

Diana, M., Melis, M., Muntoni, A. L., and Gessa, G. L. (1998). Mesolimbic dopaminergic decline after cannabinoid withdrawal. *Proc. Natl. Acad. Sci. U.S.A., 95,* 10269–10273.

Diana, M., Pistis, M., Carboni, S., Gessa, G. L., and Rossetti, Z. L. (1993). Profound decrement of mesolimbic dopaminergic neuronal activity during ethanol withdrawal syndrome in rats: Electrophysiological and biochemical evidence. *Proc. Natl. Acad. Sci. U.S.A., 90,* 7966–7969.

Diana, M., Pistis, M., Muntoni, A., and Gessa, G. (1995). Profound decrease of mesolimbic dopaminergic neuronal activity in morphine withdrawn rats. *J. Pharmacol. Exp. Ther., 272,* 781–785.

Di Ciano, P., and Everitt, B. J. (2003). The GABA(B) receptor agonist baclofen attenuates cocaine- and heroin-seeking behavior by rats. *Neuropsychopharmacology, 28,* 510–518.

Di Ciano, P., and Everitt, B. J. (2004). Contribution of the ventral tegmental area to cocaine-seeking maintained by a drug-paired conditioned stimulus in rats. *Eur. J. Neurosci., 19,* 1661–1667.

Dugast, C., Suaud-Chagny, M. F., and Gonon, F. (1994). Continuous in vivo monitoring of evoked dopamine release in the rat nucleus accumbens by amperometry. *Neuroscience, 62,* 647–654.

Dunn, A. J., and File, S. E. (1983). Cold restraint alters dopamine metabolism in frontal cortex, nucleus accumbens and neostriatum. *Physiol. Behav., 31,* 511–513.

Dunn, A. J., Gildersleeve, N. B., and Gray, H. E. (1978). Mouse brain tyrosine hydroxylase and glutamic acid decarboxylase following treatment with adrenocorticotropic hormone, vasopressin or corticosterone. *J. Neurochem., 31,* 977–982.

Dziedzicka-Wasylewska, M., Willner, P., and Papp, M. (1997). Changes in dopamine receptor mRNA expression following chronic mild stress and chronic antidepressant treatment. *Behav. Pharmacol.*, *8*, 607–618.

Einhorn, L. C., Johansen, P. A., and White, F. J. (1988). Electrophysiological effects of cocaine in the meso-accumbens dopamine system: Studies in the ventral tegmental area. *J. Neurosci.*, *8*, 100–112.

Enrico, P., Bouma, M., de Vries, J. B., and Westerink, B. H. (1998). The role of afferents to the ventral tegmental area in the handling of stress-induced increase in the release of dopamine in the medial prefrontal cortex: A dual-probe microdialysis study in the rat brain. *Brain Res.*, *779*, 205–213.

Everitt, B. J., and Wolf, M. E. (2002). Psychomotor stimulant addiction: A neural systems perspective. *J. Neurosci.*, *22*, 3312–3320.

Ewing, A. G., Wightman, R. M., and Dayton, M. A. (1982). In vivo voltammetry with electrodes that discriminate between dopamine and ascorbate. *Brain Res.*, *249*, 361–370.

Fa, M., Mereu, G., Ghiglieri, V., Meloni, A., Salis, P., and Gessa, G. L. (2003). Electrophysiological and pharmacological characteristics of nigral dopaminergic neurons in the conscious, head-restrained rat. *Synapse*, *48*, 1–9.

Fadda, F., and Liguori, G. (1981). Effect of stress and ACTH on dopamine metabolism in the nucleus accumbens and frontal cortex. *Boll. Soc. Ital. Biol. Sper.*, *57*, 454–458.

Fadda, F., Melis, M. R., and Argiolas, A. (1978). Effect of electric foot shock on dopamine and 3,4-dihydroxyphenylacetic acid (DOPAC) in different brain areas of rats. *Boll. Soc. Ital. Biol. Sper.*, *54*, 1747–1750.

Fairbrother, I. S., Arbuthnott, G. W., Kelly, J. S., and Butcher, S. P. (1990a). In vivo mechanisms underlying dopamine release from rat nigrostriatal terminals: I. Studies using veratrine and ouabain. *J. Neurochem.*, *54*, 1834–1843.

Fairbrother, I. S., Arbuthnott, G. W., Kelly, J. S., and Butcher, S. P. (1990b). In vivo mechanisms underlying dopamine release from rat nigrostriatal terminals: II. Studies using potassium and tyramine. *J. Neurochem.*, *54*, 1844–1851.

Faleiro, L. J., Jones, S., and Kauer, J. A. (2003). Rapid AMPAR/NMDAR response to amphetamine: A detectable increase in AMPAR/NMDAR ratios in the ventral tegmental area is detectable after amphetamine injection. *Ann. N. Y. Acad. Sci.*, *1003*, 391–394.

Federici, M., Geracitano, R., Bernardi, G., and Mercuri, N. B. (2005). Actions of methylphenidate on dopaminergic neurons of the ventral midbrain. *Biol. Psychiatry*, *57*, 361–365.

Feenstra, M. G., Botterblom, M. H., and van Uum, J. F. (2002). Behavioral arousal and increased dopamine efflux after blockade of NMDA-receptors in the prefrontal cortex are dependent on activation of glutamatergic neurotransmission. *Neuropharmacology*, *42*, 752–763.

Ferraro, T. N., Golden, G. T., Berrettini, W. H., Gottheil, E., Yang, C. H., Cuppels, G. R., and Vogel, W. H. (2000). Cocaine intake by rats correlates with cocaine-induced dopamine changes in the nucleus accumbens shell. *Pharmacol. Biochem. Behav.*, *66*, 397–401.

Finlay, J. M., and Zigmond, M. J. (1997). The effects of stress on central dopaminergic neurons: Possible clinical implications. *Neurochem. Res*, *22*, 1387–1394.

Finlay, J. M., Zigmond, M. J., and Abercrombie, E. D. (1995). Increased dopamine and norepinephrine release in medial prefrontal cortex induced by acute and chronic stress: Effects of diazepam. *Neuroscience*, *64*, 619–628.

Fiorillo, C. D., Tobler, P. N., and Schultz, W. (2003). Discrete coding of reward probability and uncertainty by dopamine neurons. *Science*, *299*, 1898–1902.

Floresco, S. B., West, A. R., Ash, B., Moore, H., and Grace, A. A. (2003). Afferent modulation of dopamine neuron firing differentially regulates tonic and phasic dopamine transmission. *Nat. Neurosci.*, *6*, 968–973.

Franken, I. H., Booij, J., and van den, B. W. (2005). The role of dopamine in human addiction: From reward to motivated attention. *Eur. J. Pharmacol.*, *526*, 199–206.

Freeman, A. S., Meltzer, L. T., and Bunney, B. S. (1985). Firing properties of substantia nigra dopaminergic neurons in freely moving rats. *Life Sci.*, *36*, 1983–1994.

Gambarana, C., Masi, F., Tagliamonte, A., Scheggi, S., Ghiglieri, O., and De Montis, M. G. (1999). A chronic stress that impairs reactivity in rats also decreases dopaminergic transmission in the nucleus accumbens: A microdialysis study. *J. Neurochem.*, *72*, 2039–2046.

Gariano, R. F., Tepper, J. M., Sawyer, S. F., Young, S. J., and Groves, P. M. (1989). Mesocortical dopaminergic neurons. 1. Electrophysiological properties and evidence for soma-dendritic autoreceptors. *Brain Res. Bull.*, *22*, 511–516.

Garris, P. A., Budygin, E. A., Phillips, P. E., Venton, B. J., Robinson, D. L., Bergstrom, B. P., Rebec, G. V., and Wightman, R. M. (2003). A role for presynaptic mechanisms in the actions of nomifensine and haloperidol. *Neuroscience*, *118*, 819–829.

Garris, P. A., Christensen, J. R., Rebec, G. V., and Wightman, R. M. (1997). Real-time measurement of electrically evoked extracellular dopamine in the striatum of freely moving rats. *J. Neurochem.*, *68*, 152–161.

Gerhardt, G. A., Ksir, C., Pivik, C., Dickinson, S. D., Sabeti, J., and Zahniser, N. R. (1999). Methodology for coupling local application of dopamine and other chemicals with rapid in vivo electrochemical recordings in freely-moving rats. *J. Neurosci. Methods*, *87*, 67–76.

German, D. C., Schlusselberg, D. S., and Woodward, D. J. (1983). Three-dimensional computer reconstruction of midbrain dopaminergic neuronal populations: From mouse to man. *J. Neural Transm.*, *57*, 243–254.

Gessa, G. L., Melis, M., Muntoni, A. L., and Diana, M. (1998). Cannabinoids activate mesolimbic dopamine neurons by an action on cannabinoid CB1 receptors. *Eur. J. Pharmacol.*, *341*, 39–44.

Giorgi, O., Corda, M. G., Carboni, G., Frau, V., Valentini, V., and Di Chiara, G. (1997). Effects of cocaine and morphine in rats from two psychogenetically selected lines: A behavioral and brain dialysis study. *Behav. Genet.*, *27*, 537–546.

Glick, S. D., Merski, C., Steindorf, S., Wang, S., Keller, R. W., and Carlson, J. N. (1992). Neurochemical predisposition to self-administer morphine in rats. *Brain Res.*, *578*, 215–220.

Goeders, N. E. (2002). Stress and cocaine addiction. *J. Pharmacol. Exp. Ther.*, *301*, 785–789.

Gonon, F. G. (1988). Nonlinear relationship between impulse flow and dopamine released by rat midbrain dopaminergic neurons as studied by in vivo electrochemistry. *Neuroscience*, *24*, 19–28.

Grace, A. A., and Bunney, B. S. (1983). Intracellular and extracellular electrophysiology of nigral dopaminergic neurons—1. Identification and characterization. *Neuroscience*, *10*, 301–315.

Grace, A. A., and Bunney, B. S. (1984a). The control of firing pattern in nigral dopamine neurons: Burst firing. *J. Neurosci.*, *4*, 2877–2890.

Grace, A. A., and Bunney, B. S. (1984b). The control of firing pattern in nigral dopamine neurons: Single spike firing. *J. Neurosci.*, *4*, 2866–2876.

Gratton, A., Hoffer, B. J., and Gerhardt, G. A. (1989). In vivo electrochemical studies of monoamine release in the medial prefrontal cortex of the rat. *Neuroscience*, *29*, 57–64.

Gresch, P. J., Sved, A. F., Zigmond, M. J., and Finlay, J. M. (1994). Stress-induced sensitization of dopamine and norepinephrine efflux in medial prefrontal cortex of the rat. *J. Neurochem.*, *63*, 575–583.

Grimm, J. W., Hope, B. T., Wise, R. A., and Shaham, Y. (2001). Neuroadaptation. Incubation of cocaine craving after withdrawal. *Nature*, *412*, 141–142.

Grimm, J. W., and See, R. E. (1997). Cocaine self-administration in ovariectomized rats is predicted by response to novelty, attenuated by 17-beta estradiol, and associated with abnormal vaginal cytology. *Physiol. Behav.*, *61*, 755–761.

Groenewegen, H. J., Berendse, H. W., and Haber, S. N. (1993). Organization of the output of the ventral striatopallidal system in the rat: Ventral pallidal efferents. *Neuroscience*, *57*, 113–142.

Guyenet, P. G., and Aghajanian, G. K. (1978). Antidromic identification of dopaminergic and other output neurons of the rat substantia nigra. *Brain Res.*, *150*, 69–84.

Gysling, K., and Wang, R. Y. (1983). Morphine-induced activation of A10 dopamine neurons in the rat. *Brain Res.*, *277*, 119–127.

Haber, S. N., and Fudge, J. L. (1997). The primate substantia nigra and VTA: Integrative circuitry and function. *Crit. Rev. Neurobiol.*, *11*, 323–342.

Hajos, M., and Greenfield, S. A. (1994). Synaptic connections between pars compacta and pars reticulata neurones: Electrophysiological evidence for functional modules within the substantia nigra. *Brain Res.*, *660*, 216–224.

Hamamura, T., and Fibiger, H. C. (1993). Enhanced stress-induced dopamine release in the prefrontal cortex of amphetamine-sensitized rats. *Eur. J. Pharmacol.*, *237*, 65–71.

Hamilton, M. E., Mele, A., and Pert, A. (1992). Striatal extracellular dopamine in conscious vs. anesthetized rats: Effects of chloral hydrate anesthetic on responses to drugs of different classes. *Brain Res.*, *597*, 1–7.

Harfstrand, A., Fuxe, K., Cintra, A., Agnati, L. F., Zini, I., Wikstrom, A. C., Okret, S., Yu, Z. Y., Goldstein, M., and Steinbusch, H. (1986). Glucocorticoid receptor immunoreactivity in monoaminergic neurons of rat brain. *Proc. Natl. Acad. Sci. U. S. A.*, *83*, 9779–9783.

Hedou, G., Feldon, J., and Heidbreder, C. A. (1999). Effects of cocaine on dopamine in subregions of the rat prefrontal cortex and their efferents to subterritories of the nucleus accumbens. *Eur. J. Pharmacol.*, *372*, 143–155.

Herman, J. P., Guillonneau, D., Dantzer, R., Scatton, B., Semerdjian-Rouquier, L., and Le, M. M. (1982). Differential effects of inescapable footshocks and of stimuli previously paired with inescapable footshocks on dopamine turnover in cortical and limbic areas of the rat. *Life Sci.*, *30*, 2207–2214.

Herve, D., Tassin, J. P., Barthelemy, C., Blanc, G., Lavielle, S., and Glowinski, J. (1979). Difference in the reactivity of the mesocortical dopaminergic neurons to stress in the BALB/C and C57 BL/6 mice. *Life Sci.*, *25*, 1659–1664.

Hoebel, B. G., Hernandez, L., Schwartz, D. H., Mark, G. P., and Hunter, G. A. (1989). Microdialysis studies of brain norepinephrine, serotonin, and dopamine release during ingestive behavior. Theoretical and clinical implications. *Ann. N. Y. Acad. Sci.*, *575*, 171–191.

Holsboer, F. (2001). Stress, hypercortisolism and corticosteroid receptors in depression: Implications for therapy. *J. Affect. Disord.*, *62*, 77–91.

Hooks, M. S., Colvin, A. C., Juncos, J. L., and Justice, J. B., Jr. (1992). Individual differences in basal and cocaine-stimulated extracellular dopamine in the nucleus accumbens using quantitative microdialysis. *Brain Res.*, *587*, 306–312.

Hooks, M. S., Jones, G. H., Smith, A. D., Neill, D. B., and Justice, J. B., Jr. (1991). Response to novelty predicts the locomotor and nucleus accumbens dopamine response to cocaine. *Synapse*, *9*, 121–128.

Horvitz, J. C. (2000). Mesolimbocortical and nigro-striatal dopamine responses to salient non-reward events. *Neuroscience, 96*, 651–656.

Ho-Van-Hap, A., Babineau, L. M., and Berlinguet, L. (1967). Hormonal action on monoamine oxidase activity in rats. *Can. J. Biochem., 45*, 355–362.

Huber, J. D., Darling, S. F., Park, K. K., and Soliman, K. F. (2001). The role of NMDA receptors in neonatal cocaine-induced neurotoxicity. *Pharmacol. Biochem. Behav., 69*, 451–459.

Hurd, Y. L., Kehr, J., and Ungerstedt, U. (1988). In vivo microdialysis as a technique to monitor drug transport: Correlation of extracellular cocaine levels and dopamine overflow in the rat brain. *J. Neurochem., 51*, 1314–1316.

Hurd, Y. L., Ponten, M., McGregor, A., Guix, T., and Ungerstedt, U. (1998). Dopamine efflux studies into in vivo actions of psychostimulant drugs. *Adv. Pharmacol., 42*, 1010–1013.

Hurd, Y. L., and Ungerstedt, U. (1989a). Ca2+ dependence of the amphetamine, nomifensine, and Lu 19-005 effect on in vivo dopamine transmission. *Eur. J. Pharmacol., 166*, 261–269.

Hurd, Y. L., and Ungerstedt, U. (1989b). Cocaine: An in vivo microdialysis evaluation of its acute action on dopamine transmission in rat striatum. *Synapse, 3*, 48–54.

Hyland, B. I., Reynolds, J. N., Hay, J., Perk, C. G., and Miller, R. (2002). Firing modes of midbrain dopamine cells in the freely moving rat. *Neuroscience, 114*, 475–492.

Hyytia, P., Backstrom, P., and Liljequist, S. (1999). Site-specific NMDA receptor antagonists produce differential effects on cocaine self-administration in rats. *Eur. J. Pharmacol., 378*, 9–16.

Ikemoto, S., and Panksepp, J. (1999). The role of nucleus accumbens dopamine in motivated behavior: A unifying interpretation with special reference to reward-seeking. *Brain Res. Brain Res. Rev., 31*, 6–41.

Imperato, A., Angelucci, L., Casolini, P., Zocchi, A., and Puglisi-Allegra, S. (1992a). Repeated stressful experiences differently affect limbic dopamine release during and following stress. *Brain Res., 577*, 194–199.

Imperato, A., Cabib, S., and Puglisi-Allegra, S. (1993). Repeated stressful experiences differently affect the time-dependent responses of the mesolimbic dopamine system to the stressor. *Brain Res., 601*, 333–336.

Imperato, A., Mele, A., Scrocco, M. G., and Puglisi-Allegra, S. (1992b). Chronic cocaine alters limbic extracellular dopamine. Neurochemical basis for addiction. *Eur. J. Pharmacol., 212*, 299–300.

Imperato, A., Puglisi-Allegra, S., Casolini, P., and Angelucci, L. (1991). Changes in brain dopamine and acetylcholine release during and following stress are independent of the pituitary-adrenocortical axis. *Brain Res., 538*, 111–117.

Imperato, A., Puglisi-Allegra, S., Casolini, P., Zocchi, A., and Angelucci, L. (1989). Stress-induced enhancement of dopamine and acetylcholine release in limbic structures: Role of corticosterone. *Eur. J. Pharmacol., 165*, 337–338.

Innis, R. B., and Aghajanian, G. K. (1987). Pertussis toxin blocks autoreceptor-mediated inhibition of dopaminergic neurons in rat substantia nigra. *Brain Res., 411*, 139–143.

Inoue, T., Tsuchiya, K., and Koyama, T. (1994). Regional changes in dopamine and serotonin activation with various intensity of physical and psychological stress in the rat brain. *Pharmacol. Biochem. Behav., 49*, 911–920.

Ito, R., Dalley, J. W., Robbins, T. W., and Everitt, B. J. (2002). Dopamine release in the dorsal striatum during cocaine-seeking behavior under the control of a drug-associated cue. *J. Neurosci., 22*, 6247–6253.

Iuvone, P. M., Morasco, J., and Dunn, A. J. (1977). Effect of corticosterone on the synthesis of [3H]catecholamines in the brains of CD-1 mice. *Brain Res., 120*, 571–576.

Jedema, H. P., and Moghaddam, B. (1994). Glutamatergic control of dopamine release during stress in the rat prefrontal cortex. *J. Neurochem., 63*, 785–788.

Johnson, S. W., and North, R. A. (1992). Two types of neurone in the rat ventral tegmental area and their synaptic inputs. *J. Physiol, 450*, 455–468.

Jones, S., and Bonci, A. (2005). Synaptic plasticity and drug addiction. *Curr. Opin. Pharmacol., 5*, 20–25.

Joseph, M. H., Datla, K., and Young, A. M. (2003). The interpretation of the measurement of nucleus accumbens dopamine by in vivo dialysis: The kick, the craving or the cognition? *Neurosci. Biobehav. Rev., 27*, 527–541.

Joyce, E. M., and Iversen, S. D. (1979). The effect of morphine applied locally to mesencephalic dopamine cell bodies on spontaneous motor activity in the rat. *Neurosci. Lett., 14*, 207–212.

Jung, M. C., Shi, G., Borland, L., Michael, A. C., and Weber, S. G. (2006). Simultaneous determination of biogenic monoamines in rat brain dialysates using capillary high-performance liquid chromatography with photoluminescence following electron transfer. *Anal. Chem., 78*, 1755–1760.

Justice, J. B., Jr. (1993). Quantitative microdialysis of neurotransmitters. *J. Neurosci. Methods, 48*, 263–276.

Kabbaj, M., Devine, D. P., Savage, V. R., and Akil, H. (2000). Neurobiological correlates of individual differences in novelty-seeking behavior in the rat: Differential expression of stress-related molecules. *J. Neurosci., 20*, 6983–6988.

Kalivas, P. W. (1993). Neurotransmitter regulation of dopamine neurons in the ventral tegmental area. *Brain Res. Brain Res. Rev., 18*, 75–113.

Kalivas, P. W., and Duffy, P. (1989). Similar effects of daily cocaine and stress on mesocorticolimbic dopamine neurotransmission in the rat. *Biol. Psychiatry, 25,* 913–928.

Kalivas, P. W., and Duffy, P. (1991). A comparison of axonal and somatodendritic dopamine release using in vivo dialysis. *J. Neurochem., 56,* 961–967.

Kalivas, P. W., and Duffy, P. (1995). Selective activation of dopamine transmission in the shell of the nucleus accumbens by stress. *Brain Res., 675,* 325–328.

Kalivas, P. W., and McFarland, K. (2003). Brain circuitry and the reinstatement of cocaine-seeking behavior. *Psychopharmacology (Berl), 168,* 44–56.

Kaneyuki, H., Yokoo, H., Tsuda, A., Yoshida, M., Mizuki, Y., Yamada, M., and Tanaka, M. (1991). Psychological stress increases dopamine turnover selectively in mesoprefrontal dopamine neurons of rats: Reversal by diazepam. *Brain Res, 557,* 154–161.

Kauer, J. A. (2004). Learning mechanisms in addiction: Synaptic plasticity in the ventral tegmental area as a result of exposure to drugs of abuse. *Annu. Rev. Physiol., 66,* 447–475.

Kawagoe, K. T., Garris, P. A., Wiedemann, D. J., and Wightman, R. M. (1992). Regulation of transient dopamine concentration gradients in the microenvironment surrounding nerve terminals in the rat striatum. *Neuroscience, 51,* 55–64.

Keefe, K. A., Sved, A. F., Zigmond, M. J., and Abercrombie, E. D. (1993). Stress-induced dopamine release in the neostriatum: Evaluation of the role of action potentials in nigrostriatal dopamine neurons or local initiation by endogenous excitatory amino acids. *J. Neurochem., 61,* 1943–1952.

Keller, R. W., Jr., Stricker, E. M., and Zigmond, M. J. (1983). Environmental stimuli but not homeostatic challenges produce apparent increases in dopaminergic activity in the striatum: An analysis by in vivo voltammetry. *Brain Res., 279,* 159–170.

Kelley, A. E. (2004). Memory and addiction: Shared neural circuitry and molecular mechanisms. *Neuron, 44,* 161–179.

Kita, T., Kita, H., and Kitai, S. T. (1986). Electrical membrane properties of rat substantia nigra compacta neurons in an in vitro slice preparation. *Brain Res., 372,* 21–30.

Kitai, S. T., Shepard, P. D., Callaway, J. C., and Scroggs, R. (1999). Afferent modulation of dopamine neuron firing patterns. *Curr. Opin. Neurobiol., 9,* 690–697.

Kiyatkin, E. A. (2002). Dopamine in the nucleus accumbens: Cellular actions, drug- and behavior-associated fluctuations, and a possible role in an organism's adaptive activity. *Behav. Brain Res., 137,* 27–46.

Kiyatkin, E. A., and Rebec, G. V. (1997). Activity of presumed dopamine neurons in the ventral tegmental area during heroin self-administration. *Neuroreport, 8,* 2581–2585.

Kiyatkin, E. A., and Rebec, G. V. (1998). Heterogeneity of ventral tegmental area neurons: Single-unit recording and iontophoresis in awake, unrestrained rats. *Neuroscience, 85,* 1285–1309.

Kiyatkin, E. A., and Rebec, G. V. (2001). Impulse activity of ventral tegmental area neurons during heroin self-administration in rats. *Neuroscience, 102,* 565–580.

Klein, J. F. (1992). Adverse psychiatric effects of systemic glucocorticoid therapy. *Am. Fam. Physician, 46,* 1469–1474.

Klitenick, M. A., DeWitte, P., and Kalivas, P. W. (1992). Regulation of somatodendritic dopamine release in the ventral tegmental area by opioids and GABA: An in vivo microdialysis study. *J. Neurosci., 12,* 2623–2632.

Koob, G. F., Caine, B., Markou, A., Pulvirenti, L., and Weiss, F. (1994). Role for the mesocortical dopamine system in the motivating effects of cocaine. *NIDA Res. Monogr., 145,* 1–18.

Kosaka, T., Kosaka, K., Hataguchi, Y., Nagatsu, I., Wu, J. Y., Ottersen, O. P., Storm-Mathisen, J., and Hama, K. (1987). Catecholaminergic neurons containing GABA-like and/or glutamic acid decarboxylase-like immunoreactivities in various brain regions of the rat. *Exp. Brain Res., 66,* 191–210.

Kuhr, W. G., and Wightman, R. M. (1986). Real-time measurement of dopamine release in rat brain. *Brain Res., 381,* 168–171.

Lacey, M. G., Mercuri, N. B., and North, R. A. (1987). Dopamine acts on D2 receptors to increase potassium conductance in neurones of the rat substantia nigra zona compacta. *J. Physiol., 392,* 397–416.

Lacey, M. G., Mercuri, N. B., and North, R. A. (1990). Actions of cocaine on rat dopaminergic neurones in vitro. *Br. J. Pharmacol., 99,* 731–735.

Lavielle, S., Tassin, J. P., Thierry, A. M., Blanc, G., Herve, D., Barthelemy, C., and Glowinski, J. (1979). Blockade by benzodiazepines of the selective high increase in dopamine turnover induced by stress in mesocortical dopaminergic neurons of the rat. *Brain Res., 168,* 585–594.

Leggio, B., Masi, F., Grappi, S., Nanni, G., Gambarana, C., Colombo, G., and De Montis, M. G. (2003). Sardinian alcohol-preferring and non-preferring rats show different reactivity to aversive stimuli and a similar response to a natural reward. *Brain Res., 973,* 275–284.

Leone, P., Pocock, D., and Wise, R. A. (1991). Morphine-dopamine interaction: Ventral tegmental morphine increases nucleus accumbens dopamine release. *Pharmacol. Biochem. Behav., 39,* 469–472.

Levita, L., Dalley, J. W., and Robbins, T. W. (2002). Nucleus accumbens dopamine and learned fear revisited: A review and some new findings. *Behav. Brain Res., 137,* 115–127.

Leyton, M., Boileau, I., Benkelfat, C., Diksic, M., Baker, G., and Dagher, A. (2002). Amphetamine-induced increases in extracellular dopamine, drug wanting, and novelty seeking: A PET/[11C]raclopride study in healthy men. *Neuropsychopharmacology, 27,* 1027–1035.

Lindley, S. E., Bengoechea, T. G., Schatzberg, A. F., and Wong, D. L. (1999). Glucocorticoid effects on mesotelencephalic dopamine neurotransmission. *Neuropsychopharmacology*, 21, 399–407.

Lovinger, D. M., Partridge, J. G., and Tang, K. C. (2003). Plastic control of striatal glutamatergic transmission by ensemble actions of several neurotransmitters and targets for drugs of abuse. *Ann. N. Y. Acad. Sci.*, 1003, 226–240.

Lu, Y., Peters, J. L., and Michael, A. C. (1998). Direct comparison of the response of voltammetry and microdialysis to electrically evoked release of striatal dopamine. *J. Neurochem.*, 70, 584–593.

Luine, V. N. (1994). Steroid hormone influences on spatial memory. *Ann. N. Y. Acad. Sci.*, 743, 201–211.

Luine, V. N. (1997). Steroid hormone modulation of hippocampal dependent spatial memory. *Stress*, 2, 21–36.

Luine, V. N., Spencer, R. L., and McEwen, B. S. (1993). Effects of chronic corticosterone ingestion on spatial memory performance and hippocampal serotonergic function. *Brain Res.*, 616, 65–70.

Lupien, S. J., Gaudreau, S., Tchiteya, B. M., Maheu, F., Sharma, S., Nair, N. P., Hauger, R. L., McEwen, B. S., and Meaney, M. J. (1997). Stress-induced declarative memory impairment in healthy elderly subjects: Relationship to cortisol reactivity. *J. Clin. Endocrinol. Metab.*, 82, 2070–2075.

Mangiavacchi, S., Masi, F., Scheggi, S., Leggio, B., De Montis, M. G., and Gambarana, C. (2001). Long-term behavioral and neurochemical effects of chronic stress exposure in rats. *J. Neurochem.*, 79, 1113–1121.

Mantz, J., Thierry, A. M., and Glowinski, J. (1989). Effect of noxious tail pinch on the discharge rate of mesocortical and mesolimbic dopamine neurons: Selective activation of the mesocortical system. *Brain Res.*, 476, 377–381.

Marinelli, M. (2005a). Stress and drug induced plasticity of dopamine neurons: Relevance to addiction. *Soc. Neurosci, Abs*.

Marinelli, M. (2005b). The many facets of the locomotor response to a novel environment test: Theoretical comment on Mitchell, Cunningham, and Mark (2005). *Behav. Neurosci.*, 119, 1144–1151.

Marinelli, M., Ambroggi, F., Turiault, M., Le Moal, M., Tronche, F., and Piazza, P. V. (2003a). Decreased impulse activity of midbrain dopamine neurons in mice lacking glucocorticoid receptors in the brain or in D1 dopamine receptor-expressing neurons. *Soc. Neurosci. Abs.*, 113, 12.

Marinelli, M., Aouizerate, B., Barrot, M., Le Moal, M., and Piazza, P. V. (1998). Dopamine-dependent responses to morphine depend on glucocorticoid receptors. *Proc. Natl. Acad. Sci. U. S. A.*, 95, 7742–7747.

Marinelli, M., Cooper, D. C., Baker, L. K., and White, F. J. (2003b). Impulse activity of midbrain dopamine neurons modulates drug-seeking behavior. *Psychopharmacology (Berl)*, 168, 84–98.

Marinelli, M., and Piazza, P. V. (2002). Interaction between glucocorticoid hormones, stress and psychostimulant drugs. *Eur. J. Neurosci.*, 16, 387–394.

Marinelli, M., and Piazza, P. V. (2003). Influence of environmental and hormonal factors in the sensitivity to psychostimulants. In: *Molecular basis of drug addiction* (R. Maldonado, Ed.) (pp. 133–159). Totowa, NJ: Humana Press Inc.

Marinelli, M., Rudick, C. N., Hu, X. T., and White, F. J. (2006). Excitability of dopamine neurons: Modulation and physiological consequences. *CNS Neurol. Disord. Drug Targets 5*, 79–97.

Marinelli, M., and White, F. J. (2000). Enhanced vulnerability to cocaine self-administration is associated with elevated impulse activity of midbrain dopamine neurons. *J. Neurosci.*, 20, 8876–8885.

Marsden, C. A., Joseph, M. H., Kruk, Z. L., Maidment, N. T., O'Neill, R. D., Schenk, J. O., and Stamford, J. A. (1988). In vivo voltammetry—present electrodes and methods. *Neuroscience*, 25, 389–400.

Mash, D. C., Pablo, J., Ouyang, Q., Hearn, W. L., and Izenwasser, S. (2002). Dopamine transport function is elevated in cocaine users. *J. Neurochem.*, 81, 292–300.

Mathon, D. S., Kamal, A., Smidt, M. P., and Ramakers, G. M. (2003). Modulation of cellular activity and synaptic transmission in the ventral tegmental area. *Eur. J. Pharmacol.*, 480, 97–115.

Mathon, D. S., Lesscher, H. M., Gerrits, M. A., Kamal, A., Pintar, J. E., Schuller, A. G., Spruijt, B. M., Burbach, J. P., Smidt, M. P., Van Ree, J. M., and Ramakers, G. M. (2005a). Increased GABAergic input to ventral tegmental area dopaminergic neurons associated with decreased cocaine reinforcement in mu-opioid receptor knockout mice. *Neuroscience*, 130, 359–367.

Mathon, D. S., Ramakers, G. M., Pintar, J. E., and Marinelli, M. (2005b). Decreased firing frequency of midbrain dopamine neurons in mice lacking mu opioid receptors. *Eur. J. Neurosci.*, 21, 2883–2886.

McFarland, K., and Kalivas, P. W. (2001). The circuitry mediating cocaine-induced reinstatement of drug-seeking behavior. *J. Neurosci.*, 21, 8655–8663.

Meiergerd, S. M., Schenk, J. O., and Sorg, B. A. (1997). Repeated cocaine and stress increase dopamine clearance in the rat medial prefrontal cortex. *Brain Res.*, 773, 203–207.

Melis, M., Pistis, M., Perra, S., Muntoni, A. L., Pillolla, G., and Gessa, G. L. (2004). Endocannabinoids mediate presynaptic inhibition of glutamatergic transmission in rat ventral tegmental area dopamine neurons through activation of CB1 receptors. *J. Neurosci.*, 24, 53–62.

Melis, M., Spiga, S., and Diana, M. (2005). The dopamine hypothesis of drug addiction: Hypodopaminergic state. *Int. Rev. Neurobiol.*, 63, 101–154.

Meltzer, L. T., Christoffersen, C. L., and Serpa, K. A. (1997). Modulation of dopamine neuronal activity by glutamate receptor subtypes. *Neurosci. Biobehav. Rev.*, *21*, 511–518.

Mercuri, N. B., Calabresi, P., and Bernardi, G. (1992). The electrophysiological actions of dopamine and dopaminergic drugs on neurons of the substantia nigra pars compacta and ventral tegmental area. *Life Sci.*, *51*, 711–718.

Mereu, G., Fadda, F., and Gessa, G. L. (1984). Ethanol stimulates the firing rate of nigral dopaminergic neurons in unanesthetized rats. *Brain Res.*, *292*, 63–69.

Miczek, K. A., Mutschler, N. H., van Erp, A. M., Blank, A. D., and McInerney, S. C. (1999). d-amphetamine "cue" generalizes to social defeat stress: Behavioral sensitization and attenuated accumbens dopamine. *Psychopharmacology (Berl)*, *147*, 190–199.

Mirenowicz, J., and Schultz, W. (1996). Preferential activation of midbrain dopamine neurons by appetitive rather than aversive stimuli. *Nature*, *379*, 449–451.

Mittleman, G., Blaha, C. D., and Phillips, A. G. (1992). Pituitary-adrenal and dopaminergic modulation of schedule-induced polydipsia: Behavioral and neurochemical evidence. *Behav. Neurosci.*, *106*, 408–420.

Moghaddam, B., and Bunney, B. S. (1989). Ionic composition of microdialysis perfusing solution alters the pharmacological responsiveness and basal outflow of striatal dopamine. *J. Neurochem.*, *53*, 652–654.

Moghaddam, B., Roth, R. H., and Bunney, B. S. (1990). Characterization of dopamine release in the rat medial prefrontal cortex as assessed by in vivo microdialysis: Comparison to the striatum. *Neuroscience*, *36*, 669–676.

Moore, H., Rose, H. J., and Grace, A. A. (2001). Chronic cold stress reduces the spontaneous activity of ventral tegmental dopamine neurons. *Neuropsychopharmacology*, *24*, 410–419.

Moreau, J. L., Scherschlicht, R., Jenck, F., and Martin, J. R. (1995). Chronic mild stress-induced anhedonia model of depression; sleep abnormalities and curative effects of electroshock treatment. *Behav. Pharmacol.*, *6*, 682–687.

Morrow, B. A., Clark, W. A., and Roth, R. H. (1993). Stress activation of mesocorticolimbic dopamine neurons: Effects of a glycine/NMDA receptor antagonist. *Eur. J. Pharmacol.*, *238*, 255–262.

Muller, M. B., Uhr, M., Holsboer, F., and Keck, M. E. (2004). Hypothalamic-pituitary-adrenocortical system and mood disorders: Highlights from mutant mice. *Neuroendocrinology*, *79*, 1–12.

Muma, N. A., and Beck, S. G. (1999). Corticosteroids alter G protein inwardly rectifying potassium channels protein levels in hippocampal subfields. *Brain Res.*, *839*, 331–335.

Munck, A., and Guyre, P. M. (1986). Glucocorticoid physiology, pharmacology and stress. *Adv. Exp. Med. Biol.*, *196*, 81–96.

Muscat, R., and Willner, P. (1992). Suppression of sucrose drinking by chronic mild unpredictable stress: A methodological analysis. *Neurosci. Biobehav. Rev.*, *16*, 507–517.

Newcomer, J. W., Craft, S., Hershey, T., Askins, K., and Bardgett, M. E. (1994). Glucocorticoid-induced impairment in declarative memory performance in adult humans. *J. Neurosci.*, *14*, 2047–2053.

Nieoullon, A. (2002). Dopamine and the regulation of cognition and attention. *Prog. Neurobiol.*, *67*, 53–83.

Nomikos, G. G., Damsma, G., Wenkstern, D., and Fibiger, H. C. (1990). In vivo characterization of locally applied dopamine uptake inhibitors by striatal microdialysis. *Synapse*, *6*, 106–112.

Oades, R. D., and Halliday, G. M. (1987). Ventral tegmental (A10) system: Neurobiology. 1. Anatomy and connectivity. *Brain Res*, *434*, 117–165.

Ortiz, J., DeCaprio, J. L., Kosten, T. A., and Nestler, E. J. (1995). Strain-selective effects of corticosterone on locomotor sensitization to cocaine and on levels of tyrosine hydroxylase and glucocorticoid receptor in the ventral tegmental area. *Neuroscience*, *67*, 383–397.

Osborne, P. G., O'Connor, W. T., Drew, K. L., and Ungerstedt, U. (1990). An in vivo microdialysis characterization of extracellular dopamine and GABA in dorsolateral striatum of awake freely moving and halothane anaesthetised rats. *J. Neurosci. Methods*, *34*, 99–105.

Osborne, P. G., O'Connor, W. T., Kehr, J., and Ungerstedt, U. (1991a). In vivo characterisation of extracellular dopamine, GABA and acetylcholine from the dorsolateral striatum of awake freely moving rats by chronic microdialysis. *J. Neurosci. Methods*, *37*, 93–102.

Osborne, P. G., O'Connor, W. T., and Ungerstedt, U. (1991b). Effect of varying the ionic concentration of a microdialysis perfusate on basal striatal dopamine levels in awake rats. *J. Neurochem.*, *56*, 452–456.

Oswald, L. M., Wong, D. F., McCaul, M., Zhou, Y., Kuwabara, H., Choi, L., Brasic, J., and Wand, G. S. (2005). Relationships among ventral striatal dopamine release, cortisol secretion, and subjective responses to amphetamine. *Neuropsychopharmacology*, *30*, 821–832.

Overton, P., and Clark, D. (1991). N-methyl-D-aspartate increases the excitability of nigrostriatal dopamine terminals. *Eur. J. Pharmacol.*, *201*, 117–120.

Overton, P., and Clark, D. (1992). Iontophoretically administered drugs acting at the N-methyl-D-aspartate receptor modulate burst firing in A9 dopamine neurons in the rat. *Synapse*, *10*, 131–140.

Overton, P. G., and Clark, D. (1997). Burst firing in midbrain dopaminergic neurons. *Brain Res. Brain Res. Rev.*, *25*, 312–334.

Overton, P. G., Tong, Z. Y., Brain, P. F., and Clark, D. (1996). Preferential occupation of mineralocorticoid receptors by corticosterone enhances glutamate-induced burst firing in rat midbrain dopaminergic neurons. *Brain Res.*, *737*, 146–154.

Pacchioni, A. M., Gioino, G., Assis, A., and Cancela, L. M. (2002). A single exposure to restraint stress induces behavioral and neurochemical sensitization to stimulating effects of amphetamine: Involvement of NMDA receptors. *Ann. N. Y. Acad. Sci., 965,* 233–246.

Paladini, C. A., Fiorillo, C. D., Morikawa, H., and Williams, J. T. (2001). Amphetamine selectively blocks inhibitory glutamate transmission in dopamine neurons. *Nat. Neurosci., 4,* 275–281.

Paladini, C. A., and Williams, J. T. (2004). Noradrenergic inhibition of midbrain dopamine neurons. *J. Neurosci., 24,* 4568–4575.

Papp, M., Willner, P., and Muscat, R. (1991). An animal model of anhedonia: Attenuation of sucrose consumption and place preference conditioning by chronic unpredictable mild stress. *Psychopharmacology (Berl), 104,* 255–259.

Parry, T. J., Carter, T. L., and McElligott, J. G. (1990). Physical and chemical considerations in the in vitro calibration of microdialysis probes for biogenic amine neurotransmitters and metabolites. *J. Neurosci. Methods, 32,* 175–183.

Parsons, L. H., Kerr, T. M., and Weiss, F. (1998). Simple microbore high-performance liquid chromatographic method for the determination of dopamine and cocaine from a single in vivo brain microdialysis sample. *J. Chromatogr. B Biomed. Sci. Appl., 709,* 35–45.

Parsons, L. H., Smith, A. D., and Justice, J. B., Jr. (1991). Basal extracellular dopamine is decreased in the rat nucleus accumbens during abstinence from chronic cocaine. *Synapse, 9,* 60–65.

Parvez, H., and Parvez, S. (1973). The regulation of monoamine oxidase activity by adrenal cortical steroids. *Acta Endocrinol. (Copenh), 73,* 509–517.

Paulson, P. E., and Robinson, T. E. (1994). Relationship between circadian changes in spontaneous motor activity and dorsal versus ventral striatal dopamine neurotransmission assessed with on-line microdialysis. *Behav. Neurosci., 108,* 624–635.

Paulson, P. E., and Robinson, T. E. (1995). Amphetamine-induced time-dependent sensitization of dopamine neurotransmission in the dorsal and ventral striatum: A microdialysis study in behaving rats. *Synapse, 19,* 56–65.

Peters, J. L., and Michael, A. C. (1998). Modeling voltammetry and microdialysis of striatal extracellular dopamine: The impact of dopamine uptake on extraction and recovery ratios. *J. Neurochem., 70,* 594–603.

Phillips, P. E., Robinson, D. L., Stuber, G. D., Carelli, R. M., and Wightman, R. M. (2003a). Real-time measurements of phasic changes in extracellular dopamine concentration in freely moving rats by fast-scan cyclic voltammetry. *Methods Mol. Med., 79,* 443–464.

Phillips, P. E., Stuber, G. D., Heien, M. L., Wightman, R. M., and Carelli, R. M. (2003b). Subsecond dopamine release promotes cocaine seeking. *Nature, 422,* 614–618.

Phillips, P. E., and Wightman, R. M. (2004). Extra synaptic dopamine and phasic neuronal activity. *Nat. Neurosci., 7,* 199.

Phillips, P. E., and Wightman, R. M. (2003). Critical guidelines for validation of the selectivity of in-vivo chemical microsensors. *Trends in Analytical Chemistry, 22.*

Piazza, P. V., Barrot, M., Rouge-Pont, F., Marinelli, M., Maccari, S., Abrous, D. N., Simon, H., and Le Moal, M. (1996a). Suppression of glucocorticoid secretion and antipsychotic drugs have similar effects on the mesolimbic dopaminergic transmission. *Proc. Natl. Acad. Sci. U. S. A., 93,* 15445–15450.

Piazza, P. V., Deminiere, J. M., Maccari, S., Mormede, P., Le Moal, M., and Simon, H. (1990). Individual reactivity to novelty predicts probability of amphetamine self-administration. *Behav. Pharmacol., 1,* 339–345.

Piazza, P. V., Deroche, V., Deminiere, J. M., Maccari, S., Le Moal, M., and Simon, H. (1993). Corticosterone in the range of stress-induced levels possesses reinforcing properties: Implications for sensation-seeking behaviors. *Proc. Natl. Acad. Sci. U. S. A., 90,* 11738–11742.

Piazza, P. V., and Le Moal, M. (1996). Pathophysiological basis of vulnerability to drug abuse: Role of an interaction between stress, glucocorticoids, and dopaminergic neurons. *Annu. Rev. Pharmacol. Toxicol., 36,* 359–378.

Piazza, P. V., and Le Moal, M. (1998). The role of stress in drug self-administration. *Trends Pharmacol. Sci., 19,* 67–74.

Piazza, P. V., Maccari, S., Deminiere, J. M., Le Moal, M., Mormede, P., and Simon, H. (1991a). Corticosterone levels determine individual vulnerability to amphetamine self-administration. *Proc. Natl. Acad. Sci. U. S. A., 88,* 2088–2092.

Piazza, P. V., Marinelli, M., Rouge-Pont, F., Deroche, V., Maccari, S., Simon, H., and Le, M. M. (1996b). Stress, glucocorticoids, and mesencephalic dopaminergic neurons: A pathophysiological chain determining vulnerability to psychostimulant abuse. *NIDA Res. Monogr., 163,* 277–299.

Piazza, P. V., Rouge-Pont, F., Deminiere, J. M., Kharouby, M., Le Moal, M., and Simon, H. (1991b). Dopaminergic activity is reduced in the prefrontal cortex and increased in the nucleus accumbens of rats predisposed to develop amphetamine self-administration. *Brain Res., 567,* 169–174.

Piazza, P. V., Rouge-Pont, F., Deroche, V., Maccari, S., Simon, H., and Le Moal, M. (1996c). Glucocorticoids have state-dependent stimulant effects on the mesencephalic dopaminergic transmission. *Proc. Natl. Acad. Sci. U. S. A., 93,* 8716–8720.

Pierce, R. C., and Kalivas, P. W. (1997). A circuitry model of the expression of behavioral sensitization to amphetamine-like psychostimulants. *Brain Res. Brain Res. Rev., 25*, 192–216.

Pilla, M., Perachon, S., Sautel, F., Garrido, F., Mann, A., Wermuth, C. G., Schwartz, J. C., Everitt, B. J., and Sokoloff, P. (1999). Selective inhibition of cocaine-seeking behaviour by a partial dopamine D3 receptor agonist. *Nature, 400*, 371–375.

Plihal, W., Krug, R., Pietrowsky, R., Fehm, H. L., and Born, J. (1996). Corticosteroid receptor mediated effects on mood in humans. *Psychoneuroendocrinology, 21*, 515–523.

Plotsky, P. M., Wightman, R. M., Chey, W., and Adams, R. N. (1977). Liquid chromatographic analysis of endogenous catecholamine release from brain slices. *Science, 197*, 904–906.

Pontieri, F. E., Tanda, G., and Di Chiara, G. (1995). Intravenous cocaine, morphine, and amphetamine preferentially increase extracellular dopamine in the "shell" as compared with the "core" of the rat nucleus accumbens. *Proc. Natl. Acad. Sci. U. S. A., 92*, 12304–12308.

Pothos, E. N., Creese, I., and Hoebel, B. G. (1995a). Restricted eating with weight loss selectively decreases extracellular dopamine in the nucleus accumbens and alters dopamine response to amphetamine, morphine, and food intake. *J. Neurosci., 15*, 6640–6650.

Pothos, E. N., Hernandez, L., and Hoebel, B. G. (1995b). Chronic food deprivation decreases extracellular dopamine in the nucleus accumbens: Implications for a possible neurochemical link between weight loss and drug abuse. *Obes. Res., 3* (Suppl 4), 525S–529S.

Pothos, E., Rada, P., Mark, G. P., and Hoebel, B. G. (1991). Dopamine microdialysis in the nucleus accumbens during acute and chronic morphine, naloxone-precipitated withdrawal and clonidine treatment. *Brain Res., 566*, 348–350.

Prasad, B. M., Sorg, B. A., Ulibarri, C., and Kalivas, P. W. (1995). Sensitization to stress and psychostimulants. Involvement of dopamine transmission versus the HPA axis. *Ann. N. Y. Acad. Sci., 771*, 617–625.

Puglisi-Allegra, S., Imperato, A., Angelucci, L., and Cabib, S. (1991). Acute stress induces time-dependent responses in dopamine mesolimbic system. *Brain Res., 554*, 217–222.

Puglisi-Allegra, S., Kempf, E., and Cabib, S. (1990). Role of genotype in the adaptation of the brain dopamine system to stress. *Neurosci. Biobehav. Rev., 14*, 523–528.

Ranaldi, R., French, E., and Roberts, D. C. (1996). Systemic pretreatment with MK-801 (dizocilpine) increases breaking points for self-administration of cocaine on a progressive-ratio schedule in rats. *Psychopharmacology (Berl), 128*, 83–88.

Rebec, G. V., Christensen, J. R., Guerra, C., and Bardo, M. T. (1997a). Regional and temporal differences in real-time dopamine efflux in the nucleus accumbens during free-choice novelty. *Brain Res., 776*, 61–67.

Rebec, G. V., Grabner, C. P., Johnson, M., Pierce, R. C., and Bardo, M. T. (1997b). Transient increases in catecholaminergic activity in medial prefrontal cortex and nucleus accumbens shell during novelty. *Neuroscience, 76*, 707–714.

Rebec, G. V., and Segal, D. S. (1978). Dose-dependent biphasic alterations in the spontaneous activity of neurons in the rat neostriatum produced by d-amphetamine and methylphenidate. *Brain Res., 150*, 353–366.

Redgrave, P., Prescott, T. J., and Gurney, K. (1999). Is the short-latency dopamine response too short to signal reward error? *Trends Neurosci., 22*, 146–151.

Refshauge, C., Kissinger, P. T., Dreiling, R., Blank, L., Freeman, R., and Adams, R. N. (1974). New high performance liquid chromatographic analysis of brain catecholamines. *Life Sci., 14*, 311–322.

Rice, M. E., and Nicholson, C. (1989). Measurement of nanomolar dopamine diffusion using low-noise perfluorinated ionomer coated carbon fiber microelectrodes and high-speed cyclic voltammetry. *Anal. Chem., 61*, 1805–1810.

Robbins, T. W., Granon, S., Muir, J. L., Durantou, F., Harrison, A., and Everitt, B. J. (1998). Neural systems underlying arousal and attention. Implications for drug abuse. *Ann. N. Y. Acad. Sci., 846*, 222–237.

Roberts, D. C., Andrews, M. M., and Vickers, G. J. (1996). Baclofen attenuates the reinforcing effects of cocaine in rats. *Neuropsychopharmacology, 15*, 417–423.

Robertson, M. W., Leslie, C. A., and Bennett, J. P., Jr. (1991). Apparent synaptic dopamine deficiency induced by withdrawal from chronic cocaine treatment. *Brain Res., 538*, 337–339.

Robinson, D. L., Venton, B. J., Heien, M. L., and Wightman, R. M. (2003). Detecting subsecond dopamine release with fast-scan cyclic voltammetry in vivo. *Clin. Chem., 49*, 1763–1773.

Robinson, D. L., and Wightman, R. M. (2004). Nomifensine amplifies subsecond dopamine signals in the ventral striatum of freely-moving rats. *J. Neurochem., 90*, 894–903.

Robinson, T. E., Becker, J. B., Young, E. A., Akil, H., and Castaneda, E. (1987). The effects of footshock stress on regional brain dopamine metabolism and pituitary beta-endorphin release in rats previously sensitized to amphetamine. *Neuropharmacology, 26*, 679–691.

Robinson, T. E., and Berridge, K. C. (2000). The psychology and neurobiology of addiction: An incentive-sensitization view. *Addiction, 95* (Suppl 2), S91–117.

Robinson, T. E., and Camp, D. M. (1990). Does amphetamine preferentially increase the extracellular concentration of dopamine in the mesolimbic system of freely moving rats? *Neuropsychopharmacology, 3*, 163–173.

Robinson, T. E., Jurson, P. A., Bennett, J. A., and Bentgen, K. M. (1988). Persistent sensitization of dopamine neurotransmission in ventral striatum (nucleus accumbens) produced by prior experience with (+)-amphetamine: A microdialysis study in freely moving rats. *Brain Res., 462,* 211–222.

Roitman, M. F., Stuber, G. D., Heien, M. L., Wightman, R. M., and Carelli, R. M. (2005). Subsecond dopamine release is selectively evoked by rewarding and not aversive taste stimuli. *Soc. Neurosci. Abs.*

Rossetti, Z. L., Hmaidan, Y., and Gessa, G. L. (1992a). Marked inhibition of mesolimbic dopamine release: A common feature of ethanol, morphine, cocaine and amphetamine abstinence in rats. *Eur. J. Pharmacol., 221,* 227–234.

Rossetti, Z. L., Melis, F., Carboni, S., Diana, M., and Gessa, G. L. (1992b). Alcohol withdrawal in rats is associated with a marked fall in extraneuronal dopamine. *Alcohol Clin. Exp. Res., 16,* 529–532.

Roth, R. H., Tam, S. Y., Ida, Y., Yang, J. X., and Deutch, A. Y. (1988). Stress and the mesocorticolimbic dopamine systems. *Ann. N. Y. Acad. Sci., 537,* 138–147.

Rouge-Pont, F., Deroche, V., Le Moal, M., and Piazza, P. V. (1998). Individual differences in stress-induced dopamine release in the nucleus accumbens are influenced by corticosterone. *Eur. J. Neurosci., 10,* 3903–3907.

Rouge-Pont, F., Marinelli, M., Le Moal, M., Simon, H., and Piazza, P. V. (1995). Stress-induced sensitization and glucocorticoids. II. Sensitization of the increase in extracellular dopamine induced by cocaine depends on stress-induced corticosterone secretion. *J. Neurosci., 15,* 7189–7195.

Rouge-Pont, F., Piazza, P. V., Kharouby, M., Le Moal, M., and Simon, H. (1993). Higher and longer stress-induced increase in dopamine concentrations in the nucleus accumbens of animals predisposed to amphetamine self-administration. A microdialysis study. *Brain Res., 602,* 169–174.

Saal, D., Dong, Y., Bonci, A., and Malenka, R. C. (2003). Drugs of abuse and stress trigger a common synaptic adaptation in dopamine neurons. *Neuron, 37,* 577–582.

Sabeti, J., Adams, C. E., Burmeister, J., Gerhardt, G. A., and Zahniser, N. R. (2002a). Kinetic analysis of striatal clearance of exogenous dopamine recorded by chronoamperometry in freely-moving rats. *J. Neurosci. Methods, 121,* 41–52.

Sabeti, J., Gerhardt, G. A., and Zahniser, N. R. (2002b). Acute cocaine differentially alters accumbens and striatal dopamine clearance in low and high cocaine locomotor responders: Behavioral and electrochemical recordings in freely moving rats. *J. Pharmacol. Exp. Ther., 302,* 1201–1211.

Salamone, J. D. (1992). Complex motor and sensorimotor functions of striatal and accumbens dopamine: Involvement in instrumental behavior processes. *Psychopharmacology (Berl), 107,* 160–174.

Salamone, J. D. (1994). The involvement of nucleus accumbens dopamine in appetitive and aversive motivation. *Behav. Brain Res., 61,* 117–133.

Salamone, J. D. (1996). The behavioral neurochemistry of motivation: Methodological and conceptual issues in studies of the dynamic activity of nucleus accumbens dopamine. *J. Neurosci. Methods, 64,* 137–149.

Salamone, J. D., and Correa, M. (2002). Motivational views of reinforcement: Implications for understanding the behavioral functions of nucleus accumbens dopamine. *Behav. Brain Res., 137,* 3–25.

Salamone, J. D., Cousins, M. S., and Snyder, B. J. (1997). Behavioral functions of nucleus accumbens dopamine: Empirical and conceptual problems with the anhedonia hypothesis. *Neurosci. Biobehav. Rev., 21,* 341–359.

Sandi, C. (1998). The role and mechanisms of action of glucocorticoid involvement in memory storage. *Neural Plast., 6,* 41–52.

Sandi, C., Loscertales, M., and Guaza, C. (1997). Experience-dependent facilitating effect of corticosterone on spatial memory formation in the water maze. *Eur. J. Neurosci., 9,* 637–642.

Sanghera, M. K., Trulson, M. E., and German, D. C. (1984). Electrophysiological properties of mouse dopamine neurons: In vivo and in vitro studies. *Neuroscience, 12,* 793–801.

Santiago, M., and Westerink, B. H. (1990). Characterization of the in vivo release of dopamine as recorded by different types of intracerebral microdialysis probes. *Naunyn Schmiedebergs Arch. Pharmacol., 342,* 407–414.

Sarnyai, Z., McKittrick, C. R., McEwen, B. S., and Kreek, M. J. (1998). Selective regulation of dopamine transporter binding in the shell of the nucleus accumbens by adrenalectomy and corticosterone-replacement. *Synapse, 30,* 334–337.

Schenk, S., Valadez, A., Worley, C. M., and McNamara, C. (1993). Blockade of the acquisition of cocaine self-administration by the NMDA antagonist MK-801 (dizocilpine). *Behav. Pharmacol., 4,* 652–659.

Schultz, W. (2002). Getting formal with dopamine and reward. *Neuron, 36,* 241–263.

Schultz, W., and Romo, R. (1987). Responses of nigro-striatal dopamine neurons to high-intensity somatosensory stimulation in the anesthetized monkey. *J. Neurophysiol., 57,* 201–217.

Schultz, W., Dayan, P., and Montague, P. R. (1997). A neural substrate of prediction and reward. *Science, 275,* 1593–1599.

Shaham, Y., Erb, S., and Stewart, J. (2000). Stress-induced relapse to heroin and cocaine seeking in rats: A review. *Brain Res. Brain Res. Rev., 33,* 13–33.

Shaham, Y., Shalev, U., Lu, L., de Wit, H., and Stewart, J. (2003). The reinstatement model of drug relapse: History, methodology and major findings. *Psychopharmacology (Berl), 168,* 3–20.

Shaham, Y., and Stewart, J. (1995). Stress reinstates heroin-seeking in drug-free animals: An effect mimicking heroin, not withdrawal. *Psychopharmacology (Berl)*, *119*, 334–341.

Shaham, Y., and Stewart, J. (1996). Effects of opioid and dopamine receptor antagonists on relapse induced by stress and re-exposure to heroin in rats. *Psychopharmacology (Berl)*, *125*, 385–391.

Shalev, U., Highfield, D., Yap, J., and Shaham, Y. (2000). Stress and relapse to drug seeking in rats: Studies on the generality of the effect. *Psychopharmacology (Berl)*, *150*, 337–346.

Shalev, U., Marinelli, M., Baumann, M. H., Piazza, P. V., and Shaham, Y. (2003). The role of corticosterone in food deprivation-induced reinstatement of cocaine seeking in the rat. *Psychopharmacology (Berl)*, *168*, 170–176.

Shanks, N., Griffiths, J., Zalcman, S., Zacharko, R. M., and Anisman, H. (1990). Mouse strain differences in plasma corticosterone following uncontrollable footshock. *Pharmacol. Biochem. Behav.*, *36*, 515–519.

Sharp, T., Zetterstrom, T., Ljungberg, T., and Ungerstedt, U. (1987). A direct comparison of amphetamine-induced behaviours and regional brain dopamine release in the rat using intracerebral dialysis. *Brain Res.*, *401*, 322–330.

Shepard, P. D., and Bunney, B. S. (1988). Effects of apamin on the discharge properties of putative dopamine-containing neurons in vitro. *Brain Res.*, *463*, 380–384.

Shoaib, M., Swanner, L. S., Beyer, C. E., Goldberg, S. R., and Schindler, C. W. (1998). The GABAB agonist baclofen modifies cocaine self-administration in rats. *Behav. Pharmacol.*, *9*, 195–206.

Smith, A. D., and Bolam, J. P. (1990). The neural network of the basal ganglia as revealed by the study of synaptic connections of identified neurones. *Trends Neurosci.*, *13*, 259–265.

Somogyi, P., Bolam, J. P., Totterdell, S., and Smith, A. D. (1981). Monosynaptic input from the nucleus accumbens–ventral striatum region to retrogradely labelled nigrostriatal neurones. *Brain Res.*, *217*, 245–263.

Sorg, B. A. (1992). Mesocorticolimbic dopamine systems: Cross-sensitization between stress and cocaine. *Ann. N. Y. Acad. Sci.*, *654*, 136–144.

Sorg, B. A., and Kalivas, P. W. (1991). Effects of cocaine and footshock stress on extracellular dopamine levels in the ventral striatum. *Brain Res.*, *559*, 29–36.

Sorg, B. A., and Kalivas, P. W. (1993). Effects of cocaine and footshock stress on extracellular dopamine levels in the medial prefrontal cortex. *Neuroscience*, *53*, 695–703.

Sorg, B. A., and Steketee, J. D. (1992). Mechanisms of cocaine-induced sensitization. *Prog. Neuropsychopharmacol. Biol. Psychiatry*, *16*, 1003–1012.

Steckler, T., Holsboer, F., and Reul, J. M. (1999). Glucocorticoids and depression. *Baillieres Best Pract. Res. Clin. Endocrinol. Metab.*, *13*, 597–614.

Stewart, J. (1984). Reinstatement of heroin and cocaine self-administration behavior in the rat by intracerebral application of morphine in the ventral tegmental area. *Pharmacol. Biochem. Behav.*, *20*, 917–923.

Stewart, J. (2000). Pathways to relapse: The neurobiology of drug- and stress-induced relapse to drug-taking. *J. Psychiatry Neurosci.*, *25*, 125–136.

Stoner, G. R., Skirboll, L. R., Werkman, S., and Hommer, D. W. (1988). Preferential effects of caffeine on limbic and cortical dopamine systems. *Biol. Psychiatry*, *23*, 761–768.

Strecker, R. E., and Jacobs, B. L. (1985). Substantia nigra dopaminergic unit activity in behaving cats: Effect of arousal on spontaneous discharge and sensory evoked activity. *Brain Res.*, *361*, 339–350.

Stuber, G. D., Roitman, M. F., Phillips, P. E., Carelli, R. M., and Wightman, R. M. (2005). Rapid dopamine signaling in the nucleus accumbens during contingent and noncontingent cocaine administration. *Neuropsychopharmacology*, *30*, 853–863.

Suaud-Chagny, M. F., Chergui, K., Chouvet, G., and Gonon, F. (1992). Relationship between dopamine release in the rat nucleus accumbens and the discharge activity of dopaminergic neurons during local in vivo application of amino acids in the ventral tegmental area. *Neuroscience*, *49*, 63–72.

Sullivan, R. M., and Gratton, A. (1998). Relationships between stress-induced increases in medial prefrontal cortical dopamine and plasma corticosterone levels in rats: Role of cerebral laterality. *Neuroscience*, *83*, 81–91.

Suto, N., Austin, J. D., and Vezina, P. (2001). Locomotor response to novelty predicts a rat's propensity to self-administer nicotine. *Psychopharmacology (Berl)*, *158*, 175–180.

Szabo, B., Siemes, S., and Wallmichrath, I. (2002). Inhibition of GABAergic neurotransmission in the ventral tegmental area by cannabinoids. *Eur. J. Neurosci.*, *15*, 2057–2061.

Taber, M. T., and Fibiger, H. C. (1997). Feeding-evoked dopamine release in the nucleus, accumbens: Regulation by glutamatergic mechanisms. *Neuroscience*, *76*, 1105–1112.

Thierry, A. M., Tassin, J. P., Blanc, G., and Glowinski, J. (1976). Selective activation of mesocortical DA system by stress. *Nature*, *263*, 242–244.

Thomas, M. J., Malenka, R. C., and Bonci, A. (2000). Modulation of long-term depression by dopamine in the mesolimbic system. *J. Neurosci.*, *20*, 5581–5586.

Thorre, K., Pravda, M., Sarre, S., Ebinger, G., and Michotte, Y. (1997). New antioxidant mixture for long term stability of serotonin, dopamine and their metabolites in automated microbore liquid chromatography with dual electrochemical detection. *J. Chromatogr. B Biomed. Sci. Appl.*, *694*, 297–303.

Tidey, J. W., and Miczek, K. A. (1996). Social defeat stress selectively alters mesocorticolimbic dopamine release: An in vivo microdialysis study. *Brain Res.*, *721*, 140–149.

Tidey, J. W., and Miczek, K. A. (1997). Acquisition of cocaine self-administration after social stress: Role of accumbens dopamine. *Psychopharmacology (Berl)*, *130*, 203–212.

Tran-Nguyen, L. T., Fuchs, R. A., Coffey, G. P., Baker, D. A., O'Dell, L. E., and Neisewander, J. L. (1998). Time-dependent changes in cocaine-seeking behavior and extracellular dopamine levels in the amygdala during cocaine withdrawal. *Neuropsychopharmacology*, *19*, 48–59.

Trulson, M. E., and Preussler, D. W. (1984). Dopamine-containing ventral tegmental area neurons in freely moving cats: Activity during the sleep-waking cycle and effects of stress. *Exp. Neurol.*, *83*, 367–377.

Turiault, M., Ambroggi, F., Marinelli, M., Deroche-Gamonet, V., Parnadeau, S., Milet, A., Rouzeau, J., Kretz, O., Sahly, I., Schuetz, G., Lemberger, T., Piazza, P. V., and Tronche, F. (2005). Specific inactivation of the glucocorticoid receptor in the dopaminergic system: New insights on drug addiction. *Soc. Neurosci., Abs*.

Ungless, M. A., Magill, P. J., and Bolam, J. P. (2004). Uniform inhibition of dopamine neurons in the ventral tegmental area by aversive stimuli. *Science*, *303*, 2040–2042.

Ungless, M. A., Singh, V., Crowder, T. L., Yaka, R., Ron, D., and Bonci, A. (2003). Corticotropin-releasing factor requires CRF binding protein to potentiate NMDA receptors via CRF receptor 2 in dopamine neurons. *Neuron*, *39*, 401–407.

Ungless, M. A., Whistler, J. L., Malenka, R. C., and Bonci, A. (2001). Single cocaine exposure in vivo induces long-term potentiation in dopamine neurons. *Nature*, *411*, 583–587.

Veals, J. W., Korduba, C. A., and Symchowicz, S. (1977). Effect of dexamethasone on monoamine oxidase inhibition by iproniazid in rat brain. *Eur. J. Pharmacol.*, *41*, 291–299.

Venton, B. J., Michael, D. J., and Wightman, R. M. (2003a). Correlation of local changes in extracellular oxygen and pH that accompany dopaminergic terminal activity in the rat caudate-putamen. *J. Neurochem.*, *84*, 373–381.

Venton, B. J., Seipel, A. T., Phillips, P. E., Wetsel, W. C., Gitler, D., Greengard, P., Augustine, G. J., and Wightman, R. M. (2006). Cocaine increases dopamine release by mobilization of a synapsin-dependent reserve pool. *J. Neurosci.*, *26*, 3206–3209.

Venton, B. J., Zhang, H., Garris, P. A., Phillips, P. E., Sulzer, D., and Wightman, R. M. (2003b). Real-time decoding of dopamine concentration changes in the caudate-putamen during tonic and phasic firing. *J. Neurochem.*, *87*, 1284–1295.

Vezina, P. (2004). Sensitization of midbrain dopamine neuron reactivity and the self-administration of psychomotor stimulant drugs. *Neurosci. Biobehav. Rev.*, *27*, 827–839.

Vezina, P., and Stewart, J. (1984). Conditioning and place-specific sensitization of increases in activity induced by morphine in the VTA. *Pharmacol. Biochem. Behav.*, *20*, 925–934.

Volkow, N. D., Fowler, J. S., Wang, G. J., and Goldstein, R. Z. (2002). Role of dopamine, the frontal cortex and memory circuits in drug addiction: Insight from imaging studies. *Neurobiol. Learn. Mem.*, *78*, 610–624.

Von Krosigk, M., Smith, Y., Bolam, J. P., and Smith, A. D. (1992). Synaptic organization of GABAergic inputs from the striatum and the globus pallidus onto neurons in the substantia nigra and retrorubral field which project to the medullary reticular formation. *Neuroscience*, *50*, 531–549.

Vorel, S. R., Liu, X., Hayes, R. J., Spector, J. A., and Gardner, E. L. (2001). Relapse to cocaine-seeking after hippocampal theta burst stimulation. *Science*, *292*, 1175–1178.

Wang, R. Y. (1981). Dopaminergic neurons in the rat ventral tegmental area. III. Effects of D- and L-amphetamine. *Brain Res. Brain Res. Rev.*, *3*, 153–165.

Wang, T., and French, E. D. (1993a). Electrophysiological evidence for the existence of NMDA and non-NMDA receptors on rat ventral tegmental dopamine neurons. *Synapse*, *13*, 270–277.

Wang, T., and French, E. D. (1993b). L-glutamate excitation of A10 dopamine neurons is preferentially mediated by activation of NMDA receptors: Extra- and intracellular electrophysiological studies in brain slices. *Brain Res.*, *627*, 299–306.

Wedzony, K., Mackowiak, M., Fijal, K., and Golembiowska, K. (1996). Evidence that conditioned stress enhances outflow of dopamine in rat prefrontal cortex: A search for the influence of diazepam and 5-HT1A agonists. *Synapse*, *24*, 240–247.

Weiss, F., Imperato, A., Casu, M. A., Mascia, M. S., and Gessa, G. L. (1997). Opposite effects of stress on dopamine release in the limbic system of drug-naive and chronically amphetamine-treated rats. *Eur. J. Pharmacol.*, *337*, 219–222.

Weiss, F., Maldonado-Vlaar, C. S., Parsons, L. H., Kerr, T. M., Smith, D. L., and Ben-Shahar, O. (2000). Control of cocaine-seeking behavior by drug-associated stimuli in rats: Effects on recovery of extinguished operant-responding and extracellular dopamine levels in amygdala and nucleus accumbens. *Proc. Natl. Acad. Sci. U. S. A.*, *97*, 4321–4326.

Weiss, F., Markou, A., Lorang, M. T., and Koob, G. F. (1992a). Basal extracellular dopamine levels in the nucleus accumbens are decreased during cocaine withdrawal after unlimited-access self-administration. *Brain Res.*, *593*, 314–318.

Weiss, F., Paulus, M. P., Lorang, M. T., and Koob, G. F. (1992b). Increases in extracellular dopamine in the nucleus accumbens by cocaine are inversely related to basal levels: Effects of acute and repeated administration. *J. Neurosci., 12,* 4372–4380.

White, F. J. (1996). Synaptic regulation of mesocortico-limbic dopamine neurons. *Annu. Rev. Neurosci., 19,* 405–436.

White, F. J., and Kalivas, P. W. (1998). Neuroadaptations involved in amphetamine and cocaine addiction. *Drug Alcohol Depend., 51,* 141–153.

Wiedemann, D. J., Kawagoe, K. T., Kennedy, R. T., Ciolkowski, E. L., and Wightman, R. M. (1991). Strategies for low detection limit measurements with cyclic voltammetry. *Anal. Chem., 63,* 2965–2970.

Wightman, R. M., Amatore, C., Engstrom, R. C., Hale, P. D., Kristensen, E. W., Kuhr, W. G., and May, L. J. (1988). Real-time characterization of dopamine over-flow and uptake in the rat striatum. *Neuroscience, 25,* 513–523.

Wightman, R. M., Plotsky, P. M., Strope, E., Delcore, R., Jr., and Adams, R. N. (1977). Liquid chromato-graphic monitoring of CSF metabolites. *Brain Res., 131,* 345–349.

Wilkinson, L. S., Humby, T., Killcross, A. S., Torres, E. M., Everitt, B. J., and Robbins, T. W. (1998). Dissociations in dopamine release in medial prefron-tal cortex and ventral striatum during the acquisition and extinction of classical aversive conditioning in the rat. *Eur. J. Neurosci., 10,* 1019–1026.

Williams, J., and Lacey, M. (1988). Actions of cocaine on central monoamine neurons: Intracellular record-ings in vitro. *NIDA Res. Monogr., 90,* 234–242.

Willner, P. (1997). Validity, reliability and utility of the chronic mild stress model of depression: A 10-year review and evaluation. *Psychopharmacology (Berl), 134,* 319–329.

Wise, R. A. (1998). Drug-activation of brain reward pathways. *Drug Alcohol Depend., 51,* 13–22.

Wise, R. A. (2005). Forebrain substrates of reward and motivation. *J. Comp. Neurol., 493,* 115–121.

Wolf, M. E., Sun, X., Mangiavacchi, S., and Chao, S. Z. (2004). Psychomotor stimulants and neuronal plas-ticity. *Neuropharmacology, 47* (Suppl 1), 61–79.

Wolf, M. E., White, F. J., and Hu, X. T. (1994). MK-801 prevents alterations in the mesoaccumbens dopa-mine system associated with behavioral sensitiza-tion to amphetamine. *J. Neurosci., 14,* 1735–1745.

Xi, Z. X., and Stein, E. A. (1999). Baclofen inhibits heroin self-administration behavior and mesolim-bic dopamine release. *J. Pharmacol. Exp. Ther., 290,* 1369–1374.

Xi, Z. X., and Stein, E. A. (2000). Increased mesolim-bic GABA concentration blocks heroin self-admin-istration in the rat. *J. Pharmacol. Exp. Ther., 294,* 613–619.

Zahm, D. S., and Brog, J. S. (1992). On the significance of subterritories in the "accumbens" part of the rat ventral striatum. *Neuroscience, 50,* 751–767.

Zetterstrom, T., Sharp, T., Collin, A. K., and Ungerstedt, U. (1988). In vivo measurement of extracellular dopamine and DOPAC in rat striatum after various dopamine-releasing drugs; implications for the ori-gin of extracellular DOPAC. *Eur. J. Pharmacol., 148,* 327–334.

Zuckerman, M. (1990). The psychophysiology of sensation seeking. *J. Pers., 58,* 313–345.

Endogenous Opiates, Addiction, and the Stress Response

RACHEL Y. CHONG, MAGDALENA UHART, AND GARY S. WAND

The endogenous opioid system regulates mesolimbic dopamine (DA) and the cortisol response to stress, both of which are implicated in drug and alcohol reward. A considerable body of research has highlighted the relationship between this system and alcohol addiction, and experiments have clearly demonstrated that alcohol affects endogenous opioid activity and receptors. Moreover, differences in the endogenous opioid system appear to be related to differences in alcohol and possibly cocaine consumption. Underscoring the role of this system in addiction, opioid antagonists have efficacy in reducing alcohol and, to some extent, cocaine consumption. Given that alcohol and drug use disorders have high heritability, it is possible that genetic differences in endogenous opioid tone are associated with differing vulnerabilities to alcohol and drug abuse. Indeed, β-endorphin activity and hypothalamic-pituitary-adrenal (HPA) axis response to opioid receptor antagonists and stress have been shown to differ as a function of family history of alcoholism. It has been speculated that individuals at increased familial risk for alcohol abuse have altered opioid tone that may modulate mesolimbic DA in ways that enhance reinforcement and reward, and thus addictive behaviors. These alterations may also have indirect effects on mesolimbic DA by affecting cortisol production, which itself influences the mesolimbic reward pathway. Thus, it is not surprising that there has been great interest in identifying genetic variations in this system, particularly variations in the μ-opioid receptor gene, which may contribute to alcohol and substance abuse.

I. INTRODUCTION

Endogenous opioids are peptides produced in a variety of organs but principally by the pituitary and brain. The endogenous opioid system is involved in several physiological processes, including modulation of the response to stress and painful stimuli; homeostatic functions such as temperature, food, and water regulation; pituitary function; and sexual behavior. In addition, it is important in controlling and modulating reward processes in the brain (Bodnar and Klein, 2005). In particular, it regulates mesolimbic dopamine (DA) and also modulates the hypothalamic-pituitary-adrenal (HPA) axis responses to stress, both of which are heavily implicated in drug and alcohol reward (Cowen and Lawrence, 1999; Gianoulakis, 1998).

II. THE ENDOGENOUS OPIOID SYSTEM

There are three major families of endogenous opioids: the enkephalins, the dynorphins, and the endorphins. Each family is derived from a specific precursor protein. The enkephalins—Met-enkephalin, Leu-enkephalin, Met-enkephalin-Arg^6-Gly^7-Leu^8, and Met-enkephalin-Arg^6-Phe^7—are derived from the precursor protein, proenkephalin. Enkephalins can be found widely throughout the brain, but proenkephalin mRNA is found at the highest levels in the striatum, ventral medial nucleus of the hypothalamus, and dentate gyrus of the hippocampus (Feldman et al., 1997; Mansour et al., 1988).

The dynorphins—dynorphin A-(1–17), dynorphin A-(1–8), dynorphin B, α-neoendorphin, and β-neoendorphin—are derived from prodynorphin. Like the enkephalins, dynorphins are also widely distributed in the brain and can be found in similar areas (Feldman et al., 1997; Mansour et al., 1988).

β-endorphin is derived from proopiomelanocortin (POMC). Unlike proenkephalin and prodynorphin, POMC is synthesized only in limited areas of the brain. β-endorphin neurons are located mainly in the ventromedial arcuate nucleus in the hypothalamus but project to many brain areas, including the ventral tegmental area (VTA), nucleus accumbens (NAc), amygdala, and other parts of the hypothalamus. These areas are important in drug reward and reinforcement. Other locations of POMC production include the nucleus tract solitarius, which is involved in analgesia, and the pituitary gland, where

POMC mRNA is found in highest concentration (Feldman et al., 1997; Mansour et al., 1988).

Like other neurotransmitters, endogenous opioids function by interacting with cell receptors, all of which belong to the superfamily of seven transmembrane G-protein coupled receptors (Akil et al., 1998). The three classes of opioids interact with at least three opioid receptor types: mu (μ), delta (δ), and kappa (κ) (Reisine and Bell, 1993). There are also subtypes in each of the three major classes of opioid receptors, for instance, μ1, μ2, and μ3 (Cadet, 2004; Pasternak, 1986); δ1 and δ2 ; and κ1, κ2, and κ3 (Corbett et al., 2006).

The three types of opioids have differing affinities for these cell receptors: β-endorphin has about equal affinity for δ- and μ-opioid receptors. Enkephalins have the greatest affinity for δ-receptors, with a 20-fold greater affinity for these receptors than for μ-opioid receptors. Dynorphins, on the other hand, show selective affinity for κ-receptors. The activation of δ- and μ-opioid receptors seems to produce similar patterns of neurotransmitter release, while the activation of κ-receptors seems to cause effects opposite to those mediated by δ- and μ-opioid receptors (Herz and Spanagel, 1995).

III. THE ENDOGENOUS OPIOID SYSTEM AND REWARD AND REINFORCEMENT

The mesocorticolimbic dopaminergic system, with its central component, the NAc, comprises the brain reward system circuitry and has intimate ties to the endogenous opioid system. The major components of this system modulating the reward pathway are the VTA, which contains dopaminergic cell bodies, the basal forebrain (composed of the NAc, amygdala, olfactory tubercle, and frontal and limbic cortices), the dopaminergic connections between the VTA and the basal forebrain, and the opioidergic neurons within these circuits. In addition, many neural systems interact with the VTA and the basal forebrain, including those involving γ-aminobutyric acid (GABA), glutamate, and serotonin (Koob, 1992; Leshner and Koob, 1999). Two regions are recognized in the NAc: the core and the shell. The shell is strongly connected to areas of the brain associated with the VTA and the lateral hypothalamus. Research has shown that there are μ-, δ-, and κ-opioid receptors in the NAc (Mansour et al., 1988). Also, each of the three types of endogenous opioids is present in the NAc: Enkephalins and dynorphins are synthesized in NAc neurons (Curran and Watson, Jr., 1995), and β-endorphin neurons innervate the NAc (Khachaturian et al., 1984).

The rewarding effects of most drugs of abuse have been associated with increased synaptic DA in the NAc of rodents (Tupala and Tiihonen, 2004). There is evidence that this effect also occurs in humans. For instance, positron emission tomography (PET) imaging has shown that drug euphoria and desire are related to alcohol-, amphetamine-, cocaine-, and methylphenidate-induced release of DA in the brain (Drevets et al., 2001; Leyton et al., 2002; Martinez et al., 2003; Oswald et al., 2005; Volkow et al., 1999; Yoder et al., 2005). β-endorphin and enkephalin increase DA release within the NAc via μ- and δ-opioid receptors and are thus implicated in reward and reinforcement. In contrast, dynorphin decreases DA release through κ-receptors and may counteract reinforcement (Koob, 1992). Indeed, studies have demonstrated that self-administration of selective μ- and δ-opioid receptor agonists results in reward, while administration of selective κ-agonists causes aversion (Devine and Wise, 1994; Shippenberg et al., 1992; Skoubis et al., 2005).

Different drugs of abuse may interact with the mesolimbic dopaminergic systems in different ways. For instance, stimulants, such as amphetamine and cocaine, activate dopaminergic activity in the dopaminergic synapse (Wise, 1984). Opiates have been shown to bind to μ- and possibly δ-receptors of the GABA-ergic system in the VTA and counteract the inhibition of the firing of DA neurons (Johnson and North, 1992; Wise, 1998). Ethanol is also thought to interact with the endogenous opioid system to affect the mesolimbic DA system. Extensive research has documented a link between alcohol addiction and endogenous opioids, and these data will be the focus of this chapter. The endogenous opioid system is also implicated in cocaine abuse, which will be briefly discussed.

IV. EFFECT OF ALCOHOL ON ENDOGENOUS OPIOID ACTIVITY

In vitro studies have demonstrated that ethanol acutely stimulates β-endorphin release from the hypothalamus and the pituitary (De Waele and Gianoulakis, 1993; De Waele et al., 1992; Gianoulakis, 1990; Keith et al., 1986). A rapid increase in β-endorphin is observed, lasting 10–20 minutes. This effect seems to follow an inverse U-shaped dose-response curve, with low ethanol concentrations inducing hypothalamic β-endorphin release in a dose-dependent fashion, and higher concentrations inducing less of a release (De Waele et al., 1992; Gianoulakis, 1990).

Acute alcohol consumption induces β-endorphin release not only in the pituitary and hypothalamus but also in other brain regions implicated in addiction, including in the NAc and VTA (Olive et al., 2001; Rasmussen et al., 1998). One model proposes that alcohol stimulates β-endorphin–producing neurons in the hypothalamus to increase β-endorphin release from axon terminals ending in the NAc and VTA. Ultimately, this release stimulates DA release in the NAc. This action may involve a direct effect through interaction with μ- and δ-opioid receptors on dopaminergic neurons or an indirect effect involving other neurotransmitter systems. For instance, β-endorphin neurons tonically inhibit GABA neurons, which in turn inhibit DA neurons in the VTA that project to the NAc. Hence, stimulation of β-endorphin neurons removes GABAergic inhibition of these VTA DA neurons, resulting in an increase in DA in the NAc (Jamensky and Gianoulakis, 1997). Indeed, DA release induced by alcohol can be blocked by opioid antagonists (Benjamin et al., 1993).

The increase in β-endorphin release in the NAc and VTA following acute alcohol consumption may be important for the *initiation* of drinking. However, it may not be important for the *maintenance* of alcohol consumption, since this increase is not maintained with chronic alcohol exposure. In fact, several studies have suggested that chronic alcohol exposure decreases endogenous opioid activity (Boyadjieva et al., 2001; Scanlon et al., 1992; Schulz et al., 1980; Winkler et al., 1995). The decrease in β-endorphins observed with chronic alcohol exposure, by causing feelings of discomfort, may help maintain alcohol consumption by negative reinforcement. However, findings regarding the effect of chronic alcohol on brain endorphins, particularly in the pituitary and hypothalamus, have been conflicting (Adams and Cicero, 1991; Angelogianni and Gianoulakis, 1993; Seizinger et al., 1983; Seizinger et al., 1984).

Less is known about the effect of ethanol on enkephalins and dynorphins. Some, but not all, studies have shown that acute alcohol administration increases Met-enkephalin levels in the pituitary, striatum, and hypothalamus of rats (Schulz et al., 1980; Seizinger et al., 1983). Acute ethanol has also been shown to increase proenkephalin mRNA in the NAc (Li et al., 1998). Chronic ethanol may decrease Met-enkephalin in certain regions of the brain (Schulz et al., 1980; Seizinger et al., 1983) while increasing Met-enkephalin-Arg[6]-Phe[7] in the NAc (Nylander et al., 1994). Chronic alcohol consumption has also been shown to decrease dynorphin and α-neo endorphin expression in the hypothalamus and hippocampus of rats (Seizinger et al., 1983). Still, the findings have not always been consistent, and how they relate to alcohol addiction is unclear.

V. EFFECT OF ALCOHOL ON ENDOGENOUS OPIOID RECEPTORS

Alcohol may alter not only endogenous opioid peptide levels but also the density and affinity of opioid receptors in the brain. However, the results of these studies have again been variable. Data from some *in vitro* studies have indicated that acute ethanol administration decreases δ- but not μ- or κ-receptors binding, while the results of other studies have shown that it increases μ-receptor binding (Gianoulakis, 1983; Hiller et al., 1981; Hiller et al., 1984; Hoffman et al., 1984; Levine et al., 1983; Tabakoff and Hoffman, 1983). Likewise, the effect of chronic alcohol on μ-opioid receptor binding has shown appreciable discrepancy (Gianoulakis, 1983; Hoffman et al., 1982; Khatami et al., 1987; Tabakoff and Hoffman, 1983; Tabakoff et al., 1981). The inconsistencies among these reports may be related to several factors, including the specific brain regions selected for investigation, the specific class of receptors studied, the study ligands utilized, the amount and route by which alcohol is delivered, and the types of laboratory animals used.

VI. ENDOGENOUS OPIOID ACTIVITY AND RECEPTORS AND ALCOHOL PREFERENCE

A. Experimental Animal Findings

Results of studies involving natural and selected breeds of ethanol-preferring and -nonpreferring rodents have suggested that genetic differences in endogenous opioid activity play a role in ethanol preference.

For example, levels of hypothalamic β-endorphin release and POMC mRNA expression have been shown to be greater in alcohol-preferring mice (C57BL/6) than in alcohol-avoiding mice (DBA/2); (De Waele et al., 1992; Jamensky and Gianoulakis, 1999). Likewise, selectively bred ethanol-preferring alko-alcohol (AA) rats have greater hypothalamic POMC mRNA expression than do ethanol-avoiding alko-non-alcohol (ANA) rats (Gianoulakis et al., 1992; Marinelli et al., 2000). Enkephalin and dynorphin production may differ according to alcohol preference, though the findings have not always been consistent (Jamensky and Gianoulakis, 1997; Li et al., 1998; Ng et al., 1996; Nylander et al., 1994).

Endogenous opioid activity in response to alcohol, as well as that at baseline, appears to differ according to alcohol preference. For instance, selectively bred ethanol-preferring P rats have greater ethanol-induced increases in pituitary POMC mRNA than do ethanol-avoiding NP rats (Krishnan-Sarin et al., 1998). Similarly, C57BL/6 mice produce greater amounts of hypothalamic POMC mRNA in response to alcohol than DBA/2 mice (De Waele and Gianoulakis, 1994). In addition, there is greater hypothalamic β-endorphin release in C57BL/6 mice compared with DBA/2 mice (De Waele and Gianoulakis, 1993; De Waele and Gianoulakis, 1994; De Waele et al., 1992). Furthermore, it has been shown that differences in pituitary β-endorphin correlate genetically with severity of ethanol withdrawal symptoms in 16 lines of mice (Crabbe et al., 1983).

In addition to differences in endogenous opioid activity, opioid receptor expression has been shown to vary as a function of alcohol preference in these rodent breeds. For example, as compared to ANA rats, AA rats have been shown to have a higher μ-opioid receptor density in the shell region of the NAc and prefrontal cortex but a lower κ-opioid receptor density in the ventromedial hypothalamus (Marinelli et al., 2000). Also, P rats have been shown to

have a higher density of μ-opioid receptors in some regions of the limbic system than do NP rats (McBride et al., 1998). In addition, C57BL/6 mice appear to have a higher δ-receptor density and lower κ-opioid receptor density in the NAc than do DBA/2 mice (De Waele and Gianoulakis, 1997; Jamensky and Gianoulakis, 1997).

A number of targeted gene mutation models in mice have provided further evidence of the role of endogenous opioid receptors in alcohol preference. As one might expect based on what is known about endogenous opioids and reward, C57BL/6 mice with the targeted disruption of the μ-opioid receptor have decreased ethanol preference when compared to their non-knockout counterparts (Hall et al., 2001). Since β-endorphin binds preferentially to μ-opioid receptors, it would be expected that POMC knockout mice, which lack the β-endorphin peptide, would also consume less alcohol than wild-type mice. However, experiments have not shown any difference in alcohol intake between these mice and their wild-type littermates (Grahame et al., 1998; Grisel et al., 1999). The reason for this discrepancy is unclear. Moreover, whereas δ-opioid receptor antagonists block alcohol consumption in rodents (Krishnan-Sarin et al., 1995), δ-opioid receptor knockout mice self-administer more ethanol compared to wild-type mice (Roberts et al., 2001).

Exploiting the relationship between endogenous opioids and alcohol, numerous preclinical studies have shown that a variety of nonselective opioid antagonists (namely naloxone and naltrexone); (Altshuler et al., 1980; Froehlich et al., 1990; Hubbell et al., 1991; Kornet et al., 1991; Marfaing-Jallat et al., 1983; Myers et al., 1986; Reid et al., 1991; Weiss et al., 1990) and selective μ- and δ-opioid receptors antagonists can decrease ethanol consumption (Honkanen et al., 1996; Krishnan-Sarin et al., 1995). κ-opioid receptor antagonists may also have some potential efficacy in reducing ethanol consumption (Sandi et al., 1988).

B. Findings in Humans

Consistent with preclinical research in rodents, opioid receptor availability appears to differ according to alcoholic exposure in humans. For example, PET studies using the radioligand [^{11}C]carfentenil, a potent and selective μ-opioid receptor agonist, have demonstrated that lower μ-opioid receptor availability is associated with higher craving in several brain regions: Alcoholics show lower μ-opioid receptor availability in the right dorsal lateral prefrontal cortex, the right anterior frontal cortex, and the right parietal cortex than do control subjects (Bencherif et al., 2004). Also, another PET study using the same radioligand further indicated that detoxified alcoholic patients have increased μ-opioid receptors in the ventral striatum, including the NAc, when compared to healthy individuals. Furthermore, the higher availability of μ-opioid receptors was found to correlate with alcohol-craving intensity (Heinz et al., 2005).

VII. OPIOID ANTAGONISTS IN THE TREATMENT OF ALCOHOL ADDICTION

Encouraged by preclinical findings that have demonstrated the efficacy of opioid receptor antagonists in reducing alcohol consumption in rodents, researchers conducted several trials to determine whether opioid antagonists are effective in treating alcohol use disorders in humans. In one 12-week, double-blind, placebo-controlled study of 70 alcohol-dependent veterans, oral naltrexone given as an adjunct to psychosocial therapy was associated with relapse in 23% of patients, as compared to 54% of those treated with placebo (Volpicelli et al., 1992). This drug, which acts primarily on μ-opioid receptors but also on δ- and κ-receptors, was also associated with lower craving for alcohol and fewer drinking days. In another 12-week, double-blind,

placebo-controlled trial of 97 detoxified alcohol-dependent persons, naltrexone in combination with coping skills/relapse prevention or supportive therapy, was associated with better abstinence rates, fewer drinking days, and a lower severity of alcohol-related problems (O'Malley et al., 1992). In sum, naltrexone was shown in these trials to reduce the frequency and amount of alcohol consumption and to reduce rates of complete relapse among individuals who eventually resumed drinking. A long-acting depot form of naltrexone that can be injected monthly is currently being studied (Garbutt et al., 2005). In addition, a 6-methylene analog of naltrexone, nalmefene, has shown some success in treating alcohol dependence (Mason et al., 1999).

Since the United States Food and Drug Administration has approved naltrexone for adjunctive therapy, there have been several other studies demonstrating the efficacy of this drug in diminishing relapse and alcohol consumption (Anton et al., 1999; Chick et al., 2000; Guardia et al., 2002; Morris et al., 2001; O'Malley et al., 1996). However, a study of 627 veterans, almost all of whom were male, demonstrated no benefit of short- or long-term naltrexone therapy in severe alcohol dependence (Krystal et al., 2001). Such findings, in the face of multiple previous studies showing the benefits of naltrexone, could be attributed to differences in study populations and psychosocial interventions. Also, while naltrexone may initially diminish alcohol consumption, its administration over the long term may be less effective in preventing alcohol relapse (Iso and Brush, 1991; Phillips et al., 1997). Chronic naltrexone may in fact upregulate the endogenous opioid system and increase opioid receptors and peptides, as has been shown in animal models (Chang et al., 1991; Cote et al., 1993; Tempel et al., 1985).

The mechanism responsible for the efficacy of opioid antagonists in decreasing alcohol consumption is uncertain. One possibility is that naltrexone may work by decreasing reinforcement. This theory is supported by studies indicating that among heavy drinkers and alcoholics who resumed drinking after detoxification, those that were taking naltrexone experienced decreased positive effects of and/or decreased "high" from ethanol when compared to those taking placebo (McCaul et al., 2000; Sinclair, 2001; Volpicelli et al., 1995). However, laboratory studies in humans have produced equivocal findings with regard to the effect of opioid antagonists on subjective responses to alcohol (Davidson et al., 1999; de Wit et al., 1999; McCaul et al., 2000; Swift et al., 1994). Naltrexone may be also effective in treating alcohol abuse by causing nausea (McCaul et al., 2000), but it is uncertain whether this side effect has a clinically meaningful impact on alcohol consumption.

VIII. ENDOGENOUS OPIOID ACTIVITY AND RECEPTORS AND COCAINE PREFERENCE

Cocaine is another drug that has been shown to interact with the endogenous opioid system. Cocaine exerts its psychoactive effects mainly by stimulating mesolimbic dopaminergic activity through inhibition of the presynaptic dopamine transporter (Dackis and O'Brien, 2001). However, this effect is modulated by other neurotransmitters, including endogenous opioids acting on μ-opioid receptors found on mesolimbic dopaminergic neurons (Ambrose et al., 2004).

In rodents, it has been suggested that self-administered cocaine may increase β-endorphin levels in the anterior limbic areas (Sweep et al., 1989). In addition, *in vivo* autoradiography has revealed decreased opioid receptor occupancy—probably from the release of endogenous opioids—in discrete areas of the mesocorticolimbic system, hypothalamus, and thalamus (Gerrits et al., 1999). Correspondingly, intraperitoneal cocaine has been found to increase β-endorphin in the NAc (Olive et al., 2001).

Cocaine has also been shown to increase binding to μ-opioid receptors and μ-opioid receptor mRNA expression in rodent brain reward areas (Azaryan et al., 1996; Azaryan et al., 1998; Hammer, Jr., 1989; Unterwald, 2001; Unterwald et al., 1994). Increased dynorphin mRNA expression has also been found in the dorsal striatum after cocaine administration, but only at repeated high doses. This finding implies that dynorphin may affect long-term sensitization to cocaine rather than early reinforcement (Daunais et al., 1993).

Finally, studies in humans have also suggested that the endogenous opioid system is important in cocaine abuse. Among persons addicted to cocaine, PET imaging with [^{11}C]carfentenil has demonstrated that μ-opioid receptor binding is increased in several regions of the brain when compared to those in nonaddicted individuals. Furthermore, μ-opioid receptor binding correlates with self-reported cocaine craving among cocaine users (Gorelick et al., 2005; Zubieta et al., 1996).

IX. OPIOID ANTAGONISTS IN THE TREATMENT OF COCAINE ADDICTION

Naloxone and naltrexone have been shown to decrease not only alcohol but also cocaine self-administration in laboratory animals. It has been suggested that these opioid antagonists work by decreasing cocaine-related reinforcement (DeVry et al., 1989; Kuzmin et al., 1997a; Ramsey et al., 1999). While these findings suggest that μ-opioid receptors are involved in cocaine use, other opioid receptors seem to be involved in cocaine self-administration as well. The δ-receptor antagonist naltrindole (Reid et al., 1995) and the κ-receptor agonists U50,488H and spiradoline (Glick et al., 1995; Kuzmin et al., 1997b) have also been shown to decrease cocaine consumption. In particular, treatment with U50,488H appears to shift the dose-response curve for cocaine reinforcement to the left, suggesting that activation of κ-receptor systems sensitizes rats to the reinforcing properties of cocaine (Kuzmin et al., 1997b). In sum, activation of μ- and δ-receptors appears to desensitize animals to cocaine reinforcement, while activation of κ-opioid receptors may do the opposite. In humans, naltrexone has been found to lessen the euphoria and "crash" associated with cocaine use (Kosten et al., 1992).

X. OPIOIDS AND RISK FOR ALCOHOLISM

As described above, alcohol and cocaine modulate endogenous opioid activity, which can in turn influence mesolimbic DA, reward, and possibly craving. Given that alcohol and drug use disorders have high heritability (Oroszi and Goldman, 2004; Palomo et al., 2004), it is possible that individual differences in endogenous opioid tone create a vulnerable substrate for alcohol and drug abuse, even before heavy drinking begins. To test this hypothesis, investigators have conducted studies employing a family history of alcoholism-related design. In these studies, the offspring of alcohol-dependent (family history-positive, FHP) persons were compared with the offspring of nonalcohol-dependent (family history-negative, FHN) persons before either group developed heavy alcohol consumption (Schuckit, 1994). The strategy was to detect genetic and developmental differences that distinguish the low-risk group from the high-risk group. The ability to develop markers to predict the future development of alcohol or drug abuse could lead to early interventions that target high-risk subjects.

Studies using this design indicated that basal levels of plasma β-endorphin are lower in subjects who are FHP for alcoholism than in those who are FHN (Dai et al., 2002a; Gianoulakis et al., 1989; Gianoulakis et al., 2005). Following alcohol ingestion, plasma β-endorphin levels have been shown to increase in FHP but not FHN individu-

als (Gianoulakis, 1996; Gianoulakis et al., 1989). Moreover, stress—which activates the endogenous opioid system and is thought to play a role in addiction—results in lower increases in plasma β-endorphin in FHP than in FHN individuals (Dai et al., 2002a). This study also found that alcohol administration attenuates the stress-induced increase in plasma β-endorphin to a lesser degree in FHP individuals (Dai et al., 2002a).

To test the hypothesis that FHP subjects have altered endogenous opioid activity when compared to FHN subjects, naloxone challenge has been used as an indirect technique to measure endogenous opioid tone. Following the perception of stress, corticotropin-releasing hormone (CRH) neurons in the hypothalamus receive regulatory impulses from several major neurotransmitter systems, including direct and indirect inhibitory signals from β-endorphin–producing neurons (Calogero, 1995). CRH release stimulates the synthesis and release of adrenocorticotropic hormone (ACTH), which in turn stimulates cortisol synthesis and release by the adrenal cortex. Administration of a nonselective opioid receptor antagonist such as naloxone increases the plasma concentrations of ACTH and cortisol by blocking the central inhibitory effect of endogenous opioids directed at the CRH-producing neurons. These effects are thought to result primarily from the direct blockade of opioid pathways involving β-endorphin and enkephalins from the arcuate nucleus (Bujdoso et al., 2001; Chrousos and Gold, 1992; Yajima et al., 1986) to the hypothalamic CRH neurons. A blockade of opioid inhibition of norepinephrine neurons in the locus coeruleus, which provide direct stimulatory input to hypothalamic CRH neurons, may also be involved (Grossman and Besser, 1982; Sim-Selley et al., 2000; Valentino and Van Bockstaele, 2001) (Figure 4-1).

Because developmental or inborn abnormalities in opioid activity could alter inhibitory tone on CRH neurons, an individual's HPA axis-mediated hormonal

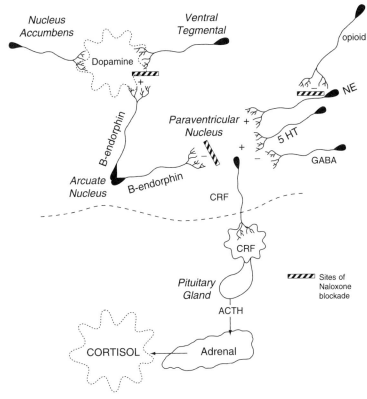

FIGURE 4-1   β-endorphin neurons in the arcuate nucleus of the hypothalamus directly inhibit CRH neurons of the hypothalamus. Opioid neurons also indirectly inhibit hypothalamic CRH neurons by inhibiting norepinephrine neurons in the locus coeruleus that stimulate hypothalamic CRH neurons. β-endorphin neurons also stimulate DA release in the NAc. GABA, γ-aminobutyric acid; NE, norepinephrine.

From Wand, G. S., Mangold, D., El, D. S., McCaul, M. E., and Hoover, D. (1998). Family history of alcoholism and hypothalamic opioidergic activity. *Arch. Gen. Psychiatry*, *55*, 1116, Fig. 1. Copyright © (1998), American Medical Association. All Rights Reserved.

response to opioid receptor blockade provides a functional assessment of hypothalamic opioid activity. Presumably, the stronger the opioidergic inhibition of CRH neurons, the higher the dose of opioid antagonist needed for disinhibition. It has been shown that lower concentrations of naloxone are needed to remove the opioid inhibitory control of the CRH neurons in FHP individuals than in FHN individuals (Wand et al., 1998). In subsequent studies, administration of naloxone and naltrexone have also resulted in higher ACTH and/or cortisol responses in FHP than FHN individuals, providing further evidence that those at increased genetic or developmen-

tal risk for alcoholism have altered HPA axis responses to opioid receptor blockade (Hernandez-Avila et al., 2002; King et al., 2002; Wand et al., 1999a; Wand et al., 1999b; Wand et al., 2001) (Figure 4-2).

These findings suggest that FHP individuals have lower central opioid tone directed at hypothalamic CRH neurons than do FHN individuals. Thus, individuals who are at high risk for excessive ethanol consumption by virtue of their family history may have an inherited or acquired deficiency in activity of the endogenous opioid system. In this regard, it has been suggested that a dysfunction in the pituitary β-endorphin system may predate the development of

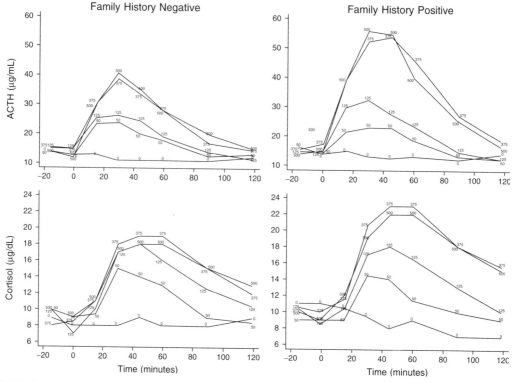

FIGURE 4-2   (Top) ACTH responses to naloxone, as a function of dose and family history of alcoholism. ACTH responses are higher in FHP than in FHN subjects at doses of 375 ($p < 0.001$) and 500 µg ($p = 0.02$), after adjusting for placebo responses. (Bottom) Cortisol responses to naloxone, as a function of dose and family history of alcoholism. Cortisol responses are higher in FHP than in FHN subjects at doses of 125 ($p = 0.004$), 375 ($p < 0.001$), and 500 µg ($p = 0.001$), after adjusting for placebo responses.

From Wand et al. (2001, Fig. 1, p. 1136).

alcoholism in FHP individuals, while it may develop following alcohol dependence in FHN individuals (Dai et al., 2005). At present, it is not known which component of the hypothalamic endogenous opioid system influences the hypoactivity. Deficits in opioid activity could be the result of decreased synaptic opioid content, reduced opioid receptor density, and/or differences in the type or binding affinities of opioid receptors in specific brain regions. Lower central opioid activity in FHP individuals may increase their vulnerability to alcoholism by diminishing basal levels of DA within the NAc and/or diminishing accumulation of DA following ethanol ingestion. Thus, FHP individuals might require higher blood ethanol levels to stimulate the opioid-mesolimbic DA cascade.

If FHP individuals have less opioid inhibitory activity directed at the hypothalamic CRH neurons when compared to FHN persons, FHP individuals would be expected to demonstrate a greater cortisol response to stress. Indeed, it has been shown that FHP subjects demonstrate higher cortisol responses to a psychological stress test than do FHN subjects (Uhart et al., 2006; Zimmermann et al., 2004). However, such differences in cortisol responses to stress have not always been reproduced (Dai et al., 2002b). It is interesting to note that no differences in cortisol response have been observed between FHP and FHN individuals after stimulation by CRH (Waltman et al., 1994) or direct adrenal stimulation by the ACTH analog, cosyntropin (Wand et al., 1999b). Also, differences have not been found in the 24-hour cortisol circadian profile (Wand et al., 1999b). Thus, the differences seen in the cortisol response to opioid antagonist and psychological stress may exist at the hypothalamic level and thus involve endogenous opioids.

The data described above suggest that individuals at increased risk for alcohol and drug use have differences in opioid tone that may modulate mesolimbic DA in ways that enhance reinforcement and reward, and therefore addictive behaviors. The data also suggest that differences in opioid tone create a more labile HPA axis. There is extensive literature indicating that stress hormones modulate mesolimbic DA and enhance drug-seeking behaviors (Piazza and Le, 1998). Therefore, alterations in endogenous opioid activity could have direct as well as indirect effects (through cortisol) on the mesolimbic reward pathway. Interestingly, naltrexone treatment modulates the HPA axis, and it has been suggested that some of the therapeutic properties of the opioid receptor antagonists are imparted through their ability to alter cortisol secretion (McCaul et al., 2001). (For a discussion of stress, cortisol, and mesolimbic dopamine, please refer to preceding chapters.)

XI. THE μ-OPIOID RECEPTOR GENE

Given the apparent importance of the endogenous opioid system in addiction, there has been great interest in identifying genes related to this neurotransmitter system that may contribute to genetic vulnerability to alcohol and substance abuse. Much of the attention has been focused on the μ-opioid receptor gene. Investigators have identified numerous polymorphisms in the μ-opioid receptor gene, such as the 118A>G SNP in exon 1. This SNP has a minor allele frequency as high as 48.9% within racial groups (rs1799971 [http://www.hapmap.org/]), and causes an asparagine-to-aspartate exchange at protein position 40 of the extracellular C-terminal portion of the receptor. The minor (G) allele of this SNP was originally associated with increased binding affinity to β-endorphin (Bond et al., 1998). More recently, research has suggested that the G allele is associated with lower production of μ-opioid receptor mRNA and protein (Zhang et al., 2005). It is still uncertain, however, whether the 118A>G SNP is truly a functional polymorphism (Beyer et al., 2004; Bond et al., 1998; Zhang et al., 2005).

While the relationship between this SNP and abuse of alcohol, opioids, and other substances has been widely studied, the findings have been conflicting: Several studies in humans have suggested that the 118A allele may be a risk factor for opiate and other drug addiction (Bond et al., 1998; Schinka et al., 2002; Tan et al., 2003; Town et al., 1999). On the other hand, however, the 118G allele has been reported to be more common in opioid-dependent (Szeto et al., 2001) and alcohol-dependent individuals (Bart et al., 2005) and is linked to heavier drinking (Kim et al., 2004). A recent study demonstrated that this minor allele was linked to more robust subjective responses to alcohol and a positive family history of alcohol use disorders among healthy subjects (Ray and Hutchison, 2004). However, other studies have found no association between this polymorphism and substance dependence (Bergen et al., 1997; Compton et al., 2003; Crowley et al., 2003; Franke et al., 2001; Gelernter et al., 1999; Hoehe et al., 2000; Ide et al., 2004; Loh et al., 2004; Luo et al., 2003; Sander et al., 1998; Shi et al., 2002). Furthermore, it has been demonstrated that while haplotypes at the μ-opioid receptor gene locus are associated with substance abuse, the 118A>G polymorphism does not contribute any further information (Luo et al., 2003).

Also of interest is the relationship between the 118A>G SNP, opioids, and the HPA axis. It has been demonstrated that persons expressing the minor allele (G) of the 118A>G MOR polymorphism have an exaggerated cortisol response to naloxone when compared to subjects expressing only the major allele (Chong et al., 2006; Hernandez-Avila et al.,

2003) (Figure 4-3a). Furthermore, subjects expressing the G allele of the SNP have been shown to have a blunted cortisol response to psychosocial stress (Chong et al., 2006) (Figure 4-3b). These results suggest that the 118A>G MOR SNP exerts not only a pharmacogenetic effect on naloxone-induced activation of the HPA axis but also an effect on HPA axis activation by stress. It may be of clinical relevance that one study has demonstrated that 12 weeks of naltrexone treatment led to significantly lower relapse rates in alcohol-dependent persons with the 118G allele, who also took longer to resume drinking than did individuals with only the 118A allele (Oslin et al., 2003).

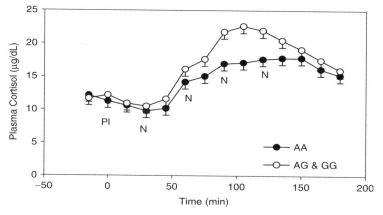

FIGURE 4-3a   Plasma cortisol response to naloxone as a function of A118G μ-opioid receptor gene genotype. Healthy subjects expressing the minor allele (G) of this polymorphism show an exaggerated cortisol response to naloxone when compared to subjects expressing only the major allele ($p = 0.046$). Values reflect means (SE) adjusted for gender, age, race, body mass index, level of education, and baseline cortisol. **Pl** denotes time of placebo (saline) administration. **N** denotes times of incremental intravenous naloxone administration.
     Adapted from Chong et al. (2006, Fig. 1, p. 208).

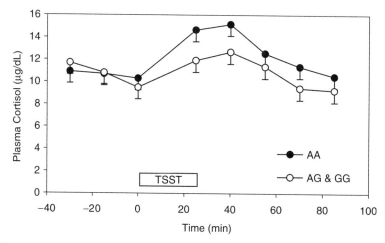

FIGURE 4-3b   Plasma cortisol response to the Trier Social Stress Test (TSST), a standardized psychological stress test, as a function of A118G μ-opioid receptor gene genotype. Healthy subjects expressing the minor allele (G) of this polymorphism show a blunted cortisol response to the TSST when compared to subjects expressing only the major allele ($p = 0.044$). Values reflect means (SE) adjusted for gender, age, race, body mass index, level of education, and baseline cortisol.
     Adapted from Chong et al. (2006, Fig. 2, p. 208).

Another variation in OPRM1 that has been studied for a possible association with alcohol and substance abuse is the 17C>T SNP in exon 1, which has a minor allele frequency of up to 7% (Bond et al., 1998; Skarke et al., 2004). It results in an alanine-to-valine change at position 6 of the extracellular portion of the receptor. It is unknown whether this SNP affects ligand binding or receptor function. It has been reported that the minor allele may be present in a greater percentage of opioid-dependent individuals compared with nondependent individuals (Bond et al., 1998). However, most studies have found no significant association with alcohol or substance abuse (Crowley et al., 2003; Gscheidel et al., 2000; Rommelspacher et al., 2001). This finding is also true for several SNPs that have been studied, such as -172G>T and IVS2-691C>G SNPs (Bergen et al., 1997; Gscheidel et al., 2000; Hoehe et al., 2000; Rommelspacher et al., 2001).

Haplotype analysis, which more comprehensively captures the variation in a gene, may provide better information regarding association with alcohol and drug abuse than single SNP analysis. Haplotypes including the -1793T>A, -1699-(-1698)insT, -1320A>G, -111C>T, and 17C>T SNPs (Hoehe et al., 2000); the 118A>G and IVS2-31G>A SNPs (Shi et al., 2002); the 118A>G and IVS2-1031C>G SNPs (Szeto et al., 2001); and the -2044C>A SNP (Luo et al., 2003) have been associated with substance dependence and drug consumption.

XII. CONCLUSIONS

The endogenous opioid system regulates the mesolimbic dopaminergic system both directly and indirectly by modulating the HPA axis response to stress. Inherent individual differences in the endogenous opioid system may contribute to drug and alcohol addiction susceptibility. Much remains to be learned about the use of opioid antagonists in alcohol and drug treatment and the specific role of the endogenous opioid system in reward and reinforcement. Further research in this area may open additional avenues for treatment and prevention of alcohol and drug abuse disorders. In particular, the use of genetic polymorphisms in the endogenous opioid system may yield the potential to identify individuals who are particularly vulnerable to addictive substances. Also, discovering genetic variants in the endogenous opioid system and HPA axis neurotransmitter system may some day help identify individuals who would be responsive to opioid antagonist and related therapies. In other words, an understanding of the genetic basis for differences in this neurotransmitter system could lead to pharmacogenetically directed therapies in the future.

REFERENCES

Adams, M. L., and Cicero, T. J. (1991). Effects of alcohol on beta-endorphin and reproductive hormones in the male rat. *Alcohol Clin. Exp. Res., 15,* 685–692.

Akil, H., Owens, C., Gutstein, H., Taylor, L., Curran, E., and Watson, S. (1998). Endogenous opioids: Overview and current issues. *Drug Alcohol Depend., 51,* 127–140.

Altshuler, H. L., Phillips, P. E., and Feinhandler, D. A. (1980). Alteration of ethanol self-administration by naltrexone. *Life Sci., 26,* 679–688.

Ambrose, L. M., Unterwald, E. M., and Van Bockstaele, E. J. (2004). Ultrastructural evidence for co-localization of dopamine D2 and micro-opioid receptors in the rat dorsolateral striatum. *Anat. Rec. A Discov. Mol. Cell Evol. Biol., 279,* 583–591.

Angelogianni, P., and Gianoulakis, C. (1993). Chronic ethanol increases proopiomelanocortin gene expression in the rat hypothalamus. *Neuroendocrinology, 57,* 106–114.

Anton, R. F., Moak, D. H., Waid, L. R., Latham, P. K., Malcolm, R. J., and Dias, J. K. (1999). Naltrexone and cognitive behavioral therapy for the treatment of outpatient alcoholics: Results of a placebo-controlled trial. *Am. J. Psychiatry, 156,* 1758–1764.

Azaryan, A. V., Clock, B. J., Rosenberger, J. G., and Cox, B. M. (1998). Transient upregulation of mu opioid receptor mRNA levels in nucleus accumbens during chronic cocaine administration. *Can. J. Physiol Pharmacol., 76,* 278–283.

Azaryan, A. V., Coughlin, L. J., Buzas, B., Clock, B. J., and Cox, B. M. (1996). Effect of chronic cocaine treatment on mu- and delta-opioid receptor mRNA levels in dopaminergically innervated brain regions. *J. Neurochem., 66,* 443–448.

Bart, G., Kreek, M. J., Ott, J., LaForge, K. S., Proudnikov, D., Pollak, L., and Heilig, M. (2005). Increased attributable risk related to a functional mu-opioid receptor gene polymorphism in association with alcohol dependence in central Sweden. *Neuropsychopharmacology, 30*, 417–422.

Bencherif, B., Wand, G. S., McCaul, M. E., Kim, Y. K., Ilgin, N., Dannals, R. F., and Frost, J. J. (2004). Mu-opioid receptor binding measured by [11C] carfentanil positron emission tomography is related to craving and mood in alcohol dependence. *Biol. Psychiatry, 55*, 255–262.

Benjamin, D., Grant, E. R., and Pohorecky, L. A. (1993). Naltrexone reverses ethanol-induced dopamine release in the nucleus accumbens in awake, freely moving rats. *Brain Res., 621*, 137–140.

Bergen, A. W., Kokoszka, J., Peterson, R., Long, J. C., Virkkunen, M., Linnoila, M., and Goldman, D. (1997). Mu opioid receptor gene variants: Lack of association with alcohol dependence. *Mol. Psychiatry, 2*, 490–494.

Beyer, A., Koch, T., Schroder, H., Schulz, S., and Hollt, V. (2004). Effect of the A118G polymorphism on binding affinity, potency and agonist-mediated endocytosis, desensitization, and resensitization of the human mu-opioid receptor. *J. Neurochem., 89*, 553–560.

Bodnar, R. J., and Klein, G. E. (2005). Endogenous opiates and behavior: 2004. *Peptides, 26*, 2629–2711.

Bond, C., LaForge, K. S., Tian, M., Melia, D., Zhang, S., Borg, L., Gong, J., Schluger, J., Strong, J. A., Leal, S. M., Tischfield, J. A., Kreek, M. J., and Yu, L. (1998). Single-nucleotide polymorphism in the human mu opioid receptor gene alters beta-endorphin binding and activity: Possible implications for opiate addiction. *Proc. Natl. Acad. Sci. U. S. A., 95*, 9608–9613.

Boyadjieva, N., Dokur, M., Advis, J. P., Meadows, G. G., and Sarkar, D. K. (2001). Chronic ethanol inhibits NK cell cytolytic activity: Role of opioid peptide beta-endorphin. *J. Immunol., 167*, 5645–5652.

Bujdoso, E., Jaszberenyi, M., Tomboly, C., Toth, G., and Telegdy, G. (2001). Behavioral and neuroendocrine actions of endomorphin-2. *Peptides, 22*, 1459–1463.

Cadet, P. (2004). Mu opiate receptor subtypes. *Med. Sci. Monit., 10*, MS28–MS32.

Calogero, A. E. (1995). Neurotransmitter regulation of the hypothalamic corticotropin-releasing hormone neuron. *Ann. N. Y. Acad. Sci., 771*, 31–40.

Chang, S. C., Lutfy, K., Sierra, V., and Yoburn, B. C. (1991). Dissociation of opioid receptor upregulation and functional supersensitivity. *Pharmacol. Biochem. Behav., 38*, 853–859.

Chick, J., Anton, R., Checinski, K., Croop, R., Drummond, D. C., Farmer, R., Labriola, D., Marshall, J., Moncrieff, J., Morgan, M. Y., Peters, T., and Ritson, B. (2000). A multicentre, randomized, double-blind, placebo-controlled trial of naltrexone in the treatment of alcohol dependence or abuse. *Alcohol Alcohol, 35*, 587–593.

Chong, R. Y., Oswald, L., Yang, X., Uhart, M., Lin, P. I., and Wand, G. S. (2006). The mu-opioid receptor polymorphism A118G predicts cortisol responses to naloxone and stress. *Neuropsychopharmacology, 31*, 204–211.

Chrousos, G. P., and Gold, P. W. (1992). The concepts of stress and stress system disorders. Overview of physical and behavioral homeostasis. *JAMA, 267*, 1244–1252.

Compton, P., Geschwind, D. H., and Alarcon, M. (2003). Association between human mu-opioid receptor gene polymorphism, pain tolerance, and opioid addiction. *Am. J. Med. Genet. B Neuropsychiatr. Genet., 121*, 76–82.

Corbett, A. D., Henderson, G., McKnight, A. T., and Paterson, S. J. (2006). 75 years of opioid research: The exciting but vain quest for the Holy Grail. *Br. J. Pharmacol., 147* (Suppl 1), S153–S162.

Cote, T. E., Izenwasser, S., and Weems, H. B. (1993). Naltrexone-induced upregulation of mu opioid receptors on 7315c cell and brain membranes: Enhancement of opioid efficacy in inhibiting adenylyl cyclase. *J. Pharmacol. Exp. Ther., 267*, 238–244.

Cowen, M. S., and Lawrence, A. J. (1999). The role of opioid-dopamine interactions in the induction and maintenance of ethanol consumption. *Prog. Neuropsychopharmacol. Biol. Psychiatry, 23*, 1171–1212.

Crabbe, J. C., Keith, L. D., Kosobud, A., and Stack, J. (1983). Ethanol dependence and the pituitary-adrenal axis in mice. I. Genotypic differences in hormone levels. *Life Sci., 33*, 1877–1887.

Crowley, J. J., Oslin, D. W., Patkar, A. A., Gottheil, E., Demaria, P. A., Jr., O'Brien, C. P., Berrettini, W. H., and Grice, D. E. (2003). A genetic association study of the mu opioid receptor and severe opioid dependence. *Psychiatr. Genet., 13*, 169–173.

Curran, E. J., and Watson, S. J., Jr. (1995). Dopamine receptor mRNA expression patterns by opioid peptide cells in the nucleus accumbens of the rat: A double in situ hybridization study. *J. Comp. Neurol., 361*, 57–76.

Dackis, C. A., and O'Brien, C. P. (2001). Cocaine dependence: A disease of the brain's reward centers. *J. Subst. Abuse Treat., 21*, 111–117.

Dai, X., Thavundayil, J., and Gianoulakis, C. (2002a). Differences in the responses of the pituitary beta-endorphin and cardiovascular system to ethanol and stress as a function of family history. *Alcohol Clin. Exp. Res., 26*, 1171–1180.

Dai, X., Thavundayil, J., and Gianoulakis, C. (2002b). Response of the hypothalamic-pituitary-adrenal axis to stress in the absence and presence of ethanol in subjects at high and low risk of alcoholism. *Neuropsychopharmacology, 27*, 442–452.

Dai, X., Thavundayil, J., and Gianoulakis, C. (2005). Differences in the peripheral levels of beta-endorphin in response to alcohol and stress as a function of alcohol dependence and family history of alcoholism. *Alcohol Clin. Exp. Res., 29*, 1965–1975.

Daunais, J. B., Roberts, D. C., and McGinty, J. F. (1993). Cocaine self-administration increases preprodynorphin, but not c-Fos, mRNA in rat striatum. *Neuroreport, 4*, 543–546.

Davidson, D., Palfai, T., Bird, C., and Swift, R. (1999). Effects of naltrexone on alcohol self-administration in heavy drinkers. *Alcohol Clin. Exp. Res., 23*, 195–203.

Devine, D. P., and Wise, R. A. (1994). Self-administration of morphine, DAMGO, and DPDPE into the ventral tegmental area of rats. *J. Neurosci., 14*, 1978–1984.

DeVry, J., Donselaar, I., and van Ree, J. M. (1989). Food deprivation and acquisition of intravenous cocaine self-administration in rats: Effect of naltrexone and haloperidol. *J. Pharmacol. Exp. Ther., 251*, 735–740.

De Waele, J. P., and Gianoulakis, C. (1993). Effects of single and repeated exposures to ethanol on hypothalamic beta-endorphin and CRH release by the C57BL/6 and DBA/2 strains of mice. *Neuroendocrinology, 57*, 700–709.

De Waele, J. P., and Gianoulakis, C. (1994). Enhanced activity of the brain beta-endorphin system by free-choice ethanol drinking in C57BL/6 but not DBA/2 mice. *Eur. J. Pharmacol., 258*, 119–129.

De Waele, J. P., and Gianoulakis, C. (1997). Characterization of the mu and delta opioid receptors in the brain of the C57BL/6 and DBA/2 mice, selected for their differences in voluntary ethanol consumption. *Alcohol Clin. Exp. Res., 21*, 754–762.

De Waele, J. P., Papachristou, D. N., and Gianoulakis, C. (1992). The alcohol-preferring C57BL/6 mice present an enhanced sensitivity of the hypothalamic beta-endorphin system to ethanol than the alcohol-avoiding DBA/2 mice. *J Pharmacol. Exp. Ther., 261*, 788–794.

de Wit, H., Svenson, J., and York, A. (1999). Non-specific effect of naltrexone on ethanol consumption in social drinkers. *Psychopharmacology (Berl), 146*, 33–41.

Drevets, W. C., Gautier, C., Price, J. C., Kupfer, D. J., Kinahan, P. E., Grace, A. A., Price, J. L., and Mathis, C. A. (2001). Amphetamine-induced dopamine release in human ventral striatum correlates with euphoria. *Biol. Psychiatry, 49*, 81–96.

Feldman, R. S., Meyer, J. S., and Quenzer, L. F. (1997). *Principles of neuropsychopharmacology.* Sunderland, MA: Sinauer Associates.

Franke, P., Wang, T., Nothen, M. M., Knapp, M., Neidt, H., Albrecht, S., Jahnes, E., Propping, P., and Maier, W. (2001). Nonreplication of association between mu-opioid-receptor gene (OPRM1) A118G polymorphism and substance dependence. *Am. J. Med. Genet., 105*, 114–119.

Froehlich, J. C., Harts, J., Lumeng, L., and Li, T. K. (1990). Naloxone attenuates voluntary ethanol intake in rats selectively bred for high ethanol preference. *Pharmacol. Biochem. Behav., 35*, 385–390.

Garbutt, J. C., Kranzler, H. R., O'Malley, S. S., Gastfriend, D. R., Pettinati, H. M., Silverman, B. L., Loewy, J. W., and Ehrich, E. W. (2005). Efficacy and tolerability of long-acting injectable naltrexone for alcohol dependence: A randomized controlled trial. *JAMA, 293*, 1617–1625.

Gelernter, J., Kranzler, H., and Cubells, J. (1999). Genetics of two mu opioid receptor gene (OPRM1) exon I polymorphisms: Population studies, and allele frequencies in alcohol- and drug-dependent subjects. *Mol. Psychiatry, 4*, 476–483.

Gerrits, M. A., Wiegant, V. M., and van Ree, J. M. (1999). Endogenous opioids implicated in the dynamics of experimental drug addiction: An in vivo autoradiographic analysis. *Neuroscience, 89*, 1219–1227.

Gianoulakis, C. (1983). Long-term ethanol alters the binding of 3H-opiates to brain membranes. *Life Sci., 33*, 725–733.

Gianoulakis, C. (1990). Characterization of the effects of acute ethanol administration on the release of beta-endorphin peptides by the rat hypothalamus. *Eur. J. Pharmacol., 180*, 21–29.

Gianoulakis, C. (1996). Implications of endogenous opioids and dopamine in alcoholism: Human and basic science studies. *Alcohol Alcohol Suppl, 1*, 33–42.

Gianoulakis, C. (1998). Alcohol-seeking behavior: The roles of the hypothalamic-pituitary-adrenal axis and the endogenous opioid system. *Alcohol Health Res. World, 22*, 202–210.

Gianoulakis, C., Beliveau, D., Angelogianni, P., Meaney, M., Thavundayil, J., Tawar, V., and Dumas, M. (1989). Different pituitary beta-endorphin and adrenal cortisol response to ethanol in individuals with high and low risk for future development of alcoholism. *Life Sci., 45*, 1097–1109.

Gianoulakis, C., Dai, X., Thavundayil, J., and Brown, T. (2005). Levels and circadian rhythmicity of plasma ACTH, cortisol, and beta-endorphin as a function of family history of alcoholism. *Psychopharmacology (Berl), 181*, 437–444.

Gianoulakis, C., De Waele, J. P., and Kiianmaa, K. (1992). Differences in the brain and pituitary beta-endorphin system between the alcohol-preferring AA and alcohol-avoiding ANA rats. *Alcohol Clin. Exp. Res., 16*, 453–459.

Glick, S. D., Maisonneuve, I. M., Raucci, J., and Archer, S. (1995). Kappa opioid inhibition of morphine and cocaine self-administration in rats. *Brain Res., 681*, 147–152.

Gorelick, D. A., Kim, Y. K., Bencherif, B., Boyd, S. J., Nelson, R., Copersino, M., Endres, C. J., Dannals, R. F., and Frost, J. J. (2005). Imaging brain mu-opioid receptors in abstinent cocaine users: Time course and relation to cocaine craving. *Biol. Psychiatry, 57*, 1573–1582.

Grahame, N. J., Low, M. J., and Cunningham, C. L. (1998). Intravenous self-administration of ethanol in beta-endorphin-deficient mice. *Alcohol Clin. Exp. Res., 22,* 1093–1098.

Grisel, J. E., Mogil, J. S., Grahame, N. J., Rubinstein, M., Belknap, J. K., Crabbe, J. C., and Low, M. J. (1999). Ethanol oral self-administration is increased in mutant mice with decreased beta-endorphin expression. *Brain Res., 835,* 62–67.

Grossman, A., and Besser, G. M. (1982). Opiates control ACTH through a noradrenergic mechanism. *Clin. Endocrinol. (Oxf), 17,* 287–290.

Gscheidel, N., Sander, T., Wendel, B., Heere, P., Schmidt, L. G., Rommelspacher, H., Hoehe, M. R., and Samochowiec, J. (2000). Five exon 1 variants of mu opioid receptor and vulnerability to alcohol dependence. *Pol. J. Pharmacol., 52,* 27–31.

Guardia, J., Caso, C., Arias, F., Gual, A., Sanahuja, J., Ramirez, M., Mengual, I., Gonzalvo, B., Segura, L., Trujols, J., and Casas, M. (2002). A double-blind, placebo-controlled study of naltrexone in the treatment of alcohol-dependence disorder: Results from a multicenter clinical trial. *Alcohol Clin. Exp. Res., 26,* 1381–1387.

Hall, F. S., Sora, I., and Uhl, G. R. (2001). Ethanol consumption and reward are decreased in mu-opiate receptor knockout mice. *Psychopharmacology (Berl), 154,* 43–49.

Hammer, R. P., Jr. (1989). Cocaine alters opiate receptor binding in critical brain reward regions. *Synapse, 3,* 55–60.

Heinz, A., Reimold, M., Wrase, J., Hermann, D., Croissant, B., Mundle, G., Dohmen, B. M., Braus, D. F., Schumann, G., Machulla, H. J., Bares, R., and Mann, K. (2005). Correlation of stable elevations in striatal mu-opioid receptor availability in detoxified alcoholic patients with alcohol craving: A positron emission tomography study using carbon 11-labeled carfentanil. *Arch. Gen. Psychiatry, 62,* 57–64.

Hernandez-Avila, C. A., Oncken, C., Van, K. J., Wand, G., and Kranzler, H. R. (2002). Adrenocorticotropin and cortisol responses to a naloxone challenge and risk of alcoholism. *Biol. Psychiatry, 51,* 652–658.

Hernandez-Avila, C. A., Wand, G., Luo, X., Gelernter, J., and Kranzler, H. R. (2003). Association between the cortisol response to opioid blockade and the Asn40Asp polymorphism at the mu-opioid receptor locus (OPRM1). *Am. J. Med. Genet. B Neuropsychiatr. Genet., 118,* 60–65.

Herz, A., and Spanagel, R. (1995). Endogenous opioids and addiction. In L. F. Tseng, Ed. *The pharmacology of opioids* (pp. 445–462). Germany: Harwood.

Hiller, J. M., Angel, L. M., and Simon, E. J. (1981). Multiple opiate receptors: Alcohol selectively inhibits binding to delta receptors. *Science, 214,* 468–469.

Hiller, J. M., Angel, L. M., and Simon, E. J. (1984). Characterization of the selective inhibition of the

delta subclass of opioid binding sites by alcohols. *Mol. Pharmacol., 25,* 249–255.

Hoehe, M. R., Kopke, K., Wendel, B., Rohde, K., Flachmeier, C., Kidd, K. K., Berrettini, W. H., and Church, G. M. (2000). Sequence variability and candidate gene analysis in complex disease: Association of mu opioid receptor gene variation with substance dependence. *Hum. Mol. Genet., 9,* 2895–2908.

Hoffman, P. L., Chung, C. T., and Tabakoff, B. (1984). Effects of ethanol, temperature, and endogenous regulatory factors on the characteristics of striatal opiate receptors. *J. Neurochem., 43,* 1003–1010.

Hoffman, P. L., Urwyler, S., and Tabakoff, B. (1982). Alterations in opiate receptor function after chronic ethanol exposure. *J. Pharmacol. Exp. Ther., 222,* 182–189.

Honkanen, A., Vilamo, L., Wegelius, K., Sarviharju, M., Hyytia, P., and Korpi, E. R. (1996). Alcohol drinking is reduced by a mu 1- but not by a delta-opioid receptor antagonist in alcohol-preferring rats. *Eur. J. Pharmacol., 304,* 7–13.

Hubbell, C. L., Marglin, S. H., Spitalnic, S. J., Abelson, M. L., Wild, K. D., and Reid, L. D. (1991). Opioidergic, serotonergic, and dopaminergic manipulations and rats' intake of a sweetened alcoholic beverage. *Alcohol, 8,* 355–367.

Ide, S., Kobayashi, H., Tanaka, K., Ujike, H., Sekine, Y., Ozaki, N., Inada, T., Harano, M., Komiyama, T., Yamada, M., Iyo, M., Ikeda, K., and Sora, I. (2004). Gene polymorphisms of the mu opioid receptor in methamphetamine abusers. *Ann. N. Y. Acad. Sci., 1025,* 316–324.

Iso, H., and Brush, F. R. (1991). Opposite effects of naltrexone on ETOH intake by Syracuse high and low avoidance rats. *Alcohol, 8,* 443–448.

Jamensky, N. T., and Gianoulakis, C. (1997). Content of dynorphins and kappa-opioid receptors in distinct brain regions of C57BL/6 and DBA/2 mice. *Alcohol Clin. Exp. Res., 21,* 1455–1464.

Jamensky, N. T., and Gianoulakis, C. (1999). Comparison of the proopiomelanocortin and proenkephalin opioid peptide systems in brain regions of the alcohol-preferring C57BL/6 and alcohol-avoiding DBA/2 mice. *Alcohol, 18,* 177–187.

Johnson, S. W., and North, R. A. (1992). Opioids excite dopamine neurons by hyperpolarization of local interneurons. *J. Neurosci., 12,* 483–488.

Keith, L. D., Crabbe, J. C., Robertson, L. M., and Kendall, J. W. (1986). Ethanol-stimulated endorphin and cortcotropin secretion in vitro. *Brain Res., 367,* 222–229.

Khachaturian, H., Lewis, M. E., Haber, S. N., Akil, H., and Watson, S. J. (1984). Proopiomelanocortin peptide immunocytochemistry in rhesus monkey brain. *Brain Res. Bull., 13,* 785–800.

Khatami, S., Hoffman, P. L., Shibuya, T., and Salafsky, B. (1987). Selective effects of ethanol on opiate receptor subtypes in brain. *Neuropharmacology, 26,* 1503–1507.

Kim, S. G., Kim, C. M., Kang, D. H., Kim, Y. J., Byun, W. T., Kim, S. Y., Park, J. M., Kim, M. J., and Oslin, D. W. (2004). Association of functional opioid receptor genotypes with alcohol dependence in Koreans. *Alcohol Clin. Exp. Res., 28*, 986–990.

King, A. C., Schluger, J., Gunduz, M., Borg, L., Perret, G., Ho, A., and Kreek, M. J. (2002). Hypothalamic-pituitary-adrenocortical (HPA) axis response and biotransformation of oral naltrexone: Preliminary examination of relationship to family history of alcoholism. *Neuropsychopharmacology, 26*, 778–788.

Koob, G. F. (1992). Drugs of abuse: Anatomy, pharmacology and function of reward pathways. *Trends Pharmacol. Sci., 13*, 177–184.

Kornet, M., Goosen, C., and van Ree, J. M. (1991). Effect of naltrexone on alcohol consumption during chronic alcohol drinking and after a period of imposed abstinence in free-choice drinking rhesus monkeys. *Psychopharmacology (Berl), 104*, 367–376.

Kosten, T., Silverman, D. G., Fleming, J., Kosten, T. A., Gawin, F. H., Compton, M., Jatlow, P., and Byck, R. (1992). Intravenous cocaine challenges during naltrexone maintenance: A preliminary study. *Biol. Psychiatry, 32*, 543–548.

Krishnan-Sarin, S., Jing, S. L., Kurtz, D. L., Zweifel, M., Portoghese, P. S., Li, T. K., and Froehlich, J. C. (1995). The delta opioid receptor antagonist naltrindole attenuates both alcohol and saccharin intake in rats selectively bred for alcohol preference. *Psychopharmacology (Berl), 120*, 177–185.

Krishnan-Sarin, S., Wand, G. S., Li, X. W., Portoghese, P. S., and Froehlich, J. C. (1998). Effect of mu opioid receptor blockade on alcohol intake in rats bred for high alcohol drinking. *Pharmacol. Biochem. Behav., 59*, 627–635.

Krystal, J. H., Cramer, J. A., Krol, W. F., Kirk, G. F., and Rosenheck, R. A. (2001). Naltrexone in the treatment of alcohol dependence. *N. Engl. J Med., 345*, 1734–1739.

Kuzmin, A. V., Gerrits, M. A., van Ree, J. M., and Zvartau, E. E. (1997a). Naloxone inhibits the reinforcing and motivational aspects of cocaine addiction in mice. *Life Sci., 60*, L-64.

Kuzmin, A. V., Semenova, S., Gerrits, M. A., Zvartau, E. E., and van Ree, J. M. (1997b). Kappa-opioid receptor agonist U50,488H modulates cocaine and morphine self-administration in drug-naive rats and mice. *Eur. J. Pharmacol., 321*, 265–271.

Leshner, A. I., and Koob, G. F. (1999). Drugs of abuse and the brain. *Proc. Assoc. Am. Physicians, 111*, 99–108.

Levine, A. S., Hess, S., and Morley, J. E. (1983). Alcohol and the opiate receptor. *Alcohol Clin. Exp. Res., 7*, 83–84.

Leyton, M., Boileau, I., Benkelfat, C., Diksic, M., Baker, G., and Dagher, A. (2002). Amphetamine-induced increases in extracellular dopamine, drug wanting, and novelty seeking: A PET/[11C]raclopride study in healthy men. *Neuropsychopharmacology, 27*, 1027–1035.

Li, X. W., Li, T. K., and Froehlich, J. C. (1998). Enhanced sensitivity of the nucleus accumbens proenkephalin system to alcohol in rats selectively bred for alcohol preference. *Brain Res., 794*, 35–47.

Loh, E. W., Fann, C. S., Chang, Y. T., Chang, C. J., and Cheng, A. T. (2004). Endogenous opioid receptor genes and alcohol dependence among Taiwanese Han. *Alcohol Clin. Exp. Res., 28*, 15–19.

Luo, X., Kranzler, H. R., Zhao, H., and Gelernter, J. (2003). Haplotypes at the OPRM1 locus are associated with susceptibility to substance dependence in European-Americans. *Am. J. Med. Genet. B Neuropsychiatr. Genet., 120*, 97–108.

Mansour, A., Khachaturian, H., Lewis, M. E., Akil, H., and Watson, S. J. (1988). Anatomy of CNS opioid receptors. *Trends Neurosci., 11*, 308–314.

Marfaing-Jallat, P., Miceli, D., and Le, M. J. (1983). Decrease in ethanol consumption by naloxone in naive and dependent rats. *Pharmacol. Biochem. Behav., 18* (Suppl 1), 537–539.

Marinelli, P. W., Kiianmaa, K., and Gianoulakis, C. (2000). Opioid propeptide mRNA content and receptor density in the brains of AA and ANA rats. *Life Sci., 66*, 1915–1927.

Martinez, D., Slifstein, M., Broft, A., Mawlawi, O., Hwang, D. R., Huang, Y., Cooper, T., Kegeles, L., Zarahn, E., bi-Dargham, A., Haber, S. N., and Laruelle, M. (2003). Imaging human mesolimbic dopamine transmission with positron emission tomography. Part II: Amphetamine-induced dopamine release in the functional subdivisions of the striatum. *J. Cereb. Blood Flow Metab. 23*, 285–300.

Mason, B. J., Salvato, F. R., Williams, L. D., Ritvo, E. C., and Cutler, R. B. (1999). A double-blind, placebo-controlled study of oral nalmefene for alcohol dependence. *Arch. Gen. Psychiatry, 56*, 719–724.

McBride, W. J., Chernet, E., McKinzie, D. L., Lumeng, L., and Li, T. K. (1998). Quantitative autoradiography of mu-opioid receptors in the CNS of alcohol-naive alcohol-preferring P and -nonpreferring NP rats. *Alcohol, 16*, 317–323.

McCaul, M. E., Wand, G. S., Eissenberg, T., Rohde, C. A., and Cheskin, L. J. (2000). Naltrexone alters subjective and psychomotor responses to alcohol in heavy drinking subjects. *Neuropsychopharmacology, 22*, 480–492.

McCaul, M. E., Wand, G. S., Stauffer, R., Lee, S. M., and Rohde, C. A. (2001). Naltrexone dampens ethanol-induced cardiovascular and hypothalamic-pituitary-adrenal axis activation. *Neuropsychopharmacology, 25*, 537–547.

Morris, P. L., Hopwood, M., Whelan, G., Gardiner, J., and Drummond, E. (2001). Naltrexone for alcohol dependence: A randomized controlled trial. *Addiction, 96*, 1565–1573.

Myers, R. D., Borg, S., and Mossberg, R. (1986). Antagonism by naltrexone of voluntary alcohol selection in the chronically drinking macaque monkey. *Alcohol, 3*, 383–388.

Ng, G. Y., O'Dowd, B. F., and George, S. R. (1996). Genotypic differences in mesolimbic enkephalin gene expression in DBA/2J and C57BL/6J inbred mice. *Eur. J. Pharmacol., 311*, 45–52.

Nylander, I., Hyytia, P., Forsander, O., and Terenius, L. (1994). Differences between alcohol-preferring (AA) and alcohol-avoiding (ANA) rats in the prodynorphin and proenkephalin systems. *Alcohol Clin. Exp. Res., 18*, 1272–1279.

O'Malley, S. S., Jaffe, A. J., Chang, G., Rode, S., Schottenfeld, R., Meyer, R. E., and Rounsaville, B. (1996). Six-month follow-up of naltrexone and psychotherapy for alcohol dependence. *Arch. Gen. Psychiatry, 53*, 217–224.

O'Malley, S. S., Jaffe, A. J., Chang, G., Schottenfeld, R. S., Meyer, R. E., and Rounsaville, B. (1992). Naltrexone and coping skills therapy for alcohol dependence. A controlled study. *Arch. Gen. Psychiatry, 49*, 881–887.

Olive, M. F., Koenig, H. N., Nannini, M. A., and Hodge, C. W. (2001). Stimulation of endorphin neurotransmission in the nucleus accumbens by ethanol, cocaine, and amphetamine. *J. Neurosci., 21*, RC184.

Oroszi, G., and Goldman, D. (2004). Alcoholism: Genes and mechanisms. *Pharmacogenomics, 5*, 1037–1048.

Oslin, D. W., Berrettini, W., Kranzler, H. R., Pettinati, H., Gelernter, J., Volpicelli, J. R., and O'Brien, C. P. (2003). A functional polymorphism of the mu-opioid receptor gene is associated with naltrexone response in alcohol-dependent patients. *Neuropsychopharmacology, 28*, 1546–1552.

Oswald, L. M., Wong, D. F., McCaul, M., Zhou, Y., Kuwabara, H., Choi, L., Brasic, J., and Wand, G. S. (2005). Relationships among ventral striatal dopamine release, cortisol secretion, and subjective responses to amphetamine. *Neuropsychopharmacology, 30*, 821–832.

Palomo, T., Kostrzewa, R. M., Beninger, R. J., and Archer, T. (2004). Gene-environment interplay in alcoholism and other substance abuse disorders: Expressions of heritability and factors influencing vulnerability. *Neurotox. Res., 6*, 343–361.

Pasternak, G. W. (1986). Multiple morphine and enkephalin receptors: Biochemical and pharmacological aspects. *Ann. N. Y. Acad. Sci., 467*, 130–139.

Phillips, T. J., Wenger, C. D., and Dorow, J. D. (1997). Naltrexone effects on ethanol drinking acquisition and on established ethanol consumption in C57BL/6J mice. *Alcohol Clin. Exp. Res., 21*, 691–702.

Piazza, P. V., and Le, M. M. (1998). The role of stress in drug self-administration. *Trends Pharmacol. Sci., 19*, 67–74.

Ramsey, N. F., Gerrits, M. A., and van Ree, J. M. (1999). Naltrexone affects cocaine self-administration in naive rats through the ventral tegmental area rather than dopaminergic target regions. *Eur. Neuropsychopharmacol., 9*, 93–99.

Rasmussen, D. D., Bryant, C. A., Boldt, B. M., Colasurdo, E. A., Levin, N., and Wilkinson, C. W. (1998). Acute alcohol effects on opiomelanocortinergic regulation. *Alcohol Clin. Exp. Res., 22*, 789–801.

Ray, L. A., and Hutchison, K. E. (2004). A polymorphism of the mu-opioid receptor gene (OPRM1) and sensitivity to the effects of alcohol in humans. *Alcohol Clin. Exp. Res., 28*, 1789–1795.

Reid, L. D., Delconte, J. D., Nichols, M. L., Bilsky, E. J., and Hubbell, C. L. (1991). Tests of opioid deficiency hypotheses of alcoholism. *Alcohol, 8*, 247–257.

Reid, L. D., Glick, S. D., Menkens, K. A., French, E. D., Bilsky, E. J., and Porreca, F. (1995). Cocaine self-administration and naltrindole, a delta-selective opioid antagonist. *Neuroreport, 6*, 1409–1412.

Reisine, T., and Bell, G. I. (1993). Molecular biology of opioid receptors. *Trends Neurosci., 16*, 506–510.

Roberts, A. J., Gold, L. H., Polis, I., McDonald, J. S., Filliol, D., Kieffer, B. L., and Koob, G. F. (2001). Increased ethanol self-administration in delta-opioid receptor knockout mice. *Alcohol Clin. Exp. Res., 25*, 1249–1256.

Rommelspacher, H., Smolka, M., Schmidt, L. G., Samochowiec, J., and Hoehe, M. R. (2001). Genetic analysis of the mu-opioid receptor in alcohol-dependent individuals. *Alcohol, 24*, 129–135.

Sander, T., Gscheidel, N., Wendel, B., Samochowiec, J., Smolka, M., Rommelspacher, H., Schmidt, L. G., and Hoehe, M. R. (1998). Human mu-opioid receptor variation and alcohol dependence. *Alcohol Clin. Exp. Res., 22*, 2108–2110.

Sandi, C., Borrell, J., and Guaza, C. (1988). Involvement of kappa type opioids on ethanol drinking. *Life Sci., 42*, 1067–1075.

Scanlon, M. N., Lazar-Wesley, E., Grant, K. A., and Kunos, G. (1992). Proopiomelanocortin messenger RNA is decreased in the mediobasal hypothalamus of rats made dependent on ethanol. *Alcohol Clin. Exp. Res., 16*, 1147–1151.

Schinka, J. A., Town, T., Abdullah, L., Crawford, F. C., Ordorica, P. I., Francis, E., Hughes, P., Graves, A. B., Mortimer, J. A., and Mullan, M. (2002). A functional polymorphism within the mu-opioid receptor gene and risk for abuse of alcohol and other substances. *Mol. Psychiatry, 7*, 224–228.

Schuckit, M. A. (1994). The 1994 Isaacson Award Lecture: A prospective study of sons of alcoholics. *Alcohol Alcohol Suppl, 2*, 1–6.

Schulz, R., Wuster, M., Duka, T., and Herz, A. (1980). Acute and chronic ethanol treatment changes endorphin levels in brain and pituitary. *Psychopharmacology (Berl), 68*, 221–227.

Seizinger, B. R., Bovermann, K., Hollt, V., and Herz, A. (1984). Enhanced activity of the beta-endorphinergic system in the anterior and neuro-intermediate lobe of the rat pituitary after chronic treatment with ethanol liquid diet. *J. Pharmacol. Exp. Ther., 230*, 455–461.

Seizinger, B. R., Bovermann, K., Maysinger, D., Hollt, V., and Herz, A. (1983). Differential effects of acute and chronic ethanol treatment on particular opioid peptide systems in discrete regions of rat brain and pituitary. *Pharmacol. Biochem. Behav., 18* (Suppl 1), 361–369.

Shi, J., Hui, L., Xu, Y., Wang, F., Huang, W., and Hu, G. (2002). Sequence variations in the mu-opioid receptor gene (OPRM1) associated with human addiction to heroin. *Hum. Mutat., 19,* 459–460.

Shippenberg, T. S., Herz, A., Spanagel, R., Bals-Kubik, R., and Stein, C. (1992). Conditioning of opioid reinforcement: Neuroanatomical and neurochemical substrates. *Ann. N. Y. Acad. Sci., 654,* 347–356.

Sim-Selley, L. J., Xiao, R., and Childers, S. R. (2000). Anatomical distribution of sodium-dependent [(3)H]naloxone binding sites in rat brain. *Synapse, 35,* 256–264.

Sinclair, J. D. (2001). Evidence about the use of naltrexone and for different ways of using it in the treatment of alcoholism. *Alcohol Alcohol, 36,* 2–10.

Skarke, C., Kirchhof, A., Geisslinger, G., and Lotsch, J. (2004). Comprehensive mu-opioid-receptor genotyping by pyrosequencing. *Clin. Chem., 50,* 640–644.

Skoubis, P. D., Lam, H. A., Shoblock, J., Narayanan, S., and Maidment, N. T. (2005). Endogenous enkephalins, not endorphins, modulate basal hedonic state in mice. *Eur. J. Neurosci., 21,* 1379–1384.

Sweep, C. G., Wiegant, V. M., De, V. J., and van Ree, J. M. (1989). Beta-endorphin in brain limbic structures as neurochemical correlate of psychic dependence on drugs. *Life Sci., 44,* 1133–1140.

Swift, R. M., Whelihan, W., Kuznetsov, O., Buongiorno, G., and Hsuing, H. (1994). Naltrexone-induced alterations in human ethanol intoxication. *Am. J. Psychiatry, 151,* 1463–1467.

Szeto, C. Y., Tang, N. L., Lee, D. T., and Stadlin, A. (2001). Association between mu opioid receptor gene polymorphisms and Chinese heroin addicts. *Neuroreport, 12,* 1103–1106.

Tabakoff, B., and Hoffman, P. L. (1983). Alcohol interactions with brain opiate receptors. *Life Sci., 32,* 197–204.

Tabakoff, B., Urwyler, S., and Hoffman, P. L. (1981). Ethanol alters kinetic characteristics and function of striatal morphine receptors. *J. Neurochem., 37,* 518–521.

Tan, E. C., Tan, C. H., Karupathivan, U., and Yap, E. P. (2003). Mu opioid receptor gene polymorphisms and heroin dependence in Asian populations. *Neuroreport, 14,* 569–572.

Tempel, A., Gardner, E. L., and Zukin, R. S. (1985). Neurochemical and functional correlates of naltrexone-induced opiate receptor up-regulation. *J. Pharmacol. Exp. Ther., 232,* 439–444.

Town, T., Abdullah, L., Crawford, F., Schinka, J., Ordorica, P. I., Francis, E., Hughes, P., Duara, R., and Mullan, M. (1999). Association of a functional mu-opioid receptor allele (+118A) with alcohol dependency. *Am. J. Med. Genet., 88,* 458–461.

Tupala, E., and Tiihonen, J. (2004). Dopamine and alcoholism: Neurobiological basis of ethanol abuse. *Prog. Neuropsychopharmacol. Biol. Psychiatry, 28,* 1221–1247.

Uhart, M., Oswald, L., McCaul, M., Chong, R., and Wand, G. (2006, In press). Hormonal responses to psychological stress and family history of alcoholism. *Neuropsychopharmacology.*

Unterwald, E. M. (2001). Regulation of opioid receptors by cocaine. *Ann. N. Y. Acad. Sci., 937,* 74–92.

Unterwald, E. M., Rubenfeld, J. M., and Kreek, M. J. (1994). Repeated cocaine administration upregulates kappa and mu, but not delta, opioid receptors. *Neuroreport, 5,* 1613–1616.

Valentino, R. J., and Van Bockstaele, E. (2001). Opposing regulation of the locus coeruleus by corticotropin-releasing factor and opioids. Potential for reciprocal interactions between stress and opioid sensitivity. *Psychopharmacology (Berl), 158,* 331–342.

Volkow, N. D., Wang, G. J., Fowler, J. S., Logan, J., Gatley, S. J., Wong, C., Hitzemann, R., and Pappas, N. R. (1999). Reinforcing effects of psychostimulants in humans are associated with increases in brain dopamine and occupancy of D(2) receptors. *J. Pharmacol. Exp. Ther., 291,* 409–415.

Volpicelli, J. R., Alterman, A. I., Hayashida, M., and O'Brien, C. P. (1992). Naltrexone in the treatment of alcohol dependence. *Arch. Gen. Psychiatry, 49,* 876–880.

Volpicelli, J. R., Watson, N. T., King, A. C., Sherman, C. E., and O'Brien, C. P. (1995). Effect of naltrexone on alcohol "high" in alcoholics. *Am. J. Psychiatry, 152,* 613–615.

Waltman, C., McCaul, M. E., and Wand, G. S. (1994). Adrenocorticotropin responses following administration of ethanol and ovine corticotropin-releasing hormone in the sons of alcoholics and control subjects. *Alcohol Clin. Exp. Res., 18,* 826–830.

Wand, G. S., Mangold, D., and Ali, M. (1999a). Adrenocorticotropin responses to naloxone in sons of alcohol-dependent men. *J. Clin. Endocrinol. Metab. 84,* 64–68.

Wand, G. S., Mangold, D., Ali, M., and Giggey, P. (1999b). Adrenocortical responses and family history of alcoholism. *Alcohol Clin. Exp. Res., 23,* 1185–1190.

Wand, G. S., Mangold, D., El, D. S., McCaul, M. E., and Hoover, D. (1998). Family history of alcoholism and hypothalamic opioidergic activity. *Arch. Gen. Psychiatry, 55,* 1114–1119.

Wand, G. S., McCaul, M. E., Gotjen, D., Reynolds, J., and Lee, S. (2001). Confirmation that offspring from families with alcohol-dependent individuals have greater hypothalamic-pituitary-adrenal axis activation induced by naloxone compared with offspring without a family history of alcohol dependence. *Alcohol Clin. Exp. Res., 25*, 1134–1139.

Weiss, F., Mitchiner, M., Bloom, F. E., and Koob, G. F. (1990). Free-choice responding for ethanol versus water in alcohol preferring (P) and unselected Wistar rats is differentially modified by naloxone, bromocriptine, and methysergide. *Psychopharmacology (Berl), 101*, 178–186.

Winkler, A., Roske, I., Furkert, J., Fickel, J., and Melzig, M. F. (1995). Effects of voluntary ethanol ingestion on the POMC gene expression in the rat pituitary and on the plasma beta-endorphin content. *Alcohol Alcohol, 30*, 231–238.

Wise, R. A. (1984). Neural mechanisms of the reinforcing action of cocaine. *NIDA Res. Monogr. 50*, 15–33.

Wise, R. A. (1998). Drug-activation of brain reward pathways. *Drug Alcohol Depend., 51*, 13–22.

Yajima, F., Suda, T., Tomori, N., Sumitomo, T., Nakagami, Y., Ushiyama, T., Demura, H., and Shizume, K. (1986). Effects of opioid peptides on immunoreactive corticotropin-releasing factor release from the rat hypothalamus in vitro. *Life Sci., 39*, 181–186.

Yoder, K. K., Kareken, D. A., Seyoum, R. A., O'Connor, S. J., Wang, C., Zheng, Q. H., Mock, B., and Morris, E. D. (2005). Dopamine D(2) receptor availability is associated with subjective responses to alcohol. *Alcohol Clin. Exp. Res., 29*, 965–970.

Zhang, Y., Wang, D., Johnson, A. D., Papp, A. C., and Sadee, W. (2005). Allelic expression imbalance of human mu opioid receptor (OPRM1) caused by variant A118G. *J. Biol. Chem., 280*, 32618–32624.

Zimmermann, U., Spring, K., Kunz-Ebrecht, S. R., Uhr, M., Wittchen, H. U., and Holsboer, F. (2004). Effect of ethanol on hypothalamic-pituitary-adrenal system response to psychosocial stress in sons of alcohol-dependent fathers. *Neuropsychopharmacology, 29*, 1156–1165.

Zubieta, J. K., Gorelick, D. A., Stauffer, R., Ravert, H. T., Dannals, R. F., and Frost, J. J. (1996). Increased mu opioid receptor binding detected by PET in cocaine-dependent men is associated with cocaine craving. *Nat. Med., 2*, 1225–1229.

Early Life Stress and Vulnerability to Addiction

THERESE A. KOSTEN AND PRISCILLA KEHOE

Early life stress is a risk factor for addiction. To better understand this association, we established a model in rats, termed neonatal isolation, and examined its immediate and enduring behavioral, neurochemical, and hormonal effects. In this procedure, pups are removed from the litter, dam, and nest and isolated individually for 1-hour per day on postnatal days 2–9. As adults, the rats exhibit enhanced acquisition, maintenance, and reinstatement of intravenous cocaine self-administration, animal models of addiction. These effects are greater in female rats. Further, estrous stage interactions on the behavioral effects of cocaine are eliminated by neonatal isolation. The mechanisms that may contribute to these effects include alterations in the mesolimbic dopamine system, a region linked to drug reinforcement, and the hypothalamic-pituitary-adrenal axis, a system also associated with self-administration behavior in rats. Neonatal isolation increases extracellular dopamine responses to psychostimulant administrations and enhances stress responsivity. Changes in maternal behavior that likely occur at post-isolation reunion may mediate these modified responses. Results from this research approach show
its validity as an animal model of early life stress and can be used to inform more effective prevention and treatment approaches for addiction.

I. INTRODUCTION

Cocaine addiction is a chronic relapsing disorder for which there are no approved treatment medications (Leshner, 1997). Close to 2 million people in the United States use cocaine (SAMHSA, 2001), but not all will develop addiction. Vulnerability to addiction has genetic components but these explain only about one-third of the overall variance. Environmental factors play a greater role in the predisposition to develop this disorder (Tsuang et al., 1998; vandenBree et al., 1998). How environmental factors contribute to initiation, maintenance, and relapse to drug use are important research goals. In rats, a valid model of ontogeny of early-onset psychiatric disorders (Unis, 1995), we show that cocaine self-administration, a valid model of addiction (Katz, 1989), is facilitated by an environmental factor of early life stress we have termed neonatal isolation (Kosten et al., 2000; Kosten et al., 2004a; Kosten et al., 2006; Zhang et al., 2005). These outcomes occur in a sex-specific manner; female rats show greater and more generalized effects compared to male rats. Importantly, these preclinical sex effects are consistent with clinical reports (Najavits et al., 1998; Wechsberg et al., 1998).

The mechanisms that contribute to the facilitation of self-administration may include alterations in the mesolimbic dopamine (DA) system, a region linked to the rewarding effects of drugs (Koob and Bloom, 1988; Wise and Rompre, 1989). Indeed, neonatal isolation increased neurochemical responses to psychostimulants in this region (Kehoe et al., 1996; Kosten et al., 2003; Kosten et al., 2005c). The purpose of this chapter is to review these preclinical data to further understand the mechanisms that contribute to the ability of early life stress to enhance the vulnerability to addiction. Ultimately, this knowledge may provide insights into developing more effective prevention and treatment programs.

We focus this review on early life stress and cocaine addiction as evidenced from animal studies. While most findings discussed in this chapter are about cocaine, many effects will likely generalize to other abused drugs. Given there is limited research conducted on early life stress in animals with other drugs, this focus provides a template for future research. First, we present an overview of the neurohormonal effects of stress and cocaine. Second, we describe animal models of addiction and early life stress with emphasis on our model, neonatal isolation. Third, we describe the neurohormonal effects of neonatal isolation in rats. Fourth, we present the neonatal isolation-induced alterations in the behavioral effects of cocaine. Fifth, we examine the sex-dependent effects of early life stress. Sixth, we discuss a current model of the mediation of early life stress effects through alterations in maternal care. Finally, we discuss the clinical relevance of the preclinical research findings.

II. NEUROHORMONAL MECHANISMS OF STRESS RELEVANT TO COCAINE ADDICTION

A. Hypothalamic-Pituitary-Adrenal Axis Effects

Stress increases limbic DA levels (Deutch et al., 1985; Kalivas and Stewart, 1991; Sorg and Kalivas, 1991; Thierry et al., 1986) and stimulates a cascade of events involving the release of corticotropin-releasing factor (CRF) from the paraventricular nucleus (PVN) of the hypothalamus. CRF leads to enhanced secretion of adrenocorticotropic hormone (ACTH) from the pituitary (Dunn and Berridge, 1990; Rivier and Plotsky, 1986). ACTH stimulates corticosterone (CORT) secretion from the adrenal cortex into the circulatory system. The hypothalamic-pituitary-adrenal (HPA) hormonal system operates on a negative feedback mechanism whereby increased levels of circulating CORT are detected causing ACTH secretion to decrease and shut down the adrenal secretion of CORT. Hippocampal glucocorticoid receptors play a large role in this negative feedback mechanism (Kim and Yoon, 1998; McEwen and Sapolsky, 1995). Like stress, cocaine activates the HPA axis via a DA-mediated mechanism (Borowsky and Kuhn, 1991). Cocaine induces ACTH and CORT secretion (Moldow and Fischman, 1987; Rivier and Vale, 1987) that involves CRF secretion from the PVN (Rivier and Vale, 1987; Sarnyai et al., 1992) as well as extra-hypothalamic areas (Sarnyai et al., 2001). Brain CRF stimulation contributes to context conditioning to cocaine (DeVries et al., 1998) but whether it is involved in cocaine self-administration is unclear (Broadbear et al., 1999; Goeders and Guerin, 2000). Yet, CRF is important for foot shock, but not cocaine-induced, reinstatement of cocaine-seeking, that involves CRF receptors in the bed nucleus of the stria terminalis (Erb et al., 1998; Erb and Stewart, 1999; Shaham et al.,

1998). Some neural mechanisms underlying drug- versus foot shock-induced reinstatement differ (Shalev et al., 2002), but they also have common neural substrates (McFarland et al., 2004).

Stress causes minimal hormonal responses in rat pups if they are in contact with the dam (Stanton et al., 1988; Suchecki et al., 1995). However, stress hormone levels increase and hypothalamic CRH mRNA levels decrease after 24 hours of separation from the dam (Smith et al., 1997). Suppressing CORT secretion pharmacologically does not alter these responses. However, these responses are reduced by tactile stimulation or feeding (vanOers et al., 1998). This demonstrates the importance of maternal behavior to suppress HPA axis activation in pups. Maternal behaviors, such as nursing and licking in the anogenital area, occur periodically under typical rearing conditions (Stern, 1989) and are stimulated by maternal separation (Pryce et al., 2001). Further, anogenital licking influences the CRF-HPA axis of adult offspring (Liu et al., 1997).

B. Mesocorticolimbic Dopamine System

Cocaine activates the mesocorticolimbic DA system (Wise and Rompre, 1989) consisting of cell bodies in the ventral tegmental area (VTA) that project to forebrain structures including the nucleus accumbens (NAc) and medial prefrontal cortex (mPFC; Fuxe et al., 1985). Cocaine increases synaptic DA levels in the NAc (Pettit and Justice, 1989) via its actions at the DA transporter (DAT) inhibiting uptake into the presynaptic terminals (Harris and Baldessarini, 1973). These effects are linked to cocaine's ability to act as a reinforcer (Bergman et al., 1989; Ritz et al., 1987) and are associated with anticipatory responses to drug delivery (Carelli and Deadwyler, 1996; DiCiano et al., 1998; Gratton and Wise, 1994; Schultz, 2000).

Other regions contribute to the behavioral effects of cocaine including the amygdala (Caine et al., 1995; McGregor and Roberts, 1993; Whitelaw et al., 1996; Wilson

et al., 1994) and the mPFC (Brown et al., 1992; Ciccocioppo et al., 2001; Goeders and Smith, 1983; Neisewander et al., 2000; Robinson et al., 2001; Schenk et al., 1991). Neuroimaging studies reveal similar brain regions are activated in response to cocaine and cues in humans (Breiter et al., 1997; Childress et al., 1999; Grant et al., 1996).

C. Gonadal Hormones and Gender Effects

Many brain areas involved in drug self-administration and stress are sexually dimorphic or show estrous stage effects (Andersen and Teicher, 2000; Becker, 1999; DeVries, 1989; Juraska, 1991; Thompson and Moss, 1997). Female and male rats differ in stress and drug responses. Foot shock induces larger CORT and ACTH responses, enhanced behavioral effects, and greater neural activity in monoamine areas in female versus male rats (Beatty and Beatty, 1970; Heinsbroek et al., 1991; Heinsbroek et al., 1990; Kosten et al., 2005a; Rivier, 1999). Cocaine induces greater ACTH (Kuhn and Francis, 1997) and activity responses (Glick and Hinds, 1984; vanHaaren and Meyer, 1991) in female rats although gender and ovarian hormones do not alter cocaine plasma levels (Bowman et al., 1999). These effects may reflect activational effects of gonadal hormones (Becker et al., 1982; Viau and Meaney, 1991), but organizational effects contribute too (Cicero et al., 2002; Kitay, 1961; Kuhn et al., 2001; McCormick et al., 2002b).

Stress hormones, the mesolimbic DA system, and cocaine behaviors are affected by estrous stage. In general, estrogen has excitatory effects on HPA function. Females have higher plasma ACTH and CORT levels during proestrus stage when estrogen levels are high (Buckingham et al., 1978). High estrogen levels are associated with greater increases in these hormone levels after acute stress (Viau and Meaney, 1991). Estrogen can also enhance NAc DA levels (Becker, 1999) and upregulate D_2-like receptor gene expression in various brain regions related to cocaine behaviors (Zhou et al., 2002).

The early life stress of maternal separation can have sex-dependent effects on the CRF-HPA axis system of adult rats (Calatayud and Belzung, 2001; Erskine et al., 1975; Weinberg et al., 1978; Weinberg and Levine, 1977). It decreases hippocampal corticosteroid receptor levels in male rats and increases these levels in female rats (Sutanto et al., 1996). Such sex-dependent effects may reflect disruptions in the influence of pup sex on maternal care seen under typical rearing conditions. That is, male pups are licked more than female pups (Moore and Chadwick-Dias, 1986; Moore and Morelli, 1979). Because maternal behavior can shape the CRF-HPA axis of adult offspring (Champagne and Meaney, 2001; Francis et al., 1999; Liu et al., 1997), the sex-dependent effects of maternal care may contribute to the sex differences seen in stress responses (Beatty and Beatty, 1970; Heinsbroek et al., 1990; Heinsbroek et al., 1991; Kosten et al., 2005a; Rivier, 1999).

III. ANIMAL MODELS

Animal models of early life stress and addiction provide several advantages to understand this risk factor for addiction. First, it allows control over the type and duration of stress exposure as well as the age at which it is experienced. Second, animal models of addiction, such as operant self-administration, have been refined over many years and are well established as indicators of abuse liability. Moreover, control over drug administration routes and exposures are possible with animals. Third, research with animals provides the opportunities to investigate underlying neural and hormonal mechanisms. Thus, although findings with animal models need to be verified with clinical work, much knowledge can be gained from this approach.

A. Addiction Models

Low to moderate cocaine doses stimulate ambulation (Scheel-Kruger et al., 1977), whereas higher doses decrease this effect and increase emission of stereotyped behaviors (Post et al., 1987). Cocaine acts as a discriminative stimulus (Colpaert, 1978), supports context conditioning (Carr et al., 1989), and is self-administered by animals, a procedure that evaluates the reinforcing properties of drugs (Katz, 1989; Koob and Goeders, 1989). Like drug addicts, rats make a voluntary response to obtain the drug intravenously, a route of administration used by addicts. Self-administered drugs serve as reinforcers (Pickens et al., 1978; Schuster and Thompson, 1969); they increase the likelihood that behaviors preceding the drug infusion occur again. More than 20 drugs self-administered by humans serve as reinforcers in animals supporting its use as a model of abuse liability (Collins et al., 1984).

Drug self-administration models various aspects of addiction. Acquisition of self-administration models vulnerability to addiction (Deminiere et al., 1989). It is affected by environmental or genetic manipulations including enhancements after stress (Carroll and Lac, 1993; Goeders and Guerin, 1994; Haney et al., 1995; Horger et al., 1990; Kosten et al., 1997; Miczek and Mutschler, 1996; Piazza et al., 1990). Drug "craving" is examined by replacing the drug with saline and measuring persistence of responding or latency to extinguish (Markou et al., 1993). After extinction, noncontingent drug infusions or foot shock reinstates responding even though the drug is not available (Ahmed and Koob, 1997; Erb et al., 1996; Piazza and LeMoal, 1998; Shaham and Stewart, 1995). Such effects may reflect increased craving that addicts report as a primary reason to relapse (Gawin and Kleber, 1986).

B. Neonatal Isolation Model of Early Life Stress

We employ a procedure of early life stress we termed *neonatal isolation* (Kehoe and

Shoemaker, 2001; Kosten and Kehoe, 2005). This involves individual pup isolation in addition to the removal from the dam and the nest. Litters are culled to 12 pups on postnatal day 1 (PN1) taking care to attempt an even sex distribution. Commencing the following day, each pup is isolated individually in a container with no bedding in a temperature-maintained room (30°C) for 1 hour/day on PN2-9 (ISO). Our typical comparison group, nonhandled (NH) rats, is also culled to 12 pups on PN1 but are not disturbed during the next 8 days.

The parameters of the neonatal isolation procedure are based on our previous work (Kehoe and Blass, 1986; Kehoe and Shoemaker, 2001; Kehoe et al., 1998b). First, isolation takes place within the first 2 weeks of life, sometimes referred to as the stress hyporesponsive period (Levine, 1994). This period is sufficient to see long-term effects on HPA axis activity (Hess et al., 1969). Second, we use a between-litter design in which the whole litter is assigned to the same treatment condition. We choose not to use a within-litter design, in which part of the litter is assigned to one treatment while the other part is not, for the following reasons. In the within-litter design, male rats in the Nonisolate condition (i.e., remain in the nest while some siblings were isolated) responded like ISO male rats, not like NH rats (Kehoe et al., 1998b). Yet, Nonisolate female rats differ from ISO female rats but not from NH female rats. We find that the between-litter procedure reduces variability in maternal behavior and variability among the pups (Kehoe and Shoemaker, 2001). Third, in the neonatal isolation procedure, each ISO pup is removed from the nest, dam, and siblings and isolated individually in a cup with no bedding. Individual isolation is used, not whole litter separation from the dam, because the pup cannot huddle and receive tactile stimulation and varying amounts of warmth in this situation. Fourth, no bedding is used during the isolation because this condition is associated with behavioral and neurochemical

responses suggestive of greater stress compared to isolation with bedding, a cue that is likely familiar (Kehoe and Blass, 1986; Kehoe and Shoemaker, 2001). Finally, we use a 1 hour isolation time because nutritional effects do not compromise it.

C. Other Early Life Stress Models

Numerous reports show that handling (~5-minute removal of dam from pups and nest) and maternal separation (≥3-hour removal) have enduring effects on brain and behavior (Anisman et al., 1998; Hall, 1998; Kehoe and Shoemaker, 2001; Lehmann and Feldon, 2000; Meaney et al., 1996). In these procedures, the dam is usually removed from the nest, and the pups remain together in a huddle. The litter may remain in a huddle in the home cage or be removed to a different cage that often contains bedding. There are many procedural differences in the manner in which maternal separation is conducted across laboratories. Separations can differ by duration, the number of times and on which postnatal days the separations occurred, and many other variables. These procedural variations likely contribute to the discrepancies and inconsistencies in results reported in the literature (Lehmann and Feldon, 2000; Pryce and Feldon, 2003).

Neonatal isolation differs in important ways from most maternal separation procedures. One difference is the length of the isolation (1 hour) versus greater lengths of separations (e.g., 3 hours or more). Also, in neonatal isolation, the pups are isolated individually in a container with no bedding, whereas in most maternal separation paradigms, the pups remain in a huddle with their littermates often in a cage with bedding. We have argued that whole litter separation is a stressor for the dam, whereas neonatal isolation is a stressor for both dam and pups (Kosten and Kehoe, 2005). In contrast to maternal separation, our work with neonatal isolation has shown relatively consistent findings as discussed below. Moreover, the effects we find are consistent with clinical observations that early life stress is a risk factor for addiction. Thus, neonatal isolation is a relevant model of early life stress that can be used to investigate mechanisms that contribute to vulnerability to addiction (Kosten and Kehoe, 2005).

IV. NEUROHORMONAL EFFECTS OF NEONATAL ISOLATION

Neonatal isolation and other early life manipulations have various neural and hormonal effects. Our studies were conducted at various ages, including in pups tested 1 day following termination of neonatal isolation (postnatal day 10), in juvenile (the prepubertal postnatal days 26–30), and in adult (postnatal day 90 or older) rats. Note that not all tests have been performed at all ages. The results of these studies are described below and summarized by age in Table 5-1.

A. Hypothalamic-Pituitary-Adrenal Axis

Pups that experience an acute episode of 1 hour of isolation showed increased CORT levels compared to pups that have not been isolated (McCormick et al., 1998). However, after 8 days of 1 hour isolations (i.e., neonatal isolation) CORT levels were greater than in those pups that received one isolation (McCormick et al., 1998). Knuth and Etgen followed up on this study and assessed plasma ACTH levels and Fos immunoreactivity in PVN as well as plasma CORT levels (Knuth and Etgen, 2005). They confirmed chronic isolation increased CORT and found enhanced ACTH, suggesting a centrally mediated effect although there was no ISO effect on Fos immunoreactivity in PVN. Interestingly, the CORT response was sexually dimorphic in this study; only females exhibited increased CORT. Juvenile ISO rats show higher CORT levels after 1 hour of restraint stress compared to NH rats (McCormick et al., 2002a). These data indicate that neonatal isolation is a stressor for the pups and that the stress effect sensitizes

TABLE 5-1   Comparison of Neonatal Isolation versus Nonhandled Experience on Neural and Hormonal Measures in Infant (PN10), Juvenile (PN26–30), and Adult (≥PN90) Rats

Measure	Infant	Juvenile	Adult
Corticosterone levels in response to stress	↑	↑	N/A
Central allopregnanolone levels	↑	=	N/A
Basal ventral striatal extracellular DA levels	=	=	=
Stimulant-induced increases in DA levels	↑	↑	↑
Stress-induced increases in DA levels	N/A	↓	N/A
Basal ventral striatal extracellular 5-HT levels	↓	N/A	=
NMDA receptor binding in ventral striatum	N/A	N/A	=
NMDA receptor binding in dorsal striatum	N/A	N/A	↑ (males) ↓ (females)
Cocaine plasma levels	N/A	N/A	=

Symbols: ↑: ISO greater than NH rats; ↓: ISO less than NH rats; =: no differences; N/A: data not available.

(i.e., becomes greater with increasing exposures). Further, the ability of neonatal isolation to enhance stress responsivity endures into the prepubertal age.

Handling and maternal separation alter plasma CORT and ACTH levels, CRF mRNA expression and content in the PVN, glucocorticoid receptor levels in hippocampus and hypothalamus, basally and after stress. Enhanced or attenuated effects are seen depending upon age, frequency, and duration of separation (Lehmann and Feldon, 2000). Compared to nonhandled rats, handled rats show decreased HPA responses to stress (Ader and Grota, 1969; Hess et al., 1969; Levine, 1962; Meaney et al., 1989; Plotsky and Meaney, 1993) and increased negative feedback sensitivity to glucocorticoids (Meaney et al., 1989; Viau et al., 1993) that may reflect increased type II glucocorticoid receptor binding in hippocampus (Meaney et al., 1989). In line with the role of hippocampus to mediate inhibitory effects over CRF synthesis, CRF mRNA expression and content are lower in PVN of handled rats (Plotsky and Meaney, 1993). Maternal separation alters CRF levels in hypothalamus, hippocampus, and amygdala and lowers glucocorticoid receptor binding in hippocampus and hypothalamus (Heim et al., 1997; Ladd et al., 1996; Plotsky and Meaney, 1993). Some reports show increased HPA response to stress (Ladd et al., 1996; Plotsky and Meaney, 1993; Rots et al., 1996) and decreased negative feedback sensitivity (Plotsky and Meaney, 1993) with maternal separation. Another reports the opposite effects (Ogawa et al., 1994). Indeed, whether maternal separation has consistent effects on brain and behavior has been called into question (Lehmann and Feldon, 2000; Marmendal et al., 2004).

B. Mesolimbic DA System

Because stress experienced in adulthood affects the mesolimbic DA system (see Section II.A), we sought to determine whether the early life stress of neonatal isolation had immediate and enduring effects on this system. Amphetamine-induced increases in extracellular ventral striatal DA levels were greater in ISO pups and juveniles compared to NH control groups (Kehoe et al., 1998a; Kehoe et al., 1996). Adult rats with maternal separation experience also showed enhanced amphetamine-induced increases in extracellular DA in NAc (Hall et al., 1999). Increased extracellular DA levels in ventral striatum occurred after cocaine administration in ISO pups and ISO adult male rats (Kosten et al., 2003; Kosten et al., 2005c). In contrast, restraint stress increased DA levels in the NAc of NH rats but failed to have this effect in ISO juvenile rats (McCormick et al., 2002a). Across all studies, no group differences were found in basal DA levels. Basal DA levels in NAc were also unaffected by maternal separation in adult rats (Hall et al., 1999; Zimmerberg and Brown, 1998). Thus, either environmental or pharmacological challenges are necessary to provoke the system to observe these effects of early life stress. Moreover, these effects are seen months after termination of the stress exposure.

C. Other Neurohormonal Effects of Neonatal Isolation

The immediate and enduring effects of neonatal isolation on other neural and hormonal systems have been investigated. Neonatal isolation altered NMDA receptor levels in dorsal, but not ventral striatum in adult rats (Sircar et al., 2001). No effect of neonatal isolation was seen in other brain regions tested, including hippocampus and medial prefrontal cortex. Interestingly, there was a sex-specific effect; NMDA receptor levels were upregulated in ISO male rats and downregulated in ISO female rats. Brain levels of the neurosteroid, allopregnanolone (3α, 5α-THP), were greater in ISO pups compared to NH pups (Kehoe et al., 2000). However, this effect did not endure in juvenile rats (McCormick et al., 2002a). Neonatal isolation decreased basal extracellular ventral striatal levels of serotonin (5-HT) in pups (Kosten et al., 2004b), but this effect was not seen in adult rats (Zhang et al., 2006). Similarly, neither maternal separation nor handling changed NAc 5-HT levels (Matthews et al., 2001; Papaioannou et al., 2002). Alterations in these systems seen immediately after the isolation stress experience may reflect altered emotional states. Both 5-HT (Golden and Gilmore, 1990) and allopregnanolone through its effect on GABAergic systems (Rupprecht, 2003) are related to affect regulation and emotion.

V. BEHAVIORAL EFFECTS OF NEONATAL ISOLATION

Neonatal isolation affects various behavioral measures. Some studies were conducted at different ages, and most were conducted in rats of both sexes. However, some procedures cannot be conducted in young rats (e.g., intravenous self-administration). Further, some studies are completed with male rats but have yet to be completed with female rats. The results

of these studies are described below and summarized by sex in Table 5-2.

A. Acute Effects of Pharmacological and Environmental Challenges

Initially, we examined the effects of neonatal isolation on amphetamine-induced locomotor activity and stereotypy in juvenile and adult rats (Kehoe et al., 1996; Kehoe et al., 1998b). ISO juvenile rats exhibited heightened locomotor activity induced by a high amphetamine dose (7.0 mg/kg) but did not differ from comparison groups at a lower dose (2.0 mg/kg). Enhanced locomotor activity may reflect that amphetamine-induced stereotypy was slower to develop in this group. Yet, there were no group differences in spontaneous activity levels. As adults, ISO rats demonstrated increased locomotor activity induced by amphetamine (1.0 and 2.0 mg/kg) relative to NH groups. Enhanced stereotypy was also seen with the 2.0 mg/kg dose and the 1.0 mg/kg in ISO female rats. In contrast, ISO juveniles showed greater suppression of locomotor activity after 60 minutes of

TABLE 5-2   Comparison of Neonatal Isolation versus Nonhandled Experience on Behavioral Measures in Male and Female Adult Rats

Measure	Male	Female
Basal locomotor activity	=	=
Amphetamine-induced locomotor activity	↑	↑
Amphetamine-induced stereotypy	=	↑
Cocaine-induced locomotor activity	=	=
Cocaine effects on schedule-controlled responding	=	=
Acquisition of cocaine self-administration	↑	↑
Maintenance of cocaine self-administration (FR)	↑ (low doses)	↑ (low doses)
Maintenance of cocaine self-administration (PR)	↑ (low doses)	↑
Acquisition of food responding	=	↑
Maintenance of food responding (FR)	↓	=
Maintenance of food responding (PR)	=	↑
Reinstatement of cocaine self-administration (drug)	=	N/A
Reinstatement of cocaine self-administration (cue)	↑	↑
Locomotor sensitization	N/A	=

Symbols: ↑: ISO greater than NH rats; ↓: ISO less than NH rats; =: no differences; N/A: data not available.

restraint relative to NH groups (McCormick et al., 2002a). Prior studies in adult rats indicate that amphetamine increases while restraint decreases locomotor activity (Kuczenski and Segal, 1989; Sudha and Pradhan, 1995). Thus, these results demonstrate that neonatal isolation exaggerates behavioral responses to pharmacological and environmental challenges.

Recently, we tested the effects of neonatal isolation on acute responses to cocaine administration in adult male and female rats (Kosten et al., 2005b; Kosten et al., 2005c). Tests included locomotor activity conducted in the same manner and using the same apparatus employed in our amphetamine studies. We also examined whether neonatal isolation would alter the ability of cocaine to disrupt responding in a schedule-controlled responding test. In this test, operant rates of responding for food (fixed-ratio 15) were assessed after acute cocaine administration across a wide dose range (0.3–30 mg/kg). Cocaine increased locomotor activity and suppressed scheduled-controlled responding as expected. In contrast to our findings with amphetamine, neonatal isolation did not alter the acute locomotor responses to cocaine (5 and 10 mg/kg) nor the effects of cocaine on scheduled-controlled responding.

The discrepancies in the results obtained with amphetamine versus cocaine could reflect differences in the neuronal effects of the drugs. Cocaine blocks DA, NE, and 5-HT transporters leading to increased synaptic levels in regions such as the NAc. While amphetamine also blocks reuptake of DA, it also causes DA release from the presynaptic terminals. There were also differences in the neonatal isolation procedure employed across these studies. The amphetamine studies utilized a mixed-litter design in which some pups were isolated and other pups remained with the mother. The cocaine studies utilized a between-litter design in which all pups in a given litter were subjected to neonatal isolation or were nonhandled. These two procedures likely have different effects on mother-pup interactions as discussed above. Nonetheless, neonatal isolation did enhance extracellular DA levels in the ventral striatum in response to both amphetamine and cocaine as described above (Section IV.B).

Other early life manipulations affect the acute locomotor responses to psychostimulants. Female, but not male rats, with maternal separation experience showed a decreased locomotor response to a low dose of amphetamine (0.5 mg/kg) but did not differ from handled rats in response to higher doses (Matthews et al., 1996a). Data from other studies suggest a lack of effect of maternal separation and handling on the locomotor response to moderate amphetamine doses (1 to 1.5 mg/kg; Campbell and Spear, 1999; Marmendal et al., 2004; Weiss et al., 2001). Thus, across studies, psychostimulant drugs, and early life manipulations, there is not a robust effect on activity responses under conditions of acute drug exposure.

B. Acquisition of Cocaine Self-Administration

Next, we investigated whether neonatal isolation facilitates cocaine self-administration in adult rats. We switched from amphetamine to cocaine because we were conducting cocaine self-administration studies in our laboratory. Our initial study examined acquisition of cocaine self-administration, a model of vulnerability to addiction (Deminiere et al., 1989), in adult male rats (Kosten et al., 2000). Under an escalating dose training procedure (Goeders and Guerin, 1994), ISO male rats self-administered cocaine at lower doses and after fewer training trials compared to NH rats. Yet, NH rats self-administered equivalent amounts of cocaine after more training trials. The facilitation of operant responding for cocaine appeared specific to the drug; there was no difference in acquisition of operant responding for food. Both cocaine and food served as reinforcers as evidenced by the rapid extinction of responding when the reinforcers were not available. Extinction responding did not differ by group. Thus, because the clinical literature shows a strong association between early life stress and vulnerability to addiction, our data suggest that neonatal isolation is a valid model of early life stress relevant to studies on the propensity to develop drug addiction (Kosten and Kehoe, 2005).

Expanding upon these results, we tested whether neonatal isolation facilitates acquisition of cocaine self-administration in female rats (Kosten et al., 2004a). Reports from the clinical literature suggested that stress was more commonly reported among female versus male addicts (Najavits et al., 1998; Wechsberg et al., 1998). Thus, we anticipated that neonatal isolation would affect female rats to a greater extent than male rats. This study included male rats that also provided a test of whether the neonatal isolation effect could be replicated. The procedure employed in this second study was similar in many ways to the initial study. However, unlike the prior study, we did not provide priming (noncontingent) cocaine infusions at the start of each session. Rather, primes were used as an experimental manipulation after the acquisition phase was completed. In the priming tests, the numbers of active and inactive lever presses were compared to the numbers of presses emitted without primes. Finally, we tested how well cocaine maintained behavior across increasing fixed ratio (FR) schedules.

The results with male rats were similar to our prior study; we replicated that neonatal isolation facilitated acquisition of cocaine self-administration. During the maintenance phase, primes were given and active lever press responses increased for both ISO and NH groups. Both groups also showed regulation of cocaine intake when the fixed ratios were changed. Further, we also replicated the lack of group differences in acquisition of food responding. Thus, this confirmation of the ability of neonatal isolation to facilitate acquisition of cocaine

self-administration in adult male rats demonstrates that it is a reliable effect.

Neonatal isolation also enhanced acquisition of cocaine self-administration in adult female rats. However, the manner in which this occurred differed from male rats. NH female rats showed high and variable levels of cocaine intake, whereas ISO female rats showed modest but increasing levels of cocaine intake across sessions and increasing doses. The response patterns of NH female rats suggested poor response learning. NH female rats showed poor lever discrimination compared to ISO female rats and to male rats because they responded on both active and inactive levers, whereas the other groups increased responding on the active lever and decreased responding on the inactive lever across sessions. NH female rats also responded more on the active lever during times this lever was inactive (i.e., infusion and time-out periods). Further, NH female rats increased responding on both levers in response to cocaine primes, whereas ISO females increased responding almost exclusively on the active lever. NH female rats performed poorly in the acquisition of food-responding task. Only 30% of NH female rats acquired the operant. However, ISO female rats show an acquisition rate (70%) that did not differ from rates shown by ISO and NH male rats. Overall, the behavioral patterns of the NH female rats whether responding for food or cocaine suggested that they showed poor response learning. Neonatal isolation enhanced this learning in female rats. Thus, we concluded that neonatal isolation facilitated acquisition of cocaine and food self-administration behaviors in female rats by enhancing response learning.

Adult rats with handling or aversive stimulation experience in the early neonatal period (PN1-10) showed altered oral cocaine consumption patterns (Marquardt et al., 2004). Compared to control rats, rats with these experiences ingested higher levels of cocaine initially and maintained this high intake level across days. Control rats, on the other hand, avoided cocaine ingestion initially and then showed great fluctuation in intake over days (i.e., binge intake). Cocaine self-administration was also enhanced in female rats that received saline injections during the second postnatal week (PN8-14) compared to control, undisturbed groups and also to rats that received saline injections during the first postnatal week (PN2-8; Flagel et al., 2003). In contrast, prolonged maternal separation (6 hours) during the postnatal period (PN5-20) attenuated acquisition of cocaine self-administration, particularly in female rats trained with low-moderate cocaine dose (~0.31 mg/kg/infusion), and in male rats trained with a low dose (~0.17 mg/kg/infusion). However, these effects were relative to rats that had experienced handling during the same postnatal period (Matthews et al., 1999). The results of the last study appear discrepant with the results of the other studies but this may reflect the comparison group (handled) used. Overall, early life stress enhances acquisition of cocaine self-administration.

C. Maintenance of Cocaine Self-Administration

The next tests were conducted after cocaine self-administration behavior was well established (i.e., maintenance). We sought to examine how well behavior was regulated in the face of pharmacological and motivational challenges by examining cocaine self-administration behavior in response to various doses and under a progressive ratio (PR) schedule of reinforcement (Kosten et al., 2006; Zhang et al., 2005). In the latter condition, rats must emit increasing numbers of active lever presses to obtain each ensuing reinforcer. Behavior under this schedule is thought to represent the amount of work the animal will perform or motivation to obtain the reinforcer (Hodos, 1961; Richardson and Roberts, 1996; Rodefer and Carroll, 1996).

Cocaine self-administration was greater in ISO male rats compared to NH male rats under low cocaine dose conditions (<0.5 mg/kg/infusion) and an FR3 schedule (Zhang et al., 2005). Responding for cocaine under the PR schedule was greater in ISO male rats but again only at low cocaine doses. Along with the findings from the acquisition studies with male rats, these data suggest neonatal isolation increases the sensitivity to the reinforcing effects of cocaine in adult male rats.

We then investigated the effects of neonatal isolation on maintenance of cocaine self-administration in female rats (Kosten et al., 2006). Overall, neonatal isolation enhanced responding for cocaine across doses under the FR3 schedule with the greater effects at low cocaine doses (<0.5 mg/kg/infusion). When a PR schedule was employed, ISO female rats showed much greater responding for cocaine even at high doses (0.5 and 1.0 mg/kg/infusion). Thus, as in the acquisition studies, neonatal isolation enhances responding for cocaine in rats of both sexes, but the manner in which this effect occurred differs by sex. For males, neonatal isolation enhances the sensitivity to the reinforcing effects of cocaine, whereas for females, it has a greater effect on motivation to obtain cocaine. The ability of neonatal isolation to facilitate cocaine self-administration behavior is likely not due to altered cocaine disposition. It does not alter cocaine plasma levels in either sex (Kosten et al., 2005b; Kosten et al., 2005c). It is also unlikely that the heightened responding for cocaine seen in ISO rats reflects increased activity levels. We consistently find no differences between ISO and NH rats in locomotor activity (Kosten et al., 2000; Kosten et al., 2004a; Kosten et al., 2005a).

We examined maintenance of operant responding for food by training rats to lever press for food pellets under an FR15 schedule of reinforcement. Tests were conducted using the same PR schedule employed in the self-administration studies. ISO male rats showed lower levels of responding under the FR schedule but did not differ from NH male rats under the PR schedule. Although there are several parametric differences between operant responding for cocaine versus food, these data suggested that the heightened responding for cocaine induced by neonatal isolation was not a generalized increase in behavior in male rats. ISO female rats did not differ in responding for food under the FR schedule compared to NH female rats. However, neonatal isolation led to heightened responding for food under the PR schedule for female rats. That neonatal isolation increased both acquisition and maintenance of operant responding for food in female rats, but not in male rats, suggests that the effect is more generalized to motivated behavior in this sex.

D. Reinstatement of Cocaine Self-Administration

Another cocaine self-administration model is the reinstatement of the behavior after extinction. This model is thought to reflect relapse to drug-seeking behavior. Behavior can be reinstated by the drug itself, foot-shock stress, or by cues associated with drug delivery. We have examined the effects of neonatal isolation on drug-induced reinstatement of cocaine-seeking behavior in adult male rats (Zhang et al., 2005). We examined drug-seeking behavior after administering a low (0.5 mg/kg IV) and a high (2.0 mg/kg IV) dose of cocaine. There were no differences in cocaine-seeking behavior between ISO and NH male rats. However, a recent study, in which a modified version of neonatal isolation was employed, reports that neonatal isolation enhances cue-induced reinstatement of cocaine-seeking behavior in rats of both sexes (Lynch and Taylor, 2005). This study also replicated our findings that neonatal isolation heightens maintenance of cocaine self-administration behavior. Whether stress-induced reinstatement of cocaine-seeking behavior is altered by neonatal isolation remains to be tested. Neonatal isolation may alter the ability of

some precipitants to induce reinstatement while not affecting the degree to which other precipitants induce reinstatement.

E. Sensitization

Behavioral sensitization is the phenomenon of increased behavioral output, usually measured as locomotor activity or stereotypy, seen after repeated intermittent administrations of psychostimulants (Kalivas and Stewart, 1991; Post et al., 1987; Robinson and Berridge, 1993). Sensitization is considered a key characteristic in the development of drug addiction and may be homologous to intensification of drug "craving" over time reported upon by drug addicts (Robinson and Berridge, 1993). Cross-sensitization is often exhibited in which prior exposure to stress facilitates the response to subsequent psychostimulant administrations (Antelman et al., 1980). Stress experienced during adulthood enhances acquisition of cocaine self-administration (Goeders and Guerin, 1994; Haney et al., 1995; Tidey and Miczek, 1997). Stress experienced during early postnatal life may cross-sensitize to the effects of cocaine and facilitate its self-administration. To test whether heightened responding to cocaine in ISO rats reflects increased sensitization, we examined the development and expression of cocaine locomotor sensitization. We utilized a threshold dose and treatment regimen that does not consistently cause locomotor sensitization unless a pharmacological or environmental manipulation is employed (Haile et al., 2001; Haile et al., 2003) because we hypothesized that neonatal isolation would enhance sensitization.

Separate sets of adult ISO and NH female rats were assigned to the cocaine administration condition (ISO: n = 9; NH: n = 11) or to the vehicle administration condition (ISO: n = 11; NH: n = 9). Rats were habituated to the locomotor apparatus for 60 minutes on two separate occasions. The development phase began on Day 1. Rats were administered cocaine (10 mg/kg; IP) or vehicle according to group assignment and immediately placed in the center of the arena under dim illumination. Locomotor activity was assessed as total distance traveled (cm) over 60 minutes. This procedure was repeated once daily for the next 4 days. A 10-day drug "wash-out" followed this development phase. The expression of cocaine locomotor sensitization was tested on Day 15 when all rats were administered cocaine.

The data from the development phase (Days 1 and 5) are shown in Figure 5-1 (left panel). As expected, locomotor activity was greater in groups administered cocaine compared to groups administered vehicle, $F(1,38) = 62.47$. There was no evidence that locomotor sensitization occurred ($p > 0.10$) and there was no effect of Treatment condition ($p > 0.10$).

A test of expression of cocaine locomotor sensitization was performed on Day 15 when all rats were administered cocaine. As seen in Figure 5-1 (right panel), there was no evidence that locomotor sensitization occurred. Groups previously administered cocaine did not differ from groups previously administered vehicle ($p > 0.10$). There

was also no effect of neonatal isolation on the expression of locomotor sensitization to cocaine ($p > 0.10$).

Thus, that neonatal isolation heightens cocaine self-administration is likely not due to stress-induced cross-sensitization to the locomotor-activating effects of cocaine. Further, such sensitization cannot explain neonatal isolation-induced increases in food self-administration in female rats because this effect occurs in rats with no prior cocaine exposure. Neonatal isolation may decrease locomotor sensitization to cocaine, an effect that was less likely to be seen under the conditions of the present study. Indeed, maternal separation decreased locomotor sensitization to cocaine (Li et al., 2003) although another study reports it does not affect amphetamine sensitization (Weiss et al., 2001) in adult female rats. Overall, the data suggest that neonatal isolation facilitates cocaine reinforcement specifically.

F. Other Behaviors

While the focus of our work has been on behaviors thought to reflect addiction and the possible neural and hormonal under-

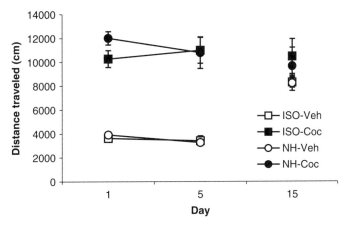

FIGURE 5-1 Mean ± S.E.M. locomotor activity levels are assessed as total distance traveled (cm) over 60-minute sessions in ISO (squares) and NH (circles) female rats administered either cocaine (Coc; 10 mg/kg; closed symbols) or vehicle (Veh; open symbols) (n's = 9–11/group). Cocaine (or vehicle) was administered for 5 consecutive days. Data are shown for Days 1 and 5 (development phase). After a 10-day drug "wash-out" period, the expression of locomotor sensitization was assessed by administering cocaine to all rats on Day 15. Under the conditions of this study, no locomotor sensitization to cocaine was observed and there was no effect of ISO (p's > 0.10).

pinnings, there is a large literature on the enduring effects of handling or maternal separation on other behaviors. Much of that research focuses on emotional and cognitive behaviors such as spatial memory, aversive conditioning, and unconditioned measures of anxiety or fear. However, some studies examined other aspects of reward-related behaviors in adult rats with early life stress. Maternal separation attenuated the consummatory contrast effects of a sucrose reinforcer and decreased Pavlovian conditioned locomotor responses to food (Matthews et al., 1996a; Matthews et al., 1996b). However, these studies compared maternally separated rats to rats with handling experience, that decreases amphetamine conditioned place preference relative to NH rats (Campbell and Spear, 1999).

VI. SEX DIFFERENCES AND ESTROUS STAGE EFFECTS OF NEONATAL ISOLATION

There are numerous sex differences and estrous stage effects on stress hormones, mesolimbic DA function, and cocaine responses (see Section II.C). Neonatal isolation shows some sex-specific effects, summarized in Table 5-2. Neonatal isolation has greater and more generalized effects in female versus male rats on behavior. That is, ISO female rats exhibit higher response levels in cocaine self-administration than NH female rats under a PR schedule (Kosten et al., 2006). Neonatal isolation also facilitates acquisition and maintenance of food responding in female rats (Kosten et al., 2004a; Kosten et al., 2006), an effect not seen in male rats (Kosten et al., 2000; Kosten et al., 2004a; Zhang et al., 2005). NMDA receptor binding in dorsal striatum was upregulated in ISO males but downregulated in ISO females (Sircar et al., 2001). And, chronic neonatal isolation increased CORT levels in female pups relative to NH female pups, but this effect was not seen in male pups (Knuth and Etgen, 2005). Interestingly, the latter

sex difference was seen prior to puberty, the onset of gonadal hormone secretions. This suggests that neonatal isolation may alter the organizational effects of gonadal hormones.

The activational effects of gonadal hormones may be affected by neonatal isolation. For example, estrous stage affects acute locomotor activity induced by cocaine (Quinones-Jenab et al., 1999; Sell et al., 2000). We confirmed and extended these findings. The behavioral effects of cocaine on locomotor activity and schedule-controlled responding differ between estrus- and proestrus-stage NH female rats. Further, this estrous stage distinction is eliminated by neonatal isolation (Kosten et al., 2005b). In addition, the pattern of basal monoamine levels in NAc varies by estrous stage, and this pattern is altered by neonatal isolation (Zhang et al., 2006). Yet, neonatal isolation does not alter estrous cyclicity (Kosten et al., 2005b) or fertility or fecundity (Kosten and Kehoe, unpublished observations). These data suggest that ovarian hormones are intact. Perhaps neonatal isolation affects the interaction of estrogen on the mesolimbic DA system to alter behavioral effects of cocaine. These data point to the importance of studying early life stress in rats of both sexes.

VII. MATERNAL CARE HYPOTHESIS

Recent research shows that the CRF-HPA axis of adult offspring is shaped by maternal behavior received (Champagne and Meaney, 2001; Francis et al., 1999; Liu et al., 1997). Offspring of dams that exhibited high amounts of pup licking and arched-back nursing show greater glucocorticoid receptor feedback and more moderate HPA axis responses to stress. Early life manipulations, such as handling and maternal separation, alter maternal behavior (Barnett and Urn, 1967; Levine, 1987; Liu et al., 1997; Marmendal et al., 2004; Pryce et al., 2001). Our preliminary investigations suggest that neonatal isolation alters maternal behaviors immediately post-reunion (Kosten and Kehoe, unpublished findings). Further, female pups receive less maternal licking than male pups (Moore and Chadwick-Dias, 1986; Moore and Morelli, 1979). This sex-dependent effect of maternal care may contribute to sex differences seen in stress responsivity (see Section II.C). The CRF-HPA axis and stress responsivity are linked to drug self-administration in animals (Goeders, 2003; Kosten and Ambrosio, 2002; Piazza and LeMoal, 1998). These effects may be related in a nonlinear manner such that low- or high-stress responsivity may associate with greater propensity to self-administer drugs (Kosten and Ambrosio, 2002). Thus, it is possible that alterations in maternal behavior induced by the early life stress may mediate the effects on cocaine self-administration behavior in the adult offspring. However, much needs to be learned about the relationship of maternal behavior to stress responsivity and the relationship of stress responsivity to drug self-administration behavior.

VIII. CONCLUSIONS AND TRANSLATION FOR CLINICAL RELEVANCE

Results from our research program indicate that neonatal isolation is a viable model for studying the risk factor of early life stress on propensity to addiction. Neonatal isolation facilitates acquisition and maintenance of operant self-administration for cocaine as well as some aspects of reinstatement of operant responding for cocaine. Moreover, research in female rats suggests that early life stress eliminates estrous stage effects, has a greater effect on cocaine self-administration, and generalizes to other reinforced behaviors. Perhaps then, early life stress may predispose females to other afflictions, such as

eating disorders, and alter menstrual phase effects. The facilitation of these behaviors suggests that early life stress enhances vulnerability to initiate, maintain, and relapse cocaine addiction. These findings are in line with clinical and epidemiological research that supports this link between early life stress and addiction proneness. Addicts are three times as likely to have a history of trauma than nondrug users (Cottler et al., 1992). Over half of female addicts have a trauma history (Najavits et al., 1997). Among adolescents, those that report physical or sexual abuse are more than twice as likely to use drugs (Harrison et al., 1997) and initiate drug use earlier (Bensley et al., 1999).

The mechanisms that contribute to the ability of early life stress to promote vulnerability to addiction likely include stress-induced alterations in the meso-limbic DA system and in CRF-HPA axis function. These effects may be mediated through alterations in maternal behavior. Although many neurohormonal and behavioral alterations endure into adulthood, some effects are only seen immediately after termination of the stress. Yet, these transient effects may help shape the enduring consequences. Future research will determine whether the enduring behavioral effects seen with cocaine generalize to other abused drugs as well as identify other neural and hormonal contributions to these behaviors. Such information will be valuable for establishing more viable prevention and treatment strategies for addiction.

ACKNOWLEDGMENTS

This research was supported by the Patrick and Catherine Weldon Donaghue Foundation (DF # 00-202), a VA Merit grant, and by the Yale IWHR Scholar Program on Women and Drug Abuse (1K12DA14038). The authors wish to thank Diane Lendroth for excellent technical assistance.

REFERENCES

Ader, R., and Grota, L. J. (1969). Effects of early experience on adrenocortical reactivity. *Physiology & Behavior, 4*, 303–305.

Ahmed, S. H., and Koob, G. F. (1997). Cocaine- but not food-seeking behavior is reinstated by stress after extinction. *Psychopharmacology, 132*, 289–295.

Andersen, S. L., and Teicher, M. H. (2000). Sex differences in dopamine receptors and their relevance to ADHD. *Neuroscience and Biobehavioral Reviews, 24*, 137–141.

Anisman, H., Zaharia, M. D., Meaney, M. J., and Merali, Z. (1998). Do early-life events permanently alter behavioral and hormonal responses to stressors? *International Journal of Developmental Neuroscience, 16*, 149–164.

Antelman, S. M., Eichler, A. J., Black, C. A., and Kocan, D. (1980). Interchangeability of stress and amphetamine in sensitization. *Science, 207*, 329–331.

Barnett, S. A., and Urn, J. B. (1967). Early stimulation and maternal behavior. *Nature, 213*, 150–152.

Beatty, W. W., and Beatty, P. A. (1970). Hormonal determinants of sex differences in avoidance behavior and reactivity to electric shock in the rat. *Journal of Comparative and Physiological Psychology, 73*, 446–455.

Becker, J. B. (1999). Gender differences in dopaminergic function in striatum and nucleus accumbens. *Pharmacology, Biochemistry and Behavior, 64*, 803–812.

Becker, J. B., Robinson, T. E., and Lorenz, D. A. (1982). Sex differences and estrous cycle variations in amphetamine-elicited rotational behavior. *European Journal of Pharmacology, 80*, 65–72.

Bensley, L. S., Spieker, S. J., VanEenwyk, J., and Schoder, J. (1999). Self-reported abuse history and adolescent problem behaviors II. Alcohol and drug use. *Journal of Adolescent Health, 24*, 173–180.

Bergman, J., Madras, B. K., Johnson, S. E., and Spealman, R. D. (1989). Effects of cocaine and related drugs in nonhuman primates. III: Self-administration by squirrel monkeys. *Journal of Pharmacology and Experimental Therapeutics, 251*, 150–155.

Borowsky, B., and Kuhn, C. M. (1991). Monoamine mediation of cocaine-induced hypothalamic-pituitary-adrenal activation. *Journal of Pharmacology and Experimental Therapeutics, 256*, 204–210.

Bowman, B. P., Vaughan, S. R., Walker, Q. D., Davis, S. L., Little, P. J., Scheffler, N. M., Thomas, B. F., and Kuhn, C. M. (1999). Effects of sex and gonadectomy on cocaine metabolism in the rat. *Journal of Pharmacology and Experimental Therapeutics, 290*, 1316–1323.

Breiter, H. C., Gollub, R. L., Weisskoff, R. M., Kennedy, D. N., Makris, N., Berke, J. D., Goodman, J. M., Kantor, H. L., Gastfriend, D. R., Riorden, J. P., Mathew, R. T., Rosen, B. R., and Hyman, S. E. (1997). Acute effects of cocaine on human brain activity and emotion. *Neuron, 19*.

Broadbear, J. H., Winger, G., and Woods, J. H. (1999) Cocaine-reinforced responding in rhesus-monkeys: Pharmacological attenuation of the hypothalamic-pituitary-adrenal axis response. *Journal of Pharmacology and Experimental Therapeutics, 290*, 1347–1355.

Brown, E. E., Robertson, G. S., and Fibiger, H. C. (1992). Evidence for conditional neuronal activation following exposures to a cocaine-paired environment: Role of forebrain limbic structures. *Journal of Neuroscience, 12*, 4112–4121.

Buckingham, J., Dohler, K., and Wilson, C. (1978). Activity of the pituitary-adrenocortical secretion and thyroid gland during the oestrous cycle of the rat. *Journal of Endocrinology, 78*, 359–366.

Caine, S. B., Heinrich, S. C., Coffin, V. L., and Koob, G. F. (1995). Effects of the dopamine D-1 antagonist SCH-23390 microinjected into the accumbens, amygdala or striatum on cocaine self-administration in the rat. *Brain Research, 692*, 47–56.

Calatayud, F., and Belzung, C. (2001). Emotional reactivity in mice, a case of nongenetic heredity? *Physiology & Behavior, 74*, 355–362.

Campbell, J., and Spear, L. P. (1999). Effects of handling on amphetamine-induced locomotor activation and conditioned place preference in the adult rat. *Psychopharmacology, 143*, 183–189.

Carelli, R. M., and Deadwyler, S. A. (1996). Dose-dependent transitions in nucleus accumbens cell firing and behavioral responding during cocaine self-administration sessions in rats. *Journal of Pharmacology and Experimental Therapeutics, 277*, 385–393.

Carr, G. D., Fibiger, H. C., and Phillips, A. G. (1989). Conditioned place preference as a measure of drug reward. In Liebman, J. and Cooper, S. (Eds). *The neuropharmacological basis of reward* (pp. 264–319). New York: Oxford University Press.

Carroll, M. E., and Lac, S. T. (1993). Autoshaping i.v. cocaine self-administration in rats: Effects of nondrug alternative reinforcers on acquisition. *Psychopharmacology, 110*, 5–12.

Champagne, F., and Meaney, M. J. (2001). Like mother, like daughter: Evidence for non-genomic transmission of parental behavior and stress responsivity. *Progress in Brain Research, 133*, 287–302.

Childress, A. R., Mozley, D., McElgin, W., Fitzgerald, J., Reivich, M., and O'Brien, C. P. (1999). Limbic activation during cue-induced cocaine craving. *American Journal of Psychiatry, 156*, 11–18.

Ciccocioppo, R., Sanna, P. P., and Weiss, F. (2001). Cocaine-predictive stimulus induces drug-seeking behavior and neural activation in limbic brain regions after multiple months of abstinence: Reversal by D1 antagonists. *Proceedings of the National Academy of Science, 98*, 1976–1981.

Cicero, T. J., Nock, B., O'Connor, L., and Meyer, E. R. (2002). Role of steroids in sex differences in morphine-induced analgesia: Activational and organization effects. *Journal of Pharmacology and Experimental Therapeutics, 300,* 695–701.

Collins, R. J., Weeks, J. R., Cooper, M. M., Good, P. I., and Russell, R. R. (1984). Prediction of abuse liability of drugs using IV self-administration by rats. *Psychopharmacology, 82,* 6–13.

Colpaert, F. C. (1978). Discriminative stimulus properties of narcotic analgesic drugs. *Pharmacology, Biochemistry and Behavior, 9,* 863–887.

Cottler, L. B., Compton, W. M., Mager, D., Spitznagel, E. L., and Janca, A. (1992). Post-traumatic stress disorder among substance users from the general population. *American Journal of Psychiatry, 149,* 664–670.

Deminiere, J. M., Piazza, P. V., LeMoal, M., and Simon, H. (1989). Experimental approach to individual vulnerability to psychostimulant addiction. *Neuroscience & Biobehavioral Reviews, 13,* 141–147.

Deutch, A. Y., Tam, S. Y., and Roth, R. H. (1985). Footshock and conditioned stress increase 3,4-dihydroxyphenylacetic acid (DOPAC) in the ventral tegmental area but not substantia nigra. *Brain Research, 616,* 89–98.

DeVries, A. C., Taymans, S. E., Sundstrom, J. M., and Pert, A. (1998). Conditioned release of corticosterone by contextual stimuli associated with cocaine is mediated by corticotropin-releasing factor. *Brain Research, 786,* 39–46.

DeVries, G. J. (1989). Review article—Sex differences in neurotransmitter systems. *Journal of Neuroendocrinology, 2,* 1–13.

DiCiano, P., Blaha, C. D., and Phillips, A. G. (1998). Conditioned changes in oxidation currents in the nucleus accumbens of rats by stimuli paired with self-administration or yoked administration of d-amphetamine. *European Journal of Neuroscience, 10,* 1121–1127.

Dunn, A. J., and Berridge, C. W. (1990). Physiological and behavioral responses to corticotropin-releasing factor administration: Is CRF a mediator of anxiety or stress responses? *Brain Research Reviews, 15,* 71–100.

Erb, S., Shaham, Y., and Stewart, J. (1996). Stress reinstates cocaine-seeking behavior after prolonged extinction and a drug-free period. *Psychopharmacology, 128,* 408–412.

Erb, S., Shaham, Y., and Stewart, J. (1998). The role of corticotropin-releasing factor and corticosterone in stress- and cocaine-induced relapse to cocaine seeking in rats. *Journal of Neuroscience, 18,* 5529–5536.

Erb, S., and Stewart, J. (1999). A role for the bed nucleus of the stria terminalis, but not the amygdala, in the effects of corticotropin-releasing factor on stress-induced reinstatement of cocaine seeking. *Journal of Neuroscience, 19,* RC35.

Erskine, M. S., Stern, J. M., and Levine, S. (1975). Effects of prepubertal handling on shock-induced fighting and ACTH in male and female rats. *Physiology and Behavior, 14,* 413–420.

Flagel, S. B., Vazquez, D. M., and Robinson, T. E. (2003). Manipulations during the second, but not the first, week of life increase susceptibility to cocaine self-administration in female rats. *Neuropsychopharmacology, 28,* 1741–1751.

Francis, D. D., Diorio, J., Liu, D., and Meaney, M. J. (1999). Nongenomic transmission across generations of maternal behavior and stress responses in the rat. *Science, 286,* 1155–1158.

Fuxe, K., Agnati, L. F., Kalia, M., Goldstein, M., Anderson, K., and Harfstrand, A. (1985). Dopaminergic systems in the brain and pituitary. In Fluckiger, E., Muller, E. E., and Thorner, M. O. (Eds), *Basic and clinical aspects of neuroscience* (pp. 11–25). Berlin: Springer-Verlag.

Gawin, F. H., and Kleber, H. D. (1986). Abstinence symptomatology and psychiatric diagnosis in cocaine abusers. *Archives of General Psychiatry, 43,* 107–113.

Glick, S. D., and Hinds, P. A. (1984). Sex differences in sensitization to cocaine-induced rotation. *European Journal of Pharmacology, 99,* 119–121.

Goeders, N. E. (2003). The impact of stress on addiction. *European Journal of Neuropsychopharmacology, 13,* 435–441.

Goeders, N. E., and Guerin, G. F. (1994). Noncontingent electric footshock facilitates the acquisition of intravenous cocaine self-administration in rats. *Psychopharmacology, 114,* 63–70.

Goeders, N. E., and Guerin, G. F. (2000). Effects of the CRH receptor antagonist CP-154,526 on intravenous cocaine self-administration in rats. *Neuropsychopharmacology, 23,* 577–586.

Goeders, N. E., and Smith, J. E. (1983). Cortical dopaminergic involvement in cocaine reinforcement. *Science, 221,* 773–775.

Golden, R. N., and Gilmore, J. (1990). Serotonin and mood disorder. *Psychiatric Annals, 20,* 580–586.

Grant, S., London, E. D., Newlin, D. B., Villemagne, V. L., Liu, X., Contoregg, C., Phillips, R. L., Kimes, A. S., and Margolin, A. (1996). Activation of memory circuits during cue-elicited cocaine craving. *Proceedings of the National Academy of Science, 93,* 12040–12045.

Gratton, A., and Wise, R. A. (1994). Drug- and behavior-associated changes in dopamine-related electrochemical signals during intravenous cocaine self-administration. *Journal of Neuroscience, 114,* 4130–4146.

Haile, C. N., During, M. J., Jatlow, P. I., Kosten, T. R., and Kosten, T. A. (2003). Disulfiram facilitates the development and expression of locomotor sensitization to cocaine in rats. *Biological Psychiatry, 54,* 915–921.

Haile, C. N., Grandpre, T. N., and Kosten, T. A. (2001). Chronic unpredictable stress, but not chronic predictable stress, enhances the sensitivity to the behavioral effects of cocaine. *Psychopharmacology, 154,* 213–220.

Hall, F. S. (1998). Social deprivation of neonatal, adolescent, and adult rats has distinct neurochemical and behavioral consequences. *Critical Reviews in Neurobiology, 12,* 129–162.

Hall, F. S., Wilkinson, L. S., Humby, T., and Robbins, T. W. (1999). Maternal deprivation of neonatal rats produces enduring changes in dopamine function. *Synapse, 32,* 37–43.

Haney, M., Maccari, S., LeMoal, M., Simon, H., and Piazza, P. V. (1995). Social stress increases the acquisition of cocaine self-administration in male and female rats. *Brain Research, 698,* 46–52.

Harris, J. E., and Baldessarini, R. J. (1973). Uptake of [^{3}H]-catecholamines by homogenates of rat corpus striatum and cerebral cortex: Effects of amphetamine analogues. *Neuropharmacology, 12,* 659–679.

Harrison, P. A., Fulkerson, J. A., and Beebe, T. J. (1997). Multiple substance use among adolescent physical and sexual abuse victims. *Child Abuse and Neglect, 21,* 529–539.

Heim, C., Owens, M. J., Plotsky, P. M., and Nemeroff, C. B. (1997). Persistent changes in corticotropin-releasing factor systems due to early life stress: Relationship to the pathophysiology of major depression and post-traumatic stress disorder. *Psychopharmacology Bulletin, 33,* 185–192.

Heinsbroek, R. P. W., vanHaaren, F., Feenstra, M. G. P., Boon, P., and vandePoll, N. E. (1991). Controllable and uncontrollable footshock and monoaminergic activity in the frontal cortex of male and female rats. *Brain Research, 551,* 247–255.

Heinsbroek, R. P. W., vanHaaren, F., Feenstra, M. G. P., VanGalen, H., Boer, G., and vandePoll, N. E. (1990). Sex differences in the effects of inescapable footshock on central catecholaminergic and serotoninergic activity. *Pharmacology, Biochemistry and Behavior, 37,* 539–550.

Hess, J. L., Denenberg, V. H., Zarrow, M. X., and Pfeifer, W. D. (1969). Modification of the corticosterone response curve as a function of handling in infancy. *Physiology & Behavior, 4,* 109–112.

Hodos, W. (1961). Progessive ratio as a measure of reward. *Science, 134,* 943–944.

Horger, B. A., Shelton, K., and Schenk, S. (1990). Preexposure sensitizes rats to the rewarding effects of cocaine. *Pharmacology Biochemistry and Behavior, 37,* 707–711.

Juraska, J. M. (1991). Sex differences in "cognitive" regions of the rat brain. *Psychoneuroendocrinology, 16,* 105–109.

Kalivas, P. W., and Stewart, J. (1991). Dopamine transmission in the initiation and expression of drug- and stress-induced sensitization of motor activity. *Brain Research Reviews, 16,* 223–244.

Katz, J. L. (1989). Drugs as reinforcers: Pharmacological and behavioral factors. In Liebman, J. and Coopers, S. (Eds), *The neuropharmacological basis of reward* (pp. 164–213). New York: Oxford University Press.

Kehoe, P., and Blass, E. M. (1986). Opioid-mediation of separation distress in 10-day-old rats: Reversal of stress with maternal stimuli. *Developmental Psychobiology, 19,* 385–398.

Kehoe, P., Mallinson, K., McMormick, C. M., and Frye, C. A. (2000). Central allopregnanolone is increased in rat pups in response to repeated, short episodes of neonatal isolation. *Developmental Brain Research, 123,* 133–136.

Kehoe, P., and Shoemaker, W. J. (2001). Infant stress, neuroplasticity, and behavior. In Blass, E. (Ed), *Developmental Psychobiology* (Vol. 13, pp. 551–585). New York: Kluwer Academic/Plenum.

Kehoe, P., Shoemaker, W. J., Arons, C., Triano, L., and Suresh, G. (1998a). Repeated isolation stress in the neonatal rat: Relation to brain dopamine systems in the 10-day-old rat. *Behavioral Neuroscience, 112,* 1466–1474.

Kehoe, P., Shoemaker, W. J., Triano, L., Callahan, M., and Rappolt, G. (1998b). Adult rats stressed as neonates show exaggerated behavioral responses to both pharmacological and environmental challenges. *Behavioral Neuroscience, 112,* 116–125.

Kehoe, P., Shoemaker, W. J., Triano, L., Hoffman, J., and Arons, C. (1996). Repeated isolation in the neonatal rat produces alterations in behavior and ventral striatal dopamine release in the juvenile following amphetamine challenge. *Behavioral Neuroscience, 110,* 1434–1444.

Kim, J. J., and Yoon, K. L. (1998). Stress: Metaplastic effects on hippocampus. *Trends in Neurosciences, 21,* 505–509.

Kitay, J. I. (1961). Sex differences in adrenal cortical secretion in the rat. *Endocrinology, 68,* 818–824.

Knuth, E. D., and Etgen, A. M. (2005). Corticosterone secretion induced by chronic isolation in neonatal rats is sexually dimorphic and accompanied by elevated ACTh. *Hormones and Behavior, 47,* 65–75.

Koob, G. F., and Bloom, F. E. (1988). Cellular and molecular mechanisms of drug dependence. *Science, 242,* 715–723.

Koob, G. F., and Goeders, N. E. (1989). Neuroanatomical substrates of drug self-administration. In Liebman, J. and Cooper, S. (Eds) *The neuropharmacological basis of reward,* (pp. 214–263). New York: Oxford University Press.

Kosten, T. A., and Ambrosio, E. (2002). HPA axis function and drug addictive behaviors: Insights from studies with Lewis and Fischer 344 inbred rats. *Psychoneuroendocrinology, 27,* 35–69.

Kosten, T. A., and Kehoe, P. (2005). Neonatal isolation is a relevant model for studying the contributions of early life stress to vulnerability to drug abuse: Response to Marmendal et al. 2004. *Developmental Psychobiology, 47,* 108–110.

Kosten, T. A., Miserendino, M. J. D., Bombace, J. C., Lee, H. J., and Kim, J. J. (2005a). Sex-selective effects of neonatal isolation on fear conditioning and foot shock sensitivity. *Behavioural Brain Research, 157*, 235–244.

Kosten, T. A., Miserendino, M. J. D., Haile, C. N., DeCaprio, J. L., Jatlow, P. I., and Nestler, E. J. (1997). Acquisition and maintenance of intravenous cocaine self-administration in Lewis and Fischer inbred rat strains. *Brain Research, 778*, 418–429.

Kosten, T. A., Miserendino, M. J. D., and Kehoe, P. (2000). Enhanced acquisition of cocaine self-administration in adult rats with neonatal isolation stress experience. *Brain Research, 875*, 44–50.

Kosten, T. A., Sanchez, H., Jatlow, P. I., and Kehoe, P. (2005b). Neonatal isolation alters estrous cycle interaction on acute behavioral effects of cocaine. *Psychoneuroendocrinology, 30*, 753–761.

Kosten, T. A., Sanchez, H., Zhang, X. Y., and Kehoe, P. (2004a). Neonatal isolation enhances acquisition of cocaine self-administration and food responding in female rats. *Behavioural Brain Research, 151*, 137–149.

Kosten, T. A., Zhang, X. Y., and Kehoe, P. (2003). Chronic neonatal isolation stress enhances cocaine-induced increases in ventral striatal dopamine levels in rat pups. *Brain Research. Developmental Brain Research, 141*, 109–116.

Kosten, T. A., Zhang, X. Y., and Kehoe, P. (2004b). Infant rats with chronic neonatal isolation experience show decreased extracellular serotonin levels in ventral striatum at baseline and in response to cocaine. *Developmental Brain Research, 152*, 19–24.

Kosten, T. A., Zhang, X.-Y., and Kehoe, P. (2005c). Neurochemical and behavioral responses to cocaine in adult male rats with neonatal isolation experience. *Journal of Pharmacology and Experimental Therapeutics, 314*, 661–667.

Kosten, T. A., Zhang, X.-Y. and Kehoe, P. (2006). Heightened cocaine and food self-administration in female rats with neonatal isolation experience. *Neuropsychopharmacology, 31*, 70–76.

Kuczenski, R., and Segal, D. S. (1989). Concomitant characterization of behavioral and striatal neurotransmitter response to amphetamine using in vivo microdialysis. *Journal of Neuroscience, 9*, 2051–2065.

Kuhn, C., and Francis, R. (1997). Gender differences in cocaine-induced HPA axis activation. *Neuropsychopharmacology, 16*, 399–407.

Kuhn, C. M., Walker, Q. D., Kaplan, K. A., and Li, S. T. (2001). Sex, steroids, and stimulant sensitivity. *Annals of the New York Academy of Sciences, 937*, 188–201.

Ladd, C. O., Owens, M. J., and Nemeroff, C. B. (1996). Persistent changes in corticotropin-releasing factor neuronal systems induced by maternal deprivation. *Endocrinology, 137*, 1212–1218.

Lehmann, J., and Feldon, J. (2000). Long-term biobehavioral effects of maternal separation in the rat: Consistent or confusing? *Reviews in Neuroscience, 11*, 383–408.

Leshner, A. I. (1997). Addiction is a brain disease, and it matters. *Science, 278*, 45–47.

Levine, S. (1962). Plasma-free corticosteroid response to electric shock in rats stimulated in infancy. *Science, 135*, 795–796.

Levine, S. (1987). Psychobiologic consequences of disruption in mother-infant relationships. In Krasneger, N., Blass, E., Hofer, M., and Smotherman, W. (Eds). *Perinatal development: A psychobiological perspective.* New York: Academic Press.

Levine, S. (1994). The ontogeny of the hypothalamic-pituitary-adrenal axis: The influence of maternal factors. *Annals of the New York Academy of Science, 746*, 275–288.

Li, Y. L., Robinson, T. E., and Bhatnagar, S. (2003). Effects of maternal separation on behavioural sensitization produced by repeated cocaine administration in adulthood. *Brain Research, 960*, 42–47.

Liu, D., Diorio, J., Tannenbaum, B., Caldji, C., Francis, D., Freedman, A., Sharma, S., Pearson, D., Plotsky, P. M., and Meaney, M. J. (1997). Maternal care, hippocampal glucocorticoid receptors, and hypothalamic-pituitary-adrenal responses to stress. *Science, 277*, 1659–1662.

Lynch, W. J., and Taylor, J. R. (2005). Neonatal isolation stress potentiates cocaine seeking behavior in adult male and female rats. *Neuropsychopharmacology, 30*, 322–329.

Markou, A., Weiss, F., Gold, L. H., Caine, S. B., Schulteis, G., and Koob, G. F. (1993). Animal models of drug craving. *Psychopharmacology, 112*, 163–182.

Marmendal, M., Roman, E., Eriksson, C. J. P., Nylander, I., and Fahlke, C. (2004). Maternal separation alters maternal care, but has minor effects on behavior and brain opioid peptides in adult offspring. *Developmental Psychobiology, 45*, 140–152.

Marquardt, A. R., Ortiz-Lemos, L., Lucion, A. B., and Barros, H. M. T. (2004). Influence of handling or aversive stimulation during rats' neonatal or adolescence periods on oral cocaine self-administration and cocaine withdrawal. *Behavioral Pharmacology, 15*, 403–412.

Matthews, K., Dalley, J. W., Matthews, C., Tsai, T. H., and Robbins, T. W. (2001). Periodic maternal separation of neonatal rats produces region- and gender-specific effects on biogenic amine content in postmortem adult brain. *Synapse, 40*, 1–10.

Matthews, K., Hall, F. S., Wilkinson, L. S., and Robbins, T. W. (1996a). Retarded acquisition and reduced expression of conditioned locomotor activity in adult rats following repeated early maternal separation: Effects of prefeeding, d-amphetamine, dopamine antagonists and clonidine. *Psychopharmacology, 126*, 75–84.

Matthews, K., Robbins, T. W., Everitt, B. J., and Caine, S. B. (1999). Repeated neonatal maternal separation alters intravenous cocaine self-administration in adult rats. *Psychopharmacology, 141*, 123–134.

Matthews, K., Wilkinson, L. S., and Robbins, T. W. (1996b). Repeated maternal separation of preweanling rats attenuates behavioral responses to primary and conditioned incentives in adulthood. *Physiology & Behavior, 59,* 99–107.

McCormick, C. M., Kehoe, P., and Kovacs, S. (1998). Corticosterone release in response to repeated, short episodes of neonatal isolation: Evidence of sensitization. *International Journal of Developmental Neuroscience, 16,* 175–185.

McCormick, C. M., Kehoe, P., Mallinson, K., Cecchi, L., and Frye, C. A. (2002a). Neonatal isolation alters stress hormone and mesolimbic dopamine release in juvenile rats. *Pharmacology, Biochemistry and Behavior, 73,* 77–85.

McCormick, C. M., Linkroum, W., Sallinen, B. J., and Miller, N. W. (2002b). Peripheral and central sex steroids have differential effects on the HPA axis of male and female rats. *Stress, 5,* 235–247.

McEwen, B. S., and Sapolsky, R. M. (1995). Stress and cognitive function. *Current Opinion in Neurobiology, 5,* 205–216.

McFarland, K., Davidge, S. B., Lapish, C. C., and Kalivas, P. W. (2004). Limbic and motor circuitry underlying footshock-induced reinstatement of cocaine-seeking behavior. *Journal of Neuroscience, 24,* 1551–1560.

McGregor, A., and Roberts, D. C. (1993). Dopaminergic antagonism within the nucleus accumbens or the amygdala produces differential effects on intravenous cocaine self-administration under fixed and progressive ratio schedules of reinforcement. *Brain Research, 624,* 245–252.

Meaney, M. J., Aitken, D. H., Viau, V., Sharma, S., and Sarrieau, A. (1989). Neonatal handling alters adrenocortical negative feedback sensitivity and hippocampal type II glucocorticoid receptor binding in the rat. *Neuroendocrinology, 50,* 597–604.

Meaney, M. J., Diorio, R., Francis, D., Widdowson, J., LaPlante, P., Caldji, C., Sharm, V., Seckl, J. R., and Plotsky, P. M. (1996). Early environmental regulation of forebrain glucocorticoid receptor gene expression: Implications for adrenocortical responses to stress. *Developmental Neuroscience, 18,* 49–72.

Miczek, K. A., and Mutschler, N. H. (1996). Activational effects of social stress on IV cocaine self-administration in rats. *Psychopharmacology, 128,* 256–264.

Moldow, R. L., and Fischman, A. J. (1987). Cocaine induced secretion of ACTH, beta-endorphin and corticosterone. *Peptides, 8,* 819–822.

Moore, C. L., and Chadwick-Dias, A. M. (1986). Behavioral responses of infant rats to maternal licking: Variations with age and sex. *Developmental Psychobiology, 19,* 427–438.

Moore, C. L., and Morelli, G. A. (1979). Mother rats interact differently with male and female offspring. *Journal of Comparative and Physiological Psychology, 93,* 667–684.

Najavits, L. M., Gastfriend, D. R., Barber, J. P., Reif, S., Muenz, L. R., Blaine, J., Frank, A., Crits-Christoph, P., Thase, M., and Weiss, R. D. (1998). Cocaine dependence with and without PTSD among subjects in the National Institute on Drug Abuse Collaborative Cocaine Treatment Study. *American Journal of Psychiatry, 155,* 214–219.

Najavits, L. M., Weiss, R. D., and Shaw, S. R. (1997). The link between substance abuse and post-traumatic stress disorder in women. *American Journal of Addictions, 6,* 273–281.

Neisewander, J. L., Baker, D. A., Fuchs, R. A., Tran-Nguyen, L. T., Palmer, A., and Marshall, J. F. (2000). Fos protein expression and cocaine-seeking behavior in rats after exposure to a cocaine self-administration environment. *Journal of Neuroscience, 20,* 798–805.

Ogawa, T., Mikuni, M., Kuroda, Y., Muneoka, K., Mori, K., and Takahashi, K. (1994). Periodic maternal deprivation alters stress response in adult offspring: Potentiates the negative feedback regulation of restraint stress-induced adrenocortical response and reduces the frequencies of open field-induced behaviors. *Pharmacology Biochemistry and Behavior, 49,* 961–967.

Papaioannou, A., Dafni, U., Alikaridis, F., Bolaris, S., and Stylianopoulou, F. (2002). Effects of neonatal handling on basal and stress-induced monoamine levels in the male and female rat brain. *Neuroscience, 114,* 195–206.

Pettit, H. O., and Justice, J. B. (1989). Dopamine in the nucleus accumbens during cocaine self-administration as studied by in vivo microdialysis. *Pharmacology, Biochemistry and Behavior, 34,* 899–904.

Piazza, P. V., Deminiere, J.-M., LeMoal, M., and Simon, H. (1990). Stress- and pharmacologically-induced behavioral sensitization increases vulnerability to acquisition of amphetamine self-administration. *Brain Research, 514,* 22–26.

Piazza, P. V., and LeMoal, M. (1998). The role of stress in drug self-administration. *Trends in Pharmacological Sciences, 19,* 67–74.

Pickens, R., Meisch, R. A., and Thompson, T. (1978). Drug self-administration: An analysis of the reinforcing effects of drugs. In Iverson, L., Iverson, S., and Snyder, S. (Eds), *Handbook of Psychopharmacology* (Vol. 12, pp. 1–37). New York: Plenum Press.

Plotsky, P. M., and Meaney, M. J. (1993). Early, postnatal experience alters hypothalamic corticotropin-releasing factor (CRF) mRNA, median eminence CRF content and stress-induced release in adult rats. *Molecular Brain Research, 18,* 195–200.

Post, R. M., Weiss, S. R. B., Pert, A., and Uhde, T. W. (1987). Chronic cocaine administration: Sensitization and kindling effects. In Fisher, S., Raskin, A., and Uhlenhuth, E. (Eds), *Cocaine: Clinical and biobehavioral aspects* (pp. 109–173). New York: Oxford University Press.

Pryce, C. R., Bettschen, D., and Feldon, J. (2001). Comparison of the effects of early handling and early deprivation on maternal care in the rat. *Developmental Psychobiology, 38,* 239–251.

Pryce, C. R., and Feldon, J. (2003). Long-term neurobehavioral impact of the postnatal environment in rats: Manipulations, effects and mediating mechanisms. *Neuroscience and Biobehavioral Reviews, 27,* 57–71.

Quinones-Jenab, V., Ho, A., Schlussman, S. D., Franck, J., and Kreek, M. J. (1999). Estrous cycle differences in cocaine-induced stereotypic and locomotor behaviors in Fischer rats. *Behavioural Brain Research*, *101*, 15–20.

Richardson, N. R., and Roberts, D. C. (1996). Progressive ratio schedules in drug self-administration studies in rats: A method to evaluate reinforcing efficacy. *Journal of Neuroscience Methods*, *66*, 1–11.

Ritz, M. C., Lamb, R. J., Goldberg, S. R., and Kuhar, M. J. (1987). Cocaine receptors on dopamine transporters are related to self-administration of cocaine. *Science*, *237*, 1219–1223.

Rivier, C. (1999). Gender, sex steroids, corticotropin-releasing factor, nitric oxide, and the HPA response to stress. *Pharmacology, Biochemistry and Behavior*, *64*, 739–751.

Rivier, C. L., and Plotsky, P. M. (1986). Mediation by corticotropin releasing factor (CRF) of adrenohypophysial hormone secretion. *Annual Review of Physiology*, *48*, 475–494.

Rivier, C. L., and Vale, W. (1987). Cocaine stimulates adrenocorticotropin (ACTH) secretion through a corticotropin-releasing (CRF)-mediated mechanism. *Brain Research*, *422*, 403–406.

Robinson, T. E., and Berridge, K. C. (1993). The neural basis of drug craving: An incentive sensitization theory of addiction. *Brain Research Reviews*, *18*, 247–291.

Robinson, T. E., Gorny, G., Mitton, E., and Kolb, B. (2001). Cocaine self-administration alters the morphology of dendrites and dendritic spines in the nucleus accumbens and neocortex. *Synapse*, *39*, 257–266.

Rodefer, J. S., and Carroll, M. E. (1996). Progressive ratio and behavioral economic evaluation of the reinforcing efficacy of orally delivered phencyclidine and ethanol in monkeys: Effects of feeding conditions. *Psychopharmacology*, *128*, 265–273.

Rots, N., deJong, J., Workel, J. O., Levine, S., Cools, A. R., and DeKloet, E. R. (1996). Neonatal maternally deprived rats have as adults elevated basal pituitary-adrenal activity and enhanced susceptibility to apomorphine. *Journal of Neuroendcrinology*, *8*, 501–506.

Rupprecht, R. (2003). Neuroactive steroids: Mechanisms of action and neuropsychopharmacological properties. *Psychoneuroendocrinology*, *28*, 139–168.

SAMHSA. (2001). National Household Survey on Drug Abuse. www.samhsa.gov/oas/NHSDA/2k1NHSDA/vol1/Chapter7.htm.

Sarnyai, Z., Biro, E., Gardi, J., Vecsernyes, M., Julesz, J., and Telegdy, G. (1992). The cocaine-induced elevation of plasma corticosterone is mediated by endogenous corticotropin-releasing factor (CRF) in rats. *Brain Research*, *589*, 154–156.

Sarnyai, Z., Shaham, Y., and Heinrichs, S. C. (2001). The role of corticotropin-releasing factor in drug addiction. *Pharmacological Reviews*, *53*, 209–243.

Scheel-Kruger, J., Baestrup, C., Nielson, M., Golembiowska, K., and Mogilnicka, E. (1977). Cocaine: Discussion on the role of dopamine in the bio-

chemical mechanisms of action. In Ellinwood, J., and Kilbey, M. (Eds), *Cocaine and Other Stimulants*. New York: Plenum Press.

Schenk, S., Horger, B. A., Peltier, R., and Shelton, K. (1991). Supersensitivity to the reinforcing effects of cocaine following 6-hydroxydopamine lesions to the medial prefrontal cortex in rats. *Brain Research*, *543*, 227–235.

Schultz, W. (2000). Multiple reward signals in the brain. *Nature Reviews*, *1*, 199–207.

Schuster, C. R., and Thompson, T. (1969). Self-administration of and behavioral dependence on drugs. *Annual Review of Pharmacology*, *9*, 483–502.

Sell, S. L., Scalzitti, J. M., Thomas, M. L., and Cunningham, K. A. (2000). Influence of ovarian hormones and estrous cycle on the behavioral response to cocaine in female rats. *Journal of Pharmacology and Experimental Therapeutics*, *293*, 879–886.

Shaham, Y., Erb, S., Leung, S., Buczek, Y., and Stewart, J. (1998). CP-154,526, a selective, non-peptide antagonist of the corticotropin-releasing factor-1 receptor attenuates stress-induced relapse to drug seeking in cocaine and heroin-trained rats. *Psychopharmacology*, *137*, 184–190.

Shaham, Y., and Stewart, J. (1995). Stress reinstates heroin-seeking in drug free animals: An effect mimicing heroin, not withdrawal. *Psychopharmacology*, *119*, 334–341.

Shalev, U., Grimm, J. W., and Shaham, Y. (2002). Neurobiology of relapse to heroin and cocaine seeking: A review. *Pharmacological Reviews*, *54*, 1–42.

Sircar, R., Mallinson, K., Goldbloom, L. M., and Kehoe, P. (2001). Postnatal stress selectively upregulates striatal N-methyl-D-aspartate receptors in male rats. *Brain Research*, *904*, 145–148.

Smith, M. A., Kim, S.-Y., VanOers, H. J. J., and Levine, S. (1997). Maternal deprivation and stress induce immediated early genes in the infant rat brain. *Endocrinology*, *138*, 4622–4628.

Sorg, B. A., and Kalivas, P. W. (1991). Effects of cocaine and footshock stress on extracellular dopamine levels in the ventral striatum. *Brain Research*, *559*, 29–36.

Stanton, M. E., Gutierrez, Y. R., and Levine, S. (1988). Maternal deprivation potentiates pituitary-adrenal stress responses in infant rats. *Behavioral Neuroscience*, *102*, 692–700.

Stern, J. M. (1989). Maternal behavior: Sensory, hormonal, and neural determinants. In Brush, F. R. and Levine, S. L. (Eds), *Psychoendocrinology* (pp. 105–226). New York: Academic Press.

Suchecki, D., Nelson, D. Y., VanOers, H., and Levine, S. (1995). Activation and inhibition of the hypothalamic-pituitary-adrenal axis of the neonatal rat: Effects of maternal deprivation. *Psychoneuroendocrinology*, *20*, 169–182.

Sudha, S., and Pradhan, N. (1995). Stress-induced changes in regional monoamine metabolism and behavior in rats. *Physiology & Behavior*, *57*, 1061–1066.

Sutanto, W., Rosenfeld, P., deKloet, E. R., and Levine, S. (1996). Long-term effects of neonatal maternal deprivation and ACTH on hippocampal mineralocorticoid and glucocorticoid receptors. *Developmental Brain Research, 92,* 156–164.

Thierry, A. M., DeDourin, C., Penit, J., Ferron, A., and Glowinski, J. (1986). Variation in the ability of neuroleptics to block the inhibitory influence of dopaminergic neurons on the activity of cells in the rat medial prefrontal cortex. *Brain Research Bulletin, 16,* 155–160.

Thompson, T. L., and Moss, R. L. (1997). Modulation of mesolimbic dopaminergic activity over the rat estrous cycle. *Neuroscience Letters, 229,* 145–148.

Tidey, J. W., and Miczek, K. A. (1997). Acquisition of cocaine self-administration after social stress: Role of accumbens dopamine. *Psychopharmacology, 130,* 203–212.

Tsuang, M. T., Lyons, M. J., Meyers, J. M., Doyle, T., Eisen, S. A., Goldberg, J., True, W., Lin, N., Toomey, R., and Eaves, L. (1998). Co-occurrence of abuse of different drugs in men: The role of drug-specific and shared vulnerabilities. *Archives of General Psychiatry, 55,* 967–972.

Unis, A. S. (1995). Developmental molecular psychopharmacology in early-onset psychiatric disorder: From models to mechanisms. *Child and Adolescent Psychiatric Clinics of North America, 4,* 41–57.

vandenBree, M. B. M., Johnson, E. O., Neale, M. C., and Pickens, R. W. (1998). Genetic and environmental influences on drug use and abuse/dependence in male and female twins. *Drug and Alcohol Dependence, 52,* 231–241.

vanHaaren, F., and Meyer, M. E. (1991). Sex differences in locomotor activity after acute and chronic cocaine administration. *Pharmacology Biochemistry and Behavior, 39,* 923–927.

vanOers, H. J. J., deKloet, E. R., Whelan, T., and Levine, S. (1998). Maternal deprivation effect on the infant's neural stress markers is reversed by tactile stimulation and feeding but not by suppressing corticosterone. *Journal of Neuroscience, 18,* 10171–10179.

Viau, V., and Meaney, M. J. (1991). Variations in the hypothalamic-pituitary-adrenal response to stress during the estrous cycle in the rat. *Endocrinology, 129,* 2503–2511.

Viau, V., Sharma, S., Plotsky, P. M., and Meaney, M. J. (1993). Increased plasma ACTH responses to stress in nonhandled compared with handled rats require basal levels of corticosterone and are associated with increased levels of ACTH secretagogues in the median eminence. *Journal of Neuroscience, 13,* 1097–1105.

Wechsberg, W. M., Craddock, S. G., and Hubbard, R. L. (1998). How are women who enter substance abuse treatment different than men? A gender comparison from the Drug Abuse Treatment Outcome Study (DATOS). *Drugs & Society, 13,* 97–115.

Weinberg, J., Krahn, E. A., and Levine, S. (1978). Differential effects of early handling on exploration in male and female rats. *Developmental Psychobiology, 11,* 251–259.

Weinberg, J., and Levine, S. (1977). Early handling influences on behavioral and physiological responses during active avoidance. *Developmental Psychobiology, 10,* 161–169.

Weiss, I. C., Domeney, A. M., Heidbreder, C. A., Moreau, J. L., and Feldon, J. (2001). Early social isolation, but not maternal separation, affects behavioral sensitization to amphetamine in male and female adult rats. *Pharmacology, Biochemistry & Behavior, 70,* 397–409.

Whitelaw, R. B., Markou, A., Robbins, T. W., and Everitt, B. J. (1996). Excitotoxic lesions of the basolateral amygdala impair the acquisition of cocaine-seeking behaviour under a second-order schedule of reinforcement. *Psychopharmacology, 127,* 213–224.

Wilson, J. M., Nobrega, J. N., Corrigall, W. A., Coen, K. M., Shannak, K., and Kish, S. J. (1994). Amygdala dopamine levels are markedly elevated after self- but not passive-administration of cocaine. *Brain Research, 668,* 39–45.

Wise, R. A., and Rompre, P. P. (1989). Brain dopamine and reward. In Rosenzweig, M. R. and Porter, L. W. (Eds), *Annual review of psychology,* (Vol. 40, pp. 191–225). Palo Alto, CA: Annual Reviews Inc.

Zhang, X. Y., Kosten, T. A., and Kehoe, P. (2006). Neonatal isolation alters estrous cycle effects on ventral striatal extracellular monoamine levels. *Progress in Neuro-Psychopharmacology & Biological Psychiatry. 30,* 504–511.

Zhang, X. Y., Sanchez, H., Kehoe, P., and Kosten, T. A. (2005). Neonatal isolation enhances maintenance but not reinstatement of cocaine self-administration in adult male rats. *Psychopharmacology, 177,* 391–399.

Zhou, W., Cunningham, K. A., and Thomas, M. L. (2002). Estrogen regulation of gene expression in the brain: A possible mechanism altering the response to psychostimulants in female rats. *Molecular Brain Research, 100,* 75–83.

Zimmerberg, B., and Brown, R. C. (1998). Prenatal experience and postnatal stress modulate the adult neurosteroid and catecholaminergic stress responses. *International Journal of Developmental Neuroscience, 16,* 217–228.

6

Genetics, Stress, and the Risk for Addiction

MARY-ANNE ENOCH

The risk for addiction is almost equally divided between genetic and environmental vulnerability factors. Animal models have shown that environmental stressors experienced at an early stage of development permanently alter the expression of glucocorticoid and neurotransmitter receptor genes, particularly in the hippocampus, resulting in aberrant stress responses and therefore perhaps vulnerability to addiction. In human and nonhuman primates, interactions between common gene variants and stressors have been shown to be important in the development of addiction and comorbid disorders. There is significant overlap in genetic origins between the commonest addictive disorders, alcohol and nicotine addiction, and among the group of illicit abused drugs; however, heritability studies indicate that there is a genetic component that is common to all addictions. This is likely to derive from genetic variation in the two interacting systems that are fundamental to positive and negative reinforcement: The stress response system and the dopamine "reward" pathway, consisting primarily of the ventral tegmentum, the nucleus accumbens, the limbic system, and the orbitofrontal cortex. Addictive drugs modulate both systems. Baseline cortisol and cortisol response to stress show heritable interindividual variation, and this itself may be a vulnerability factor for addiction. Genetic vulnerability to addiction and variability in the stress response are likely to be due to interacting variation in numerous genes, each with small to modest effects, in many neurobiological pathways. This chapter will focus on known common functional genetic variants in systems that are important links between the reward pathway and stress response, for example, the opioid system.

I. INTRODUCTION

Addiction has been graphically described as the relentless cycling of preoccupation and anticipation, binge/intoxication, and withdrawal/negative affect (Koob, 2003). The essential features of addiction are loss of control over consumption, obsessional thoughts about the drug, and continuation of use despite knowledge of negative health and social consequences (American Psychiatric Association, 1994). Both positive (euphoric) and negative (anxiolytic, antidysphoric) reinforcement are features of addiction, the latter often predominating over the former as the disease progresses.

Stress and Addiction: Biological and Psychological Mechanisms
Edited by **Mustafa al'Absi, Ph.D.**

Stress and addiction are intimately entwined; coping mechanisms for stress can result in maintained drug use and the altered homeostasis subsequent to addiction results in stress upon drug withdrawal (Merikangas et al., 1998a, Wand, 2005). Although impulsivity has been associated with initiation of alcohol, tobacco, and drug use in humans, numerous studies have shown that addiction may result from excessive stress-related use; for example, premorbid anxiety/dysphoria is associated with use of alcohol and nicotine (Thomas et al., 2003), although not cannabis, as coping mechanisms (Stewart et al., 1997). Certainly, alcohol and drugs of abuse relieve anxiety in laboratory animals (Pandey et al., 2005b).

A complex mix of gene-stress interactions is likely to underlie addiction vulnerability and development. Certain stressors may be more likely to precipitate addiction; for example, both aggression and social defeat produce similar stress responses in rats; however, social defeat results in increased cocaine self-administration (Covington et al., 2005). Severe childhood stressors, especially emotional, physical, and sexual abuse, have been associated with increased vulnerability to addiction, especially in women in whom childhood sexual abuse is associated with a fourfold increase in the lifetime prevalence of both alcoholism and other drug abuse (Wilsnack et al., 1997; Winfield et al., 1990). Among female drug users, 70% report childhood sexual abuse (NIDA, 1994). However, not all stressed children develop addiction; for example, Caspi et al. (2002) showed that it was an interaction between maltreatment (physical/sexual abuse, rejection) and a genotype conferring low levels of expression of the monoamine-oxidase A (MAOA) gene that predicted adult antisocial behavior, often associated with addiction, and another study (Foley et al., 2004) showed that MAOA genotype interacted with family adversity (interparental violence, neglect) to predict childhood conduct disorder, often an antecedent for addiction.

II. THE EXTENT OF THE PROBLEM: PREVALENCE OF ADDICTION

Nicotine and alcohol addiction are by far the most common drugs of abuse. A recent, very large national epidemiological survey (NESARC) of *DSM-IV* psychiatric disorders has shown that the 12-month prevalence for nicotine dependence is 12.8% and for substance use disorders (abuse plus dependence) is alcohol, 8.5%; cannabis, 1.5%; opioids, 0.4%; cocaine, 0.3%; and amphetamines, sedatives, tranquilizers, hallucinogens, 0.1–0.2% (Grant et al., 2004).

Individuals are frequently addicted to more than one substance; joint addiction to alcohol and nicotine is common: among current alcoholics, 35% are also nicotine dependent, whereas 23% of individuals with nicotine dependence have alcohol use disorders (Grant et al., 2004). There is also comorbidity with other drugs of abuse; 13% of current alcoholics have a current drug use disorder, predominantly cannabis (10%) and cocaine or opioids (2.5%); (Stinson et al., 2005). In contrast, the prevalence of current alcohol use disorders among individuals with a current drug use disorder is 55%. The prevalence of alcoholism in drug-dependent individuals is even higher: 100% for hallucinogens, 90% for cocaine, 78% for amphetamines, 74% for opioids, 68% for cannabis (Stinson et al., 2005). Fifty-two percent of individuals with a drug use disorder (69% with dependence) are also nicotine dependent (Grant et al., 2004). This suggests that among drug abusers there may be a substantial shared vulnerability to addiction.

III. HERITABILITY OF ADDICTION

Both alcoholism and drug disorders are familial; alcoholism in a parent predicts alcoholism in his/her offspring (OR = 1.7; Kendler et al., 1997). Among female drug users, more than 80% had at least one parent addicted to alcohol or drugs (NIDA, 1994). Two large studies have shown that relatives of drug-dependent (alcohol, opioids, cocaine, and cannabis) probands had an increased risk of drug disorders; however, although a common risk factor for dependence was identified, alcoholism and the different drug disorders tended to aggregate independently in families, suggesting substance-specific transmission factors (Bierut et al., 1998; Merikangas et al., 1998b).

The familial transmission of substance dependence may result from genetic and/or environmental factors. Alcoholism and other drug abuse disorders are heterogeneous diseases in which the expression of genetic vulnerability is modified by environmental factors that can be shared within the family or are uniquely experienced by the individual (nonshared).

Many very large population-based twin studies have used multivariate twin analysis to investigate the heritability (the measure of the genetic component of variance in interindividual vulnerability) of drug dependence and have found that the genetic risk for alcoholism, nicotine addiction, and psychoactive substance dependence is substantial, with heritability ranging from 40–60% (reviewed in Goldman et al., 2005). Thus genetic vulnerability and environmental stressors are equally important in the development of addiction. Within alcoholism, the nonshared environment contributes 50% of the vulnerability to development of the disease (Knopik et al., 2004). Cannabis, more than other drugs, is influenced by family environmental factors (20–30%); (True et al., 1999a; Tsuang et al., 1998). Family environment appears to be important for substance initiation (Kendler et al., 2000) particularly in adolescents (Rhee et al., 2003), whereas shared environmental factors are important for substance use.

A. General Versus Substance-Specific Heritability

The common psychiatric disorders are influenced by two major genetic risk factors

that load onto internalizing disorders (anxiety disorders, major depression) and externalizing disorders (alcoholism, drug abuse/dependence, adult antisocial behavior and conduct disorder) (Hicks et al., 2004; Kendler et al., 2003b; Kruger, 1999). Two large twin studies found that alcohol dependence and drug abuse/dependence (not specified) had substantial disorder-specific genetic loading (13–14% and 19–21% of the variance, respectively) (Hicks et al., 2004; Kendler et al., 2003b). Cannabis dependence has been shown to have a 36% specific contribution and an 8% contribution from genes common with alcohol dependence (True et al., 1999a). However, within the illicit substance group (cannabis, cocaine, hallucinogens, sedatives, stimulants, opiates), one common genetic factor was found to have a strong influence on risk for use, abuse, and dependence for all six classes, and shared environmental risk factors for use, abuse, and dependence were also nonspecific (Kendler et al., 2003a; Tsuang et al., 2001).

There is strong evidence from twin studies for shared, as well as specific, genetic vulnerability for alcohol and nicotine addiction. Approximately 50% of the genetic effects for nicotine dependence are shared with alcoholism, whereas 15–26% of the genetic effects for alcoholism are shared with nicotine addiction (Hettema et al., 1999; Swan et al., 1997; True et al., 1999b). A heavy smoking–heavy alcohol genetic factor accounted for 45% of the heritable variance in heavy drinking and 35% of the heritable variance in heavy smoking (Swan et al., 1997).

B. Origins of Shared Genetic Vulnerability to Addiction: "Reward" Pathway and Stress Response System

Addictive substances have two common features that result in positive and negative reinforcement: They interact with the "reward" pathway, consisting primarily of the ventral tegmentum, the nucleus accumbens, the limbic system, and the orbitofrontal cortex, and they also alter the physiological response to stress.

The three components of the stress response system that are of interest in addiction vulnerability are the hypothalamic-pituitary-adrenal (HPA) axis, the limbic behavioral stress response system, and the locus coeruleus (LC)-norepinephrine (NE) system. Short-term activation is advantageous and indeed is essential for survival; however, chronic hyperactivity can lead to dysregulation of the HPA axis plus structural and physiological alterations in the hippocampus resulting in deleterious effects on a wide range of physiological systems, including mood and cognition.

Genetic vulnerability for addictive disorders is likely to be due to numerous interacting genetic variants with small to modest effects. This genetic variation in neurobiological pathways, including stress-response systems, may mean that some individuals are more vulnerable to the development of long-term or permanent neurological changes in response to heavy drug use. Likewise, genetic variation may determine increased vulnerability to relapse in response to stressors.

IV. HPA AXIS

Regulation of HPA axis responsiveness is complex and is dependent on the nature of the stressor. Exposure to acute stress results in activation of the HPA axis. Corticotropin-releasing factor/hormone (CRF), located in the paraventricular nucleus of the hypothalamus, stimulates the release of adrenocorticotropic hormone (ACTH) from the anterior pituitary. ACTH then stimulates the release of glucocorticoid hormones, from the adrenal cortex: predominantly cortisol in humans and corticosterone in rodents. Cortisol is responsible for negative feedback inhibition of the pituitary, hypothalamus, and hippocampus. CRF also increases the release of β-endorphin in the anterior pituitary. The HPA axis is under tonic inhibitory control

by the μ-opioid receptor and by endogenous cannabinoids acting via centrally located CB1 receptors (Barna et al., 2004).

A. HPA Axis and Addiction

Addictive substances acutely activate the HPA axis, and this has been implicated in both positive and negative reinforcement of drug use. Animal studies have shown that prolonged drug exposure results in potentially pathological neuroadaptation in the HPA axis and in the behavioral stress response. This altered homeostasis, or "allostasis," is thought to increase the risk of stress-induced relapse (Adinoff et al., 2005; Koob, 2003).

It is not known whether the blunted HPA axis stress response seen in some abstinent alcoholics (Adinoff et al., 2005) is due to allostatis or is a marker for vulnerability to alcoholism—or both. However, a blunted stress response has been found in the following groups: non-alcoholics and alcoholics from families with a strong history of alcoholism (Dai et al., 2005); boys with persistent antisocial behavior, a predictor for adult substance abuse (Snoek et al., 2004); women with high neuroticism, a vulnerability factor for psychopathology including alcoholism (Oswald et al., 2006). Thus a blunted stress response may indicate vulnerability to addiction.

B. Heritability of Basal and Stimulated HPA Activity

Basal and stimulated HPA axis activity shows interindividual variability; however, there has been little research on genetic influences. The free cortisol response soon after awakening is a stable, consistent measure of HPA activity with a significant heritability of 40–60% (Bartels et al., 2003; Wust et al., 2000). Genetic variation in the negative feedback mechanism involving glucocorticoid (GR) receptors throughout the brain might contribute to individual variation in diurnal cortisol profiles (reviewed in Bartels et al., 2003). Results from studies investigating the heritability of the HPA axis in response to stress are mixed (reviewed in Federenko et al., 2004) but one twin study has suggested high heritability (>97%) for sustained stress (Federenko et al., 2004).

C. Gene-Environment Interactions in HPA Axis Variabliity

The GR mediates many of the effects of glucocorticoids on gene transcription by directly binding to hormone-responsive elements within DNA regions or by interacting with transcription factors such as AP-1 or NF-κB (Wust et al., 2004). Thus GR gene polymorphisms may be implicated in HPA axis variation. The GR gene structure is complex with several copies of exon 1, each with its own promoter, and alternative splicing resulting in cell-specific GR expression (DeRijk and de Kloet, 2005). Several polymorphisms have been described (DeRijk and de Kloet, 2005). Of these, an Asn363Ser exon 2 variant has been associated with increased salivary cortisol response to acute psycho-

social stress in healthy men, whereas a BclI variant has been associated with diminished cortisol response (Wust et al., 2004).

Studies in primates and rodents have established that naturally occurring variation in maternal behavior influences the development of individual differences in behavioral and HPA responses to stress in offspring, and this can be transmitted across generations (Higley et al., 1991; Liu et al., 1997; Meaney, 2001; Weaver et al., 2004). A recent longitudinal study in children showed that significant maternal anxiety in late pregnancy was associated with higher basal cortisol levels in the child at age 10 years (O'Connor et al., 2005). The magnitude of the HPA axis response to stress in rats can be modified by GR expression in the hippocampus; these receptors are implicated in HPA feedback regulation in response to acute stress. Poor maternal contact in early life results in reduced GR expression, diminished glucocorticoid feedback sensitivity, greater HPA axis activation, and increased fear in response to

TABLE 6-1   Genetic Polymorphisms Associated with Anxiety, Addiction, and Comorbid Behaviors

Gene	Polymorphism	Behavioral / Physiological Associations
Monoamine oxidase	MAOA VNTR functional, promoter	antisocial behavior G X E
Catechol-O-methyltransferase	COMT Val158Met functional, coding sequence	anxiety, addiction
Serotonin transporter	5-HTTLPR: S and L alleles functional, promoter insertion/ deletion	depression, anxiety, alcoholism G X E
μ-Opioid receptor	OPRM1 Asn40Asp functional, coding sequence	cortisol response to stressors; addiction treatment response
γ-Aminobutyric acid A receptor α2 subunit	GABRA2 haplotypes	alcoholism, anxiety
γ-Aminobutyric acid A receptor α6 subunit	GABRA6 Pro385Ser coding sequence	low response to alcohol and benzodiazepines
Glucocorticoid receptor	GR Asn63Ser, coding sequence GR BclI	cortisol response to acute stress
Neuropeptide Y	NPY -C485T, NPY Leu7Pro functional, promoter	increased social drinking, alcoholism
Cannabinoid receptor 1	CNR1 haplotypes	substance abuse
Galanin	GAL haplotypes	alcoholism, anxiety

VNTR: variable number of tandem repeats.

G X E: gene x environment interactions.

stress (reviewed in Weaver et al., 2005). The long-term maternal programming of the offspring's response to stress in adulthood has been shown to be due to reduced gene transcription caused by hypermethylation of a GR exon 1_7 promoter region associated with altered histone acetylation and reduced binding to nerve growth factor-inducible protein-A (NGF1-A; Weaver et al., 2004). A recent intriguing study suggests that this epigenetic phenomenon may be reversible in adult rats (Weaver et al., 2005).

V. THE "REWARD" PATHWAY OF ADDICTION: INTERACTION WITH STRESS

The mesolimbic dopamine (DA) system is implicated in the development of all addictions and is also stimulated by stress. It is fundamental to the drug-induced sensation of pleasure that acts as positive reinforcement. This "reward" pathway originates in the ventral tegmental area (VTA) of the midbrain and projects to the nucleus accumbens (NAc), the limbic system and the orbitofrontal cortex. The amygdala, hippocampus, and medial prefrontal cortex send excitatory projections to the NAc. The feeling of euphoria subsequent to drug ingestion is associated with increased synaptic DA in the NAc and elsewhere in the reward pathway that is entwined with complex changes in numerous neurotransmitters implicated in stress response including opioid peptides, cannabinoids, GABA, glutamate, and serotonin (5-HT). 5-HT neurons originating in the dorsal and median raphe nuclei project to mesolimbic structures, including the VTA and NAc, and may inhibit DA release by acting on NAc receptors: 5-HT1B, 5-HT2C, 5-HT3, 5-HT4, and 5-HT6 (see Table 6-2 for key to acronyms).

Transcription factor cAMP response element binding protein (CREB) is a component of many neurotransmitter signaling cascades that regulate expression of many genes in the reward pathway. Alcohol-preferring, anxious "P" rats have decreased CREB function and neuropeptide Y in the central and medial amygdala compared with nonalcohol preferring "NP" rats (Pandey et al., 2005b). Cocaine, morphine, alcohol, and several other drugs of abuse as well as stress activate CREB through phosphorylation at a specific site: Ser133. Chronic exposure to drugs and stress causes sustained activation of CREB that is associated with adaptation in the addictive process: reduction in reward (tolerance) and reduced sensitivity to stress (Barrot et al., 2002; Wand, 2005). CREB is also activated in relapse but in different parts of the brain depending on whether relapse is stress induced (amygdala) or drug (cocaine) induced (VTA) (Pandey et al., 2005a).

Unlike other addictive drugs that are more specific, alcohol has widespread effects throughout the brain. Alcohol acts at a variety of targets within cell membranes and in intracellular signal transduction, inducing effects on neurotransmitter and neurohormone membrane receptors and receptor-gated and voltage-activated ion channels. Alcohol alters the balance between GABA,

TABLE 6-2   Key to Acronyms

HPA axis	hypothalamic-pituitary-adrenal axis
LC-NE	locus coeruleus-norepinephrine system
CRF/H	corticotropin-releasing factor/hormone
ACTH	adrenocorticotropic hormone
GR	glucocorticoid receptor
VTA	ventral tegmental area
NAc	nucleus accumbens
OFC	orbitofrontal cortex
DA	dopamine
5-HT	serotonin
GABA	γ-aminobutyric acid
NMDA receptor	N-methyl-D-aspartate receptor
CREB	transcription factor cAMP response element binding protein

the major inhibitory neurotransmitter, and glutamate, the major excitatory neurotransmitter. Alcohol enhances GABA activity, and ingestion of large quantities leads to inhibition of glutamatergic neurotransmission, especially at the level of the postsynaptic N-methyl-D-aspartate (NMDA) receptor. Acute disruption of NMDA function may account for blackouts, whereas sensitization of NMDA receptors during chronic alcohol abuse may contribute to the neurotoxic effects of alcohol withdrawal and alcoholic brain injury (Tsai and Coyle, 1998).

VI. REWARD PATHWAY AND STRESS RESPONSE: KEY NEUROTRANSPORTER SYSTEMS

A. The Opioid System

The opioid system plays a key role in addiction and stress. Three endogenous opioid receptors—μ, δ, and κ—are the targets of the major opioid peptides, β-endorphin, enkephalins, and dynorphins. Heroin, morphine, and other exogenous opiates primarily interact with μ-opioid receptors that have several functions including response to pain, reward, and HPA stress responsivity (Kreek et al., 2005). Human and animal studies implicate the opioid system, particularly β-endorphin and the μ-opioid receptor, in sensitivity to the rewarding or reinforcing effects of opiates and alcohol. It has been shown that in nondrug-dependent rodents opiates can produce their acute rewarding effects through a dopamine-independent system mediated through brainstem reward circuits (Laviolette et al., 2004); however, in addicted animals the motivational effects of opiates derive from the mesolimbic DA system (Laviolette et al., 2002; Nader et al., 1997). $GABA_A$ receptors in the VTA control this bidirectional reward signaling; chronic opiate exposure and withdrawal induces CREB phosphorylation in a discrete population of rat VTA $GABA_A$ receptors that switches their functional conductance properties from an inhibitory to an excitatory signaling mode (Laviolette et al., 2004). This switching system (see Figure 6-1) has been shown to have considerable plasticity in rats, and it may have implications for the switch from controllable heavy drug use to addiction in humans.

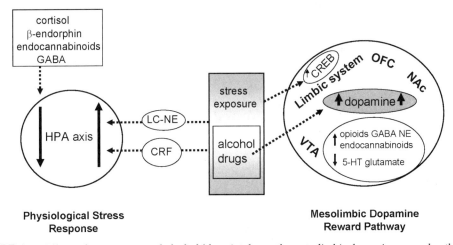

Physiological Stress Response

Mesolimbic Dopamine Reward Pathway

FIGURE 6-1 Effects of acute stress and alcohol/drug intake on the mesolimbic dopamine reward pathway and the physiological stress response system. These effects are modified after chronic stress or chronic alcohol/drug abuse.

Ethanol stimulates short-term β-endorphin release from the hypothalamus and pituitary (Oswald and Wand, 2004); however, chronic alcohol consumption results in decreased β-endorphin release and may be a factor in craving or negative reinforcement (Gianoulakis, 2001; Oswald and Wand, 2004). Alcohol self-administration is reduced in μ-opioid receptor knockout (KO) mice (Roberts et al., 2000). Abstinent alcoholics have increased densities of μ-opioid receptors in the ventral striatum including the NAc; densities correlate with severity of alcohol craving (Heinz et al., 2005b). μ-opioid receptor mRNA expression is elevated in rats subjected to repeated social defeat stress (Nikulina et al., 2005).

Although nicotinic acetylcholine receptors (nAchRs) in the NAc and VTA are the primary site of action of nicotine and are also involved in mediating ethanol-induced DA release in the NAc, CREB phosphorylation and upregulation of μ-opioid receptors is necessary for nicotine-conditioned reward (Berrendero et al., 2002; Walters et al., 2005).

Cocaine primarily acts through the inhibition of presynaptic DA transporters (DAT) as well as 5-HT and NE transporters, but it also modulates the endogenous opioid system, especially μ-opioid receptors. Selective disruption of genes has shown that the μ-opioid receptor gene, but not the DAT gene, is essential for cocaine self-administration (reviewed in Kreek et al., 2005).

A functional polymorphism, Asn40Asp (+118A/G), in the μ-opioid receptor gene (OPRM1) has frequencies ranging from 0.02 in African Americans, 0.12 in Caucasians, and 0.45 in Asians (Kreek et al., 2005). The Asp40 variant is associated with a threefold increase in β-endorphin binding affinity and potency, thereby theoretically increasing the inhibitory tone on CRF neurons (Bond et al., 1998). Thus the two alleles might be expected to show differences in HPA axis stress reactivity. Indeed, studies have shown that healthy men with the OPRM1 Asp40 variant had lower cortisol responses to psychological stressors than men with the Asn40 allele (Chong et al., 2006). There is supporting evidence from rhesus monkeys that have a functional polymorphism analogous to Asn40Asp; the variant allele is associated with lower basal and ACTH-stimulated plasma cortisol levels (Miller et al., 2004).

There have been many case-control studies that have looked at the association between opioid dependence and the Asp40 variant, other rarer OPRMI variants, and haplotypes, and nearly all have been negative (reviewed in Kreek et al., 2005). Some studies have found associations of the Asp40 variant with alcohol dependence (Bart et al., 2005; Schinka et al., 2002). However, other large studies in several different ethnic groups had negative results (Bergen et al., 1997; Schinka et al., 2002). A recent meta-analysis of 28 distinct samples and over 8,000 participants found no association with substance dependence (Arias et al., 2005). However, the relevance of this polymorphism may be in differential sensitivity to the drug and to relapse. The Asp40 variant has been associated with increased levels of subjective intoxication and higher levels of alcohol-induced sedation, and thus it could be protective against alcoholism severity (Ray and Hutchison, 2004). In general, alcoholics show reduced central dopaminergic sensitivity that is also associated with poor treatment outcome; however, alcoholics with the Asp40 variant have been shown to have significantly greater central dopaminergic receptor sensitivity after one week of abstinence compared with alcoholics without this variant, and this difference is not seen before detoxification or at 3 months of abstinence (Smolka et al., 1999). Administration of naltrexone, an opioid receptor antagonist acting primarily at the μ-opioid receptor, results in HPA axis activation and higher cortisol levels that are negatively correlated with intensity of alcohol craving (O'Malley et al., 2002). Individuals with the Asp40 variant have greater HPA activation in response to pharmacological blockade of μ-opioid receptors (Chong et al., 2006; Hernandez-Avila et al., 2003; Wand et al., 2002). Predictably, naltrexone-treated alcoholics with one or two copies of the Asp40 allele have significantly lower relapse rates and take longer to return to heavy drinking than Asn40 homozygotes (Oslin et al., 2003). In addition, the Asp40 variant has been associated with greater success with nicotine replacement therapy in smoking cessation treatment (Lerman et al., 2004).

B. Cannabinoids

The endocannabinoid signaling system has only recently been implicated in drug addiction, reward mechanisms, and stress. In the CNS this system consists of several endogenous ligands (endocannabinoids) including 2-arachidonoylglycerol (2-AG) and anandamide (arachidonoylethanolamide, AEA) that bind to G-protein–coupled CB1 receptors that are widely expressed in brain, including areas implicated in the processing of fear and emotion: amygdala, hippocampus, hypothalamus, and ventral striatum (Basavarajappa and Hungund, 2005). Most of the cells that highly express CB1 receptors are GABAergic interneurons.

Preclinical data suggest that endocannabinoids interacting with the CB1 receptor are involved in an animal's response to acute, repeated, and variable stress (reviewed in Carrier et al., 2005). It has been shown that blockade of endocannabinoid degradation is anxiolytic in mice (Kathuria et al., 2003), and endocannabinoid release in the hypothalamus inhibits HPA axis function in a context-dependent manner (Di et al., 2003; Pagotta et al., 2006; Patel et al., 2004). Although neither was sufficient on its own, environmental stress and CB1 agonist administration acted synergistically to produce activation within the central amygdala and this interaction could be important in understanding emotional and affective changes induced by cannabis intoxication (Patel et al., 2005).

Chronic alcohol consumption leads to increased synthesis of AEA and 2-AG and downregulation of CB1 receptors (Basavarajappa and Hungund, 2005). CB1 antagonists have been shown to reduce ethanol consumption in a wide variety of experimental paradigms (Manzanares et al., 2005). CB1 KO mice do not show ethanol-induced DA release in the NAc; likewise, treatment of wild-type mice with the CB1 antagonist SR141716 prior to alcohol ingestion blocks DA release in the NAc (Hungund et al., 2003). CB1 KO mice do not show alcohol withdrawal symptoms nor stress-induced alcohol consumption (Racz et al., 2003). The CB1 antagonist SR141716 has also been shown to reduce nicotine self-administration and nicotine-seeking behavior in rats several weeks after nicotine withdrawal (Cohen et al., 2005). A thorough analysis of potentially functional polymorphisms, including several start and splice variants, in the human CBI receptor gene (Cnr1), has recently been undertaken (Zhang et al., 2004). These investigators found significant differences in two haplotypes with differing mRNA expression levels between substance abusers and controls from three independent ethnic groups.

C. Serotonin (5-hydroxytryptamine, 5-HT)

HPA hyperactivity can lead to attenuation of central 5-HT transmission in a complex interaction, not yet fully understood. Variation in 5-HT function has been associated with negative mood states such as anxiety and depression. Pathologically low levels of 5-HT have been implicated in behavioral disinhibition disorders such as antisocial personality disorder and early onset male alcoholism (Linnoila et al., 1994).

The serotonin transporter (5-HTT) is largely responsible for terminating the synaptic actions of 5-HT and is the target of selective serotonin reuptake inhibitors (SSRIs) that are used to treat depression, anxiety, and comorbid alcoholism. In early abstinence (4 weeks) clinical depression has been associated with increased stress hormone activation and reduced 5-HTT levels in male but not female alcoholics (Heinz et al., 2002).

5-HTTLPR (genetic locus SLC6A4) is a common, variable number of tandem repeats polymorphism (44-base pair insertion/deletion) in the 5-HTT promoter region that alters transcription such that the less common, short "S" allele is associated with an approximately 50% reduction in 5-HTT availability and concomitant increase in synaptic 5-HT (Lesch et al., 1996). The promoter region of the 5-HTT gene contains a glucocorticoid response element, and this is a gateway for response to stress-induced changes in HPA axis activity; furthermore, the S variant shows an attenuated response to the synthetic glucocorticoid dexamethasone compared with the L variant (Glatz et al., 2003).

The S allele has been fairly consistently associated with increased anxiety and neuroticism (Lesch et al., 1996, Mazzanti et al., 1998). This may be partially mediated through the amygdala since individuals with the S allele show greater amygdala neuronal activity in response to fearful stimuli (Hariri et al., 2005). Also, extinction of negative affect is dependent on tight coupling of a feedback circuit between the amygdala and the perigenual cingulate; S allele carriers show uncoupling of this circuit, and the degree of uncoupling accounts for 30% of the variance in anxious temperament (Pezawas et al., 2005). Conversely, S allele carriers show greater coupling between the amygdala and the ventromedial prefrontal cortex (Heinz et al., 2005a), a limbic brain area implicated in major depression (Drevets, 2003). This greater coupling may reflect a lower resilience to negative emotions when stressed; for example, in a longitudinal cohort study the S allele was shown to significantly increase the risk for depression and suicide but only in individuals who had experienced stressful life events (Caspi et al., 2003). In a population-based twin study, individuals with the SS genotype were shown to have increased sensitivity to the depressogenic effects of common, low-threat events (Kendler et al., 2005).

Although in rhesus macaque monkeys, 82% of the variance in alcohol intake can be explained by 5-HTT availability (Heinz et al., 2003), there have been inconsistent results for the association of 5-HTTLPR with alcoholism in humans. The L allele has been associated with an increased subjective high upon drinking alcohol (Fromme et al., 2004) as well as a low response to the sedating effects of alcohol in alcohol-naïve humans (Hu et al., 2005) and rhesus macaque monkeys (Barr et al., 2003) and thus might increase vulnerability to addiction. However a recent meta-analysis of 17 published studies showed that the S allele increased the odds of an alcoholism diagnosis by at least 18% and increased the odds of alcoholism with comorbid psychopathology or early onset or more severe disease by 34% (Feinn et al., 2005). Possible reasons for the discrepancy in results are emerging. It has recently been reported that there are functional subtypes within 5-HTTLPR that may be masking findings (Hu et al., 2006). In addition, there may be sexually dimorphic effects, and phenotypic expression may be dependent upon the interaction of genotype and environment. For example, female macaque monkeys with the S allele that had experienced early-life stress consumed more alcohol, with progressive increase in consumption over time (Barr et al., 2004). There has been no association between 5-HTTLPR and cocaine abuse (Manelli et al., 2005), or with other drugs of abuse.

D. γ-Aminobutyric acid (GABA)

GABA inhibits, whereas glutamate activates, the HPA axis responses to stress (Herman et al., 2004). Acute stress immediately reduces GABA-stimulated chloride influx in the frontal cortex and amygdala (Martijena et al., 2002). $GABA_A$ receptors are the site of action of benzodiazepines that diminish HPA axis responsivity. $GABA_A$ receptors are affected by acute and chronic ethanol consumption and are implicated in ethanol self-administration, tolerance, and dependence.

Early life stress permanently alters $GABA_A$ receptor subunit expression in the hippocampus such that $GABA_A\alpha 2$ predominates in the stressed animals, whereas $GABA_A\alpha 1$ predominates in emotionally healthy animals (Hsu et al., 2003). The $GABA_A\alpha 2$ subunit gene (*GABRA2*) appears to mediate the anxiolytic effects of benzodiazepines (Low et al., 2000); mice with a *GABRA2* knockin point mutation are insensitive to benzodiazepines' anxiolytic effects (Low et al., 2000). *GABRA2* may therefore play an important role in mediating stress and anxiety responses. Indeed, GABRA2 haplotypes have been associated with alcoholism (Covault et al., 2004; Edenberg et al., 2004) as well as alcoholism mediated by anxiety (Enoch et al., 2006).

The Pro385Ser substitution in the $GABA_A\alpha 6$ subunit gene, GABRA6, has been associated with a lower level of response to the sedating effects of alcohol (Hu et al., 2005), and with reduced sensitivity to the effects of diazepam in children of alcoholics (Iwata et al., 1999). In addition, several studies have found associations between this GABRA6 polymorphism and alcohol dependence (Radel et al., 2005).

VII. LIMBIC REGULATION OF RESPONSE TO STRESS

The limbic behavioral stress response system plays a major role in stress-induced relapse in rodents. During acute stress, HPA axis regulation is dominated by signals from the limbic system and prefrontal system; chronic alcohol and nicotine use can modify these interactions and may account for the blunting of HPA responses seen in addiction (Lovallo, 2006). Anxiety, mood disturbances, and negative affect are common in abstinence and can persist for many months. CRF is thought to be important in stress-related anxiety, whereas neuropep-

tide Y (NPY) is anxiolytic. It is thought that CRF and NPY maintain a state of emotional homeostasis via the amygdala that may be altered in addiction. In addition, it has recently been shown that another neuropeptide may be involved in the balancing of behaviors; galanin acting in the central amygdala counteracts the anxiogenic effects of NE in response to severe stress.

A. Corticotropin-Releasing Factor (CRF)

CRF is a 41-amino acid peptide with binding sites in the anterior pituitary, amygdala, cerebral cortex, and the hippocampus. When CRF is centrally administered to rats, it increases anxiety-like behavior across a wide range of paradigms (Bruijnzeel and Gold, 2005). It is a key regulator of the HPA axis via the CRF1 receptor. Drugs of abuse induce the release of ACTH and corticosterone via a CRF-receptor dependent mechanism (Bruijnzeel and Gold, 2005). Drug withdrawal activates limbic CRF (Rodriguez de Fonseca et al., 1997). CRF is thought to contribute to stress-induced relapse via its actions on extrahypothalamic sites (Le et al., 2000). CRF is localized and cosynthesized within GABAergic neurons in the central amygdala, and in this location CRF1 receptors have been shown to mediate ethanol enhancement of GABAergic synaptic transmission (Nie et al., 2004). The CRF1 receptor has been implicated in anxiety and the modulation of ethanol, heroin, cocaine, and morphine intake and withdrawal in rodents: The selective CRF1 antagonist CP-154,526 has been shown to decrease stress-induced relapse in rats (Le et al., 2000; Wang et al., 2005). Moreover, Antalarmin, a selective CRF1 antagonist, reduces levels of voluntary ethanol consumption and ethanol preference in pretreated rats (Lodge and Laurence, 2003). In humans, CRF1 genotype predicted binge drinking and increased alcohol consumption (Treutlin et al 2006), but not anxious temperament, in alcoholics (Soyka et al., 2004). ACTH and corticosterone responses to alcohol are significantly blunted in CRF1-deficient mice (Lee et al., 2001). Unstressed CRF1-deficient mice do not differ in alcohol intake from wild-type mice; however, they respond to repeated stress by a progressive increase in alcohol consumption that persists throughout life and is associated with upregulation of the NMDA receptor subunit NR2B, an ethanol-sensitive site (Nagy, 2004) that is also influenced by stress (Sillaber et al., 2002). The results of Sillaber et al.'s study suggest that the interaction of stress with dysregulation of the CRF1 gene and/or changes in NR2B subunits could predispose to alcoholism. There is a known functional polymorphism, -200T>G(rs1019385), in the NR2B gene, but the few human studies that have been done have shown no association with alcoholism, possibly because stress was not included as a factor.

B. Neuropeptide Y (NPY)

NPY is a 36 amino acid neuropeptide that is widely expressed in the brain and is thought to be involved in the regulation of stress-related behaviors, appetite, reward, and voluntary alcohol consumption in rodents (Pandey et al., 2003). In humans, acute stress activates NPY, cortisol, and NE release (Morgan et al., 2002). NPY levels are negatively correlated with psychological distress during stress suggesting that NPY is anxiolytic (Morgan et al., 2002). Exogenous NPY has been shown to diminish experimental anxiety in a wide range of animal models, acting via central NPY Y1 receptors (Heilig and Thorsell, 2002; Pandey et al., 2003). Blockade of central NPY Y2 receptors, thought to be presynaptic autoreceptors that inhibit NPY release, reduces ethanol self-administration in rats (Thorsell et al., 2002). The anxiolytic actions of NPY can be reproduced by Y1 receptor agonists or Y2 receptor antagonists (Heilig, 2004). Decreased CREB phosphorylation and NPY expression in the central amygdala might be associated with ethanol withdrawal-induced anxiety (Pandey et al., 2003). Studies in

humans have so far identified a functional promoter polymorphism, -C485T, and a coding sequence polymorphism, Leu7Pro (T1128C), in the preproNPY gene. The Pro7 allele has been associated with increased (34%) social drinking in a large population sample of ethnically homogeneous middle-aged Finnish men (Kauhanen et al., 2000b). One study of U.S. Caucasian men and women has shown an association with alcoholism (Lappalainen et al., 2002), but another large study of Finnish and Swedish male alcoholics with carefully ethnically matched controls found no relationship (Zhu et al., 2003). A recent haplotype-based analysis found an association with alcohol dependence (Mottagui-Tabar et al., 2005).

C. Galanin (GAL)

GAL is a 30 amino acid neuropeptide that is widely expressed in the CNS. GAL coexists with 5-HT in dorsal raphe neurons and NE in LC neurons and inhibits the release of these neurotransmitters (Yoshitake et al., 2004). There is a complex interaction between GAL and NE in the behavioral stress response. Under conditions of high stress but not mild stress, GAL is released in the central amygdala and has an anxiolytic effect (Khoshbouei et al., 2002). GAL has been implicated in alcoholism and anxiety in animal studies (reviewed in Belfer et al., 2006). A recent study in two ethnically diverse human populations has found a haplotype association with alcoholism, possibly mediated by anxiety (Belfer et al., 2006).

VIII. THE LOCUS COERULEUS (LC)-NOREPINEPHRINE (NE) SYSTEM

The LC is activated by a variety of stressors, both intrinsic and extrinsic, resulting in increased NE release in CNS regions implicated in the regulation of emotionality such as the prefrontal cortex, the amygdala, and the hippocampus (Charney, 2004). The LC-

NE system is instrumental in stress-induced relapse in rodents. NE plays an important role in regulating the HPA axis stress response; indeed, ACTH response to a stressor has been correlated with average basal NE activity (Young et al., 2005). Although NE influences the magnitude of the HPA axis response to stress in healthy individuals, in depressed individuals HPA axis activation appears to be independent of NE influence (Young et al., 2005). Animal studies have shown that release of prefrontal NE is essential for morphine-induced reward and DA release in the NAc (Ventura et al., 2005). Alpha-2 adrenoceptors that influence NE activity are known to be involved in stress-induced reinstatement of heroin, cocaine, and alcohol seeking in rodents (Le et al., 2005). The NE transporter (NET) mediates re uptake and is a target for tricyclic antidepressants and psychostimulants. The NET gene has been shown to influence ethanol sensitivity in inbred long-sleep and short-sleep mice (Haughey et al., 2005). Several functional variants have been identified in humans, but as yet no published study has looked at associations with stress or addiction (Hahn et al., 2005).

Catechol-O-methyltransferase (COMT) plays an important role in the metabolism of CNS NE and DA (Huotari et al., 2002). A common COMT polymorphism, Val158Met, confined to humans, is responsible for a three- to fourfold variation in enzyme activity (Chen et al., 2004; Weinshilboum et al., 1999). The lower activity Met158 allele has been associated with greater activation in emotion-modulating brain regions, including the limbic system and connected prefrontal areas, in response to unpleasant visual stimuli (Smolka et al., 2005). The Met158 allele is also associated with a more anxious, cautious personality (Enoch et al., 2003; Olsson et al., 2005; Zubiéta et al., 2003). Met158 homozygous individuals have regionally diminished μ-opioid binding potential in the NAc, increased sensitivity to pain, and greater HPA axis response to μ-opioid receptor blockade (Oswald et al., 2004; Zubieta et al., 2003).

Thus COMT genotype may play an important role in the balance between emotional resilience and vulnerability toward stress.

COMT Val158Met has been linked with addiction. The Val158 allele has been found to be more abundant in drug abusers (Horowitz et al., 2000; Li et al., 2004; Vandenbergh et al., 1997) and also in Native American alcoholics with a binge pattern of drinking (Enoch et al., 2006). Val158 has been associated with the development of adult psychosis in adolescent cannabis users (Caspi et al., 2005). Conversely, in European men Met158 has been associated with late onset alcoholism (Hallikainen et al., 2000; Tiihonen et al., 1999) as well as increased alcohol intake in male social drinkers (Kauhanen et al., 2000a). In women, Met158 has been found to be protective against smoking and is associated with increased likelihood of smoking cessation (Colilla et al., 2005; Enoch et al., 2006).

IX. CONCLUSIONS

Genetic vulnerability for the development of addiction, for stress associated with addiction, and for stress-induced relapse is complex. It is likely to be due to additive and nonadditive (epistatic) interactions of multiple gene variants with small to modest effects. These genetic variants will be found in neurobiological pathways and signal transduction systems within, and linking, the dopamine reward pathway and the stress response system. Stress-influenced neurodevelopmental alterations in gene expression that increase vulnerability to further stress and hence addiction are also likely to be important.

REFERENCES

Adinoff, B., Junghanns, K., Kiefer, F., and Krishnan-Sarin, S. (2005). Suppression of the HPA axis stress-response: Implications for relapse. *Alcohol Clin Exp Res, 29,* 1351–1355.

American Psychiatric Association. (1994). *Diagnostic and statistical manual of mental disorders* (4th ed.). Washington, DC: Author.

Arias, A., Feinn, R., and Kranzler, H. R. (2006, December 29). Association of an Asn40Asp (A118G) polymorphism in the mu-opioid receptor gene with substance dependence: A meta-analysis. *Drug Alcohol Depend 83,* 262–268.

Barna, I., Zelena, D., Arszovszki, A. C., and Ledent, C. (2004). The role of endogenous cannabinoids in the hypothalamo-pituitary-adrenal axis regulation: In vivo and in vitro studies in CB1 receptor knockout mice. *Life Sci, 75,* 2959–2970.

Barr, C. S., Newman, T. K., Becker, M. L., Champoux, M., Lesch, K. P., Suomi, S. J., Goldman, D., and Higley, J. D. (2003). Serotonin transporter gene variation is associated with alcohol sensitivity in rhesus macaques exposed to early-life stress. *Alcohol Clin Exp Res, 27,* 812–817.

Barr, C. S., Newman, T. K., Lindell, S., Shannon, C., Champoux, M., Lesch, K. P., Suomi S. J., Goldman, D., and Higley, J. D. (2004). Interaction between serotonin transporter gene variation and rearing condition in alcohol preference and consumption in female primates. *Arch Gen Psychiatry, 61,* 1146–1152.

Barrot, M., Olivier, J. D., Perrotti, L. I., DiLeone, R. J., Berton, O., Eisch, A. J., Impey, S., Storm, D. R., Neve, R. L., Yin, J. C., Zachario, V., and Nestler, E. J. (2002). CREB activity in the nucleus accumbens shell controls gating of behavioral responses to emotional stimuli. *Proc Natl Acad Sci U S A, 99,* 11430–11440.

Bart, G., Kreek, M. J., Ott, J. F., LaForge, K. S., Proudnikov, D., Pollak, L., and Heilig, M. (2005). Increased attributable risk related to a functional mu-opioid receptor gene polymorphism in association with alcohol dependence in central Sweden. *Neuropsychopharmacology, 30,* 417–422.

Bartels, M., de Geus, E. J., Kirschbaum, C., and Sluyter, F. (2003). Heritability of daytime cortisol levels in children. *Behav Genet, 33,* 421–433.

Basavarajappa, B. S., and Hungund, B. L. (2005). Role of the endocannabinoid system in the development of tolerance to alcohol. *Alcohol Alcohol, 40,* 15–24.

Belfer, I., Hipp, H., McKnight, C., Evans, C., Buzas, B., Bollettino, A., Albaugh, B., Virkkunen, M., Yuan, Q., Max, M. B., Goldman, D., and Enoch, M. A. (2006). Association of galanin haplotypes with alcoholism and anxiety in two ethnically distinct populations. *Mol Psychiatry, 11,* 301–311.

Bergen, A. W., Kokoszka, J., Peterson, R., Long, J. C., Virkkunen, M., Linnoila, M., and Goldman, D. (1997). Mu opioid receptor gene variants: Lack of association with alcohol dependence. *Mol Psychiatry, 2,* 490–494.

Berrendero, F., Kieffer, B. L., and Maldonado, R. (2002). Attenuation of nicotine-induced antinociception, rewarding effects, and dependence in mu-opioid receptor knock-out mice. *J Neurosci, 22,* 10935–10940.

Bierut, L. J., Dinwiddie, S. H., Begleiter, H., Crowe, R. R., Hesselbrock., V., Nurnberger, J. I., Porjesz, B., Schuckit, M. A., and Reich, T. (1998). Familial transmission of substance dependence: Alcohol, marijuana, cocaine and habitual smoking. *Arch Gen Psychiatry, 55,*982–988.

Bond, C., LaForg, K. S., Tian, M., Melia, D., Zhang, S., Borg, L., Gong, J., Schluger, J., Strong, J. A., Leal, S. M., Tischfield, J. A., Kreek, M. J., and Yu, L. (1998). Single-nucleotide polymorphism in the human mu opioid receptor gene alters beta-endorphin binding and activity: Possible implications for opiate addiction. *Proc Natl Acad Sci U S A, 95,* 9608–9613.

Bruijnzeel, A. W., and Gold, M. S. (2005). The role of corticotropin-releasing factor-like peptides in cannabis, nicotine, and alcohol dependence. *Brain Res Rev, 49,* 505–528.

Carrier, E. J., Patel, S., and Hillard, C. J. (2005). Endocannabinoids in neuroimmunology and stress. *Curr Drug Targets CNS Neurol Disord, 4,* 657–665.

Caspi, A., McClay, J., Moffitt, T. E., Mill, J., Martin, J., Craig, I. W., Taylor, A., and Poulton, R. (2002). Role of genotype in the cycle of violence in maltreated children. *Science, 297,* 851–853.

Caspi, A., Moffitt, T. E., Cannon, M., McClay, J., Murray, R., Harrington, H., Taylor, A., Arseneault, L., Williams, B., Braithwaite, A., Poulton, R., and Craig, I. W. (2005). Moderation of the effect of adolescent-onset cannabis use on adult psychosis by a functional polymorphism in the catechol-O-methyltransferase gene: Longitudinal evidence of a gene X environment interaction. *Biol Psychiatry, 57,* 1117–1127.

Caspi, A., Sugden, K., Moffitt, T. E., Taylor, A., Craig, I. W., Harrington, H., McClay, J., Mill, J., Martin, J., Braithwaite, A., and Poulton, R. (2003). Influence of life stress on depression: Moderation by a polymorphism in the 5-HTT gene. *Science, 301,* 386–389.

Charney, D. S. (2004). Psychobiological mechanisms of resilience and vulnerability: Implications for successful adaptation to extreme stress. *Am J Psychiatry, 161,* 195–216.

Chen, J., Lipska, B. K., Halim, N., Ma, Q. D., Matsumoto, M., Melhem, S., Kolachana, B. S., Hyde, T. M., Herman, M. M., Apud, J., Egan, M. F., Kleinman, J. E., and Weinberger, D. R. (2004). Functional analysis of genetic variation in catechol-O-methyltransferase (COMT): Effects on mRNA, protein, and enzyme activity in postmortem human brain. *Am J Hum Genet, 75,* 807–821.

Chong, R. Y., Oswald, L., Yang, X., Uhart, M., Lin, P. I., and Wand, G. S. (2006). The mu-opioid receptor polymorphism A118G predicts cortisol responses to naloxone and stress. *Neuropsychopharmacology, 31,* 204–211.

Cohen, C., Perrault, G., Griebel, G., and Soubrie, P. (2005). Nicotine-associated cues maintain nicotine-seeking behavior in rats several weeks after nicotine withdrawal: Reversal by the cannabinoid

(CB1) receptor antagonist, rimonabant (SR141716). *Neuropsychopharmacology, 30,* 145–155.

Colilla, S., Lerman, C., Shields, P. G., Jepson, C., Rukstalis, M., Berlin, J., DeMichele, A., Bunin, G., Strom, B. L., and Rebbeck, T. R. (2005). Association of catechol-O-methyltransferase with smoking cessation in two independent studies of women. *Pharmacogenet Genomics, 15,* 393–398.

Covault, J., Gelernter, J., Hesselbrock, V., Nellissery, M., and Kranzler, H. R. (2004). Allelic and haplotypic association of GABRA2 with alcohol dependence. *Am J Med Genet (Neuropsychiatr Genet), 129B,* 104–109.

Covington, H. E. 3rd, and Miczek, K. A. (2005). Intense cocaine self-administration after episodic social defeat stress, but not after aggressive behavior: Dissociation from corticosterone activation. *Psychopharmacology (Berl), 183,* 331–340.

Dai, X., Thavundayil, J., and Gianoulakis, C. (2005). Differences in the peripheral levels of beta-endorphin in response to alcohol and stress as a function of alcohol dependence and family history of alcoholism. *Alcohol Clin Exp Res, 29,* 1965–1975.

DeRijk, R., and de Kloet, E. R. (2005). Corticosteroid receptor genetic polymorphisms and stress responsivity. *Endocrine, 28,* 263–270.

Di, S., Malcher-Lopes, R., Halmos, K. C., and Tasker, J. G. (2003). Nongenomic glucocorticoid inhibition via endocannabinoid release in the hypothalamus: A fast feedback mechanism. *J Neurosci, 23,* 4850–4857.

Drevets, W. C. (2003). Neuroimaging abnormalities in the amygdala in mood disorders. *Ann N Y Acad Sci, 985,* 420–444.

Edenberg, H. J., Dick, D. M., Xuei, X., Tian, H., Almasy, L., Bauer, L. O., Crowe, R. R., Goate, A., Hesselbrock, V., Jones, K., Kwon, J., Li, T. K., Nurnberger, J. I. Jr, O'Connor, S. J., Reich, T., Rice, J., Schuckit, M. A., Porjesz, B., Foroud, T., and Begleiter, H. (2004). Variations in GABRA2, encoding the alpha 2 subunit of the GABA(A) receptor, are associated with alcohol dependence and with brain oscillations. *Am J Hum Genet, 74,* 705–714.

Enoch, M. A., Schwartz, L., Albaugh, B., Virkkunen, M., Goldman, D. (In press). Dimensional anxiety mediates linkage of GABRA2 haplotypes with alcoholism. *AM J Med Genet Neuropsychiatr Genet.*

Enoch, M. A., Waheed, J., Harris, C. R., Albaugh, B., and Goldman, D. (2006). Sex differences in the influence of COMT Val158Met on alcoholism and smoking in Plains American Indians. *Alcohol Clin Exp Res, 30,* 399–406.

Enoch, M. A., Xu, K., Ferro, E., Harris, C. R., and Goldman, D. (2003). Genetic origins of anxiety in women: A role for a functional catechol-O-methyltransferase polymorphism. *Psychiatr Genet, 13,* 33–41.

Federenko, I. S., Nagamine, M., Hellhammer, D. H., Wadha, P. D., and Wust, S. (2004). The heritability of hypothalamus pituitary adrenal axis responses to psychosocial stress is context dependent. *J Clin Endocrinol Metab, 89,* 6244–6250.

Feinn, R., Nellissery, M., and Kranzler, H. R. (2005). Meta-analysis of the association of a functional serotonin transporter promoter polymorphism with alcohol dependence. *Am J Med Genet B Neuropsychiatr Genet, 133,* 79–84.

Foley, D. L., Eaves, L. J., Wormley, B., Silberg, J. L., Maes, H. H., Kuhn, J., and Riley, B. (2004). Childhood adversity, monoamine oxidase a genotype, and risk for conduct disorder. *Arch Gen Psychiatry, 61,* 738–744.

Fromme, K., de Wit, H., Hutchison, K. E., Ray, L., Corbin, W. R., Cook, T. A., Wall, T. L., and Goldman, D. (2004). Biological and behavioral markers of alcohol sensitivity. *Alcohol Clin Exp Res, 28,* 247–256.

Gianoulakis, C. (2001). Influence of the endogenous opioid system on high alcohol consumption and genetic predisposition to alcoholism. *J Psychiatry Neurosci, 26,* 304–318.

Glatz, K., Mossner, R., Heils, A., and Lesch, K. P. (2003). Glucocorticoid-regulated human serotonin transporter (5-HTT) expression is modulated by the 5-HTT gene-promoter–linked polymorphic region. *J Neurochem, 86,* 1072–1078.

Goldman, D., Oroszi, G., and Ducci, F. (2005). The genetics of addictions: Uncovering the genes. *Nat Rev Genet, 6,* 521–532.

Grant, B. F., Hasin, D. S., Chou, S. P., Stinson, F. S., and Dawson, D. A. (2004). Nicotine dependence and psychiatric disorders in the United States: Results from the national epidemiologic survey on alcohol and related conditions. *Arch Gen Psychiatry, 61,* 1107–1115.

Hahn, M. K., Mazei-Robison, M. S., and Blakely, R. D. (2005). Single nucleotide polymorphisms in the human norepinephrine transporter gene affect expression, trafficking, antidepressant interaction, and protein kinase C regulation. *Mol Pharmacol, 68,* 457–466.

Hallikainen, T., Lachman, H., Saito, T., Volavka, J., Kauhanen, J., Salonen, J. T., Ryynanen, O., Koulu, M., Karvonen, M. K., Pohjalainen, T., Syvalahti, E., Hietala, J., and Tiihonen, J. (2000). Lack of association between the functional variant of the catechol-o-methyltransferase (COMT) gene and early-onset alcoholism associated with severe antisocial behavior. *Am J Med Genet, 96,* 348–352.

Hariri, A. R., Drabant, E. M., Munoz, K. E., Kolachana, B. S., Mattay, V. S., Egan, M. F., and Weinberger, D. R. (2005). A susceptibility gene for affective disorders and the response of the human amygdala. *Arch Gen Psychiatry, 62,* 146–152.

Haughey, H. M., Kaiser, A. L., Johnson, T. E., Bennett, B., Sikela, J. M., and Zahniser, N. R. (2005). Norepinephrine transporter: A candidate gene for initial ethanol sensitivity in inbred long-sleep and short-sleep mice. *Alcohol Clin Exp Res, 29,* 1759–1768.

Heilig, M. (2004). The NPY system in stress, anxiety and depression. *Neuropeptides, 38,* 213–224.

Heilig, M., and Thorsell, A. (2002). Brain neuropeptide Y (NPY) in stress and alcohol dependence. *Rev Neurosci, 13,* 85–94.

Heinz, A., Braus, D. F., Smolka, M. N., Wrase, J., Puls, I., Hermann, D., Klein, S., Grusser, S. M., Flor, H., Schumann, G., Mann, K., and Buchel, C. (2005a). Amygdala-prefrontal coupling depends on a genetic variation of the serotonin transporter. *Nat Neurosci, 8,* 20–21.

Heinz, A., Jones, D. W., Bissette, G., Hommer, D., Ragan, P., Knable, M., Wellek, S., Linnoila, M., and Weinberger, D. R. (2002). Relationship between cortisol and serotonin metabolites and transporters in alcoholism. *Pharmacopsychiatry, 35,* 127–134.

Heinz, A., Jones, D. W., Gorey, J. G., Bennet, A., Suomi, S. J., Weinberger, D. R., and Higley, J. D. (2003). Serotonin transporter availability correlates with alcohol intake in non-human primates. *Mol Psychiatry, 8,* 231–234.

Heinz, A., Reimold, M., Wrase, J., Hermann, D., Croissant, B., Mundle, G., Dohmen, B. M., Braus, D. F., Schumann, G., Machulla, H. J., Bares, R., and Mann, K. (2005b). Correlation of stable elevations in striatal μ-opioid receptor availability in detoxified alcoholic patients with alcohol craving: A positron emission tomography study using carbon 11-labeled carfentanil. *Arch Gen Psychiatry, 62,* 57–64.

Herman, J. P., Mueller, N. K., and Figueiredo, H. (2004). Role of GABA and glutamate circuitry in hypothalamo-pituitary-adrenocortical stress integration. *Ann N Y Acad Sci, 1018,* 35–45.

Hernandez-Avila, C. A., Wand, G., Luo, X., Gelernter, J., and Kranzler, H. R. (2003). Association between the cortisol response to opioid blockade and the Asn40Asp polymorphism at the mu-opioid receptor locus (OPRM1). *Am J Med Genet B Neuropsychiatr Genet, 118,* 60–65.

Hettema, J. M., Corey, L. A., and Kendler, K. S. (1999). A multivariate genetic analysis of the use of tobacco, alcohol and caffeine in a population-based sample of male and female twins. *Drug Alcohol Depend, 57,* 69–78.

Hicks, B. M., Krueger, R. F., Iacono, W. G., McGue, M., and Patrick, C. J. (2004). Family transmission and heritability of externalizing disorders: A twin-family study. *Arch Gen Psychiatry, 61,* 922–928.

Higley, J. D., Hasert, M. F., Suomi, S. J., and Linnoila, M. (1991). Nonhuman primate model of alcohol abuse: Effects of early experience, personality, and stress on alcohol consumption. *Proc Natl Acad Sci U S A, 88,* 7261–7265.

Horowitz, R., Kotler, M., Shufman, E., Aharoni, S., Kremer, I., Cohen, H., and Ebstein, R. P. (2000). Confirmation of an excess of the high enzyme activity COMT val allele in heroin addicts in a family-based haplotype relative risk study. *Am J Med Genet, 96,* 599–603.

Hsu, F. C., Zhang, G. J., Raol, Y. S., Valentino, R. J., Coulter, D. A., and Brooks-Kayal, A. R. (2003). Repeated neonatal handling with maternal separation permanently alters hippocampal GABAA receptors and behavioral stress responses. *Proc Natl Acad Sci U S A, 100,* 12213–12218.

Hu, X., Oroszi, G., Chun, J., Smith, T. L., Goldman, D., and Schuckit, M. A. (2005). An expanded evaluation of the relationship of four alleles to the level of response to alcohol and the alcoholism risk. *Alcohol Clin Exp Res, 29,* 8–16.

Hu. X. Z., Lipsky, R. H., Zhu, G., Akhtar, L. A., Taubman, J., Greenberg, B. D., Xu, K., Arnold, P. D., Richter, M. A, Kennedy, J. L., Murphy, D. L., and Goldman, D. (2006). Serotonin transporter promoter gain-of-function genotypes are linked to obsessive-compulsive disorder. *Am J Hum Genet, 78,* 815-826.

Hungund, B. L., Szakall, I., Adam, A., Basavarajappa, B. S., and Vadasz, C. (2003). Cannabinoid CB1 receptor knockout mice exhibit markedly reduced voluntary alcohol consumption and lack alcohol-induced dopamine release in the nucleus accumbens. *J Neurochem, 84,* 698–704.

Huotari, M., Gogos, J. A., Karayiorgou, M., Koponen, O., Forsberg, M., Raasmaja, A., Hyttinen, J., and Mannisto, P. T. (2002). Brain catecholamine metabolism in catechol-O-methyltransferase (COMT)-deficient mice. *Eur J Neurosci, 15,* 246–256.

Iwata, N., Cowley, D. S., Radel, M., Roy-Byrne, P. P., and Goldman, D. (1999). Relationship between a $GABA_{Aa6}$ Pro385Ser substitution and benzodiazepine sensitivity. *Am J Psychiatry, 156,* 1447–1449.

Kauhanen, J., Hallikainen, T., Tuomainen, T. P., Koulu, M., Karvonen, M. K., Salonen, J. T., and Tiihonen, J. (2000a). Association between the functional polymorphism of catechol-O-methyltransferase gene and alcohol consumption among social drinkers. *Alcohol Clin Exp Res, 24,* 135–139.

Kauhanen, J., Karvonen, M. K., Pesonen, U., Koulu, M., Tuomainen, T. P., Uusitupa, M. I., and Salonen, J. T. (2000b). Neuropeptide Y polymorphism and alcohol consumption in middle-aged men. *Am J Med Genet, 93,* 117–121.

Kathuria, S., Gaetani, S., Fegley, D., Valino, F., Duranti, A., Tontini, A., Mor, M., Tarzia, G., La Rana, G., Calignano, A., Giustino, A., Tattoli, M., Palmery, M., Cuomo, V., and Piomelli, D. (2003). Modulation of anxiety through blockade of anandamide hydrolysis. *Nat Med, 9,* 76–81.

Kendler, K. S., Davis, C. G., and Kessler, R. C. (1997) The familial aggregation of common psychiatric and substance abuse disorders in the National Comorbidity Survey: A family history study. *Br J Psychiatry, 170,* 541–548.

Kendler, K. S., Jacobson, K. C., Prescott, C. A., and Neale, M. C. (2003a). Specificity of genetic and environmental risk factors for use and abuse/dependence of cannabis, cocaine, hallucinogens, sedatives, stimulants, and opiates in male twins. *Am J Psychiatry, 160,* 687–695.

Kendler, K. S., Karkowski, L. M., Neale, M. C., and Prescott, C. A. (2000). Illicit psychoactive use, heavy use, abuse, and dependence in a US population-based sample of male twins. *Arch Gen Psychiatry, 57,* 261–269.

Kendler, K. S., Kuhn, J. W., Vittum, J., Prescott, C. A., and Riley, B. (2005). The interaction of stressful life events and a serotonin transporter polymorphism in the prediction of episodes of major depression: A replication. *Arch Gen Psychiatry, 62,* 529–535.

Kendler, K. S., Prescott, C. A., Myers, J., and Neale, M. C. (2003b). The structure of genetic and environmental risk factors for common psychiatric and substance use disorders in men and women. *Arch Gen Psychiatry, 60,* 929–937.

Khoshbouei, H., Cecchi, M., Dove, S., Javors, M., and Morilak, D. A. (2002). Behavioral reactivity to stress: Amplification of stress-induced noradrenergic activation elicits a galanin-mediated anxiolytic effect in central amygdala. *Pharmacol Biochem Behav, 71,* 407– 417.

Knopik, V. S., Heath, A. C., Madden, P. A., Bucholz, K. K., Slutske, W. S., Nelson, E. C., Statham, D., Whitfield. J. B. and Martin, N. G (2004). Genetic effects on alcohol dependence risk: Re-evaluating the importance of psychiatric and other heritable risk factors. *Psychol Med, 34,* 1519–1530.

Koob, G. F. (2003). Alcoholism: Allostasis and beyond. *Alcohol Clin Exp Res, 27,* 232–243.

Kreek, M. J., Bart, G., Lilly, C., Laforge, K. S., and Nielsen, D. A. (2005). Pharmacogenetics and human molecular genetics of opiate and cocaine addictions and their treatments. *Pharmacol Rev, 57,* 1–26.

Kruger, R. F. (1999). The structure of common mental disorders. *Arch Gen Psychiatry, 56,* 921–926.

Lappalainen, J., Kranzler, H. R., Malison, R., Price, L. H., Van Dyck, C., Rosenheck, R. A., Cramer, J., Southwick, S., Charney, D., Krystal, J., and Gelernter, J. (2002). A functional neuropeptide Y Leu7Pro polymorphism associated with alcohol dependence in a large population sample from the United States. *Arch Gen Psychiatry, 59,* 825–831.

Laviolette, S. R., Gallegos, R. A., Henriksen, S. J., and van der Kooy, D. (2004). Opiate state controls bidirectional reward signaling via GABAA receptors in the ventral tegmental area. *Nat Neurosci, 7,* 160–169.

Laviolette, S. R., Nader, K., and van der Kooy, D. (2002). Motivational state determines the functional role of the mesolimbic dopamine system in the mediation of opiate reward processes. *Behav Brain Res, 129,* 17–29.

Le, A. D., Harding, S., Juzytsch, W., Funk, D., and Shaham, Y. (2005). Role of alpha-2 adrenoceptors in stress-induced reinstatement of alcohol seeking and alcohol self-administration in rats. *Psychopharmacology (Berl), 179,* 366–373.

Le, A. D., Harding, S., Juzytsch, W., Watchus, J., Shalev, U., and Shaham, Y. (2000). The role of corticotropin-releasing factor in stress-induced relapse to alcohol-seeking behavior in rats. *Psychopharmacology (Berl), 150,* 317–324.

Lee, S., Smith, G. W., Vale, W., Lee, K. F., and Rivier, C. (2001). Mice that lack corticotropin-releasing factor (CRF) receptors type 1 show a blunted ACTH response to acute alcohol despite up-regulated constitutive hypothalamic CRF gene expression. *Alcohol Clin Exp Res, 25,* 427–433.

Lerman, C., Wileyto, E. P., Patterson, F., Rukstalis, M., Audrain-McGovern, J., Restine, S., Shields, P. G., Kaufmann, V., Redden, D., Benowitz, N., and Berrettini, W. H. (2004). The functional mu opioid receptor (OPRM1) Asn40Asp variant predicts short-term response to nicotine replacement therapy in a clinical trial. *Pharmacogenomics J, 4,* 184–192.

Lesch, K. P., Bengel, D., Heils, A., Sabol, S. Z., Greenberg, B. D., Petri, S., Benjamin, J., Muller, C. R., Hamer, D. H., and Murphy, D.L. (1996). Association of anxiety-related traits with a polymorphism in the serotonin transporter gene regulatory region. *Science, 274,* 1527–1531.

Li, T., Chen, C. K., Hu, X., Ball, D., Lin, S. K., Chen, W., Sham, P. C., Loh, el-W., Murray, R. M., and Collier, D. A. (2004). Association analysis of the DRD4 and COMT genes in methamphetamine abuse. *Am J Med Genet B Neuropsychiatr Genet, 129B,* 120–124.

Linnoila, M., Virkkunen, M., George, T., Eckardt, M., Higley, J. D., Nielsen, D., and Goldman, D. (1994). Serotonin, violent behavior and alcohol. *EXS, 71,* 155–163.

Liu, D., Diorio, J., Tannenbaum, B., Caldji, C., Francis, D., Freedman, A., Sharma, S., Pearson, D., Plotsky, P. M., and Meaney, M. J. (1997). Maternal care, hippocampal glucocorticoid receptors, and hypothalamic-pituitary-adrenal responses to stress. *Science, 277,* 1659–1662.

Lodge, D. J., and Lawrence, A. J. (2003). The CRF1 receptor antagonist antalarmin reduces volitional ethanol consumption in isolation-reared fawn-hooded rats. *Neuroscience, 117,* 243–247.

Lovallo, W. R. (2006). Cortisol secretion patterns in addiction and addiction risk. *Int J Psychophysiol, 59,* 195–202.

Low, K., Crestani, F., Keist, R., Benke, D., Brunig, I., Benson, J. A., Fritschy, J. M., Rulicke, T., Bluethmann, H., Mohler, H., and Rudolph U. (2000). Molecular and neuronal substrate for the selective attenuation of anxiety. *Science, 290,* 131–134.

Mannelli, P., Patkar, A. A., Murray, H. W., Certa, K., Peindl, K., Mattila-Evenden, M., and Berrettini, W. H. (2005). Polymorphism in the serotonin transporter gene and response to treatment in African American cocaine and alcohol-abusing individuals. *Addict Biol, 10,* 261–268.

Manzanares, J., Ortiz, S., Oliva, J. M., Perez-Rial, S., and Palomo, T. (2005). Interactions between cannabinoid and opioid receptor systems in the mediation of ethanol effects. *Alcohol Alcohol, 40,* 25–34.

Martijena, I. D., Rodriguez Manzanares, P. A., Lacerra, C., and Molina, V. A. (2002). Gabaergic modulation of the stress response in frontal cortex and amygdala. *Synapse, 45,* 86–94.

Mazzanti, C. M., Lappalainen, J., Long, J. C., Bengel, D., Naukkarinen, H., Eggert, M., Virkkunen, M., Linnoila, M., and Goldman, D. (1998). Role of the serotonin transporter promoter polymorphism in anxiety-related traits. *Arch Gen Psychiatry, 55,* 936–940.

Meaney, M. J. (2001). Maternal care, gene expression, and the transmission of individual differences in stress reactivity across generations. *Annu Rev Neurosci, 24,* 1161–1192.

Merikangas, K. R., Mehta, R. L., Molnar, B. E., Walters, E. E., Swendsen, J. D., Aguilar-Gaziola, S., Bijl, R., Borges, G., Caraveo-Anduaga, J. J., DeWit, D. J., Kolody, B., Vega, W. A., Wittchen, H. U., and Kessler, R. C. (1998a). Comorbidity of substance use disorders with mood and anxiety disorders: Results of the International Consortium in Psychiatric Epidemiology. *Addict Behav, 23,* 893–907.

Merikangas, K. R., Stolar, M., Stevens, D. E., Goulet, J., Preisig, M. A., Fenton, B., Zhang, H., O'Malley, S. S., and Rounsaville, B. J. (1998b). Familial transmission of substance use disorders. *Arch Gen Psychiatry, 55,* 973–979.

Miller, G. M., Bendor, J., Tiefenbacher, S., Yang, H., Novak, M. A., and Madras, B. K. (2004). A mu-opioid receptor single nucleotide polymorphism in rhesus monkey: Association with stress response and aggression. *Mol Psychiatry, 9,* 99–108.

Morgan, C. A. 3rd, Rasmusson, A. M., Wang, S., Hoyt, G., Hauger, R. L., and Hazlett, G. (2002). Neuropeptide-Y, cortisol, and subjective distress in humans exposed to acute stress: Replication and extension of previous report. *Biol Psychiatry, 52,* 136–142.

Mottagui-Tabar, S., Prince, J. A., Wahlestedt, C., Zhu, G., Goldman, D., and Heilig, M. (2005). A novel single nucleotide polymorphism of the neuropeptide Y (NPY) gene associated with alcohol dependence. *Alcohol Clin Exp Res, 29,* 702–707.

Nader, K., and van der Kooy, D. (1997). Deprivation state switches the neurobiological substrates mediating opiate reward in the ventral tegmental area. *J Neurosci, 17,* 383–390.

Nagy, J. (2004). The NR2B subtype of NMDA receptor: A potential target for the treatment of alcohol dependence. *Curr Drug Targets CNS Neurol Disord, 3,* 169–179.

NIDA (National Institute on Drug Abuse). (1994). Capsules, women and drug abuse, *6,* 2.

Nie, Z., Schweitzer, P., Roberts, A. J., Madamba, S. G., Moore, S. D., and Siggins, G. R. (2004). Ethanol augments GABAergic transmission in the central amygdala via CRF1 receptors. *Science, 303,* 1512–1514.

Nikulina, E. M., Miczek, K. A., and Hammer, R. P. (2005). Prolonged effects of repeated social defeat stress on mRNA expression and function of mu-opioid receptors in the ventral tegmental area of rats. *Neuropsychopharmacology, 30,* 1096–1103.

O'Connor, T., Ben-Shlomo, Y., Heron, J., Golding, J., Adams, D., and Glover, V. (2005). Prenatal anxiety predicts individual differences in cortisol in pre-adolescent children. *Biol Psychiatry, 58,* 211–217.

Olsson, C. A., Anney, R. J., Lotfi-Miri, M., Byrnes, G. B., Williamson, R., and Patton, G. C. (2005). Association between the COMT Val158Met polymorphism and propensity to anxiety in an Australian population-based longitudinal study of adolescent health. *Psychiatr Genet, 15,* 109–115.

O'Malley, S. S., Krishnan-Sarin, S., Farren, C., Sinha, R., and Kreek, M. J. (2002). Naltrexone decreases craving and alcohol self-administration in alcohol-dependent subjects and activates the hypothalamo-pituitary-adrenocortical axis. *Psychopharmacology (Berl), 160,* 19–29.

Oslin, D. W., Berrettini, W., Kranzler, H. R., Pettinati, H., Gelernter, J., Volpicelli, J. R., and O'Brien, C. P. (2003). A functional polymorphism of the mu-opioid receptor gene is associated with naltrexone response in alcohol-dependent patients. *Neuropsychopharmacology, 28,* 1546–1552.

Oswald, L. M., McCaul, M., Choi, L., Yang, X., and Wand, G. S. (2004). Catechol-O-methyltransferase polymorphism alters hypothalamic-pituitary-adrenal axis responses to naloxone: A preliminary report. *Biol Psychiatry, 55,* 102–105.

Oswald, L. M., and Wand, G. S. (2004). Opioids and alcoholism. *Physiol Behav, 81,* 339–358.

Oswald, L. M., Zandi, P., Nestadt, G., Potash, J. B., Kalaydjian, A. E., and Wand, G. S. (2006, 11). Relationship between cortisol responses to stress and personality. *Neuropsychopharmacology. 31,* 1583–1591.

Pagotto, U., Marsicano, G., Cota, D., Lutz, B., and Pasquali, R. (2006). The emerging role of the endocannabinoid system in endocrine regulation and energy balance. *Endocr Rev, 27,* 73–100.

Pandey, S. C., Carr, L. G., Heilig, M., Ilveskoski, E., and Thiele, T. E. (2003). Neuropeptide Y and alcoholism: Genetic, molecular, and pharmacological evidence. *Alcohol Clin Exp Res, 27,* 149–154.

Pandey, S. C., Chartoff, E. H., Carlezon, W. A. Jr., Zou, J., Zhang, H., Kreibich, A. S., Blendy, J. A., and Crews, F. T. (2005a). CREB gene transcription factors: Role in molecular mechanisms of alcohol and drug addiction. *Alcohol Clin Exp Res, 29,* 176–184.

Pandey, S. C., Zhang, H., Roy, A., and Xu, T. (2005b). Deficits in amygdaloid cAMP-responsive element-binding protein signaling play a role in genetic predisposition to anxiety and alcoholism. *J Clin Invest, 115,* 2762–2773.

Patel, S., Cravatt, B. F., and Hillard, C. J. (2005). Synergistic interactions between cannabinoids and environmental stress in the activation of the central amygdala. *Neuropsychopharmacology, 30,* 497–507.

Patel, S., Roelke, C. T., Rademacher, D. J., Cullinan, W. E., and Hillard, C. J. (2004). Endocannabinoid signaling negatively modulates stress-induced activation of the hypothalamic-pituitary-adrenal axis. *Endocrinology, 145,* 5431–5438.

Pezawas, L., Meyer-Lindenberg, A., Drabant, E. M., Verchinski, B. A., Munoz, K. E., Kolachana, B. S., Egan, M. F., Mattay, V. S., Hariri, A. R., and Weinberger, D. R. (2005). 5- HTTLPR polymorphism impacts human cingulate-amygdala interactions: A genetic susceptibility mechanism for depression. *Nat Neurosci, 8,* 828–834.

Racz, I., Bilkei-Gorzo, A., Toth, Z. E., Michel, K., Palkovits, M., and Zimmer, A. (2003). A critical role for the cannabinoid CB1 receptors in alcohol dependence and stress-stimulated ethanol drinking. *J Neurosci, 23,* 2453–2458.

Radel, M., Vallejo, R. L., Iwata, N., Aragon, R., Long, J. C., Virkkunen, M., and Goldman, D. (2005). Haplotype-based localization of an alcohol dependence gene to the 5q34 {gamma}aminobutyric acid type A gene cluster. *Arch Gen Psychiatry, 62,* 47–55.

Ray, L. A., and Hutchison, K. E. (2004). A polymorphism of the mu-opioid receptor gene (OPRM1) and sensitivity to the effects of alcohol in humans. *Alcohol Clin Exp Res, 28,* 1789–1795.

Rhee, S. H., Hewitt, J. K., Young, S. E., Corley, R. P., Crowley, T. J., and Stallings, M. C. (2003). Genetic and environmental influences on substance initiation, use, and problem use in adolescents. *Arch Gen Psychiatry, 60,* 1256–1264.

Roberts, A. J., McDonald, J. S., Heyser, C. J., Kieffer, B. L., Matthes, H. W., Koob, G. F., and Gold, L. H. (2000). Mu-opioid receptor knockout mice do not self-administer alcohol. *J Pharmacol Exp Ther, 293,* 1002–1008.

Rodriguez de Fonseca, F., Carrera, M. R., Navarro, M., Koob, G. F., and Weiss, F. (1997). Activation of corticotropin-releasing factor in the limbic system during cannabinoid withdrawal. *Science, 276,* 2050–2054.

Schinka, J. A., Town, T., Abdullah, L., Crawford, F. C., Ordorica, P. I., Francis, E., Hughes, P., Graves, A. B., Mortimer, J. A., and Mullan, M. (2002). A functional polymorphism within the mu-opioid receptor gene and risk for abuse of alcohol and other substances. *Mol Psychiatry, 7,* 224–228.

Sillaber, I., Rammes, G., Zimmermann, S., Mahal, B., Zieglgansberger, W., Wurst, W., Holsboer, F., and Spanagel, R. (2002). Enhanced and delayed stress-induced alcohol drinking in mice lacking functional CRH1 receptors. *Science, 296,* 931–933.

Smolka, M., Sander, T., Schmidt, L. G., Samochowiec, J., Rommelspacher, H., Gscheidel, N., Wendel, B., and Hoche, M. R. (1999). Mu-opioid receptor variants and dopaminergic sensitivity in alcohol withdrawal. *Psychoneuroendocrinology, 24,* 629–638.

Smolka, M. N., Schumann, G., Wrase, J., Grusser, S. M., Flor, H., Mann., K., Braus, D. F., Goldman, D., Buchel, C., and Heinz, A. (2005). Catechol-O-methyltransferase val158met genotype affects processing of emotional stimuli in the amygdala and prefrontal cortex. *J Neurosci, 25,* 836–842.

Snoek, H., Van Goozen, S. H., Matthys, W., Buitelaar, J. K., and van Engeland, H. (2004). Stress responsivity in children with externalizing behavior disorders. *Dev Psychopathol, 16,* 389–406.

Soyka, M., Preuss, U. W., Koller, G., Zill, P., Hesselbrock, V., and Bondy, B. (2004). No association of CRH1 receptor polymorphism haplotypes, harm avoidance and other personality dimensions in alcohol dependence: Results from the Munich gene bank project for alcoholism. *Addict Biol, 9,* 73–79.

Stewart, S. H., Karp, J., Pih, R. O., and Peterson, R. A. (1997). Anxiety sensitivity and self-reported reasons for drug use. *J Subst Abuse, 9,* 223–240.

Stinson, F. S., Grant, B. F., Dawson, D. A., Ruan, W. J., Huang, B., and Saha, T. (2005). Comorbidity between DSM-IV alcohol and specific drug use disorders in the United States: Results from the National Epidemiologic Survey on Alcohol and Related Conditions. *Drug Alcohol Depend, 80,* 105–116.

Swan, G. E., Carmelli, D., and Cardon, L. R. (1997). Heavy consumption of cigarettes, alcohol and coffee in male twins. *J Stud Alcohol, 58,* 182–190.

Thomas, S. E., Randall, C. L., and Carrigan, M. H. (2003). Drinking to cope in socially anxious individuals: A controlled study. *Alcohol Clin Exp Res, 27,* 1937–1943.

Thorsell, A., Rimondini, R., and Heilig, M. (2002). Blockade of central neuropeptide Y (NPY) Y2 receptors reduces ethanol self-administration in rats. *Neurosci Lett, 332,* 1–4.

Tiihonen, J., Hallikainen, T., Lachman, H., Saito, T., Volavka, J., Kauhanen, J., Salonen, J. T., Ryynanen, O. P., Koulu, M., Karvonen, M. K., Pohjalainen, T., Syvalahti, E., and Hietala, J. (1999). Association between the functional variant of the catechol-O-methyltransferase (COMT) gene and type 1 alcoholism. *Mol Psychiatry, 4,* 286–289.

Treutlein, J., Kissling, C., Frank, J., Wiemann, S., Dong L., Depner, M., Saam, C., Lascorz, J., Soyka, M., Preuss, U.W., Rujescu, D., Skowronek, M.H., Rietschel, M., Spaangel, R., Heinz, A., Laucht, M., Mann, K., Schumann, G. (2006.) Genetic association of the human corticotropin releasing hormone receptor 1 (CRHR1) with binge drinking and alcohol intake patterns in two independent samples. *Mol Psychiatry, 11,* 594–602.

True, W. R., Heath, A. C., Scherrer, J. F., Xian, H., Lin, N., Eisen, S. A., Lyons, M. J., Goldberg, J., and Tsuang, M. T. (1999a). Interrelationship of genetic and environmental influences on conduct disorder and alcohol and marijuana dependence symptoms. *Am J Med Genet, 88,* 391–397.

True, W. R., Xian, H., Scherrer, J. F., Madden, P. A., Bucholz, K. K., Heath, A. C., Eisen, S. A., Lyons, M. J., Goldberg, J., and Tsuang, M. (1999b). Common genetic vulnerability for nicotine and alcohol dependence in men. *Arch Gen Psychiatry, 56,* 655–661.

Tsai, G., and Coyle, J. T. (1998). The role of glutamatergic neurotransmission in the pathophysiology of alcoholism. *Annu Rev Med, 49,* 173–184.

Tsuang, M. T., Bar, J. L., Harley, R. M., and Lyons, M. J. (2001). The Harvard twin study of substance abuse: What we have learned. *Harvard Rev Psychiatry, 9,* 267–279.

Tsuang, M.T., Lyons, M. J., Meyer, J. M., Doyle, T., Eisen, S. A., Goldberg, J., True, W., Lin, N., Toomey, R., and Eaves, L. (1998). Co-occurrence of abuse of different drugs in men: The role of drug-specific and shared vulnerabilities. *Arch Gen Psychiatry, 55,* 967–972.

Vandenbergh, D. J., Rodriguez, L. A., Miller, I. T., Uhl, G. R., and Lachman, H. M. (1997). High-activity catechol-O-methyltransferase allele is more prevalent in polysubstance abusers. *Am J Med Genet, 74,* 439–442.

Ventura, R., Alcaro, A., and Puglisi-Allegra, S. (2005). Prefrontal cortical norepinephrine release is critical for morphine-induced reward, reinstatement and dopamine release in the nucleus accumbens. *Cereb Cortex, 15,* 1877–1886.

Walters, C. L., Cleck, J. N., Kuo, Y.-C., and Blendy, J. A. (2005). Mu-opioid receptor and CREB activation are required for nicotine reward. *Neuron, 46,* 933–943.

Wand, G. (2005). The anxious amygdala: CREB signaling and predisposition to anxiety and alcoholism. *J Clin Invest, 115,* 2697–2699.

Wand, G. S., McCaul, M., Yang, X., Reynolds, J., Gotjen, D., Lee, S., and Ali, A. (2002). The mu-opioid receptor gene polymorphism (A118G) alters HPA axis activation induced by opioid receptor blockade. *Neuropsychopharmacology, 26,* 106–114.

Wang, J., Fang, Q., Liu, Z., and Lu, L. (2006). Region-specific effects of brain corticotropin-releasing factor receptor type 1 blockade on footshock-stress- or drug-priming–induced reinstatement of morphine conditioned place preference in rats. *Psychopharmacology (Berl), 185,* 19–28.

Weaver, I. C., Cervoni, N., Champagne, F. A., D'Alessio, A. C., Sharma, S., Seckl, J. R., Dymov, S., Szyf, M., and Meaney, M. J. (2004). Epigenetic programming by maternal behavior. *Nat Neurosci, 7,* 847–854.

Weaver, I. C., Champagne, F. A., Brown, S. E., Dymov, S., Sharma, S., Meaney, M. J., and Szyf, M. (2005). Reversal of maternal programming of stress responses in adult offspring through methyl supplementation: Altering epigenetic marking later in life. *J Neurosci, 25,* 11045–11054.

Weinshilboum, R. M., Otterness, D. M., and Szumlanski, C. L. (1999). Methylation pharmacogenetics: Catechol-O-methyltransferase, thiopurine methyl transferase, and histamine N-methyltransferase. *Annu Rev Pharmacol Toxicol, 39,* 19–52.

Wilsnack, S. C., Vogeltanz, N. D., Klassen, A. D., and Harris, T. R. (1997). Childhood sexual abuse and women's substance abuse: National survey findings. *J Stud Alcohol, 58,* 264–271.

Winfield, I., George, L. K., Swartz., M., and Blazer, D. G. (1990). Sexual assault and psychiatric disorders among a community sample of women. *Am J Psychiatry, 147,* 335–341.

Wust, S., Federenko, I., Hellhammer, D. H., and Kirschbaum, C. (2000). Genetic factors, perceived chronic stress, and the free cortisol response to awakening. *Psychoneuroendocrinology, 25,* 707–720.

Wust, S., van Rossum, E. F., Federenko, I. S., Koper, J. W., Kumsta, R., and Hellhammer, D. H. (2004). Common polymorphisms in the glucocorticoid receptor gene are associated with adrenocortical responses to psychosocial stress. *J Clin Endocrinol Metab, 89,* 565–573.

Yoshitake, T., Wang, F. H., Kuteeva, E., Holmberg, K., Yamaguchi, M., Crawley, J. N., Steiner, R., Bartfai, T., Ogren, S. O., Hokfelt, T., and Kehr, J. (2004). Enhanced hippocampal noradrenaline and serotonin release in galanin-overexpressing mice after repeated forced swimming test. *Proc Natl Acad Sci U S A, 101,* 354–359.

Young, E. A., Abelson, J. A., and Cameron, O. G. (2005). Interaction of brain noradrenergic system and the hypothalamic-pituitary-adrenal (HPA) axis in man. *Psychoneuroendocrinology, 30,* 807–814.

Zhang, P. W., Ishiguro, H., Ohtsuki, T., Hess, J., Carillo, F., Walther, D., Onaivi, E. S., Arinami, T., and Uhl, G. R. (2004). Human cannabinoid receptor 1: 5′ exons, candidate regulatory regions, polymorphisms, haplotypes and association with polysubstance abuse. *Mol Psychiatry, 9,* 916–931.

Zhu, G., Pollak, L., Mottagui-Tabar, S., Wahlestedt, C., Taubman, J., Virkkunen, M., Goldman, D., and Heilig, M. (2003). NPY leu7pro and alcohol dependence in Finnish and Swedish populations. *Alcohol Clin Exp Res, 27,* 19–24.

Zubieta, J. K., Heitzeg, M. M., Smith, Y. R., Bueller, J. A., Xu, K., Xu, Y., Koeppe, R. A., Stohler, C. S., and Goldman, D. (2003). COMT val158met genotype affects mu-opioid neurotransmitter responses to a pain stressor. *Science, 299,* 1240–1243.

CHAPTER

7

Neurobiology of Stress and Risk for Relapse

SUZANNE ERB

In recent years, there has been considerable interest in characterizing the nature of the relationship between stress and relapse to drug use. To this end, animal models of relapse, known as reinstatement procedures, have been used extensively to study the neurobiology and phenomenology of relapse to drug seeking following prolonged drug-free periods. The focus of this chapter is on experiments conducted in laboratory animals to study the effects of exposure to environmental stressors on relapse to psychostimulant, opiate, and alcohol seeking, and on the neurobiological mechanisms mediating those effects. Two commonly used animal models of relapse, so-called reinstatement procedures, are described, and a summary of the types of stressors that have been found to effectively induce relapse to drug seeking using procedures based on these models is provided. In addition, studies aimed at uncovering the neurobiological underpinnings of stress-induced relapse are reviewed. Finally, recent work demonstrating that a history of drug exposure can produce long-lasting changes in the responsivity of the central nervous system to stressors is discussed with respect to its potential implications for understanding the relationship between stress and relapse to drug seeking.

I. OVERVIEW

Relapse to drug use is one of the most debilitating long-term effects of addiction and one of the greatest challenges for treatment. There are many correlational studies implicating life stress as an important factor contributing to increased rates of drug and alcohol use, and as a trigger for relapse in individuals with substance abuse disorders (Brown et al., 1995; Kosten et al., 1986; Ludwig et al., 1974; McFall et al., 1992; McKay et al., 1995; see Sinha, 2001). A relationship between stress and relapse in drug addicts has also been studied under controlled laboratory conditions. For example, the induction of psychological stress, using a guided imagery procedure involving recall of personalized stress situations, was found to increase subjective reports of cocaine and alcohol craving in recently abstinent cocaine-dependent subjects seeking treatment (Fox et al., 2005; Sinha et al., 1999). Moreover, using these procedures, stress-induced cocaine craving reportedly predicted the incidence of cocaine relapse following inpatient treatment (see Fox et al., 2005).

Stress and Addiction: Biological and Psychological Mechanisms
Edited by **Mustafa al'Absi, Ph.D.**

147

Although mechanisms of negative reinforcement, including overcoming negative affect, are often cited as explanations for why stress might elicit increases in drug craving and relapse (e.g., Ahmed and Koob, 2005; Childress et al., 1994), there are studies to suggest that this relationship is less than clear (e.g., Hall et al., 1990). Indeed, our current understanding of the mechanisms mediating the putative relationship between stress and relapse is still evolving. Over the past decade, however, considerable work has been done to clarify the link between stress and relapse and to identify the behavioral and neurobiological mechanisms mediating relapse to drug seeking triggered by stress. To a large extent, this work has been carried out at a basic research level, using behavioral, pharmacological, and neurochemical techniques in laboratory animals.

The focus of this chapter will be on experiments conducted in, primarily, laboratory rodents, to study the effects of exposure to environmental stressors on relapse to psychostimulant, opiate, and alcohol seeking, and on the neurobiological mechanisms mediating those effects. The chapter will be divided into three major sections. In the first section, two commonly used animal models of relapse will be described, and a summary of the types of stressors that have been found to effectively induce relapse to drug seeking using procedures based on these models will be provided. In the second section, studies aimed at uncovering the neurobiological underpinnings of stress-induced relapse to drug seeking, in particular relapse to drug seeking triggered by foot-shock stress in laboratory rats, will be reviewed. This review will focus on work demonstrating a particularly important role for the stress-related neuropeptide, corticotropin-releasing factor (CRF), and its possible interactions with other systems that have also been implicated in the effects of stress on relapse; other systems include noradrenaline (NA), dopamine (DA), and glutamate. Finally, recent work demon-strating that a history of drug exposure can produce long-lasting changes in the responsivity of the central nervous system to CRF will be described. This work will be discussed with respect to its potential implications for understanding the nature of CRF involvement in relapse to drug seeking following prolonged drug-free periods.

II. ANIMAL MODELS FOR STUDYING THE EFFECTS OF STRESS ON RELAPSE TO DRUG SEEKING: THE REINSTATEMENT PROCEDURE

Animal models of relapse, known as reinstatement procedures, have been used extensively to study the neurobiology and phenomenology of relapse to drug use. From a historical perspective, the most conventional reinstatement procedures are based on the drug self-administration (SA) model, in which animals are trained to perform an operant response for drug reinforcement (e.g., de Wit and Stewart, 1981; Shaham and Stewart, 1995; Stewart and de Wit, 1987; Stretch et al., 1971). However, more recently, a reinstatement procedure was developed that is based on the conditioned place preference (CPP) paradigm, a widely used measure of the rewarding properties of drugs of abuse (e.g., Lu et al., 2002a; Lu et al., 2002b; Mueller et al., 2002; Mueller and Stewart, 2000; Parker and McDonald, 2000; Wang et al., 2001). Using both types of reinstatement procedures, various physical and pharmacological stressors have been found to trigger relapse to, or the reinstatement of, drug seeking after prolonged drug-free periods. Next, the SA and CPP reinstatement procedures will be described, followed by a summary of the types of stressors that have been shown to effectively induce reinstatement of the respective drug-related behaviors and the types of conditions under which the stressors are effective.

A. The Self-Administration (SA) Reinstatement Procedure

A generalized schematic of the SA reinstatement procedure is presented in Figure 7-1A. In this procedure, animals are trained to perform an operant response, such as lever pressing or nose poking, to obtain intravenous infusions of a psychostimulant (e.g., amphetamine, cocaine, nicotine) or opiate (e.g., heroin, morphine), or oral access to alcohol. Following training, extinction of the drug-reinforced behavior is accomplished by no longer reinforcing the behavior; that is, the operant response is either without consequence or results in an infusion of saline. Once the behavior is extinguished (i.e., responding is reduced to a low baseline level), animals are tested for the reinstatement of drug seeking induced by a specific triggering stimulus or event, such as a priming injection of the drug, presentation of a drug-paired cue, or exposure to an environmental stressor. Under testing conditions, responding continues to be nonreinforced. Thus, the reinstatement of drug seeking is defined, operationally, as an increase above baseline in the number of occurrences of the previously reinforced behavior (e.g., number of lever presses on the previously reinforced lever) in response to the presentation of a triggering stimulus, after a period of extinction.

Reinstatement procedures based on the SA method were developed originally to study in rats and monkeys the ability of acute noncontingent exposure to drugs to reinstate drug seeking (de Wit, 1996; Shaham et al., 2000a). Using several variations of the SA reinstatement procedure, priming injections of the previously self-administered drug, or one with similar pharmacological actions, have been found to reliably reinstate drug seeking in rats, mice, and monkeys trained to self-administer a variety of drugs of abuse (De Vries et al., 1998; see also de Wit, 1996; Shaham et al., 2003). The idea that a small amount of drug can prime desire for more drug is supported by parallel studies conducted in human subjects, in which priming injections of an abused drug are associated with increases on measures such as desire for drug, craving for drug, and willingness to work for more drug (e.g., Bigelow et al., 1977; Breiter et al., 1997; Jaffe et al., 1989; Kumor et al., 1989; Ludwig and Wikler, 1974; Meyer and M, 1979; Preston et al., 1992).

Clearly, events other than re-exposure to drugs provoke relapse episodes; in fact, after a period of abstinence, drug seeking is antecedent to drug taking. This notion has led in recent years to the extensive use of SA reinstatement procedures to study the role of environmental stimuli, including drug-related cues and exposure to environmental stressors, in relapse to drug seeking (see Shaham et al., 2000a; Shalev et al., 2002). Studies aimed at exploring the relationship between stress and the reinstatement of drug seeking using the SA procedure are

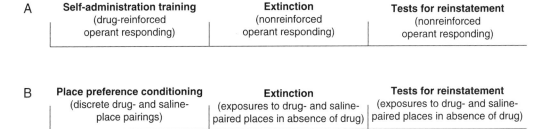

FIGURE 7-1   (A) Generalized schematic of the self-administration (SA) reinstatement procedure: Reinstatement of an operant conditioned response. (B) Generalized schematic of the conditioned place preference (CPP) reinstatement procedure: Reinstatement of a Pavlovian CPP.

reviewed below in Section II.C and are a primary focus of the present chapter.

B. The Conditioned Place Preference (CPP) Reinstatement Procedure

As mentioned, procedures based on the CPP paradigm were recently developed to study the reinstatement of an extinguished preference for a previously drug-paired environment (Lu et al., 2002a; Lu et al., 2002b; Mueller et al., 2002; Mueller and Stewart, 2000; Parker and McDonald, 2000; Wang et al., 2001). A generalized schematic of the CPP reinstatement procedure is presented in Figure 7-1B.

CPP training is a Pavlovian conditioning procedure that involves discrete pairings of a drug, such as amphetamine, cocaine, or morphine, with a distinct environmental context and pairings of saline/vehicle with a different environmental context. At test, the animal is allowed to freely explore both contexts in a drug-free state. Evidence of a CPP is demonstrated by the animal spending more time in the drug- than saline-paired context, or relatively more time in the drug-paired context after than before the conditioning phase.

In experiments aimed at studying the reinstatement of an extinguished CPP, extinction is accomplished by either repeatedly pairing saline (Lu et al., 2002a; Lu et al., 2002b; Mueller et al., 2002; Mueller and Stewart, 2000) with the previously drug-paired environment or giving repeated CPP tests (Mueller and Stewart, 2000; Parker and McDonald, 2000). In the latter case, each test constitutes an extinction trial, since it occurs in the absence of drug. Following the completion of extinction, testing for reinstatement is conducted by presenting the animals with a triggering stimulus, such as a noncontingent priming injection of the drug or exposure to an acute stressor, prior to providing the animal with free access to both of the previously drug- and saline-paired environments. In this case, reinstatement is defined operationally, as a proportionately greater amount of time spent in the previously drug- relative to saline-paired context after a period of extinction. Studies aimed at exploring the relationship between stress and the reinstatement of drug seeking using the CPP procedure are reviewed in the next section.

C. Stress and Reinstatement

To date, much of the work that has been done to explore the effects of stress on the reinstatement of drug seeking has used intermittent exposure to mild, electric foot shocks as the stress manipulation. In an initial study, Shaham and Stewart (1995) showed that following 7–10 days of extinction in rats that had been trained to self-administer heroin, 10 minutes of exposure to brief intermittent electric foot shock effectively reinstated drug seeking; in these animals, foot shock was still effective in inducing reinstatement after an additional 4- to 6-week drug-free period. In subsequent experiments, the effect of foot shock on the reinstatement of heroin seeking was replicated and extended to animals with histories of cocaine, alcohol, and nicotine self-administration (see Bossert et al., 2005; Buczek et al., 1999; Erb et al., 1996; Lê et al., 2003; Shaham et al., 2000a; Shaham et al., 2003; Shalev et al., 2002).

Since the initial experiments establishing foot-shock stress as an effective stimulus for provoking the reinstatement of drug seeking in animals with a variety of drug histories, several studies have been done to further characterize the effect of foot shock on reinstatement. In one study, it was revealed that the stressor is effective in inducing the reinstatement of drug seeking only if it is administered in the environment in which animals had previously self-administered the drug and subsequently undergone extinction; that is, foot shock did not reinstate drug seeking if exposure to the stressor occurred in a novel context, suggesting an important interaction between the stressor and drug environment in its effects on reinstatement

(Shalev et al., 2000). In another study, it was shown that the magnitude of the effect of foot-shock stress on reinstatement can be affected by the duration of daily access to drug during the self-administration phase. Specifically, it was reported that rats given 11 hours of access to intravenous heroin per day during training showed a greater level of responding to foot shock during tests for reinstatement than did animals given 1 hour of daily access to the drug (Ahmed et al., 2000).

The phenomenon of foot-shock–induced reinstatement appears to be quite specific to the reinstatement of drug-reinforced behaviors. For example, foot shock does not reinstate extinguished responding previously maintained by food pellets (Ahmed and Koob, 1997), sucrose pellets, or sucrose solution (Shaham et al., 2000a; Shalev et al., 2000). Interestingly, however, foot-shock stress is capable of reinstating responding for brain stimulation reward (BSR). In animals trained to lever press for electrical stimulation to the septal region, and subsequently subject to extinction of the operant response, 5 and 15 minutes of exposure to foot-shock stress reinstated responding for septal stimulation to a level comparable to that observed in animals with a history of drug self-administration (Shalev et al., 2000). Based on the findings that foot shock reinstates responding for drug and BSR, but not natural nondrug reinforcers such as food and sucrose, it has been suggested that the stressor facilitates pathways compatible with general approach behaviors, but not with motivational behaviors that have evolutionary significance, such as behaviors maintained by food and sex (see Shaham et al., 2000a, for a discussion).

Although the effects of foot shock on reinstatement are relatively specific to animals with a history of drug self-administration, they do generalize to the reinstatement of other drug-related behaviors. Specifically, under similar parameters to those used in the SA experiments, foot shock has been found to reactivate extinguished CPPs induced by

morphine and cocaine after drug-free periods of more than 1 month (Lu et al., 2001; Lu et al., 2002b; Wang et al., 2001). In addition, a conditioned stimulus previously paired with footshock has been found to reinstate an extinguished CPP induced by cocaine (Sanchez et al., 2003; Sanchez and Sorg, 2001). Interestingly, conditioned stimuli previously paired with foot shock are ineffective in inducing the reinstatement of heroin or cocaine self-administration. It has been suggested that the discrepancy in the effects of the conditioned stressor on reinstatement of CPP versus SA may be due to the conditioned stressor inducing conditioned freezing, a response elicited unconditionally by foot shock stress and incompatible with performance of an operant behavior (Lu et al., 2003).

In addition to generalizing to the CPP procedure, the effects of foot shock on reinstatement using the SA procedure have been found to generalize to certain other types of stressors. One stressor that has been found to be particularly effective in inducing the reinstatement of drug seeking is acute food deprivation. Shalev et al., (2000) reported that 21 hours of food deprivation was a highly effective condition for inducing the reinstatement of both heroin and cocaine seeking; in fact, levels of responding induced by this manipulation were comparable to those induced by foot-shock stress. In addition to food deprivation, various pharmacological stressors have been found to induce the reinstatement of drug seeking. For example, ICV injections of the stress-related neuropeptide, CRF, reinstates heroin (Shaham et al., 1997), cocaine (Erb et al., 2006), and alcohol (Lê et al., 1998) seeking, and injections of CRF into the bed nucleus of the stria terminalis (BNST), a brain region critically involved in the effects of CRF on stress-induced reinstatement (see below), reinstates cocaine seeking (Erb and Stewart, 1999). Likewise, systemic injections of the corticosterone synthesis inhibitor, metyrapone, reinstate heroin seeking, presumably by acting acutely to reduce negative feedback in the hypothalamus and pituitary (Shaham et al., 1997). Finally, central injections of the alpha-2 antagonist, yohimbine, reinstates responding in animals trained to self-administer alcohol (Lê et al., 2005), methamphetamine (Shepard et al., 2004), or cocaine (Lee et al., 2004).

III. THE NEUROBIOLOGY OF STRESS-INDUCED REINSTATEMENT OF DRUG SEEKING

The search for neurobiological mechanisms underlying the reinstatement of drug seeking by stress has focused to a large extent on the foot-shock reinstatement model. An emerging neural circuitry of foot-shock–induced reinstatement, based on pharmacological and neurochemical experiments carried out in the past decade, is presented in Figure 7-2. The reader is referred to this figure as a point of reference for the circuitry discussed in this section.[1]

Briefly, some of the initial experiments exploring the neurobiology of foot-shock–induced reinstatement of drug seeking identified the actions of the stress-related neuropeptide, CRF, within the extended amygdala circuitry as a critical component of the neurobiology of foot-shock–induced reinstatement (Erb et al., 2001b). The extended amygdala is a neuronal continuum that stretches from the shell of the nucleus accumbens (NAs), through the BNST and sublentricular substantia innominata to the central

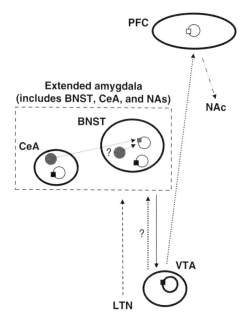

FIGURE 7-2   An emerging neural circuitry of foot-shock–induced reinstatement of drug seeking. BNST, bed nucleus of the stria terminalis; CeA, central nucleus of the amygdala; CRF, corticotropin-releasing factor; DA, dopamine; LTN, lateral tegmental nuclei; NA, noradrenaline; NAc, nucleus accumbens core; NAs, nucleus accumbens shell; PFC, prefrontal cortex; VTA, ventral tegmental area; ·······, CRFergic; ······, DAergic; –··–, Glutamatergic; -----, NAergic; ——, Unidentified; ○, cell body, identify unknown or inconclusive; ●, CRF cell body; ■, CRF receptor; ❑, DA receptor; ■, NA receptor, R, role in foot-shock–induced reinstatement unverified.

nucleus of the amygdala (CeA; Alheid et al., 1995; Alheid and Heimer, 1988; de Olmos and Heimer, 1999). In addition, the ventral NA projection, arising from cell bodies in the lateral tegmentum and projecting to the extended amygdala, has been shown to play an important role in foot-shock–induced reinstatement (Shaham et al., 2000b), possibly via a direct interaction with CRF cell bodies in the BNST and/or CeA. Subsequent to activation of the extended amygdala, this circuitry has recently been extended to include activation of the DA projection originating in the ventral tegmental area (VTA) and terminating in the prefrontal cortex (PFC); in turn, a glutamatergic projection from the PFC to the core of the nucleus accumbens (NAc) and a projection from the NAc to the ventral pal-

---

[1] This section is not intended to provide a comprehensive overview of the current state of knowledge regarding the neurobiology of stress-induced reinstatement of drug seeking. The basic literature on stress-induced reinstatement includes the involvement of additional systems, including serotonin and GABA, a growing interest in the molecular basis of foot-shock–induced reinstatement of drug seeking, and investigations of the neurobiological systems involved in the reinstatement of drug seeking by other stressors, such as food deprivation stress (see Bossert et al., 2005, for a recent review).

TABLE 7-1   Table of Abbreviations

BNST	Bed nucleus of the stria terminalis
BSR	Brain stimulation reward
CeA	Central nucleus of the amygdala
CPP	Conditioned place preference
CRF	Corticotropin-releasing factor
CRF-BP	Corticotropin-releasing factor binding protein
DA	Dopamine
HPA	Hypothalamic-pituitary-adrenal
ICV	Intracerebroventricular
NA	Noradrenaline
NAc	Nucleus accumbens, core
NAs	Nucleus accumbens, shell
PFC	Prefrontal cortex
SA	Self-administration
TTX	Tetradotoxin
VTA	Ventral tegmental area
6-OHDA	6-Hydroxydopamine

lidum have been identified as components of a final motor output circuitry common to all stimuli that trigger reinstatement of operant responding (Kalivas and McFarland, 2003; McFarland et al., 2004). (See Table 7-1 for abbreviations.)

A. A Role for CRF in Stress-Induced Reinstatement That Is Independent of Its Effects on the Pituitary and Adrenal

One major focus of the relationship between stress and substance abuse has been on the role that the hypothalamic-pituitary-adrenal (HPA) axis, known to be involved in the response to stressful events, plays in the behavioral and physiological effects of drugs of abuse (Piazza et al., 1996b; Sarnyai et al., 2001). Considerable work has been done, for example, to explore a role for glucocorticoids in drug-related behaviors. In studies carried out in rats, corticosterone has been found to facilitate the initiation of self-administration of low doses of psychostimulants (Goeders and Guerin, 1996; Piazza et al., 1991; Piazza et al., 1996a; Piazza

et al., 1996b) and to play a role in cocaine (Goeders and Guerin, 1996) and alcohol (Fahlke et al., 1994) self-administration during the maintenance phase.

In contrast to the established role that glucocorticoids play in the initiation and maintenance of drug self-administration, the preponderance of evidence suggests that they do not mediate responding during the relapse phase (Sarnyai et al., 2001; Shaham et al., 2000a). In some of the first studies aimed at determining the neurobiological basis of foot-shock–induced reinstatement of drug seeking, my colleagues and I reported that stress-induced rises in glucocorticoids were not responsible for the effects of foot-shock stress. For example, in animals trained to self-administer heroin or alcohol, pharmacological and/or surgical adrenalectomy failed to interfere in the ability of foot-shock stress to reinstate drug-seeking behavior (Lê et al., 2000; Shaham et al., 1997). Interestingly, in animals with a history of cocaine self-administration, adrenalectomy was effective in blocking the ability of foot-shock stress to induce reinstatement; however, this effect of adrenalectomy was completely reversed when basal levels of corticosterone were restored with corticosterone pellet implants and corticosterone in the drinking water (Erb et al., 1998). That is, in animals that were adrenalectomized but given corticosterone replacement, foot-shock stress induced levels of responding during the tests for reinstatement that were comparable to those observed in animals given a sham surgery. These results suggest that glucocorticoids play a permissive role in the stress-induced reinstatement of cocaine seeking that is not reliant on a stress-induced rise in corticosterone.

There is one recent report that is inconsistent with the conclusion that stress-induced rises in corticosterone are not responsible for the effects of foot-shock stress on the reinstatement of cocaine seeking (Mantsch and Goeders, 1999). In this study, cocaine-trained rats were tested for the reinstatement of cocaine seeking by foot-shock stress following pretreat- ment with ketoconazole, an antifungal agent that acts as a corticosterone synthe- sis inhibitor and glucocorticoid receptor antagonist. Ketoconazole was effective in blocking the foot-shock–induced reinstate- ment of cocaine seeking, suggesting a role for corticosterone in the effect. As noted in a recent review by Sarnyai et al. (2001), however, ketoconazole is known to act on several neurochemical systems in addition to corticosterone (including GABA, hista- mine, and testosterone), making the mech- anism by which it acts to interfere in the effects of foot-shock stress on reinstatement unclear.

Whereas activation of the HPA axis has been found to be, at the very least, noncen- tral to the effects of foot-shock stress on the reinstatement of drug seeking, activa- tion of CRF receptors plays a critical role (Sarnyai et al., 2001; Shaham et al., 2000a). Thus, although CRF is a primary instiga- tor of HPA activation in response to stress, its role in stress-induced reinstatement of drug seeking occurs through its actions as a neurotransmitter at extrahypothalamic brain sites that are independent of its neu- roendocrine effects. In experiments carried out in heroin- (Shaham et al., 1997), cocaine- (Erb et al., 1998), and alcohol-trained rats (Lê et al., 1998), ICV administration of CRF receptor antagonists significantly attenu- ated foot-shock–induced reinstatement of heroin and alcohol seeking and com- pletely blocked foot-shock–induced rein- statement of cocaine seeking. Moreover, in cocaine-trained animals that were sub- sequently adrenalectomized and given corticosterone replacement, ICV injec- tions of CRF receptor antagonists were effective in blocking the reinstatement of cocaine seeking (Erb et al., 1998). Finally, ICV administration of CRF, itself, induced the reinstatement of heroin (Shaham et al., 1997), alcohol (Lê et al., 2000), and cocaine (Erb et al., 1998) seeking, at least partially mimicking the effects of foot-shock stress on reinstatement.

B. Anatomical Localization of the Central Effects of CRF on Stress-Induced Reinstatement

In attempting to determine which brain circuitry mediates the effect of CRF on stress-induced reinstatement of drug seeking, a series of studies were conducted that focused on the BNST and CeA, primary structures of the extended amygdala (de Olmos and Heimer, 1999). Both the BNST and CeA are known to contain CRF cell bodies and termi- nals (Swanson et al., 1983); however, whereas CRF receptors are abundant in the BNST, comparatively few receptors are localized in the CeA (Chalmers et al., 1995; Potter et al., 1994). Both the CeA and BNST have been implicated in a number of physiological and behavioral responses to stress, including fear and anxiety responses (see Lee and Davis, 1997), and in a variety of general approach behaviors, including maternal behavior, sex, and feeding (e.g., Everitt et al., 1989; Numan and Numan, 1996; Numan and Numan, 1997). There is also evidence that CRF recep- tors in the CeA are directly involved in medi- ating the anxiogenic and aversive symptoms of opioid, cocaine, and alcohol withdrawal (Koob, 1999; Sarnyai et al., 2001) and that NA in the ventral BNST is critical in the media- tion of opiate withdrawal-induced aver- sion (Delfs et al., 2000), conceivably via an interaction with CRF receptors in the region (see Erb et al., 2001b). The BNST has also been implicated in drug self-administration behavior in heroin-dependent rats (Walker et al., 2000a).

In a set of reinstatement experiments carried out in cocaine-trained animals, phar- macological manipulations of CRF receptors in both the BNST and CeA were made (Erb et al., 2001b). In two initial experiments, differ- ent groups of animals were pretreated with the CRF-receptor antagonist, D-Phe CRF$_{12-41}$, injected bilaterally into either the ventrolat- eral division of the BNST (0, 10, or 50 ng/ side) or the CeA (50 or 500 ng/side), prior to being tested for foot-shock–induced rein- statement. In two additional experiments, the effects of central injections of CRF on reinstatement of cocaine-seeking were examined. Groups of animals were pretreated with CRF, which was injected bilaterally into either the BNST (0, 100, and 300 ng/side) or CeA (0 and 300 ng/side); subsequently, animals were tested for reinstatement in the absence of foot shock. At doses 10-fold lower than those that were effective when injected ICV (Erb et al., 1998), injections of the CRF receptor antagonist into the BNST blocked foot-shock–induced reinstatement of cocaine seeking, while injections of CRF into the BNST, in the absence of shock, induced reinstatement. Blockade of CRF receptors in the CeA did not affect foot-shock–induced reinstatement, nor did injections of CRF into this site produce reinstatement on its own. These results suggest that activation of CRF receptors in the BNST, but not CeA, is critical for stress-induced reinstatement of cocaine seeking (see Figure 7-2).

In a subsequent experiment, it was determined that although activation of CRF receptors in the CeA is not responsible for the effects of foot-shock stress on reinstatement of cocaine seeking, CRF cells originating in the CeA and projecting to the BNST (Sakanaka et al., 1986) provide at least one source of CRF that is of functional importance in mediating the effects of CRF on foot-shock–induced reinstatement (see Figure 7-2). In this experiment, an asymmetric lesion procedure (e.g., Easton et al., 2001; Parker and Gaffan, 1998) was used to functionally disconnect the CRF-containing pathway from the CeA to the BNST. This was achieved by injecting tetrodotoxin [TTX; a sodium channel blocker that acts reversibly to inhibit neuronal transmission (Brozek et al., 1996; Narahashi et al., 1992)] into the CeA in one hemisphere while, at the same time, injecting the CRF receptor antagonist, D-Phe CRF_{12-41}, into the BNST in the opposite hemisphere. It was reasoned that if the CRF-containing projection from the CeA to the BNST is involved in stress-induced reinstatement, then interruption of neurotransmission from the CeA in one hemisphere, while blocking CRF receptors in the BNST

in the opposite hemisphere, should interfere with stress-induced reinstatement of drug seeking. The outcome of the experiment supported a role for the CeA-BNST CRF pathway in the foot-shock–induced reinstatement of cocaine seeking. It was found that functional inactivation of the pathway significantly reduced foot-shock–induced reinstatement of responding compared to the effects seen when only one hemisphere was manipulated. Importantly, however, the manipulation did not completely block foot-shock–induced reinstatement of cocaine seeking, suggesting that the CeA does not provide the only source of CRF to the BNST involved in mediating the effects of foot shock on reinstatement. Another likely source of CRF contributing to the effects of foot shock on reinstatement is local release from cells within the BNST (see Figure 7-2). Although their role in stress-induced reinstatement has not yet been verified, it is known that CRF-containing cells within the BNST do provide local release of the peptide (Veinante et al., 1997).

More recently, the role of CRF receptors in the foot-shock–induced reinstatement of cocaine seeking has been extended to the VTA (Wang et al., 2005). The VTA, like the CeA and BNST, has been identified as an important brain region contributing to the effects of foot-shock stress on the reinstatement of drug seeking (Kalivas and McFarland, 2003; McFarland et al., 2004). In addition, the role of CRF in the VTA in stress-induced reinstatement is of interest because the peptide has been found to produce neuroadaptations in VTA DA neurons, in a manner similar to that of drugs of abuse (e.g., Ungless et al., 2001). In two of a series of experiments, Wang et al. (2005) determined the effects of intra-VTA perfusions of a CRF-receptor antagonist, alpha-helical CRF, on foot-shock–induced reinstatement of cocaine seeking and intra-VTA perfusions of CRF, itself, on reinstatement. Both manipulations produced effects consistent with a role for CRF receptor activation in the VTA in mediating stress-induced reinstatement; local blockade of CRF receptors interfered in the foot-shock–induced reinstatement of cocaine seeking, and local activation of the receptors induced reinstatement (see Figure 7-2).

In summary, there is strong evidence that activation of CRF receptors within the BNST, CeA, and VTA is a critical component of the neurobiology of stress-induced reinstatement. In the next section, characterization of the neurobiology of foot-shock–induced reinstatement of drug seeking will be expanded upon to include consideration of the involvement of neurotransmitter systems in addition to CRF and the possible interaction of CRF with these systems.

C. Roles for NA and DA, and Their Possible Interaction with CRF, in Mediating Foot-Shock–Induced Reinstatement of Drug Seeking

1. The Role of NA and Possible Interactions with CRF

A role for NA in foot-shock–induced reinstatement of drug seeking was initially established in three sets of experiments carried out in heroin- (Shaham et al., 2000b) and cocaine-trained rats (Erb et al., 2000) and rats trained with a heroin-cocaine mixture (Highfield et al., 2001). In these experiments, it was found that systemic injections of alpha-2 adrenoceptor agonists, including clonidine and lofexidine, at doses that inhibit NA cell firing and terminal release of NA, attenuated foot-shock–induced reinstatement of drug seeking. The effects of the agonists were determined to be centrally mediated because intraventricular injections of clonidine also attenuated foot-shock-induced reinstatement in heroin-trained animals (Shaham et al., 2000b), and systemic injections of the alpha-2 adrenoceptor agonist ST-91, a charged analogue of clonidine that crosses the blood-brain barrier minimally (Scriabine et al., 1977), were without effect on the reinstatement of cocaine seeking by foot-shock stress (Erb, 2000).

More recently, the effects of systemic injections of yohimbine on the reinstatement of

drug seeking have been studied. Yohimbine is an alpha-2 adrenoceptor antagonist that produces stress-like responses. Yohimbine was found to reinstate methamphetamine (Shepard et al., 2004) and alcohol seeking (Lê et al., 2005) in rats and cocaine seeking in monkeys (Lee et al., 2004). Since these effects are consistent with those of the alpha-2 adrenoceptor agonists on foot-shock–induced reinstatement, it is possible that yohimbine acts, at least in part, to mimic the effects of foot-shock stress on reinstatement.

NA projections to the forebrain arise from two groups of cells: one originating in the locus coeruleus and giving rise to the dorsal NA pathway, and the other originating in the lateral tegmental nuclei and giving rise to the ventral NA pathway (Moore and Bloom, 1979). Whereas the dorsal pathway provides the sole source of NA input to the hippocampus and frontal cortex, the BNST and CeA are major projection targets of the ventral pathway (Aston-Jones et al., 1995; Aston-Jones et al., 1999; Moore and Bloom, 1979). Studies carried out to identify which NA neurons are involved in the effects of stress on reinstatement have identified a role for the ventral (see Figure 7-2), but not dorsal, pathway. In one experiment, interference in transmission of the dorsal pathway was accomplished via local injections of clonidine or ST-91 into the locus coeruleus. These manipulations were without effect on the foot-shock–induced reinstatement of heroin seeking. In contrast, a selective 6-hydroxydopamine (6-OHDA) lesion of the ventral pathway, which reduced NA levels in the BNST by 60–70%, significantly attenuated the reinstatement of heroin seeking by foot shock.

More recently, findings consistent with those just described have been obtained using the CPP reinstatement procedure. Following extinction of a morphine CPP, disruption of neurotransmission in the ventral, but not dorsal, NA pathway significantly reduced the stress-induced reactivation of the CPP. In addition, local injections of clonidine in the BNST significantly attenuated foot-shock–induced reinstatement of a morphine CPP (Wang et al., 2001). Consistent with this latter finding, bilateral injections of beta adrenergic antagonists into either the CeA or BNST have been found to significantly attenuate the foot-shock–induced reinstatement of responding for a previously cocaine-reinforced behavior (Leri et al., 2002). Taken together, these results provide support for the idea that the ventral NA pathway, originating in the lateral tegmental nuclei and projecting to brain regions including the CeA and BNST, provides a functionally important source of NA in mediating the effects of foot shock on relapse.

Although, to date, experiments have not been carried out to directly address the possibility that NA and CRF systems interact within the BNST and/or CeA to mediate the effects of foot-shock stress on reinstatement, there are neuroanatomical data to support the idea that they may. Hornby and Piekut (1989), for example, showed that surrounding the CRF-IR cell bodies in the ventral region of the BNST (the region in which CRF has an important role in reinstatement) there is a massive network of fibers immunoreactive for dopamine-beta hydroxylase. Even more compelling is the work of Phelix et al. (1992, 1994) who, using combined light and electron microscopy, demonstrated the existence of direct synaptic interactions between NA axons and the dendrites of CRF-containing cell bodies in the ventrolateral BNST. In future studies, it would be of interest to explore directly the extent to which NA and CRF systems interact within the extended amygdala to mediate the effects of stress on the reinstatement of drug seeking.

2. The Role of DA and Possible Interactions with CRF

In studies examining the relationship between stress and relapse to drug seeking, the initial findings that exposure to intermittent foot-shock stress reinstated heroin and cocaine seeking as effectively as did priming injections of the self-administered drugs led to the hypothesis that foot-shock stress induces reinstatement by mimicking the drug effects, presumably via an effect on midbrain DA systems (Shaham and Stewart, 1995). This hypothesis was soon challenged, however, by the finding that injections of D1- or D2-like DA receptor antagonists, which effectively blocked the reinstatement of heroin seeking induced by a priming injection of the drug, had no effect on the reinstatement of heroin seeking induced by foot shock (Shaham and Stewart, 1996). Although Shaham and Stewart (1996) showed that the pathways underlying reinstatement by priming injections of drug and foot-shock stress are not identical, they did not rule out altogether a role for DA in foot-shock–induced reinstatement. In fact, they reported that administration of a mixed D1/D2-like receptor antagonist, flupenthixol, did block the ability of foot-shock stress to induce reinstatement of heroin seeking, suggesting that at least a basal tone of DA is necessary for the manifestation of stress-induced reinstatement.

The idea that DA does in fact play an important role in stress-induced reinstatement of drug seeking has been substantiated in more recent studies. For example, Capriles et al. (2003) reported that administration of a D1-like antagonist into the PFC selectively interfered in the effects of foot-shock stress on the reinstatement of cocaine seeking. McFarland et al. (2004) likewise identified a role for DA in foot-shock–induced reinstatement of cocaine seeking. Based in part on their findings that temporary inactivation of neuronal transmission in the VTA and blockade of DA receptors in the dorsal PFC interfere in foot-shock–induced reinstatement, they have argued that the effects of footshock on reinstatement involve activation of a DA projection from the VTA to the dorsal PFC (see Figure 7-2).

Consistent with these findings, Wang et al. (2005) recently demonstrated an important role for DA activation in the VTA in mediating the effects of foot-shock stress on the reinstatement of cocaine seeking. In this study, the role of DA in the VTA was shown to involve an interaction with local CRF and glutamatergic systems. Based on the results of a comprehensive series of reinstatement and corresponding *in vivo* microdialysis experiments, the authors argued that the reinstatement of cocaine seeking by foot-shock stress involves CRF release in the VTA (possibly via a CRF projection originating in the CeA or BNST), triggering glutamate release in the VTA and, in turn, DA activation.

In addition to the VTA, the BNST and CeA are possible sites in which DA may act, and possibly interact with CRF, in mediating the effects of foot-shock stress on reinstatement. In fact, both the BNST and CeA receive a substantial DA input from the VTA (see Figure 7-2), and it has been reported that a number of drugs of abuse (cocaine, morphine, nicotine, and alcohol) increase DA levels in the BNST, an effect hypothesized to be related to their reinforcing effects (Carboni et al., 1989). Although a role for neither CeA nor BNST DA in foot-shock–induced reinstatement has been established, it has been suggested that DA tone in the extended amygdala may affect its ability to activate the VTA and subsequent motor circuitry responsible for initiating the behaviors involved in relapse (McFarland et al., 2004). As for the possibility of a DA-CRF interaction in the extended amygdala being involved in the effects of foot-shock stress on reinstatement, results from electron microscopy experiments have identified a direct interaction between DA terminals and CRF cell bodies in at least the BNST (Phelix et al., 1992, 1994). In much the same way that an interaction between NA and CRF in the extended amygdala may underlie the effects of foot-shock stress on reinstatement, so too may an interaction between DA and CRF in these regions. This is a hypothesis that awaits exploration.

IV. LONG-LASTING CHANGES IN THE RESPONSIVITY OF THE CENTRAL NERVOUS SYSTEM TO CRF: BEHAVIORAL AND NEUROANATOMICAL STUDIES WITH POTENTIAL IMPLICATIONS FOR REINSTATEMENT

As mentioned, laboratory studies of the neurobiological mechanisms underlying stress-induced reinstatement of drug seeking suggest that the effect of foot-shock stress on reinstatement is specific to animals with a history of drug self-administration; that is, animals trained to self-administer non-drug reinforcers such as food or sucrose do not evidence stress-induced reinstatement (Shaham et al., 2000a). The implications of these findings are that prior experience with a drug of abuse may produce specific neuroadaptations that change animals' subsequent responses to stressors. The specific nature of these adaptations, however, is not clear. Although identification of the neuroadaptations that arise from a history of repeated drug exposure has been an active focus of research for many years, the specific neuroadaptations that may render an organism vulnerable to the effects of stress over time are a comparatively new area of investigation.

Given the important role that CRF has been found to play in the reinstatement of drug and alcohol seeking induced by stress, it is possible that a history of prior drug exposure produces persistent changes in the function of CRF systems and that these changes may make former users more vulnerable to the effects of stress over time. There is in fact accumulating evidence that although repeated exposure to drugs does not produce persistent changes in the basal activity of CRF systems (e.g., Erb et al., 2003a), it does produce persistent changes in the responsivity of the central nervous system to CRF itself and to other stressors (e.g., Erb et al., 2003b; Erb et al., 2005; Wang et al., 2005). This work will be the focus of the present discussion.

Until recently, studies of CRF systems following termination of drug exposure have focused on the early withdrawal period. It has been reported, for example, that behavioral anxiety exhibited 48 hours after withdrawal from cocaine is accompanied by reductions in tissue levels of CRF immunoreactivity in the amgydala, hypothalamus, and basal forebrain, suggesting increased release of the peptide in these regions (Sarnyai et al., 1995). It has likewise been shown that up to 48 hours after an acute "binge" pattern of cocaine administration, CRF mRNA levels are enhanced in the hypothalamus and amygdala (Zhou et al., 1996). Similarly, decreases in CRF receptor binding in the amgydala, also suggesting increased release in this region, have been observed immediately, but not 10 days, following a chronic cocaine administration regimen (Ambrosia et al., 1997). Finally, in the 12-hour period following a 12-hour cocaine self-administration session, dialysate concentrations of CRF are markedly elevated in the amygdala (Richter and Weiss, 1999). Likewise, in the 12 hours following withdrawal from a 2–3 week liquid diet containing ethanol, dialysate concentrations of CRF are elevated, both in the amygdala (Merlo Pich et al., 1995) and in the BNST (Olive et al., 2002).

Consistent with previous findings, my collaborators and I recently reported enhanced expression of CRF mRNA in the CeA 24 hours after termination of repeated intermittent exposure to cocaine, but not following extended withdrawal periods of 3–42 days. In addition, we reported an absence of change in the expression of CRF mRNA in the BNST, a region not previously examined for the effects of repeated drug exposure on CRF mRNA, at any of the timepoints assessed (Erb et al., 2003a).

In the study just mentioned, we were also interested in determining whether persistent changes in the expression of the CRF binding protein (BP) might occur as a consequence of prior exposure to cocaine, even in the absence of persistent changes in the peptide itself. The CRF BP is a modulator of CRF in the CNS (Heinrichs and De Souza, 1999; Seasholtz et al., 2002), whose role in the effects of abused drugs had not previously been explored. Although CRF is generally considered to positively regulate its BP (Heinrichs and De Souza, 1999; Kemp et al., 1998; Seasholtz et al., 2002), there is evidence that, following activation of the CRF systems, levels of the BP can remain elevated after CRF levels return to baseline (e.g., Smith et al., 1997). Thus, it seemed conceivable that persistent changes in the activity of the BP would occur following repeated drug exposure, even though the preponderance of evidence suggests that changes in the activity of the peptide itself do not persist. Consistent with the outcome of the CRF mRNA analyses, however, CRF-BP mRNA levels were not elevated in the CeA beyond a post-treatment time of 24 hours (Erb et al., 2003a). Taken together with previous results, these data suggest that a prior history of drug exposure, or at least cocaine exposure, does not produce persistent changes in the basal activity of CRF or its BP within brain regions known to be key mediators of effects of CRF on relapse to drug seeking.

The majority of the recent evidence suggests that although basal changes in CRF systems induced by drug exposure are transient (but see Zorrilla et al., 2001), changes in the responsivity of the central nervous system to CRF persist long after termination of drug exposure. Indeed, it has been reported that 10–15 weeks following a 6-week exposure to ethanol vapor, rats show enhanced electroencephalogram and event-related potential recordings in response to ICV injections of CRF (Slawecki et al., 1999). Furthermore, when injected into the VTA, CRF selectively increases local glutamate release in cocaine self-administering, as compared with control, animals up to 3 weeks after termination of self-administration (Wang et al., 2005). Finally, we recently reported that repeated intermittent exposure to cocaine produces an augmented locomotor response to ICV injections of CRF following drug-free periods of up to 4 weeks (Erb et al., 2003b; Erb et al., 2005). Rats injected with 30 mg/kg, (i.p.) cocaine once daily for 7 days exhibited a higher level of locomotor activity in response to an ICV injection of CRF (0.5 to 5.0 µg) than did rats given daily saline injections; this augmented locomotor response was observed 10 and 28 days post-treatment (Erb et al., 2003b). Likewise, rats injected with 45 mg/kg cocaine (given in 2 daily injections separated by 90 minutes) for 1 or 3 days exhibited a higher level of CRF-induced locomotor activity than did saline-injected animals; in this experiment, animals were tested 28 days post-treatment (unpublished findings). Taken together, these findings suggest that a history of cocaine exposure produces a form of sensitization within CRF systems, or those systems on which CRF acts, that might result in persistent reactivity to the effects of stressors over time.

Recently, my colleagues and I reported that, under conditions that produce an augmented locomotor response to ICV CRF, repeated cocaine exposure also results in augmented, or sensitized, neuronal responses to acute stressors in brain regions known to play an important role in the effects of stress on the reinstatement of drug seeking (Erb et al., 2004; Erb et al., 2005). In one study, expression of c-Fos mRNA, an immediate early gene that is used as a generalized marker of neuronal activation (Cullinan et al., 1995), was measured in the CeA and BNST following exposure to acute foot-shock stress, 21 days after the last cocaine injection (Erb et al., 2004). In another study, expression of c-Fos mRNA was measured in the CeA and BNST following exposure to an ICV injection of CRF (0.5 µg) 10 days after the last injection (Erb et al., 2005). In both studies, repeated exposure to cocaine produced a potentiated c-Fos mRNA response to the stressor in the CeA, but not in the BNST.

The fact that repeated cocaine exposure resulted in a similar potentiated c-Fos mRNA response to both foot-shock stress and ICV CRF in the CeA is interesting in light of observations that both stressors induce reinstatement of drug seeking (Shaham et al., 2000a) and that the effects of foot-shock stress on reinstatement are mediated, in part, via the CeA (Erb et al., 2001a). It is, therefore, tempting to speculate that foot shock and ICV CRF activate the same population of neurons in the CeA of cocaine pre-exposed animals and that the population of neurons that is activated contains CRF.

Somewhat surprising was the finding that neither foot-shock stress nor ICV CRF induced an enhanced c-Fos mRNA response in the BNST of cocaine pre-exposed rats, although foot-shock stress did induce c-Fos mRNA expression to a similar degree in cocaine and saline pre-exposed animals. Although anatomical and functional differences between the BNST and CeA have been described (Davis et al., 1997), a strong interconnection and anatomical and functional similarities between the two structures have also been reported (Alheid et al., 1995). Moreover, the BNST, like the CeA, has been found to play an important role in a number of stress- and drug-related effects (Delfs et al., 2000; Sarnyai et al., 2001; Walker et al., 2000b). Most notably, activation of CRF receptors in the BNST has been shown to be critical for stress-induced reinstatement of drug seeking (Erb and Stewart, 1999). (See Erb et al., 2004; Erb et al., 2005 for a discussion of these issues.)

In addition to the CeA, it is conceivable that the neuroadaptive changes produced by repeated cocaine exposure within midbrain DA systems, including the VTA and several of its terminal regions, render an organism more vulnerable to the effects of stress over time. Indeed, a circuit of DA and glutamatergic interconnections between the VTA and terminal regions of the mesotelencephalic DA system, including NAc and PFC, are considered responsible for the manifestation of psychostimulant sensitization (Vanderschuren and Kalivas, 2000). Furthermore, this circuitry has been implicated in the cross-sensitizing effects of psychostimulants and environmental stressors (Kalivas and Stewart, 1991; Prasad et al., 1998), and some of these effects have been found to be mediated, at least in part, by CRF (Cole et al., 1990). In addition, CRF is known to act in the VTA to affect behaviors that are also affected by psychostimulant drugs (Cador et al., 1993). For example, CRF injected into the VTA increases spontaneous locomotor activity (Kalivas et al., 1987) and, as mentioned previously, intra-VTA perfusions of CRF selectively increase local glutamate release in cocaine-experienced animals after drug-free periods of up to 3 weeks; likewise, intra-VTA perfusions of CRF induce the reinstatement of cocaine seeking (Wang et al., 2005). These findings, in combination with the postulation that neuroadaptations in glutamatergic control over VTA DA neurons contributes to the long-term plasticity underlying the effects of cocaine (Kalivas, 2004; Wolf, 1998), leads to speculation that an interaction between CRF, glutamate, and DA in the VTA contributes to behavioral sensitization to cocaine and increased vulnerability to the effects of stressors as a consequence of prior drug exposure.

Although the majority of work reviewed in this section has been conducted in animals with a history of repeated exposure to cocaine, the limited data in heroin and alcohol pre-exposed animals is corroborative (e.g., Shalev et al., 2001). In summary, recent findings suggest that a history of exposure to drugs of abuse can produce long-lasting changes in the responsivity of central CRF systems, or the systems upon which they act. These changes are manifest in both behavior and in neuronal activity and may be part of a mechanism whereby former drug users remain vulnerable to the effects of stress and relapse after prolonged drug-free periods.

V. CONCLUSIONS

The reinstatement model has proved to be a powerful tool for studying the neurobiological and behavioral mechanisms underlying the effects of stress on drug seeking. Data generated using variations of the reinstatement procedure, in combination with data from studies using other methodologies, have led to considerable progress in clarifying the relationship between stress and relapse and in elucidating the neurobiological mechanisms that render former drug users vulnerable to the effects of stress over time.

Studies aimed specifically at exploring the neurobiology of stress-induced reinstatement point to central CRF and NA systems as viable targets for medications development. It is therefore of interest that pharmacological compounds with clinical utility, because of their ability to be effective when injected systemically, have been found to interfere in stress-induced reinstatement of drug seeking. For example, systemic injections of a non-peptide CRF receptor antagonist have been found to interfere in the foot-shock–induced reinstatement of cocaine and heroin seeking, as have systemic injections of the alpha-2 adrenoceptor agonists, clonidine and lofexidine. In a recent review that included an update on the current status of clinical trials for medications development in the treatment of relapse, it was suggested that because of results such as these, CRF receptor antagonists are likely to be used in clinical trials with human addicts, once they become available for that purpose (Bossert et al., 2005). Furthermore, it was noted in that review that results from reinstatement studies in laboratory rats have led to a study using lofexidine in opiate-dependent patients that has generated promising preliminary data to support the use of lofexidine as a treatment for relapse prevention (Sinha et al., 2003).

In conclusion, considerable progress is being made toward understanding the nature of the relationship between stress and the long-lasting effects that drugs of abuse have on the brain and behavior. A great deal of the progress in the past several years has been made in delineating the neuroanatomical circuitry underlying the effects of stress on reinstatement of drug seeking and in characterizing the role of specific neurochemical systems within that circuitry. In addition, progress has been made toward understanding the nature of the changes that occur in response to the administration of drugs of abuse within systems found to be critical in mediating the effects of stress on relapse.

REFERENCES

Ahmed, S. H., and Koob, G. F. (1997). Cocaine- but not food-seeking behavior is reinstated by stress after extinction. *Psychopharmacology (Berl), 132,* 289–295.

Ahmed, S. H., and Koob, G. F. (2005). Transition to drug addiction: A negative reinforcement model based on an allostatic decrease in reward function. *Psychopharmacology (Berl), 180,* 473–490.

Ahmed, S. H., Walker, J. R., and Koob, G. F. (2000). Persistent increase in the motivation to take heroin in rats with a history of drug escalation. *Neuropsychopharmacology, 22,* 413–421.

Alheid, G. F., de Olmos, J. S., and Beltramino, C. A. (1995). Amygdala and extended amygdala. In Paxinos, G. (Ed), *The rat nervous system.* pp. 495–578. San Diego: Academic Press, Inc.

Alheid, G. F., and Heimer, L. (1988). New perspectives in basal forebrain organization of special relevance for neuropsychiatric disorders: The striatopallidal, amygdaloid, and corticipetal components of substantia innominata. *Neuroscience, 27,* 1–39.

Ambrosia, E., Sharpe, L., and Pilotte, N. (1997). Regional binding to corticotropin releasing factor receptors in brain of rats exposed to chronic cocaine and cocaine withdrawal. *Synapse, 25,* 272–276.

Aston-Jones, G., Delfs, J. M., Druhan, J., and Zhu, Y. (1999). The bed nucleus of the stria terminalis. A target site for noradrenergic actions in opiate withdrawal. *Ann N Y Acad Sci, 877,* 486–498.

Aston-Jones, G., Shipley, M. T., and Grzanna, R. (1995). The locus coeruleus, A5 and A7 noradrenergic cell groups. In Paxinos, G. (Ed), *The rat nervous system.* pp. 183–213. San Diego, Academic.

Bigelow, G. E., Griffiths, R. R., and Liebson I. A. (1977). Pharmacological influences upon human ethanol self-administration. In Gross, M. M. (Ed), *Alcohol intoxication and withdrawal.* pp. 523–538. New York, Plenum Press.

Bossert, J. M., Ghitza, U. E., Lu, L., Epstein, D. H., and Shaham Y. (2005). Neurobiology of relapse to heroin and cocaine seeking: An update and clinical implications. *Eur J Pharmacol, 526,* 36–50.

Breiter, H. C., Gollub, R. L., Weisskoff, R. M., Kennedy, D. N., Makris, N., Berke J. D., Goodman, J. M., Kantor, H. L., Gastfriend, D. R., Riorden, J. P., Mathew R. T., Rosen, B. R., and Hyman, S. E. (1997). Acute effects of cocaine on human brain activity and emotion. *Neuron, 19,* 591–611.

Brown, S., Vik, P., Patterson, T., Grant, I., and Schuckit, M. (1995). Stress, vulnerability and adult alcohol relapse. *J Stud Alcohol, 56,* 538–545.

Brozek, G., Zhuravin, I. A., Megirian, D., and Bures J. (1996). Localization of the central rhythm generator involved in spontaneous consummatory licking in rats: Functional ablation and electrical brain stimulation studies. *Proc Natl Acad Sci U S A, 93,* 3325–3329.

Buczek, Y., Lê, A. D., Wang, A., Stewart, J., and Shaham, Y. (1999). Stress reinstates nicotine seeking but not sucrose solution seeking in rats. *Psychopharmacology (Berl), 144,* 183–188.

Cador, M., Cole, B. J., Koob, G. F., Stinus, L., and Le Moal, M. (1993). Central administration of corticotropin releasing factor induces long-term sensitization to d-amphetamine. *Brain Research, 606,* 181–186.

Capriles, N., Rodaros, D., Sorge, R. E., and Stewart, J. (2003). A role for the prefrontal cortex in stress- and cocaine-induced reinstatement of cocaine seeking in rats. *Psychopharmacology (Berl), 168,* 66–74.

Carboni, E., Imperato, A., Perezzani, L., and Di Chiara, G. (1989). Amphetamine, cocaine, phencyclidine and nomifensine increase extracellular dopamine concentrations preferentially in the nucleus accumbens of freely moving rats. *Neuroscience, 28,* 653–661.

Chalmers, D., Lovenberg, T., and De Souza, E. (1995). Localization of novel corticotropin-releasing factor receptor (CRF2) mRNA expression to specific subcortical nuclei in rat brain: Comparison with CRF1 receptor mRNA expression. *Neurosci, 15,* 6340–6350.

Childress, A. R., Ehrman, R., McLellan, A. T., MacRae J., Natale, M., and O'Brien, C. P. (1994). Can induced moods trigger drug-related responses in opiate abuse patients? *J Subst Abuse Treat, 11,* 17–23.

Cole, B. J., Cador, M., Stinus, L., Rivier, J., Vale, W., Koob, G. F., and Le Moal, M. (1990). Central administration of CRF antagonist blocks the development of stress-induced behavioral sensitization. *Brain Research, 512,* 343–346.

Cullinan, W., Herman, J., Battaglia, D., Akil, H., and Watson, S. (1995). Pattern and time course of immediate early gene expression in rat brain following acute stress. *Neuroscience, 64,* 477–505.

Davis, M., Walker, D., and Lee, Y. (1997). Amygdala and bed nucleus of the stria terminalis: Differential roles in fear and anxiety measured with the acoustic startle reflex. Philos. *Trans R Soc Lond B Biol Sci, 352*, 1675–1687.

Delfs, J. M., Zhu, Y., Druhan, J. P., and Aston-Jones, G. (2000). Noradrenaline in the ventral forebrain is critical for opiate withdrawal-induced aversion. *Nature, 403*, 430–434.

de Olmos, J. S., and Heimer, L. (1999). The concepts of the ventral striatopallidal system and extended amygdala. *Ann N Y Acad Sci, 877*, 1–32.

De Vries, T., Schoffelmeer, A., Binnekade, R., Mulder, A., and Vanderschuren, L. (1998). Drug-induced reinstatement of heroin- and cocaine-seeking behaviour following long-term extinction is associated with expression of behavioural sensitization. *Eur J Neurosci, 10*, 3563–3571.

de Wit, H. (1996). Priming effects with drugs and other reinforcers. *Experimental and Clinical Psychopharmacology, 4*, 5–10.

de Wit, H., and Stewart, J. (1981). Reinstatement of cocaine-reinforced responding in the rat. *Psychopharmacology, 75*, 134–143.

Easton, A., Parker, A., and Gaffan, D. (2001). Crossed unilateral lesions of medial forebrain bundle and either inferior temporal or frontal cortex impair object recognition memory in Rhesus monkeys. *Behav Brain Res, 121*, 1–10.

Erb, S. (2000). Stress-induced relapse to cocaine seeking in the rat: Contributions of central nervous system corticotropin-releasing factor and noradrenaline. PhD Dissertation, Concordia University.

Erb, S., Borkowski, S., Funk, D., Watson, Jr, S. J., and Akil, H. (2003a). Effects of chronic cocaine on CRH and CRH-BP mRNA expression in the extended amygdala following drug-free periods of up to 28 days. Abstract for the Meeting of the Society for Neuroscience.

Erb, S., Funk, D., and Lê, A. D. (2003b). Prior, repeated exposure to cocaine potentiates locomotor responsivity to central injections of corticotropin-releasing factor (CRF) in rats. *Psychopharmacology, 170*, 383–389.

Erb, S., Funk, D., and Lê, A. D. (2005). Cocaine pre-exposure enhances CRF-induced expression of c-Fos mRNA in the central nucleus of the amygdala: An effect that parallels the effects of cocaine pre-exposure on CRF-induced locomotor activity. *Neurosci Lett, 383*, 209–214.

Erb, S., Hitchcott, P. K., Rajabi, H., Mueller, D., Shaham, Y., and Stewart J. (2000). Alpha-2 adrenergic receptor agonists block stress-induced reinstatement of cocaine seeking. *Neuropsychopharmacology, 23*, 138–150.

Erb, S., Lopak, V., and Smith, C. (2004). Cocaine pre-exposure produces a sensitized and context-specific c-Fos mRNA response to footshock stress in the central nucleus of the amygdala. *Neuroscience, 129*, 719–725.

Erb, S., Petrovic, A., Yi D., and Kayyali, H. (2006). Central injections of CRF reinstate cocaine seeking in rats after post-injection delays of up to 3 hours: An influence of time and environmental context. *Psychopharmacology, 187*, 112–20.

Erb, S., Salmaso, N., Rodaros, D., and Stewart, J. (2001a). A role for the CRF-containing pathway from central nucleus of the amygdala to bed nucleus of the stria terminalis in the stress-induced reinstatement of cocaine seeking in rats. *Psychopharmacology, 158*, 360–365.

Erb, S., Shaham, Y., and Stewart., J. (1996). Stress reinstates Cocaine - Seeking behavior after prolonged extinction and a drug-free period. Psychopharmacology, *128*, 408–12.

Erb, S., Shaham, Y., and Stewart, J. (1998). The role of corticotropin-releasing factor and corticosterone in stress- and cocaine-induced relapse to cocaine seeking in rats. *J Neurosci, 18*, 5529–5536.

Erb, S., Shaham, Y., and Stewart, J. (2001b). Stress-induced relapse to drug seeking in the rat: Role of the bed nucleus of the stria terminalis and amygdala. *Stress, 4*, 289–303.

Erb, S., and Stewart, J. (1999). A role for the bed nucleus of the stria terminalis, but not the amygdala, in the effects of corticotropin-releasing factor on stress-induced reinstatement of cocaine seeking. *J Neurosci, 19*, RC35, 1–6.

Everitt, B. J., Cador, M., and Robbins T. W. (1989). Interactions between the amygdala and ventral striatum in stimulus-reward associations: Studies using a second-order schedule of sexual reinforcement. *Neuroscience, 30*, 63–75.

Fahlke, C., Hård, E., Thomasson, R., Engel, J. A., and Hansen, S. (1994). Metyrapone-induced suppression of corticosterone synthesis reduces ethanol consumption in high-preferring rats. *Pharmacology Biochemistry and Behavior, 48*, 977–981.

Fox, H. C., Talih, M., Malison, R., Anderson, G. M., Kreek, M. J., and Sinha, R. (2005). Frequency of recent cocaine and alcohol use affects drug craving and associated responses to stress and drug-related cues. *Psychoneuroendocrinology, 30*, 880–891.

Goeders, N., and Guerin, G. (1996). Effects of surgical and pharmacological adrenalectomy on the initiation and maintenance of intravenous cocaine self-administration in rats. *Brain Research, 722*, 145–152.

Hall, S. M, E, H. B., and A, W. D. (1990). Commitment to abstinence and acute stress in relapse to alcohol, opiates and nicotine. *Journal of Consulting and Clinical Psychology, 58*, 175–181.

Heinrichs, S. C., and De Souza E. B., (1999). Corticotropin-releasing factor antagonists, binding-protein and receptors: Implications for central nervous system disorders. *Bailliere's Clinical Endocrinology and Metabolism, 13*, 541–554.

Highfield, D., Yap, J., Grimm J. W., Shalev U., and Shaham, Y. (2001). Repeated lofexidine treatment attenuates stress-induced, but not drug cues-induced reinstatement of a heroin-cocaine mixture (speedball) seeking in rats. *Neuropsychopharmacology, 25*, 320–331.

Hornby, P., and Piekut, D. (1989). Opiocortin and catecholamine input to CRF-immunoreactive neurons in rat forebrain. *Peptides, 10*, 1139–1146.

Jaffe, J. H., Cascell, N. G., Kumor, K. M., and Sherer, M. A. (1989). Cocaine-induced cocaine craving. *Psychopharmacology, 97*, 59–64.

Kalivas, P., and Stewart, J. (1991). Dopamine transmission in the initiation and expression of drug- and stress-induced sensitization of motor activity. *Brain Research Reviews, 16*, 223–244.

Kalivas, P. W. (2004). Glutamate systems in cocaine addiction. *Curr Opin Pharmacol, 4*, 23–29.

Kalivas P. W., Duffy, P., and Latimer, G. (1987). Neurochemical and behavioral effects of corticotropin-releasing factor in the ventral tegmental area of the rat. *J Pharmacol Exp Ther, 242*.

Kalivas, P. W., and McFarland, K. (2003). Brain circuitry and the reinstatement of cocaine-seeking behavior. *Psychopharmacology, 168*, 44–56.

Kemp, C., Woods, R., and Lowry, P. (1998). The corticotropin-releasing factor-binding protein: An act of several parts. *Peptides, 19*, 1119–1128.

Koob, G. F. (1999). Corticotropin-releasing factor, norepinephrine, and stress. *Biological Psychiatry, 46*, 1167–1180.

Kosten, T. R., Rounsaville, B. J., and Kleber, H. D. (1986). A 2.5-year follow-up of depression, life crises, and treatment effects on abstinence among opioid addicts. *Archives of General Psychiatry, 43*, 733–739.

Kumor, K. M., Sherer, M. A., Gomez, J., Cone E., and Jaffe, J. H. (1989). Subjective response during continuous infusion of cocaine. *Pharmacology Biochemistry and Behavior, 33*, 443–452.

Lê, A. D., Harding, S., Juzytsch, W., Funk, D., and Shaham Y. (2005). Role of alpha-2 adrenoceptors in stress-induced reinstatement of alcohol seeking and alcohol self-administration in rats. *Psychopharmacology (Berl), 179*, 366–373.

Lê, A. D., Harding, S., Juzytsch, W., Watchus, J., Shalev, U., and Shaham Y. (2000). The role of corticotropin-releasing factor in stress-induced relapse to alcohol-seeking behavior in rats. *Psychopharmacology, 150*, 317–324.

Lê, A., D., Quan, B., Juzystch, W., Fletcher, P. J., Joharchi, N, and Shaham, Y. (1998). Reinstatement of alcohol-seeking by priming injections of alcohol and exposure to stress in rats. *Psychopharmacology, 135*, 169–174.

Lê, A. D., Wang, A., Harding, S., Juzytsch, W., and Shaham, Y. (2003). Nicotine increases alcohol self-administration and reinstates alcohol seeking in rats. *Psychopharmacology (Berl), 168*, 216–221.

Lee, B., Tiefenbacher, S., Platt, D. M., and Spealman, R. D. (2004). Pharmacological blockade of alpha2-adrenoceptors induces reinstatement of cocaine-seeking behavior in squirrel monkeys. *Neuropsychopharmacology, 29*, 686–693.

Lee, Y., and Davis, M. (1997). Role of the hippocampus, the bed nucleus of the stria terminalis and the amygdala in the excitatory effect of corticotropin-releasing hormone on the acoustic startle reflex. *J Neurosci, 17*, 6434–6440.

Leri, F., Flores, J., Rodaros, D., and Stewart, J. (2002). Blockade of stress-induced but not cocaine-induced reinstatement by infusion of noradrenergic antagonists into the bed nucleus of the stria terminalis or the central nucleus of the amygdala. *J Neurosci, 22*, 5713–5718.

Lu, L., Liu, D., and Ceng, X. (2001). Corticotropin-releasing factor receptor type 1 mediates stress-induced relapse to cocaine-conditioned place preference in rats. *European Journal of Pharmacology, 415*, 203–208.

Lu, L., Shepard, J. D., Scott Hall, F., and Shaham, Y. (2003). Effect of environmental stressors on opiate and psychostimulant reinforcement, reinstatement and discrimination in rats: A review. *Neurosci Biobehav Rev, 27*, 457–491.

Lu, L., Xu, N.-J., Ge. X., Yue, W., Su, W.-J., Pei, G., and Ma, L. (2002a). Reactivation of morphine conditioned place preference by drug priming: Role of environmental cues and sensitization. *Psychopharmacology, 159*, 125–132.

Lu, L., Zhang, B., Liu, Z., and Zhang, Z. (2002b). Reactivation of cocaine conditioned place preference induced by stress is reversed by cholecystokinin-B receptors antagonist in rats. *Brain Res, 954*, 132–140.

Ludwig, A. M., A. W., and H S. L. (1974). The first drink: Psychobiological aspects of craving. *Archives of General Psychiatry, 30*, 539–547.

Ludwig, A. M., and Wikler, A. (1974). "Craving" and relapse to drink. *Quarterly Journal of Studies in Alcohol, 35*, 108–130.

Mantsch, J., and Goeders, N. (1999). Ketoconazole blocks the stress-induced reinstatement of cocaine-seeking behavior in rats: Relationship to the discriminative stimulus effects of cocaine. *Psychopharmacology, 142*, 399–407.

McFall, M. E., Mackay, P. W., and Donovan, D. M. (1992). Combat-related posttraumatic stress disorder and severity of substance abuse in Vietnam veterans. *J Stud Alcohol, 53*, 357–363.

McFarland, K., Davidge, S. B., Lapish, C. C., and Kalivas, P. W. (2004). Limbic and motor circuitry underlying footshock-induced reinstatement of cocaine seeking behavior. *Journal of Neuroscience, 24*, 1551–1560.

McKay, J. R., Rutherford, M. J., Alterman, A. I., Cacciola, J. S., and Kaplan M. R. (1995). An examination of the cocaine relapse process. *Drug and Alcohol Dependence, 38*, 35–43.

Merlo Pich, E., Lorang, M., Yeganeh, M., Rodriguez de Fonseca, F., Raber, J., Koob, G. F., and Weiss, F. (1995). Increase of extracellular corticotropin-releasing factor-like immunoreactivity levels in the amygdala of awake rats during restraint stress and ethanol withdrawal as measured by microdialysis. *Journal of Neuroscience, 15*, 5439–5447.

Meyer, R., and M, M. S. (1979). *The heroin stimulus: Implications for a theory of addiction.* New York: Plenum.

Moore, R., and Bloom, F. (1979). Central catecholamine neuron systems: Anatomy and physiology of the norepinephrine and epinephrine systems. *Ann Rev Neurosci, 2,* 113–168.

Mueller, D., Perdikaris, D., and Stewart, J. (2002). Persistence and drug-induced reinstatement of a morphine-induced conditioned place preference. *Behav Brain Res, 136,* 389–397.

Mueller, D., and Stewart, J. (2000). Cocaine-induced conditioned place preference: Reinstatement by priming injections of cocaine after extinction. *Behav Brain Res, 115,* 39–47.

Narahashi, T., Frey, J. M., Ginsburg, K. S., and Roy, M. L. (1992). Sodium and GABA-activated channels as the targets of pyrethroids and cyclodienes. *Toxicol Lett, 64–65* (Spec No) 429–436.

Numan, M., and Numan, M. (1996). A lesion and neuroanatomical tract-tracing analysis of the role of the bed nucleus of the stria terminalis in retrieval behavior and other aspects of maternal responsiveness in rats. *Dev Psychobiol, 29,* 23–51.

Numan, M., and Numan, M. (1997). Projection sites of medial preoptic area and ventral bed nucleus of the stria terminalis neurons that express Fos during maternal behavior in female rats. *J Neuroendocrinol, 9,* 369–384.

Olive, M., Koenig, H., Nannini, M., and Hodge, C. (2002). Elevated extracellular CRF levels in the bed nucleus of the stria terminalis during ethanol withdrawal and reduction by subsequent ethanol intake. *Pharmacology Biochemistry and Behavior, 72,* 213–220.

Parker, A., and Gaffan, D. (1998). Memory after frontal/temporal disconnection in monkeys: Conditional and non-conditional tasks, unilateral and bilateral frontal lesions. *Neuropsychologia, 36,* 259–271.

Parker, L. A., and McDonald, R. V., (2000). Reinstatement of both a conditioned place preference and a conditioned place aversion with drug primes. *Pharmacol Biochem Behav, 66,* 559–561.

Phelix, C. F., Liposits, Z., and Paull, W. K. (1992). Monoamine innervation of bed nucleus of stria terminalis: An electron microscopic investigation. *Brain Research Bulletin, 28,* 949–965.

Phelix, C. F., Liposits, Z., and Paull, W. K. (1994). Catecholamine-CRF synaptic interaction in a septal bed nucleus: Afferents of neurons in the bed nucleus of the stria terminalis. *Brain Research Bulletin, 33,* 109–119.

Piazza, P., Barrot, M., Rouge-Pont, F., Marinelli, M., Maccari, S., Abrous, D., Simon, H., and Le Moal, M. (1996a). Suppression of glucocorticoid secretion and antipsychotic drugs have similar effects on the mesolimbic dopaminergic transmission. *Proc Natl Acad Sci U S A, 93,* 15445–15450.

Piazza, P., Marinelli, M., Rouge-Pont, F., Deroche, V., Maccari, S., Simon, H., and Le Moal, M. (1996b). Stress, glucocorticoids, and mesencephalic dopaminergic neurons: A pathophysiological chain determining vulnerability to psychostimulant abuse. *NIDA Res Monogr, 163,* 277–299.

Piazza, P. V., Deminiere, J. M., Maccari, S., Le Moal, M., Mormede, P., and Simon, H. (1991). Individual vulnerability to drug-self-administration action of corticosterone on dopaminergic systems as possible pathophysiological mechanism. In Willner P, and Scheel-Kruger, J, (Eds), *The mesolimbic dopaminergic system: From motivation to action* (pp. 473–495). New York: Wiley.

Potter, E., Sutton, S., Donaldson, C., Chen, R., Perrin, M., Lewis, K., Sawchenko, P., and Vale, W. (1994). Distribution of corticotropin-releasing factor receptor mRNA expression in the rat brain and pituitary. *Proc Natl Acad Sci U S A, 91,* 8777–8781.

Prasad, B., Ulibarri, C., and Sorg, B. (1998). Stress-induced cross-sensitization to cocaine: Effect of adrenalectomy and corticosterone after short- and long-term withdrawal. *Psychopharmacology, 136,* 24–33.

Preston, K. L., Sullivan, J. T., Strain, E. C., and Bigelow, G. E. (1992). Effects of cocaine alone and in combination with bromocriptine in human cocaine abusers. *The Journal of Pharmacology and Experimental Therapeutics, 262,* 279–291.

Richter, R., and Weiss, F. (1999). In vivo CRF release in rat amygdala is increased during cocaine withdrawal in self-administering rats. *Synapse, 32,* 254–261.

Sakanaka, M., Shibasaki, T., and Lederis, K. (1986). Distribution and efferent projections of corticotropin-releasing factor-like immunoreactivity in the rat amygdaloid complex. *Brain Res, 382,* 213–238.

Sanchez, C. J., Bailie, T. M., Wu, W. R., Li, N., and Sorg, B. A. (2003). Manipulation of dopamine d1-like receptor activation in the rat medial prefrontal cortex alters stress- and cocaine-induced reinstatement of conditioned place preference behavior. *Neuroscience, 119,* 497–505.

Sanchez, C. J., and Sorg, B. A. (2001). Conditioned fear stimuli reinstate cocaine-induced conditioned place preference. *Brain Res, 908,* 86–92.

Sarnyai, Z., Biro, E., Gardi, J., Vecsernyés, M., Julesz, J., and Telegdy, G. (1995). Brain cortiocotropin-releasing factor mediates 'anxiety-like' behavior induced by cocaine withdrawal in rats. *Brain Res, 657,* 89–97.

Sarnyai, Z., Shaham, Y., and Heinrichs, S. C. (2001). The role of corticotropin-releasing factor in drug addiction. *Pharmacological Review, 53,* 209–243.

Scriabine, A., Sweet, C. S., Ludden, C. T., Stavorski, J. M., Wenger, H. C., and Bohidar, N. R. (1977). Some cardiovascular effects of ST-91 and clonidine. *Eur J Pharmacol, 43,* 333–341.

Seasholtz, A. F., Valverde, R. A., and Denver, R. J. (2002). Corticotropin-releasing hormone-binding protein: Biochemistry and function from fishes to mammals. *Journal of Endocrinology, 175*, 89–97.

Shaham, Y., Erb, S., and Stewart, J. (2000a). Stress-induced relapse to heroin and cocaine seeking in rats: A review. *Brain Research Reviews, 33*, 13–33.

Shaham, Y., Funk, D., Erb, S., Brown, T., Walker, C-D., and Stewart, J. (1997). Corticotropin-releasing factor, but not corticosterone, is involved in stress-induced relapse to heroin-seeking in rats. *Journal of Neuroscience, 17*, 2605–2614.

Shaham, Y., Highfield, D., Delfs, J., Leung, S., and Stewart, J. (2000b). Clonidine blocks stress-induced reinstatement of heroin seeking in rats: An effect independent of the locus coeruleus noradrenergic neurons. *Eur J Neurosci, 12*, 292–302.

Shaham, Y., Shalev, U., Lu, L., De Wit, H., and Stewart, J. (2003). The reinstatement model of drug relapse: History, methodology and major findings. *Psychopharmacology, 168*, 3–20.

Shaham, Y., and Stewart, J. (1995). Characterization of stress- and heroin-primed relapse to heroin-seeking behavior in rats. *Abst Soc Neurosci, 21*, 725.

Shaham, Y., and Stewart, J. (1996). Effects of opioid and dopamine receptor antagonists on relapse induced by stress and re-exposure to heroin in rats. *Psychopharmacology, 125*, 385–391.

Shalev, U., Grimm, J. W., and Shaham, Y. (2002). Neurobiology of relapse to heroin and cocaine seeking: A review. *Pharmacological Review, 54*, 1–42.

Shalev, U., Highfield, D., Yap, J., and Shaham, Y. (2000). Stress and relapse to drug seeking in rats: Studies on the generality of the effect. *Psychopharmacology (Berl), 150*, 337–346.

Shalev, U., Morales, M., Hope, B., Yap, J., and Shaham, Y. (2001). Time dependent changes in extinction behavior and stress-induced reinstatement of drug seeking during heroin withdrawal. *Psychopharmacologia, 156*, 98–107.

Shepard, J. D., Bossert, J. M., Liu, S. Y., and Shaham, Y. (2004). The anxiogenic drug yohimbine reinstates methamphetamine seeking in a rat model of drug relapse. *Biol Psychiatry, 55*, 1082–1089.

Sinha R. (2001). How does stress increase risk of drug abuse and relapse? *Psychopharmacology (Berl), 158*, 343–359.

Sinha, R., Catapano, D., and O'Malley, S. (1999). Stress-induced craving and stress response in cocaine dependent individuals. *Psychopharmacology, 142*, 343–351.

Sinha, R., Fuse, T., Aubin, L. R., and O'Malley, S. S. (2000). Psychological stress, drug related cues and cocaine craving. *Psychopharmacology, 152*, 140–148.

Sinha, R., Holtzman, K., Hogan, I., Meandizija, B., Kimmerling, A., Scanley, B., and Kosten, T. (2003). Lofexidine: Enhancing naltrexone treatment to prevent stress related opiate relapse. Proc Annu Meeting College Problems Drug Dependence.

Slawecki, C., Somes, C., and Ehlers, C. L. (1999). Effects of chronic ethanol exposure on neurophysiological responses to corticotropin-releasing factor and neuropeptide Y. *Alcohol Alcohol, 34*, 289–299.

Smith, M., Weiss, S., Berry, R., Zhang, L., Clark, M., Massenburg, G., and Post, R. (1997). Amygdala-kindled seizures increase the expression of corticotropin-releasing factor (CRF) and CRF-binding protein in GABAergic interneurons of the dentate hilus. *Brain Res, 745*, 248–256.

Stewart, J., and de Wit, H. (1987). Reinstatement of drug-taking behavior as a method of assessing incentive motivational properties of drugs. In Bozarth, MA (Ed), *Methods of assessing the reinforcing properties of abused drugs* (pp. 211–227). New York: Springer-Verlag.

Stretch, R., Gerber, G. J., and Wood, S. M. (1971). Factors affecting behavior maintained by response-contingent intravenous infusions of amphetamine in squirrel monkeys. *Canadian Journal of Physiology and Pharmacology, 49*, 581–589.

Swanson, L., Sawchenko, P., Rivier, J., and Vale, W. (1983). Organization of ovine corticotropin releasing factor immunoreactive cells and fibers in the rat brain: An immunohistochemical study. *Neuroendocrinology, 36*, 165–186.

Ungless, M. A., Whistler, J. L., Malenka, R. C., and Bonci, A. (2001). Single cocaine exposure in vivo induces long-term potentiation in dopamine neurons. *Nature, 411*, 583–587.

Vanderschuren, L. J., and Kalivas, P. W. (2000). Alterations in dopaminergic and glutamatergic transmission in the induction and expression of behavioral sensitization: A critical review of preclinical studies. *Psychopharmacology (Berl), 151*, 99–120.

Veinante, P., Stoekel, M-E., and Freund-Mercier, M-J. (1997). GABA- and peptide-immunoreactivities co-localize in the rat central extended amygdala. *NeuroReport, 8*, 2985–2989.

Walker, J. R., Ahmed, S. H., Gracy, K. N., and Koob, G. F. (2000a). Microinjections of an opiate receptor antagonist into the bed nucleus of the stria terminalis suppress heroin self-administration in dependent rats. *Brain Research, 854*, 85–92.

Walker, J. R., Ahmed, S. H., Gracy, K. N., and Koob, G. F. (2000b). Microinjections of an opiate receptor antagonist into the bed nucleus of the stria terminalis suppress heroin self-administration in dependent rats. *Brain Res, 854*, 85–92.

Wang, B., Shaham, Y., Zitzman, D., Azari, S., Wise, R. A., and You Z. B. (2005). Cocaine experience establishes control of midbrain glutamate and dopamine by corticotropin-releasing factor: A role in stress-induced relapse to drug seeking. *J Neurosci, 25*, 5389–5396.

Wang, X., Cen, X., and Lu, L. (2001). Noradrenaline in the bed nucleus of the stria terminalis is critical for stress-induced reactivation of morphine-conditioned place preference in rats. *Eur J Pharmacol, 432*, 153–161.

Wolf, M. (1998). The role of excitatory amino acids in behavioral sensitization to psychomotor stimulants. *Progress in Neurobiology, 54*, 679–720.

Zhou, Y., Spangler, R., LaForge, K., Maggos, C., Ho, A., and Kreek, M. (1996). Corticotropin-releasing factor and type 1 corticotropin-releasing factor receptor messenger RNAs in rat brain and pituitary during "binge"-pattern cocaine administration and chronic withdrawal. *Journal of Pharmacololgy and Experimental Therapeutics, 279,* 351–358.

Zorrilla, E. P., Valdez, G. R., and Weiss, F. (2001). Changes in levels of regional CRF-like-immunoreactivity and plasma corticosterone during protracted drug withdrawal in dependent rats. *Psychopharmacology, 158,* 374–381.

PSYCHOSOCIAL PROCESSES RELATED TO STRESS AND ADDICTION

8

Negative Affect and Addiction

*JON D. KASSEL, JENNIFER C. VEILLEUX, MARGARET C. WARDLE,
MARISA C. YATES, JUSTIN E. GREENSTEIN, DANIEL P. EVATT,
AND LINDA L. ROESCH*

The idea that negative affect and addiction are inextricably linked is as old as the ages. Indeed, there is a wealth of both anecdotal and empirical evidence to suggest that this association has merit. Nonetheless, we present the case that a thorough understanding of the relationship between negative affect and addiction must be guided by careful analysis of several important yet conceptually distinct questions. First, the very notion of what comprises *negative affect* must be clearly understood. We believe that a great deal of drug addiction research has treated negative affect from a somewhat atheoretical stance. Correspondingly, we review several influential theoretical models of drug addiction, all of which make a strong case for the important role played by negative affect in promoting addictive substance use. We then consider the potentially important role played by expectancies in shaping and influencing the relationship between affect and drug use. Next, we argue that a meaningful delineation of the complex relationship between negative affect and drug addiction must, at the very least, consider the following three questions: (1) From a between-subjects level of analysis, do drug users experience heightened negative affect relative to non-users? (2) At the level of within-subject analysis, does negative affect genuinely prompt, or cue, drug self-administration? and (3) Does drug use genuinely assuage negative affect? We maintain that the answers to any or all of these questions may vary depending on where an individual falls on the drug use continuum (ranging from drug initation through relapse). Finally, we offer our thoughts regarding future directions for this important area of theoretical and clinical inquiry.

"What are you doing there?" [the Little Prince] asked the drunkard, whom he found sunk in silence before a collection of empty bottles and also a collection of full ones.

"Drinking," replied the drunkard, with a gloomy expression.

"Why are you drinking?" the little prince asked.

"To forget," replied the drunkard. "To forget what?" inquired the little prince, who was already feeling sorry for him.

Stress and Addiction: Biological and Psychological Mechanisms
Edited by **Mustafa al'Absi, Ph.D.**

"To forget that I'm ashamed," confessed the drunkard, hanging his head.

"What are you ashamed of?" inquired the little prince, who wanted to help.

"Of drinking!" concluded the drunkard, withdrawing into silence for good.

— *The Little Prince* (Saint-Exupéry, 1943)

I. INTRODUCTION

As exemplified in the quote above from The *Little Prince*, the idea goes something like this: Those individuals who are prone to experiencing NA are more likely to engage in various addictive behaviors as a way of assuaging such aversive feelings. Indeed, perhaps the oldest and most influential model of addiction posits that NA lies at the very core of such compulsive behaviors. Once an individual has crossed the line at which withdrawal symptomatology emerges in the *absence* of drug self-administration, that person is deemed addicted; his/her drug use is now believed to be motivated predominantly by the need to stave off the uncomfortable symptoms of withdrawal, which almost universally—across virtually all drugs of abuse and even nonpharmacological addictive behaviors—include various forms of NA.

According to stress-coping (Wills and Shiffman, 1985) and self-medication (Khantzian, 1997) models of substance abuse, drugs are thought to serve a coping function whereby they facilitate general mood regulation. Across a diverse array of psychoactive drugs, including alcohol (Cooper, Russell, Skinner, and Windle, 1992), cocaine (Jaffe and Kilbey, 1994), marijuana (Schafer and Brown, 1991), and tobacco (Ikard, Green, and Horn, 1969), there is reason to believe that some—perhaps even most—people use these substances as a means of regulating their mood and coping with stress and NA.[1] Drawing upon ciga-

rette smoking as an example, virtually all smokers attribute their smoking, at least in part, to its alleged anxiolytic and sedative properties (Frith, 1971; Spielberger, 1986; see Leventhal and Cleary, 1980). As described by Pomerleau and Pomerleau (1991, p. 599), "The relationship between stress and smoking, and a corresponding link between smoking and anxiety reduction, are so well entrenched in the lore concerning cigarette smoking that they have assumed the status of truisms." Indeed, smokers reliably report that they smoke more when they are stressed or angry or anxious or sad (e.g., Ikard et al., 1969; Russell, Peto, and Patel, 1974; see Shiffman, 1993), and hold the expectation that smoking will alleviate these negative moods (Brandon and Baker, 1991; Copeland, Brandon, and Quinn, 1995). At the same time, the fact that individuals *believe* that drug use helps to reduce NA does not, in and of itself, render this a valid conceptualization. Clearly, a more thorough assessment must be undertaken to truly grasp the relationship between NA and drug self-administration.

It is also important to remember that the pathways to becoming addicted are, no doubt, complex (Kassel, Weinstein, Skitch, Veilleux, and Mermelstein, 2005). However, of the numerous factors believed to heighten vulnerability both to drug use initiation and subsequent development of addiction, the role played by various forms of psychopathology and emotional distress appears particularly critical. That is, numerous studies have reliably found higher rates of drug use among selected populations of individuals with mental illness. For example, drawing upon a large, nationally representative sample in the United

---

[1] Whereas we do not view the constructs of stress and NA as synonymous (see Kassel et al., 2003), they are used somewhat interchangeably throughout this chapter. In the present context, then, stress might be best viewed as falling under the overall rubric of NA. Also, the construct of NA is rarely invoked within the animal literature, where stress is the preferred term, in great part, because it has been operationalized by reliable behavioral indices.

States, Lasser and colleagues (2000) found that individuals with a lifetime history of any psychiatric disorder had higher rates of lifetime and current smoking compared to those individuals who had never suffered from mental illness. Indeed, other investigations have reported similar findings, demonstrating strong and reliable associations between psychiatric disorders and cigarette smoking among adults (Breslau, Kilbey, and Andreski, 1991; Covey, Glassman, and Stetner, 1998; Degenhardt and Hall, 2001), and to a lesser extent, adolescents (Brown, Lewinsohn, Seeley, and Wagner, 1996; Rohde, Lewinsohn, Brown, Gau, and Kahler, 2003). Similar associations, both cross-sectional and longitudinal, have been reported for other drugs of abuse, such as alcohol (Currie et al., 2005; Hasin, Goodwin, Stinson, and Grant, 2005), cocaine (Watkins et al., 2004), and marijuana (Fu et al., 2002).

And it is these correlational observations—individuals who experience height-ened NA are at increased risk to use and abuse drugs—that really form the foundation of the assertion that NA and addiction are inextricably linked. But as we have argued elsewhere in some detail (Kassel and Hankin; In press; Kassel, Stround, and Paronis, 2003), it is important to remember that the association between NA and substance use is perhaps more complex than it may first seem. Indeed, we believe that a thorough understanding of the relationship between NA and substance abuse requires asking, at the very least, the following distinct but frequently blurred questions (see Figure 8-1): (1) Does NA actually promote drug use? More specifically, are there valid and reliable associations between affective distress and (a) drug use status (drug user versus nonuser) and (b) actual cueing (prompting) of substance use? Second, even if it were established that NA is linked to drug self-administration (at either or both of these levels of analysis), this does not

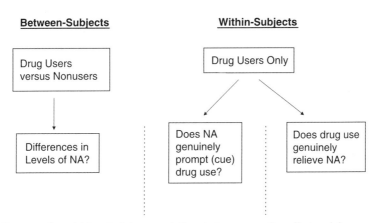

FIGURE 8-1   Conceptual model for studying associations between negative affect and drug use.

necessarily mean that substance use *relieves* NA. Hence, this often ignored point leads to another, very different, question: (2) Does drug use genuinely reduce symptoms of NA? Moving beyond the self-report of drug users, what do controlled experimental or field studies reveal regarding the influence of drug use on NA? Whereas space constraints render an exhaustive literature review impossible, we nonetheless provide a cursory overview, highlighting selected representative studies in the hope of providing a snapshot of what is ultimately a most complex relationship between addiction and NA.

We also believe it critical that an examination of relationships between drug use and NA take into account individuals' stage on the developmental continuum of drug use behavior. Drug users have been shown to proceed through a relatively well-defined developmental sequence of drug use behavior (e.g., Agrawal, Neale, Jacobson, Prescott, and Kendler, 2005; Flay, Hu, and Richardson, 1998; Mayhew, Flay, and Mott, 2000). Furthermore, factors governing substance use appear to vary across developmental stage (Flay et al., 1998; Hirschman Leventhal, and Glynn, 1984). Finally, recent research suggests that behavioral responsivity to drugs may change from adolescence to adulthood (Faraday, Elliott, and Grunberg, 2001). It is likely, then, that NA and drug use may influence one another in different ways at different stages of substance use. Thus, we will briefly examine drug use/NA relationships across the stages of initiation, maintenance, and relapse.

We begin with a consideration of just what NA is and how it is has been conceptualized. We then review several influential models of the role played by NA in promoting drug use and addictive behaviors. Next, we regard the potentially important role played by expectancy effects in shaping drug use/NA relationships. We then provide a brief overview of the relationship between substance use and NA across the initiation, maintenance, and relapse stages.

We conclude with recommendations for future research in this important area.

II. PRECISELY WHAT IS NEGATIVE AFFECT?

We believe that the majority of research on substance use has treated NA from a somewhat atheoretical stance, implicitly treating as synonymous a variety of negative emotions, such as anxiety, anger, and sadness. Correspondingly, some researchers have included measures of low positive affect (PA), or anhedonia, in their conceptualization of NA. Ultimately, though, such methodological groupings may not be desirable from the perspective of certain theories of emotion. Indeed, we maintain that a clear theoretical understanding of the various conceptualizations of NA should influence every stage of research on addiction and emotions, from design implementation and measures chosen, to prediction and evaluation of evidence.

Dimensional models of affect and emotion represent one influential theoretical perspective with respect to delineating the structure of affect. These models share the premise that two "basic" dimensions of affect create a circumplex that can capture and describe all emotional experiences (Russell, 1979, 1980). However, there are at least two alternate views with respect to how these basic dimensions operate (Carroll, Yik, Russell, and Feldman Barrett 1999; Tellegen, Watson, and Clark, 1999). The valence/arousal model posits two independent dimensions of affective valence (pleasant versus unpleasant) and affective arousal (aroused versus calm; Yik, Russell, and Feldman Barrett, 1999), whereas the PA/NA model argues for the existence of independent dimensions of PA and NA (Watson, Wiese, Vaidya, and Tellegen, 1999).

The primary difference between these conceptualizations lies in the understanding of the relationship between pleasant and unpleasant affect. The pleasantness/arousal model asserts that pleasant and unpleasant emotional states are inversely correlated (Green et al., 1993). Hence, according to this conceptualization, reduction of NA and enhancement of PA are manifestations of the same phenomenon. In contrast, the PA/NA model contends that PA and NA are independent, such that increases in NA do not necessarily lead to decreases in PA, and vice versa (Watson et al., 1999). Evidence from multiple sources supports the independence of PA and NA under some circumstances (Gross and Levenson, 1995; Ito, Caccioppo, and Lang, 1998). As such, this evidence has led most researchers to conclude that PA and NA likely have separate neural substrates (Caccioppo, Gardner, and Berntson, 1999; Lang, 1995). In support of such a contention, substance use researchers should note that, for example, both morphine and benzodiazepine have been shown to influence PA and NA separately, leading to a decrease in the punishment value of negative stimuli without an increase in the reward value of positive stimuli (Gomita and Ueki, 1981; Ichitani and Iwasaki, 1986). Moreover, there is reason to believe that different aspects of drug use may be differentially mediated by the PA and NA systems. For example, lesions of the amygdala (typically conceptualized as a critical aspect of the NA system) appear to decrease the impact of aversive withdrawal symptoms from opiates without enhancing the rewarding influences of opiate administration (Kelsey and Arnold, 1994).

Although the PA/NA model views PA and NA as separate constructs, it still subsumes a variety of aversive mood states, including anger, contempt, disgust, guilt, fear, and nervousness, under the rubric of NA (Watson, Clark, and Tellegen, 1988). A second major class of emotion theories proposes that emotions are ultimately not reducible to a small set of common dimensions. As such, both the *basic* and *appraisal* views of emotions posit a number of specified emotional states (e.g., happiness, sad-

ness, anger, disgust, and fear), in lieu of two overarching affective dimensions. The basic emotions view conceives of a limited number of evolutionarily determined and biologically based emotions, each linked to distinct neural substrates. Indeed, there is growing evidence in support of basic-emotion-specific brain activity (Murphy, Nimmo-Smith, and Lawrence, 2003; Phan, Wager, Taylor, and Liberzon, 2004). This raises the intriguing possibility that particular drugs of abuse might be found to differentially affect these distinct negative emotion substrates.

In addition to positing a number of specific emotional states, appraisal theory proposes a cognitive mechanism that ostensibly differentiates among these states (Lazarus, 1991). Thus, according to the tenets of this theory, the subjective meaning assigned to an event, or the appraisal of such an event, can vary along several dimensions, such as goal conduciveness, certainty, and novelty of the event, with each emotion elicited by its own distinct pattern of appraisals. One important contribution of this theory has been in specifying the effect of particular emotions on decision making. Although PA/NA theory might predict that two negative emotions would influence decisions similarly, appraisal theorists have demonstrated that this is not necessarily the case. For example, the negative emotions of anger and fear differ on the key appraisal of controllability, with the effect that angry individuals tend to be more willing to take risks than fearful individuals. In fact, angry individuals bear greater resemblance to happy individuals than they do fearful individuals in their willingness to take risks (Lerner and Keltner, 2000, 2001). Although to date, this model has received relatively scant attention with respect to better understanding decisions to use drugs, it would seem important for substance use researchers to carefully consider the potentially important role played by affect (be it of a positive or negative nature) in governing decisions to self-administer drugs of abuse.

In summary, it is important to keep these different conceptualizations of affect and emotion in mind when considering how researchers have typically assessed both NA and PA in the context of substance use and abuse. Depending on the theoretical orientation chosen, very different outcomes might be expected with regard to the relationship between NA and substance use. Additionally, it is important that we not ignore the possible independent role played by manifestations of PA, and to consider that initiation, maintenance, and relapse may actually be mediated by different affective systems, even for a single substance of abuse. Finally, some might argue that the construct of NA confounds separate emotions that may actually have distinct neural substrates, as well as differentially influence the decision to use substances.

III. HISTORICAL PERSPECTIVES ON THE ROLE OF WITHDRAWAL, NEGATIVE AFFECT, AND SUBSTANCE ABUSE

Withdrawal is thought to result from neuroadaptation to repeated administrations of a drug. This disruption of homeostasis leads to physiological dependence and is defined by the emergence of physical and psychological symptoms that occur in the absence of drug taking. All drugs with addictive liability ostensibly hold the potential to produce a withdrawal syndrome. Whereas the manifestations of withdrawal differ across substances—alcohol withdrawal symptoms may include convulsions, tremor, and auditory hallucinations, while cocaine, opiate, and nicotine withdrawal symptoms may include fatigue, agitation, depression, and anxiety—all such symptoms are generally experienced as unpleasant. Important, too, is the observation that although different drugs may manifest different withdrawal syndromes, NA appears to be the common denominator

to withdrawal syndromes across all addictive substances (Baker, Piper, McCarthy, Majeskie, and Fiore, 2004).

Drawing upon what is known about cigarette smoking, for example, we can thus conclude the following: It has been fairly well established that (a) physical dependence often plays a significant role in smoking (USDHHS, 1988); (b) NA states, including anxiety, dysphoria, and irritability, are among the hallmark symptoms of nicotine withdrawal (Hughes, Higgins, and Hatsukami, 1990); (c) there is marked variability in the experience and time course of withdrawal across individuals (Piasecki, Fiore, and Baker, 1998; Piasecki et al., 2000); (d) nicotine appears to often relieve these withdrawal symptoms (Hughes et al., 1984); and (e) many studies assessing subjective effects of smoking have simply compared groups of nicotine-deprived and nondeprived smokers (e.g., Fleming and Lombardo, 1987). Hence, it becomes difficult to ascertain whether observed differences in NA between nicotine-deprived and nondeprived smokers are due to withdrawal adversely affecting deprived smokers or to smoking genuinely improving mood over normal levels (see Hughes, 1991; Kalman, 2002; West, 1993). Although one could reasonably argue that the source of NA—be it from nicotine deprivation or other, more naturally occurring emotional events—does not really matter when delineating drug/ NA relationships, we agree with Hughes (1991) and others (West, 1993; Kalman, 2002) that differentiating withdrawal reversal from genuine affect enhancement effects (independent of withdrawal) is important to both theory development and intervention efforts.

We also believe, however, that these important issues, though derived from research specifically conducted with nicotine and tobacco, are pertinent to understanding withdrawal syndromes across all drugs of abuse. The bottom line is that withdrawal symptomatology, comprised as it is primarily of various manifestations of NA, serves as a potent motivating force in maintaining addictive substance use.

As such, it is probably fair to assert that most models of addiction, and models of substance abuse in particular, have always emphasized the importance of negative reinforcement processes in understanding the development and maintenance of such behavior. One influential conceptualization is Wikler's withdrawal-relief model, which asserts that addicted individuals self-administer drugs as a means to escape or avoid aversive withdrawal symptoms (Jellinek, 1960; Wikler, 1980). This perspective also posits that avoiding or escaping withdrawal symptomatology through the use of drugs increases the addicted individual's likelihood of engaging in future drug use. As such, NA ostensibly plays a crucial role in the maintenance of drug use, at least with respect to drug use motivated by withdrawal relief.

There have certainly been other models put forth that have similarly examined the relationship between NA, negative reinforcement, and substance abuse. For instance, according to Solomon's opponent-process model (Solomon, 1977; Solomon and Corbit, 1974), the initial effects of many drugs are often pleasurable because the drug temporarily reduces the individual's reward threshold (Koob and Le Moal, 1997). Hence, this process results in events that were previously experienced as only mildly rewarding now experienced as highly rewarding. Over time, internal processes increase the reward threshold in order to return the individual to his or her predrug homeostatic state. As drug administration continues and dependence develops, the individual's homeostatic reward threshold subsequently increases. Thus, in the absence of drug, events that the individual previously experienced as rewarding are now viewed as relatively "neutral," whereas events that were neutral are now perceived as unpleasant. Moreover, because of this change in reward threshold, the individual may also develop tolerance to the

drug, requiring increasingly greater doses of drug to offset this NA resting state.

According to Siegel's model of compensatory response (1983), the direct effect of a drug on the addicted individual serves as the unconditioned stimulus (UCS), whereas individuals' attempts to "defend" themselves against the drug's effect on their state of homeostasis is viewed as the unconditioned response (UCR). Thus, a stimulus frequently paired with the UCS becomes the conditioned stimulus (CS). This CS acts as a warning sign to the homeostatic regulatory system, indicating that a UCS is imminent and allows the regulatory system to prepare itself with a defensive response (CR). Through repeated episodes of drug use, this link between the UCS and the CS becomes stronger. Eventually, the CS can elicit a CR in the absence of the UCS. This CR may then affect the individual's homeostatic state, causing withdrawal symptoms, craving, and future drug use.

Although numerous empirical studies have yielded findings in support of models emphasizing the role of negative reinforcement as the primary motivating factor governing substance use, such conceptualizations have not been without their critics. Indeed, some have argued that the appetitive or incentive-sensitization effects of drugs are often given short shrift, noting that individuals self-administer drugs for reasons other than just withdrawal relief (Robinson and Berridge, 2003; Stewart, de Wit, and Eikelboom, 1984). Some researchers have also asserted that the role of negative reinforcement has been overblown, citing results demonstrating that relapse often occurs when withdrawal symptoms should have long since abated.

Recently, Baker and colleagues proposed a reformulation of the negative reinforcement models of addiction, in part, as a way of addressing some of these criticisms. According to their affective model of drug motivation (Baker et al., 2004), NA represents the motivational core of the withdrawal syndrome. As such, the model proposes that, over time, the addicted individual becomes sensitive to internal cues that signal NA through repeated withdrawal/drug-use cycles. When drug levels begin to fall in the addicted individual's body, the individual begins to experience low levels of NA. However, the detection of these NA cues may occur outside the individual's conscious awareness. Hence, this preconscious detection of NA cues biases response options, increasing the likelihood that previously reinforced responses will be performed (i.e., drug use). Thus, for the addicted individual who has access to drugs, the motivational processes leading up to drug use often occur outside the realm of conscious awareness. If the individual does not have access to drugs, or experiences stress unrelated to withdrawal, NA should increase to a point whereby the individual does become consciously aware of the affect. Such increases in NA may influence "hot" information processing, biasing attentional and response selection processes toward response options that have previously proven effective at decreasing NA (i.e., drug use), and away from alternative responses that are not as effective at diminishing NA (at least in the short term). Furthermore, increased NA may also influence "cold" information processing by decreasing the influence (and accessibility) of both declarative knowledge and controlled cognitive processing, resulting in the enhanced likelihood that the individual will engage in drug use.

In summary, the affective model of drug motivation asserts that at low levels of NA, the addicted individual is unaware that he/she is experiencing NA and engages in drug use because the behavior has become an almost automatic response to coping with NA (cf. Tiffany, 1990). By contrast, at high levels of NA, the individual is likely aware that he/she is experiencing NA. But because the NA increases the incentive value of drug use and reduces the influence of declarative knowledge and controlled processing, the individual is less able to effectively cope with the NA and is more likely to engage in drug use. Finally, and importantly, the model also posits that when NA is experienced at more moderate levels, individuals may then be able to access controlled cognitive processes in order to decide whether drug use is, indeed, the preferable option.

IV. DRUG EXPECTANCY EFFECTS AND NA

Given the widely held notion—both by those who use drugs and those who do not—that most substances do alleviate NA, we briefly examine the research base on drug expectancies. A large literature, particularly within the area of alcohol consumption, has shown that individuals' expectations of drug effects can have profound effects on motivational and drug-seeking processes (e.g., Cox and Klinger, 1988; Goldman, Del Boca, and Darkes, 1999). According to this perspective, it is conceivable that the association between drug use and NA is simply epiphenomenal, steeped in the belief, but not necessarily the reality, that drug use assuages NA. On the other hand, there is ample reason to believe that some expectancies are clearly shaped by experience. Moreover, expectancies have demonstrated predictive validity across a variety of different drugs. For example, Bauman and Chenoweth (1984) assessed the expected consequences from smoking cigarettes among 1,400 adolescents, only a small proportion of whom had ever smoked. Analyses revealed that the negative physical and social consequences factor predicted smoking initiation, whereas the pleasure factor (e.g., "smoking will make me feel more relaxed") predicted both initiation and increased smoking among those who were smokers at the study's onset. Chassin, Presson, Sherman, and Edwards (1991) found that strong positive beliefs about the psychological consequences of smoking predicted smoking onset during both adolescence and adulthood. Moreover, expectation of NA reduction, as assessed by the Smoking Consequences Questionnaire (Brandon and Baker, 1991; Copeland et al., 1995), was found to be a potent predictor of end-of-treatment outcome (Wetter et al., 1994).

With respect to alcohol use, a wealth of research points to consistent relationships between alcohol expectancies and alcohol consumption, alcohol addiction, and behavior while drinking (Brown, Christiansen, and Goldman, 1987). Indeed, positive expectancies for alcohol—particularly the expectation that alcohol will alleviate NA—appear meaningfully related to expectancies of future substance use (e.g., marijuana use), and to measures of problem drug use and resistance to peer influence (Willner, 2001). Similar findings have been reported for cocaine as well. Greater urges to use cocaine correlate positively with expected positive effects, specifically with expecting enhanced well-being and NA reduction (Rohsenow, Sirota, Martin, and Monti, 2004).

In sum, a wealth of both anecdotal and self-report questionnaire data suggests that most drug users believe that drug use will help to reduce NA. Hence, even in the absence of genuine NA-reducing properties (see Kassel et al., 2003; Steele and Josephs, 1990), this expectancy is one possible mechanism through which the link between substance use and NA may be instantiated. Furthermore, expectations of NA reduction could potentially explain drug use across the initiation, maintenance, and relapse stages.

V. INITIATION STAGE: DRUG USE AND NA

Experimentation with drugs, particularly alcohol and cigarettes, is a relatively common occurrence among youth. Indeed, more than 75% of adolescents have tried cigarettes or alcohol by the time they graduate from high school (Johnston, O'Malley, Bachman, and Schulenberg, 2004; Kandel and Logan, 1984; Wills and Stoolmiller,

2002). Significant, though smaller, numbers of high school students have also tried "harder" drugs, such as marijuana, cocaine, and ecstasy. Of these adolescents, however, only a handful actually become addicted, and it is thus important for future intervention and prevention programs to determine for whom, as well as when, dependence is most likely to develop.

Propensity to experience higher levels of NA is considered a fairly stable personality variable (Watson and Clark, 1984), evidenced in children as one facet of temperament. Temperament is often described as a biologically based precursor to later personality, and a host of research has been conducted linking temperament variables to substance abuse (Henderson, Galen, and DeLuca, 1998; Wills, Sandy, and Yeager, 2000; Wills and Stoolmiller, 2002). Specifically, behavioral disinhibition and negative affectivity are among the strongest personality predictors of adolescent substance use (Myers, Aarons, Tomlinson, and Stein, 2003; Tarter et al., 1999), such that those who tend to be more behaviorally and emotionally volatile are more likely to initiate problematic drug use at a younger age (Henderson et al., 1998; Wills et al., 2000) and manifest higher frequency of use (Henderson et al., 1998; Myers et al., 2003).

Several cross-sectional studies have demonstrated a link between psychopathology marked by NA—particularly depression—and adolescent drug use (Brown et al., 1996; Patton et al., 1996). These studies indicate that depression precedes substance use and therefore may be considered a risk factor. Other studies, however, have shown either no temporal relationship between depression and substance use (Rohde, Lewinsohn, and Seeley, 1996), or a reciprocal relationship such that substance use actually precedes—perhaps causally—the development of depression (Brown, Lewinsohn, Seeley, and Wagner, 1996).

Studies examining the relationship between another predominant manifestation of NA, anxiety, and substance use are less common, and yield findings that are equivocal. For example, some investigations report that adolescents experiencing anxiety are more likely to initiate drug use (Patton et al., 1996; Zimmerman et al., 2004), whereas a recent study found that social anxiety acted as a protective influence against substance use involvement, ostensibly because anxiety elicits avoidance rather than enabling approach behaviors (Myers et al., 2003). Correspondingly, a number of well-designed prospective investigations have found that anxiety disorders do not reliably predict the onset of cigarette smoking during adolescence (Costello, Erkanli, Federman, and Angold, 1999; Dierker, Avenevoli, Merikangas, Flaherty, and Stolar, 2001; McGee, Williams, and Stanton, 1998) or adulthood (Johnson, et al., 2000). Moreover, at least one study has suggested that anxiety disorders may actually be prophylactic, at least in the sense that they delay the onset of smoking among adolescents (Costello et al., 1999). However, whereas the relationship between anxiety disorders and smoking onset appears tenuous, the relationship between anxiety and nicotine dependence (even among teenagers) appears robust (Dierker et al., 2001; Johnson et al., 2000). Thus, the importance of differentiating among levels of drug use becomes clear (Kassel, 2000a). Finally, as was observed in the relationship between drug use and depressive symptomatology, emerging evidence similarly suggests that drug use in adolescence may predict the subsequent development of anxiety disorders (Johnson et al., 2000).

Because the majority of drug initiation studies have been conducted cross-sectionally and/or retrospectively, little is known about the daily fluctuations in adolescents' moods that may influence decisions to self-administer drugs. Recent use of ecological momentary assessment (EMA), a real-time data collection tool utilizing hand-held computers, may help untangle momentary affect from more stable affective traits (Stone and Shiffman, 1994). For instance, whereas initial reports indicate that teenagers who experiment with smoking tend to do so when experiencing NA, adolescents who progress to nicotine addiction do not show consistent patterns of smoking following any particular emotional state (Turner, Mermelstein, and Flay, 2004). Finally, as discussed earlier, other methodological problems stem from using a variety of mood measurements and distinctly different operational definitions of NA. For example, some studies designed to test how drugs influence affect consider PA and NA as opposite ends of a single bipolar dimension (e.g., Trimmel and Wittberger, 2004), whereas others consider them as independent constructs (e.g., Conklin & Perkins, 2005; Perkins et al., 2003).

In sum, regarding the initiation stage of drug use, many questions remain unanswered with respect to understanding the role played by NA. Although NA, particularly dispositional tendencies to experience NA, is very likely related to initial drug experimentation, more work is needed to elucidate mediating and moderating variables (self-control, behavioral dysregulation) in models of NA and early drug use. Also, some research indicates that young people experience reductions in NA after smoking or drinking (DiFranza et al., 2004; Stanton et al., 1993); rigorous field and laboratory studies are sorely needed to determine whether drugs actually do assuage NA for those in the initiation stage and whether individuals in the throes of acute NA are more likely to self-administer drugs.

VI. MAINTENANCE STAGE: DRUG USE AND NA

Evidence clearly shows that, relative to nonusers, individuals in the maintenance stage of drug use are far more likely to meet diagnostic criteria for numerous manifestations of psychopathology, and virtually any disorder that is exemplified by increased NA (e.g., Bowden-Jones et al., 2004; Breslau,

Kilbey, and Andreski, 1993; Dawson, Grant, Stinson, and Chou, 2005). From such a between-subjects level of analysis, then, the association between NA and addictive use of substances is incontrovertible, although establishing the direction of causality can prove difficult.

A host of studies have examined the extent to which NA appears to cue, or prompt, drug use. For instance, Park, Armeli, and Tennen (2004) used a daily diary study to show that college students drank more alcohol on days where both stress levels and NA were relatively high, while at the same time, adaptive coping strategies were underutilized. Thus, lack of effective coping coupled with NA led to a greater reliance on alcohol to cope with NA. Similarly, Hussong, Galloway, and Feagans (2005) found that college students with an increased tendency to use maladaptive techniques to cope (i.e., drinking to cope with NA) were more likely to use alcohol on days when they experienced heightened fear or shyness, but used alcohol less often on days characterized by increased feelings of sadness. Such findings highlight the problem of lumping all types of negative emotions (i.e., fear, sadness, shyness, anger, anxiety) under the rubric of NA; different negative emotions may, indeed, exert different motivational influences on drug use.

Although such findings suggest a linear relationship between NA and drug use, such that an increase in NA will reliably lead to an increase in drug use, the relationship between drug use and NA may not actually be that clear. Rodgers et al. (2000) reported a U-shaped association between alcohol use and NA, suggesting that while greater alcohol consumption and alcohol-related problems were associated with high NA scores, those individuals who also endorsed little or no drinking also evidenced increased levels of both depression and anxiety (see also Shedler and Block, 1990).

Conner et al. (2005) examined the link between certain genotypes and various substance use disorders and showed that a particular genotype, the A1-super (+) allele, was associated with the greater use of both alcohol and other substances, an earlier age of initiation for the use of marijuana, and the greater likelihood for the development of tobacco dependence. Among boys with the A1-super (+) allele, increased severity of substance use was also associated with trait NA. Correspondingly, using a college sample, Randall and Cox (2001) found that high-risk (family history positive for substance abuse) subjects experienced NA more strongly than low-risk subjects following the same mood induction procedure, and drank more nonalcoholic beer following the mood induction. The authors argue that this illustrates not only the heightened reactivity of high-risk subjects to NA situations, but also their increased motivation to use substances following such aversive events.

Finally, it is worth noting that the relationship between NA (stress) and drug intake has received attention in animal models of drug abuse, and there is a burgeoning literature on the effects of stress on drug self-administration in animals. The acquisition and reinstatement of cocaine or heroin self-administration in rats can be increased by exposure to stressors such as foot shock or injections of corticosterone, and these effects are blocked by glucocorticoid receptor antagonists, suggesting involvement of the HPA axis in psychomotor stimulant self-administration (Goeders and Guerin, 1994; Shaham, Erb, Leung, Buczek, and Stewart, 1998). Correspondingly, foot-shock stress will reinstate nicotine- but not sucrose-seeking behavior (Buczek, Le, Wong, Stewart, and Shaham, 1999). Importantly, the effects of foot-shock stress on nicotine-seeking behavior are not unique. Similar results have been reported for reinstatement of alcohol, heroin, and cocaine self-administration (Ahmed and Koob, 1997; Lê et al., 1998; Shaham, Erb, and Stewart, 2000). Likewise, food-deprivation has been shown to increase self-administration of nicotine as well as d-amphetamine and cocaine (de la Garza and Johanson, 1987).

In summary, the supposition that NA prompts drug use receives modest support from the literature. Clearly, however, much more research is needed in order to better understand such processes. As discussed above, such effects may vary across both different classes of drugs and different negative emotions. The extent to which drugs genuinely alleviate NA proves an even more difficult question to answer. Indeed, there is reason to believe that few drugs exert reliable, direct effects on emotional response. Rather, such effects appear to be moderated and mediated by factors such as environmental context, personality variables, and drug dose (e.g., Gilbert, 1995; Kassel et al., 2003; Sayette, 1999; Steele and Josephs, 1990).

VII. RELAPSE STAGE: DRUG USE AND NA

Across virtually all drugs of abuse, the modal outcome among those trying to quit is relapse. A host of potential mechanisms explaining this unfortunate outcome have been considered (see, e.g., Brigham, Henningfield, and Stitzer, 1991; Spealman et al., 2004; Stewart, 2004). Yet, across the various stages of drug use, the association between NA and relapse has probably received the strongest empirical support. Simply put, across both human and animal studies, there is strong reason to believe that NA is a frequently observed precipitant of reinstatement of drug use following a period of abstinence (Kreek and Koob, 1998).

Elevated levels of NA both prior to (Covey, 1999) and following (Cohen and Lichtenstein, 1990; Covey, 1999; Hall, Muñoz, Reus, and Sees, 1993) cessation are predictive of relapse. This link is supported by retrospective (e.g., Brandon, Tiffany, Obremski, and Baker, 1990; Shiffman, 1982) and, more importantly, real-time (Shiffman, Paty, Gnys, Kassel, and Hickox, 1996) data collection revealing elevated levels of NA just prior to lapses. Correspondingly, relapse to alcohol has been shown to be similarly associated with elevated levels of stress and NA during abstinence attempts (Brown, Irwin, and Schuckit, 1991; Brown et al., 1990; Sinha, 2001). Moreover, drinkers often report relapsing in order to cope with heightened levels of NA (LaBounty, Hatsukami, Morgan, and Nelson, 1992).

A recent study using ecological momentary assessment of mood (Shiffman and Waters, 2004; see also Shiffman, 2005) indicates that, whereas day-to-day changes in NA did not predict lapse risk, more proximal changes in affect were associated with lapses. Indeed, many lapses were marked by intense NA and by NA increases in the preceding hours. Such findings highlight the utility of assessing mood and target behaviors (e.g., drug lapse) in real time, as well as the importance of assessing dynamic changes in background conditions and in immediate affective states with respect to their influence on lapses and relapse.

Turning briefly to the animal literature, a large number of studies have investigated stress-induced reinstatement (relapse) across both a number of different drugs and animals. For instance, rat studies have typically utilized inescapable foot shock to induce a presumably stress-like state of NA. Overall, this type of NA appears to induce reliable reinstatement of drug seeking. Indeed, the observed drug-taking levels subsequent to stress exceed those observed after administration of priming doses of drug (Ahmed and Koob, 1997; Sutton, Karanian, and Self, 2000). More work needs to address NA inductions that perhaps better mirror the types of stressors and NA faced by animals (and humans) in their natural environment (Spealman et al., 2004).

VIII. CONCLUSIONS AND FUTURE DIRECTIONS

Noting that virtually all drug users attribute their use to its purported ability to assuage NA, we reviewed the empirical literature in an effort to try to address the veracity of this claim. Overall, we observed consistent between-person associations between drug use status and various indices of NA across the initiation and maintenance stages of smoking. Thus, based on a population-level of analysis, substance abusers generally experience more NA than do abstainers. However, these associations cannot speak to causality (Kassel, 2000b). In spite of this disclaimer, however, many have made the leap from correlation to causation, asserting that such between-group differences support various stress-coping, self-medication, or tension-reduction hypotheses of drug use behavior. Indeed, Leonard and Blane (1999, p. 5) observe, "As a field, we seem to have accepted the notion that alcohol is reinforcing because it reduces tension, and we have been undaunted in our pursuit of evidence of this basic precept, even in the face of a body of literature that is, at best, equivocal." Although between-person, correlational data justifiably invite interpretation, only through careful laboratory and field investigation can we begin to understand the processes underlying the observed association between drug abuse and NA.

Moving to the realm of within-person observation (e.g., do drug users self-administer drugs *on occasions* marked by heightened NA?), the findings provide no clear answer with respect to the initiation stage, a tentative "Yes" for those in the maintenance stage, and a clearer "Yes" for those experiencing a lapse or relapse after a period of abstinence. At the same time, it is important to reiterate that methodological rigor must be implemented in order to truly establish causal links between NA and drug use behavior.

The question of whether drugs actually alleviate NA yields an equally complex picture, with some studies demonstrating genuine anxiolytic effects, others finding no effect of drugs on NA, and others reporting an actual exacerbation of NA (e.g., File, Kenny, and Ouagazzal, 1998; Kassel and Unrod, 2000). As we have discussed elsewhere (Kassel and Hankin, In press;

Kassel et al., 2003), such variable findings suggest that the critical question is not *whether* drugs of abuse reliably alleviate NA, but rather *for whom*, under *what conditions*, and for *which specific affective outcomes* do *which specific* drugs relieve NA (Gilbert and Gilbert, 1998; Zinberg, 1984)? From this perspective, we believe it imperative that future research address these questions from both a contextual and transdisciplinary framework in order to truly shed light on the processes subserving drug effects on NA, as well as the influence of NA on drug self-administration.

Whereas our intention was to provide an overview of the admittedly complex association between NA and drugs of abuse, we acknowledge that such an endeavor is rife with theoretical, methodological, and operational challenges and conundrums. For instance, as discussed throughout this chapter, the very notion of NA is troublesome. There is reason to believe that although some drugs may influence response to depressive or anxiety symptoms, they may not alter symptoms of anger. Correspondingly, whereas alcohol and nicotine may assuage feelings of anxiety, they may only do so under circumscribed contextual conditions (Kassel and Shiffman, 1997; Steele and Josephs, 1990).

With respect to methodological limitations of this literature, we noted that the majority of human studies have relied upon self-report measures that frequently incorporate retrospective recall. Ecological momentary assessment (EMA) employs the use of hand-held computers and relies on repeated assessments of subjects' momentary states in their natural environments (Shiffman and Stone, 1998). Drawing upon event-contingent sampling strategies (during which subjects enter data linked to some specified behavior, e.g., injecting heroin) and signal-contingent sampling (where subjects enter data in response to a randomly presented, external signal), this methodology allows for determination of true antecedents and consequences of specified behaviors (Paty et al., 1992). Put simply, such an approach is uniquely suited to answer the question: For whom, under what conditions, and for which specific affect-related outcomes do drugs genuinely relieve NA (Delfino et al., 2001)? Recent application of this sophisticated methodological approach to drug use appears to hold much promise (e.g., Armeli, Todd, and Mohr, 2005; Shiffman et al., 2002; Simons, Gaher, Oliver, Bush, and Palmer, 2005).

We conclude with a comment from Panskepp and colleagues (2004, p. 93), who ask: "Would individuals exhibit addictive behaviors if there were no affective payoffs? We suspect an answer of 'no' for both humans and other species...." And with this opinion, we wholeheartedly concur. But the charge of delineating the precise nature of this affective payoff, the behavioral and neurophysiological processes that subserve it, and the conditions under which it is experienced, present daunting challenges to researchers. Yet, given the ultimate importance of understanding the reinforcing mechanisms that govern addictive behaviors, we must meet this call head on, and in doing so, draw up strong theoretical bases and sound methodologies in order to unravel the mysteries surrounding the relationship between drug addiction and NA.

ACKNOWLEDGMENTS

The writing of this chapter was made possible, in part, by grant #1PO1CA98262 from the National Cancer Institute, and by grant 5RO1AA12240-04 from the National Institute on Alcohol Abuse and Alcoholism.

REFERENCES

Agrawal, A., Neale, M. C., Jacobson, K. C., Prescott, C. A., and Kendler, K. S. (2005). Illicit drug use and abuse/dependence: Modeling of two-stage variables using the CCC approach. *Addictive Behaviors, 30,* 1043–1048.

Ahmed, S. H., and Koob, G. F. (1997). Cocain- but not food-seeking behavior is reinstated by stress after extinction. *Psychopharmacology, 132,* 289–295.

Armeli, S., Todd, M., and Mohr, C. (2005). A daily process approach to individual differences in stress-related alcohol use. *Journal of Personality, 73,* 1657–1686.

Baker, T. B., Piper, M. E., McCarthy, D. E., Majeskie, M. R., and Fiore, M. C. (2004). Addiction motivation reformulated: An affective processing model of negative reinforcement. *Psychological Review, 111,* 33–51.

Bauman, K. E., and Chenoweth, R. L. (1984). The relationship between the consequences adolescents expect from smoking and their behavior: A factor analysis with panel data. *Journal of Applied Social Psychology, 14,* 28–41.

Bowden-Jones, O., Iqbal, M. A., Tyrer, P., Seivewright, N., Cooper, S., Judd, A., et al. (2004). Prevalence of personality disorder in alcohol and drug services and associated comorbidity. *Addiction, 99,* 1306–1314.

Brandon, T. H., and Baker, T. B. (1991). The smoking consequences questionnaire: The subjective expected utility of smoking in college students. *Psychological Assessment, 3,* 484–491.

Brandon, T. H., Tiffany, S. T., Obremski, K. M., and Baker, T. B. (1990). Postcessation cigarette use: The process of relapse. *Addictive Behaviors, 15,* 105–114.

Breslau, N., Kilbey, M. M., and Andreski, P. (1991). Nicotine dependence, major depression, and anxiety in young adults. *Archives of General Psychiatry, 48,* 1069–1074.

Breslau, N., Kilbey, M., and Andreski, P. (1993). Nicotine dependence and major depression: New evidence from a prospective investigation. *Archives of General Psychiatry, 50,* 31–35.

Brigham, J., Henningfield, J. E., and Stitzer, M. L. (1991). Smoking relapse: A review. *International Journal of the Addictions, 25,* 1239–1255.

Brown, R. A., Lewinsohn, P. M., Seeley, J. R., and Wagner, E. F. (1996). Cigarette smoking, major depression, and other psychiatric disorders among adolescents. *Journal of the American Academy of Child and Adolescent Psychiatry, 35,* 1602–1610.

Brown, S. A., Christiansen, B. A., and Goldman, M. S. (1987). The Alcohol Expectancy Questionnaire: An instrument for the assessment of adolescent and adult alcohol expectancies. *Journal of Studies on Alcohol, 48,* 483–491.

Brown, S. A., Irwin, M., and Schuckit, M. A. (1991). Changes in anxiety among abstinent male alcoholics. *Journal of Studies on Alcohol, 52,* 55–61.

Brown, S. A., Mott, M. A., and Myers, M. G. (1991). Adolescent alcohol and drug treatment outcome. In Watson, Ronald R. (Ed.), *Drug and alcohol abuse prevention. Drug and alcohol abuse reviews* (pp. 373–403).

Buczek, J., Le, A. D., Wong, A., Stewart, J., and Shaham, Y. (1999). Stress reinstates nicotine seeking but not sucrose solution seeking in rats. *Psychopharmacology, 144*, 183–188.

Cacioppo, J. T., Gardner, W. L., and Berntson, G. G. (1999). The affect system has parallel and integrative processing components: Form follows function. *Journal of Personality and Social Psychology, 76*, 839–855.

Carroll, J. M., Yik, M. S. M., Russell, J. A., and Feldman Barrett, L. (1999). On the psychometric principles of affect. *Review of General Psychology, 3*, 14–22.

Chassin, L., Presson, C. C., Sherman, S. J., and Edwards, D. A. (1991). Four pathways to young-adult smoking status: Adolescent social-psychological antecedents in a midwestern community sample. *Health Psychology, 10*, 409–418.

Cohen, S., and Lichtenstein, E. (1990). Perceived stress, quitting smoking, and smoking relapse. *Health Psychology, 9*, 466–478.

Conklin, C. A., and Perkins, K. A. (2005). Subjective and reinforcing effects of smoking during negative mood induction. *Journal of Abnormal Psychology, 114*, 153–164.

Conner, B. T., Ernest, P., Berman, S. M., Ozkaragoz, T., Ritchie, T., Antolin, T., et al. (2005). DRD2 genotypes and substance use in adolescent children of alcoholics. *Drug and Alcohol Dependence, 79*, 379–387.

Cooper, M. L., Russell, M., Skinner, J. B., and Windle, M. (1992). Development and validation of a three-dimensional measure of drinking motives. *Psychological Assessment, 4*, 123–132.

Copeland, A. L., Brandon, T. H., and Quinn, E. P. (1995). The Smoking Consequences Questionnaire—Adult: Measurement of smoking outcome expectancies of experienced smokers. *Psychological Assessment, 7*, 484–494.

Costello, E., Erkanli, A., Federman, E., and Angold, A. (1999). Development of psychiatric comorbidity with substance abuse in adolescents: Effects of timing and sex. *Journal of Clinical Child Psychology, 28*, 298–311.

Covey, L. S. (1999). Tobacco cessation among patients with depression. *Primary Care, 26*, 691–706.

Covey, L. S., Glassman, A. H., and Stetner, F. (1998). Cigarette smoking and major depression. *Journal of Addictive Diseases, 17*, 35–46.

Cox, W. M., and Klinger, E. (1988). A motivational model of alcohol use. *Journal of Abnormal Psychology, 97*, 168–180.

Currie, S. R., Patten, S. B., Williams, J. V., Wang, J., Beck, C. A., el-Guebaly, N., et al. (2005). Comorbidity of major depression with substance use disorders. *Canadian Journal of Psychiatry, 50*, 660–666.

Dawson, D. A., Grant, B. F., Stinson, F. S., and Chou, P. S. (2005). Psychopathology associated with drinking and alcohol use disorders in the college and general adult populations. *Drug and Alcohol Dependence, 77*, 139–150.

Degenhardt, L., and Hall, W. (2001). The relationship between tobacco use, substance-use disorders and mental health: Results from the National Survey of Mental Health and Well-being. *Nicotine and Tobacco Research, 3*, 225–234.

de la Garza, R., and Johanson, C. E. (1987). Discriminative stimulus properties of intragastrically administered d-amphetamine and pentobarbital in rhesus monkeys. *Journal of Pharmacology and Experimental Therapeutics, 243*, 955–962.

Delfino, R. J., Jamner, L. D., and Whalen, C. K. (2001). Temporal analysis of the relationship of smoking behavior and urges to mood states in men versus women. *Nicotine and Tobacco Research, 3*, 235–248.

Dierker, L. C., Avenevoli, S., Merikangas, K. R., Flaherty, B. P., and Stolar, M. (2001). Association between psychiatric disorders and the progression of tobacco use behaviors. *Journal of the American Academy of Child and Adolescent Psychiatry, 40*, 1159–1167.

DiFranza, J. R., Savageau, J. A., Fletcher, K., Ockene, J. K., Rigotti, N. A., and McNeill, A. D. (2004). Recollections and repercussions of the first inhaled cigarette. *Addictive Behaviors, 29*, 261–272.

Faraday, M. M., Elliott, B. M., and Grunberg, N. E. (2001). Adult vs. adolescent rats differ in biobehavioral responses to chronic nicotine administration. *Pharmacology, Biochemistry and Behavior, 70*, 475–489.

File, S. E., Kenny, P. J., and Ouagazzal, A. M. (1998). Biomodal modulation by nicotine of anxiety in the social interaction test: Role of the dorsal hippocampus. *Behavioral Neuroscience, 112*, 1423–1429.

Flay, B. R., Hu, F. B., and Richardson, J. (1998). Psychosocial predictors of different stages of cigarette smoking among high school students. *Preventive Medicine, 27*, A9–A18.

Fleming, S. E., and Lombardo, T. W. (1987). Effects of cigarette smoking on phobic anxiety. *Addictive Behaviors, 12*, 195–198.

Frith, C. D. (1971). Smoking behaviour and its relation to the smoker's immediate experience. *British Journal of Social and Clinical Psychology, 10*, 73–78.

Fu, Q., Heath, A. C., Bucholz, K. K., Nelson, E., Goldberg, J., Lyons, M. J., et al. (2002). Shared genetic risk of major depression, alcohol dependence, and marijuana dependence: Contribution of antisocial personality disorder in men. *Archives of General Psychiatry, 59*, 1125–1132.

Gilbert, D. G. (1995). *Smoking: Individual differences, psychopathology, and emotion.* Washington, D.C.: Taylor and Francis.

Gilbert, D. G., and Gilbert, B. O. (1998). Nicotine and the Situation by Trait Adaptive Response (STAR) model: Emotional states and information processing. In J. Snel and M. M. Lorist (Eds.), *Nicotine, caffeine and social drinking: Behaviour and brain function* (pp. 131–149). Amsterdam, Netherlands: Harwood Academic Publishers.

Goeders, N. E., and Guerin, G. F. (1994). Non-contingent electric footshock facilitates the acquisition of intravenous cocaine self-administration in rats. *Psychopharmacology, 114,* 63–70.

Goldman, M. S., Del Boca, F. K., and Darkes, J. (1999). Alcohol expectancy theory: The application of cognitive neuroscience. In K. E. Leonard and H. T. Blane (Eds.), *Psychological theories of drinking and alcoholism* (pp. 203–246). New York: Guilford Press.

Gomita, Y., and Ueki, S. (1981). "Conflict" situation based on intracranial self-stimulation behavior and the effect of benzodiazepines. *Pharmacology Biochemistry and Behavior, 14,* 219–222.

Green, D. P., Goldman, S. L., and Salovey, P. (1993). Measurement error masks bioplarity in affect ratings. *Journal of Personality and Social Psychology, 64,* 1029–1041.

Gross, J. J., and Levenson, R. W. (1995). Emotion elicitation using films. *Cognition and Emotion, 9,* 87–108.

Hall, S. M., Munoz, R. F., Reus, V. I., and Sees, K. L. (1993). Nicotine, negative affect, and depression. *Journal of Consulting and Clinical Psychology, 61,* 761–767.

Hasin, D. S., Goodwin, R. D., Stinson, F. S., and Grant, B. F. (2005). Epidemiology of major depressive disorder: Results from the National Epidemiologic Survey on alcoholism and related conditions. *Archives of General Psychiatry, 62,* 1097–1106.

Henderson, M. J., Galen, L. W., and DeLuca, J. W. (1998). Temperament style and substance abuse characteristics. *Substance Abuse, 19,* 61–70.

Hirschman, R. S., Leventhal, H., and Glynn, K. (1984). The development of smoking behavior: Conceptualization and supportive cross-sectional survey data. *Journal of Applied Social Psychology, 14,* 184–206.

Hughes, J. R. (1991). Distinguishing withdrawal relief and direct effects of smoking. *Psychopharmacology, 104,* 409–410.

Hughes, J. R., Hatsukami, D. K., Pickens, R. W., Krahn, D., Malin, S., and Luknic, A. (1984). Effect of nicotine on the tobacco withdrawal syndrome. *Psychopharmacology, 83,* 82–87.

Hughes, J. R., Higgins, S. T., and Hatsukami, D. (1990). Effects of abstinence from tobacco: A critical review. In L. T. Kozlowski, H. M. Annis, H. D. Cappell, F. B. Glaser, M. S. Goodstat, Y. Israel, H. Kalant, E. M. Seelera, and E. R. Vingilis (Eds.), *Research advances in alcohol and drug problems* (vol. 10, pp. 317–398). New York: Plenum Publishing.

Hussong, A. M., Galloway, C. A., and Feagans, L. A. (2005). Coping motives as a moderator of daily mood-drinking covariation. *Journal of Studies on Alcohol, 66,* 344–353.

Ichitani, Y., and Iwasaki, T. (1986). Approach and escape responses to mesencephalic central gray stimulation in rats: Effects of morphine and naloxone. *Behavioural Brain Research, 22,* 63–73.

Ikard, F. F., Green, P. E., and Horn, D. (1969). A scale to differentiate between types of smoking as related to the management of affect. *International Journal of the Addictions, 4,* 649–659.

Ito, T. A., Cacioppo, J. T., and Lang, P. J., (1998). Eliciting affect using the International Affective Picture System: Trajectories through evaluative space. *Personality and Social Psychology Bulletin, 24,* 855–879.

Jaffe, A. J., and Kilbey, M. M., (1994). The Cocaine Expectancy Questionnaire (CEQ): Construction and predictive utility. *Psychological Assessment, 6,* 18–26.

Jellinek, E. M. (1960). *The disease concept of alcoholism.* New Brunswick, NJ: Hillhouse Press.

Johnson, J. G., Cohen, P., Pine, D. S., Klein, D. F., Kasen, S., and Brook, J. S. (2000). Association between cigarette smoking and anxiety disorders during adolescence and early adulthood. *Journal of the American Medical Association, 284,* 2348–2351.

Johnston, L. D., O'Malley, P. M., Bachman, J. G., and Schulenberg, J. E. (2004). *Monitoring the future national results on adolescent drug use: Overview of key findings, 2004.* Bethesda, MD: National Institute on Drug Abuse.

Kalman, D. (2002). The subjective effects of nicotine: Methodological issues, a review of experimental studies, and recommendations for future research. *Nicotine and Tobacco Research, 4,* 25–70.

Kandel, D. B., and Logan, J. A. (1984). Patterns of drug use from adolescence to young adulthood: I. Periods of risk for initiation, continued use, and discontinuation. *American Journal of Public Health, 74,* 660–666.

Kassel, J. D. (2000a). Are adolescent smokers addicted to nicotine? The suitability of the nicotine dependence construct as applied to adolescents. *Journal of Child and Adolescent Substance Abuse, 9,* 27–49.

Kassel, J. D. (2000b). Smoking and stress: Correlation, causation, and context. *American Psychologist, 55,* 1155–1156.

Kassel, J. D., and Hankin, B. L. (In press). Smoking and depression. In A. Steptoe (Ed.), *Depression and physical illness.* Cambridge, England: Cambridge University Press.

Kassel, J. D., and Shiffman, S. (1997). Attentional mediation of cigarette smoking's effect on anxiety. *Health Psychology, 16(4),* 359–368.

Kassel, J. D., Stroud, L. R., and Paronis, C. A. (2003). Smoking, stress, and negative affect: Correlation, causation, and context across stages of smoking. *Psychological Bulletin, 129,* 270–304.

Kassel, J. D., and Unrod, M. (2000). Smoking, anxiety, and attention: Support for the role of nicotine in attentionally mediated anxiolysis. *Journal of Abnormal Psychology, 109,* 161–166.

Kassel, J. D., Weinstein, S., Skitch, S. A., Veilleux, J., and Mermelstein, R. (2005). The development of substance abuse in adolescence. In B. L. Hankin and J. R. Abela (Eds.), *Development of psychopathology: A vulnerability-stress perspective* (pp. 355–384). Thousand Oaks, CA: Sage Publications.

Kelsey, J. E., and Arnold, S. R. (1994). Lesions of the dorsomedial amygdala, but not the nucleus accumbens, reduce the aversiveness of morphine withdrawal in rats. *Behavioural Neuroscience, 108*, 1119–1127.

Khantzian, E. J. (1997). The self-medication hypothesis of substance use disorders: A reconsideration and recent applications. *Harvard Review of Psychiatry, 4*, 231–244.

Koob, G. F., and Le Moal, M. (1997). Drug abuse: Hedonic homeostatic dysregulation. *Science, 278*, 52–58.

Kreek, M. J., and Koob, G. F. (1998). Drug dependence: Stress and dysregulation of brain reward pathways. *Drug and Alcohol Dependence, 51*, 23–47.

LaBounty, L. P., Hatsukami, D., Morgan, S. F., and Nelson, L. (1992). Relapse among alcoholics with phobic and panic symptoms. *Addictive Behaviors, 17*, 9–15.

Lang, P. J. (1995). The emotion probe. Studies of motivation and attention. *American Psychologist, 50*, 372–385.

Lasser, K., Boyd, J. W., Woolhandler, S., Himmelstein, D. U., McCormick, D., and Bor, D. H. (2000). Smoking and mental illness: A population-based prevalence study. *JAMA: Journal of the American Medical Association, 284*, 2606–2610.

Lazarus, R. S. (1991). Progress on a cognitive-motivational-relational theory of emotion. *American Psychologist, 46*, 819–834.

Le, A. D., Quan, B., Juzytch, W., Fletcher, P. J., Joharchi, N., and Shaham, Y. (1998). Reinstatement of alcohol-seeking by priming injections of alcohol and exposure to stress in rats. *Psychopharmacology, 135*, 169–174.

Leonard, K. E., and Blane, H. T. (1999). Introduction. In K. E. Leonard and H. T. Blane (Eds.), *Psychological theories of drinking and alcoholism* (pp. 1–13). New York: Guilford Press.

Lerner, J. S., and Keltner, D. (2000). Beyond valence: Toward a model of emotion-specific influences on judgment and choice. *Cognition and Emotion, 14*, 473–493.

Lerner, J. S., and Keltner, D. (2001). Fear, anger, and risk. *Journal of Personality and Social Psychology, 81*, 146–159.

Leventhal, H., and Cleary, P. D. (1980). The smoking problem: A review of the research and theory in behavioral risk modification. *Psychological Bulletin, 88*, 370–405.

Mayhew, K. P., Flay, B. R., and Mott, J. A. (2000). Stages in the development of adolescent smoking. Drug and Alcohol Dependence, 59 (Supplement 1), S61–S81.

McGee, R., Williams, S., and Stanton, W. (1998). Is mental health in childhood a major predictor of smoking in adolescence? *Addiction, 93*, 1869–1874.

Murphy, F. C., Nimmo-Smith, I., and Lawrence, A. D. (2003). Functional neuroanatomy of emotions: A meta-analysis. *Cognitive, Affective and Behavioral Neuroscience, 3*, 207–233.

Myers, M. G., Aarons, G. A., Tomlinson, K., and Stein, M. B. (2003). Social anxiety, negative affectivity, and substance use among high school students. *Psychology of Addictive Behaviors, 17*, 277–283.

Panskepp, J., Nocjar, C., Burgdorf, J., Panksepp, J. B., and Huber, R. (2004). The role of emotional systems in addiction: A neuroethological perspective. *Nebraska Symposium on Motivation, 50*, 85–126.

Park, C. L., Armeli, S., and Tennen, H. (2004). The daily stress and coping process and alcohol use among college students. *Journal of Studies on Alcohol, 65*, 126–135.

Patton, G. C., Hibbert, M., Rosier, M. J., Carlin, J. B., Caust, J., and Bowes, G. (1996). Is smoking associated with depression and anxiety in teenagers? *American Journal of Public Health, 86*, 225–230.

Paty, J., Kassel, J., and Shiffman, S. (1992). The importance of assessing base rates for clinical studies: An example of stimulus control of smoking. In M. deVries (Ed.), *The experience of psychopathology: Investigating mental disorders in their natural settings* (pp. 347–352). New York: Cambridge University Press.

Perkins, K. A., Jetton, C., and Keenan, J. (2003). Common factors across acute subjective effects of nicotine. *Nicotine and Tobacco Research, 5*, 869–875.

Phan, K., Wager, T. D., Taylor, S. F., and Liberzon, I. (2004). Functional neuroanatomy of emotion: A meta-analysis of emotion activation studies in PET and fMRI. *Neuroimage, 16*, 331–348.

Piasecki, T. M., Fiore, M. C., and Baker, T. B. (1998). Profiles in discouragement: Two studies of variability in the time course of smoking withdrawal symptoms. *Journal of Abnormal Psychology, 107*, 238–251.

Piasecki, T. M., Niaura, R., Shadel, W. G., Abrams, D., Goldstein, M., Fiore, M. C., et al. (2000). Smoking withdrawal dynamics in unaided quitters. *Journal of Abnormal Psychology, 109*, 74–86.

Pomerleau, O. F., and Pomerleau, C. S. (1991). Research on stress and smoking: Progress and problems. *British Journal of Addictions, 86(5)*, 599–603.

Randall, D. M., and Cox, W. M. (2001). Experimental mood inductions in persons at high and low risk for alcohol problems. *American Journal of Drug and Alcohol Abuse, 27*, 183–187.

Robinson, T. E., and Berridge, K. C. (2003). Addiction. *Annual Review of Psychology, 54*, 25–53.

Rodgers, B., Korten, A. E., Jorm, A. F., Jacomb, P. A., Christensen, H., and Henderson, A. S. (2000). Nonlinear relationships in associations of depression and anxiety with alcohol use. *Psychological Medicine, 30*, 421–432.

Rohde, P., Lewinsohn, P. M., Brown, R. A., Gau, J. M., and Kahler, C. W. (2003). Psychiatric disorders, familial factors and cigarette smoking: I. Associations with smoking initiation. *Nicotine and Tobacco Research, 5*, 85–98.

Rohde, P., Lewinsohn, P. M., and Seeley, J. R. (1996). Psychiatric comorbidity with problematic alcohol use in high school students. *Journal of the American Academy of Child and Adolescent Psychiatry, 35,* 101–109.

Rohsenow, D. J., Sirota, A. D., Martin, R. A., and Monti, P. M. (2004). The Cocaine Effects Questionnaire for patient populations: Development and psychometric properties. *Addictive Behaviors, 29,* 537–553.

Russell, J. A. (1979). Affective space is bipolar. *Journal of Personality and Social Psychology, 37,* 345–356.

Russell, J. A. (1980). A circumplex model of affect. *Journal of Personality and Social Psychology, 39,* 1161–1178.

Russell, M. A. H., Peto, J., and Patel, U. A. (1974). The classification of smoking by factorial structure of motives. *Journal of the Royal Statistical Society Series A, 137,* 313–333.

Saint-Exupéry, A. D. (1943). *The Little Prince.* New York: Harcourt, Inc.

Sayette, M. A. (1999). Cognitive theory and research. In K. E. Leonard and H. T. Blane (Eds.), *Psychological theories of drinking and alcoholism* (vol. 2, pp. 247–291). New York: Guilford Press.

Schafer, J., and Brown, S. A. (1991). Marijuana and cocaine effect expectancies and drug use patterns. *Journal of Consulting and Clinical Psychology, 59,* 558–565.

Shaham, Y., Erb, S., Leung, S., Buczek, Y., and Stewart, J. (1998). CP-154,526, a selective, non-peptide antagonist of the corticotropin-releasing factor, receptor attenuates stress-induced relapse to drug seeking in cocaine- and heroin-trained rats. *Psychopharmacology, 137,* 184–190.

Shaham, Y., Erb, S., and Stewart, J. (2000). Stress-induced relapse to heroin and cocaine seeking in rats: A review. *Brain Research: Brain Research Review, 33,* 13–33.

Shedler, J., and Block, J. (1990). Adolescent drug use and psychological health: A longitudinal inquiry. *American Psychologist, 45,* 612–630.

Shiffman, S. (1982). Relapse following smoking cessation: A situational analysis. *Journal of Consulting and Clinical Psychology, 50,* 71–86.

Shiffman, S. (1993). Assessing smoking patterns and motives. *Journal of Consulting and Clinical Psychology, 61,* 732–742.

Shiffman, S. (2005). Dynamic influences on smoking relapse process. *Journal of Personality, 73,* 1715–1748.

Shiffman, S., Gwaltney, C. J., Balabanis, M. H., Liu, K. S., Paty, J. A., Kassel, J. D., et al. (2002). Immediate antecedents of cigarette smoking: An analysis from ecological momentary assessment. *Journal of Abnormal Psychology, 111,* 531–545.

Shiffman, S., Paty, J. A., Gnys, M., Kassel, J. A., and Hickcox, M. (1996). First lapses to smoking: Within-subjects analysis of real-time reports. *J Consult Clin Psychol, 64(2),* 366–379.

Shiffman, S., and Stone, A. A. (1998). Ecological momentary assessment: A new tool for behavioral medicine research. In D. S. Krantz and A. Baum (Eds.), *Technology and methods in behavioral medicine* (pp. 117–131). Mahwah, NJ: Lawrence Erlbaum.

Shiffman, S., and Waters, A. J. (2004). Negative affect and smoking lapses: A prospective analysis. *Journal of Consulting and Clinical Psychology, 72,* 192–201.

Siegel, S. (1983). Classical conditioning, drug tolerance, and drug dependence. In R. G. Smart, F. B. Glaser, Y. Israel, H. Kalant, and R. E. Popham (Eds.), *Research advances in alcohol and drug problems* (vol. 7). New York: Plenum.

Simons, J. S., Gaher, R. M., Oliver, M. N. I., Bush, J. A., and Palmer, M. A. (2005). An experience sampling study of associations between affect and alcohol use and problems among college students. *Journal of Studies on Alcohol, 66,* 459–469.

Sinha, R. (2001). How does stress increase risk of drug abuse and relapse? *Psychopharmacologia, 158,* 343–359.

Solomon, R. L. (1977). An opponent-process theory of acquired motivation: The affective dynamics of addiction. In J. D. Maser and M. E. P. Seligman (Eds.), *Psychopathology: Experimental models* (pp. 66–103). San Francisco: W.H. Freeman.

Solomon, R. L., and Corbit, J. D. (1974). An opponent-process theory of motivation: I. Temporal dynamics of affect. *Psychological Review, 81,* 119–145.

Spealman, R. D., Lee, B., Tiefenbacher, S., Platt, D. M., Rowlett, J. K., and Khroyan, T. V. (2004). Triggers of relapse: Nonhuman primate models of reinstated cocaine seeking. *Nebraska Symposium on Motivation, 50,* 57–84.

Spielberger, C. D. (1986). Psychological determinants of smoking behavior. In R. D. Tollison (Ed.), *Smoking and society: Toward a more balanced assessment* (pp. 89–134). Lexington, MA: Heath and Co.

Stanton, W. R., Mahalski, P. A., McGee, R., and Silva, P. A. (1993). Reasons for smoking or not smoking in early adolescence. *Addictive Behaviors, 18,* 321–329.

Steele, C. M., and Josephs, R. A. (1990). Alcohol myopia: Its prized and dangerous effects. *American Psychologist, 45,* 921–933.

Stewart, J. (2004). Pathways to relapse: Factors controlling the reinitiation of drug seeking after abstinence. *Nebraska Symposium on Motivation, 50,* 197–234.

Stewart, J., de Wit, H., and Eikelboom, R. (1984). Role of unconditioned and conditioned drug effects in the self-administration of opiates and stimulants. *Psychological Review, 91,* 251–268.

Stone, A. A., and Shiffman, S. (1994). Ecological momentary assessment in behavioral medicine. *Annals of Behavioral Medicine, 16,* 199–202.

Sutton, M. A., Karanian, D. A., and Self, D. W. (2000). Factors that determine a propensity for relapse to cocaine-seeking behavior in rats. *Neuropsychopharmacology, 22,* 626–641.

Tarter, R. E., Vanyukov, M., Giancola, P., Dawes, M., Blackson, T., and Mezzich, A. (1999). Etiology of early age onset substance use disorder: A maturational perspective. *Development and Psychopathology, 11,* 657–683.

Tellegen, A., Watson, D., and Clark, L. A. (1999). On the dimensional and hierarchical structure of affect. *Psychological Science, 10,* 297–303.

Tiffany, S. T. (1990). A cognitive model of drug urges and drug-use behavior: Role of automatic and non-automatic processes. *Psychological Review, 97(2),* 147–168.

Trimmel, M., and Wittberger, S. (2004). Effects of transdermally administered nicotine on aspects of attention, task load, and mood in women and men. *Pharmacology Biochemistry and Behavior, 78,* 639–645.

Turner, L., Mermelstein, R., and Flay, B. R. (2004). Individual and contextual influences on adolescent smoking. *Annals of the New York Academy of Sciences, 1021,* 175–197.

United States Department of Health and Human Services. (1988). *The health consequences of smoking: Nicotine addiction. A report of the surgeon general (DHHS Publication No. CDC8u8-8406).* Atlanta, GA: Public Health Service, Centers for Disease Control and Prevention, National Center for Chronic Disease Prevention and Health Promotion, Office on Smoking and Health.

Watkins, K. E., Hunter, S. B., Wenzel, S. L., Tu, W., Paddock, S. M., Griffin, A., et al. (2004). Prevalence and characteristics of clients with co-occurring disorders in outpatient substance abuse treatment. *America Journal of Drug and Alcohol Abuse, 30,* 749–764.

Watson, D., and Clark, L. A. (1984). Negative affectivity: The disposition to experience aversive emotional states. *Psychological Bulletin, 96,* 465–490.

Watson, D., Clark, L. A., and Tellegen, A. (1988). Development and validation of brief measures of positive and negative affect: The PANAS scales. *Journal of Personality and Social Psychology, 54,* 1063–1070.

Watson, D., Wiese, D., Vaidya, J., and Tellegen, A. (1999). The two general activation systems of affect: Structural findings, evolutionary considerations, and psychobiological evidence. *Journal of Personality and Social Psychology, 76,* 820–838.

West, R. (1993). Beneficial effects of nicotine: Fact or fiction? *Addiction, 88,* 589–590.

Wetter, D. W., Smith, S. S., Kenford, S. L., Jorenby, D. E., et al. (1994). Smoking outcome expectancies: Factor structure, predictive validity, and discriminant validity. *Journal of Abnormal Psychology, 103,* 801–811.

Wikler, A. (1980). *Opioid dependence: Mechanisms and treatment.* New York: Plenum.

Wills, T. A., Sandy, J. M., and Yaeger, A. (2000). Temperament and adolescent substance use: An epigenetic approach to risk and protection. *Journal of Personality, 68,* 1127–1151.

Wills, T. A., and Shiffman, S. (1985). Coping and substance use: A conceptual framework. In S. Shiffman and T. A. Wills (Eds.), *Coping and substance use* (pp. 3–24). New York: Academic Press.

Wills, T. A., and Stoolmiller, M. (2002). The role of self-control in early escalation of substance use: A time-varying analysis. *Journal of Consulting and Clinical Psychology, 70,* 986–997.

Wilner, P. (2001). A view through the gateway: Expectancies as a possible pathway from alcohol to cannabis. *Addiction, 96,* 691–703.

Yik, M. S. M., Russell, J. A., and Feldman Barrett, L. (1999). Structure of self-reported current affect: Integration and beyond. *Journal of Personality and Social Psychology, 77,* 600–619.

Zimmerman, D. M., Sehnert, S. S., Epstein, D. H., Pickworth, W. B., Robinson, M. L., and Moolchan, E. T. (2004). Smoking topography and trajectory of asthmatic adolescents requesting cessation treatment. *Preventive Medicine, 39,* 940–942.

Zinberg, N. E. (1984). *Drug, set and setting: The basis for controlled intoxicant use.* New Haven: Yale University Press.

Stress and Impulsive Behaviors

CHRISTOPHER B. DONAHUE AND JON E. GRANT

This chapter explores the complex relationship between stress, impulsivity, and substance use disorders (SUDs). A representative sample of individual impulse control disorders is reviewed, to include pathological gambling (PG), trichotillomania (TTM), and intermittent explosive disorder (IED) and categorized as problems of reward seeking (PG), habit (TTM), and a lack of premeditation (IED). Factors that mediate the disorders include tension reduction and affective regulation and can be further complicated by, and hold many similarities to, SUDs. Individuals with impulse control disorders can engage in the problem behavior as a means to immediately reduce tension or urge intensity and also seek to regulate affective states, particularly negative states (e.g., depression, boredom, anxiety), which there is low tolerance for. Individuals with impulse control disorders suffer numerous negative psychosocial stressors as a result of their acting on the impulses. Impulsivity, aggression, and sensation seeking are common features of SUD and impulse control disorders (PG, IED) leading to problems in managing either comorbid disorders. Treatment of the differing impulse control problems require multimodal approaches (psychosocial, behavioral, pharmacological) in order to address unique qualities of each problem. Promising psychological treatment approaches include components of cognitive behavioral therapy (CBT) such as cognitive retraining, behavioral modification, cue exposure, and self-control training, requiring further research.

I. INTRODUCTION

Impulsivity has been defined as a predisposition toward rapid, unplanned reactions to either internal or external stimuli without regard for negative consequences (Moeller, Barratt, Dougherty, Schmitz, and Swann, 2001), but this definition may not adequately characterize the complex range of behaviors regarded as impulsive. Although certain disorders are formally classified as impulse control disorders, impulsivity is a key element of many psychiatric disorders (for example, substance use disorders, bipolar disorder, personality disorders, attention deficit hyperactivity disorder). In *DSM-IV-TR*, the category of Impulse Control Disorders Not

Stress and Addiction: Biological and Psychological Mechanisms
Edited by **Mustafa al'Absi, Ph.D.**

Elsewhere Classified currently includes pathological gambling, trichotillomania, intermittent explosive disorder, kleptomania, and pyromania (American Psychiatric Association, 2000). Although all of these disorders are considered impulsive behaviors, the extent to which these disorders share clinical, genetic, phenomenological, and biological features is incompletely understood.

Research suggests that there is significant heterogeneity within the impulse control disorders, and the concept of "impulsivity" may include distinct subtypes of impulsive behaviors. Because rigorous research is limited on most impulse control disorders, this chapter will focus on pathological gambling, trichotillomania, and intermittent explosive disorder, three impulse control disorders that have received significant research attention and reflect the heterogeneity of these impulsive behaviors. In addition, these disorders represent three distinct, yet not absolute, subtypes of impulsivity: reward-seeking behavior (pathological gambling), habitual behavior (trichotillomania), and behavior characterized by a lack of premeditation (intermittent explosive disorder). We recognized that the subtypes do not completely define the selected or nonselected impulse control problems, with some overlap. This chapter will examine the complex relationship of these disorders to stress, tension reduction, affective regulation, and substance use (drug and alcohol) disorders (SUDs).

II. IMPULSE CONTROL AND SUBSTANCE USE DISORDERS

Individuals with impulse control disorders are found to be at an increased risk for substance use disorders (SUDs). Studies (Lejoyeux, Feuche, Solomon, and Andes, 1999) have reported prevalence rates of 38% for individuals with impulse control disorders receiving in-patient treatment for SUDs. Individuals with early onset alco-

holism relative to late onset have reported higher levels of impulsivity and sensation seeking, as well as heightened symptom severity ratings for SUDs (Dom, Hulstijn, and Sabbe, 2006). Of the impulse control disorders reviewed in this chapter, pathological gambling has been reported as having the highest rate of comorbid SUDs (Lejoyeux et al., 1999). The constructs of impulsivity, risk taking, and novelty seeking, which are characteristic of the impulse control disorders, among other psychiatric disorders, can contribute to the initiation of drug and alcohol use, as well as transitions from initial use to regular use to addiction (Kreek, Nielsen, Butelman, and LaForge, 2005). Kreek and colleagues (2005) argued that impulsivity and risk taking contribute most to the initiation of drug use and the progression of regular drug use. Subsequent changes once the addictive process is initiated are attributed to substantial changes in the brain as a result of repeated exposure to drug or alcohol abuse. We will explore in this chapter the commonalities between SUDs and impulse control disorders, as well as abnormal stress response. Table 9-1, on page 194; provides a summary of the complex relationships between the impulse control disorders reviewed and stress.

III. REWARD-SEEKING BEHAVIOR: PATHOLOGICAL GAMBLING (PG)

How does tension reduction and affective regulation relate to gambling? Is stress a driving factor that contributes to or precipitates the impulse to gamble? Individuals who struggle with PG are preoccupied with wagering, and the amount of the wager increases in order for the person to achieve a greater sense of excitement. When the individual attempts to refrain from gambling, or even reduce the amount of gambling, he/she may become irritable. In many individuals, gambling becomes a means of escaping from negative moods

CASE VIGNETTE

B.G., a 40-year-old married Caucasian male, reports the following symptoms. "I come home from work and I feel stressed out and have this need to blow off some steam. When I gamble it gives me an initial rush and I don't really think about anything while gambling except gambling and I don't consider the consequences of my gambling. All I want to do is forget about my other problems but the gambling usually ends in me feeling worse rather than happy regardless of whether I win or lose. I have had several times in my life when I have felt depressed and my family has commented that my depression has worsened lately. My alcohol use and gambling tend to feed off each other, with one worsening the other. My gambling has gotten so out of control that I am currently in serious financial trouble, taking a second mortgage, gambling away my son's college fund, problems at work, and most importantly, my wife threatening divorce. The problems that have resulted from my gambling seem to far out weigh any benefit that I have received, yet I can't stop gambling."

(e.g., anxiety, depression). Whiteside and Lynam (2001) made an effort to broadly define impulse control problems, with a sense of urgency involving individuals experiencing strong impulses under conditions of negative affect. Sensation seeking is one additional aspect of impulse control problems, including PG, which involves the pursuit of activities that are exciting and being open to new experiences that may or may not be dangerous (Whiteside and Lynam, 2001). As seen in the case of BG, individuals with PG may also report co-occurring alcohol and drug use problems, with the problems becoming mutually reinforcing. PG has been found to have many similarities with substance use disorders (e.g., tolerance, telescoping; Taveres, Zilberman, Beites, and Gentil, 2001), as well as high rates of comorbidity with substance use disorders (Cunningham-Williams, Cottler, Compton, and Spitznagel, 1998), prompting Potenza, Fiellin, Heninger, Rounsaville, and Mazurc (2002) to categorize gambling as an addictive disorder.

A. Tension Reduction

An individual's need for tension reduction has been described as a mediating factor in substance addiction and a possible contributing characteristic of problem gambling. A study of New Zealand university students found that individuals who suffered from problem gambling were more depressed and impulsive compared to their nonproblem gambling peers (Clarke, 2004). Motivations reported by problem gamblers in this study were reducing tension, experiencing guilt, and feeling compelled to prove themselves to others. Those students with problem gambling were unable to recognize a connection between their behavior and gambling outcomes, reporting an external versus internal locus of control (Clarke, 2004). The need for tension reduction may be better conceptualized, in some pathological gamblers, as an urge to engage in the problem behavior, which can be reinforcing. Individuals experience a "craving" or an urge to engage in gambling, and as seen in cases of SUD, engaging in the behavior may be considered the only alternative to alleviate that tension. We will review physiological and neurological studies to better understand the changes that occur during gambling and similarities with SUD.

Neuroimaging studies have reported abnormalities in the brain functioning of pathological gamblers (Goldstein and Carlton, 1988; Potenza et al., 2003;

TABLE 9-1   Impulse Control Disorders and Moderating Variables

Moderators	PG (Reward)	TTM (Habit)	IED (Lack of Premeditation)
Tension Reduction	Gambling urge =/> SUD related urge. Tension/stress change pre, during, postgamble. Goal = Reward (e.g., winning, chasing losses and avoidance of distress). Autonomic arousal. Delayed hemispheric activation.	Tension increase and release not characteristic of all TTM cases. Decreased pain sensitivity in hair-pulling site. Poor tolerance for discomfort. Goal = Reduction of distress. Urge unique to location/type of hair pulled. Autonomic arousal.	Unplanned, uncontrolled aggressive outbursts (tension), followed by remorse + tension reduction. Goal = tension reduction. High autonomic arousal. Reduced central serotonin function.
Affective Regulation	Abnormal reactivity to stressors. Comorbid mood and affective disorders. Gambling negatively reinforced (avoid/escape negative affect). Risk-taking temperament.	Abnormal reactivity to stressors. Boredom significant motivator. Comorbid mood and affective disorders. Affective experience serves as cue for and reinforces hair pulling (reduces unpleasant affective state).	Rapid onset of brief, "manic-like" symptoms followed by depressed mood, fatigue, and sometimes pleasure. Comorbid mood and affective disorders. Poor distress tolerance.
Treatment	Revise erroneous gambling cognitions. Motivational interview. Modify environmental cues. Cue Exposure. Coping Skills training. SSRI Opioid antagonist (Naltrexone)	Behavioral modification (habit reversal). Modify environmental cues. Coping Skills Training. Cognitive Therapy. SSRI (Fluoxetine) Opioid antagonist (Naltraxone)	Limited CBT research. Population reluctant to seek treatment. Cue exposure, relaxation training, and cognitive therapy +. Future research: mindfulness and self-control training. SSRI (Fluoxetine) + Valproate semisodium +.
SUD	Comorbid Alcohol (73%) Comorbid Drug (38%)	Comorbid SUD (22%)	Comorbid SUD (48%)

PG = pathological gambling, TTM = trichotillomania, IED = intermittent explosive disorder, SUD = substance use disorder, CBT = cognitive behavior therapy, (+) = significant research outcomes.

Stojanov et al., 2003). Goldstein and Carlton (1988) through EEG studies found significant delays in hemispheric activation, implying inflexibility in brain shifting ability or perseverative tendencies during gambling tasks regardless of negative consequences. Stojanov and colleagues (2003) found evidence of increased arousal levels or startle response, while Potenza and colleagues (2003) reported increased activation in the right middle frontal gyrus during a gambling scenario. Potenza and colleagues concluded their findings were evidence that pathological gamblers have similar brain pathways as those experiencing drug cravings, or the need for tension reduction. The experience of stress before, during, and after problem gambling has been considered a "moderating factor." Studies have investigated "stress related" changes in problem gamblers, finding autonomic arousal and immune system changes before, during, and after gambling (Brown, Rodda, and Phillips, 2004; Shinohara, Yanagisawa, and Kagota, 1999); higher levels of nor-adrenergic metabolites in males with PG (Roy, Adinoff, and Roehrich, 1988); and higher epinephrine and cortisol levels and blood pressure differences on days focused on gambling (Schmitt, Harrison, and Spargo, 1998). Additional physiological studies of pathological gamblers have found higher skin conductance levels during gambling (Sharpe, Tarrier, Schotte, and Spence, 1995); lower diastolic blood pressure throughout a gambling task (Carrol and Huxley, 1994); and higher heart rates (Blanchard, Wulfert, Freidenberg, and Malta, 2000). Another conclusion proposed by Goudriaan, Oosterlaan, de Beurs, and Van den Brink (2004) for differences in brain functioning was an abnormal reaction to stressors, with pathological gamblers presenting with different response patterns compared to nonpathological gamblers.

Individuals who develop PG appear to have deficits in shifting attention and have a diminished capacity to consider the negative consequences of their actions. Their focus is solely on the short-term urge to gamble, focusing only on the immediate consequences—that is, the need for tension reduction. The need for tension reduction or urge to gamble is experienced once the decision has been made to gamble, which may have been cued by any number of internal or external stimuli. PGs have been shown to have a greater "craving" to gamble or need for tension reduction, and are more impulsive in comparison to individuals with SUD (Castellani and Rugle, 1995; Tavares, Zilberman, Hodgins, and el-Guebaly, 2005). As noted by Goudrian and colleagues (2004), individuals who develop PG problems appear to have abnormal reactions to stress, which is also characteristic of individuals with comorbid mood, affective disorders, and SUDs. We will review problematic affective states resulting from an inability to cope with stressors, which can potentially initiate the urge to gamble.

B. Affective Regulation

Pathological gamblers have demonstrated high rates of co-occurring mood disorders, and this may suggest that the gambling behavior is associated with impairment in affective regulation. An individual's inability to cope with significant life stressors or a lack of the requisite coping skills can lead to the development of affective disorders. Individuals receiving inpatient psychiatric care (McCormick, Russo, Ramirez, et al., 1984) with PG have exhibited elevated rates of co-occurring major depressive disorder (76%) and hypomanic episodes, while outpatient populations have also reported comorbid major depressive disorder (28%) as well as elevated rates of anxiety (28%) and bipolar (24%) disorders (Linden, Pope, and Jonas, 1986). There has been limited longitudinal study as to the order of onset of these comorbid disorders. As noted by Petry, Stinson, and Grant (2005), anxiety and mood disorders may predispose individuals to develop gambling problems, or PG may lead to the development of anxiety disorders. The national epidemiological survey on alcohol and related conditions found that individuals with PG had elevated rates of comorbid alcohol use disorders (73%), any drug use disorder (38.10%), any mood disorder (49.62%), any anxiety disorder (41.30%), and any personality disorder (60.82%). The high comorbid rates with the aforementioned psychiatric and SUDs may imply diagnostic overlap. PG can be considered an escape or avoidance from problems or a means of relieving an aversive affective state, which is characteristic of mood, anxiety, and SUD. Petry and colleagues reported one gender difference, with women reporting higher rates of generalized anxiety and major depressive disorder, which could imply that women have an increased likelihood to develop PG in an effort to alleviate anxious and depressed mood than men (p. 571). Additional studies have reported on negative affective states in pathological gamblers.

Brown et al. (2004) reported greater "negative pre-gambling valence" for problem gamblers, which dramatically decreased if the gambler lost and did not significantly improve after winning. The gambling behavior is thereby negatively reinforced, in avoidance of negative affect or distress (Clarke, 2004). A number of internally mediated factors contribute to problem gambling, while external factors can also contribute substantially. Common risk factors identified for adolescent pathological gamblers that are predictive of this problem behavior include family problems, having conduct problems, addiction to drug or alcohol, and being male (Hardoon, Gupta, and Derevensky, 2004). Individuals experiencing stress from problematic and unsupportive home lives can subsequently lead to maladaptive strategies to reduce negative mood states and manage stress. Impulsivity and emotional distress have been found to influence risk taking in gamblers, especially young gamblers (Martins, Taveres, de Sliva Lobo, Galetti, and Gentil, 2004).

According to the St. Louis Personality, Health, and Lifestyle Study (SLPHL; Cunningham-Williams et al., 2005), factors found to be most predictive of PG included personality traits (high novelty-seeking temperament) and character styles (e.g., low cooperativeness, low self-directedness) indicating immature development, which are characteristics often associated with alcohol and substance use disorders. These findings reflect the fact that, while stress plays a significant role in PG, there is also the influence of having a risk-taking temperament.

SUD and PG both share similar traits, including compulsivity, impaired control, tolerance, and interpersonal problems (Grant, Kushner, and Kim, 2002; Petry et al., 2005). Additional commonalities between PG and alcohol and substance

use disorders include novelty-seeking tendencies and stress-related changes before, during, and after engaging in the problem behavior. One potential difference between PG and SUD is the finding that alcoholics use alcohol to deal with negative affect, particularly anxiety, whereas individuals with PG turn to gambling as a way to cope with depressive feelings and a lack of positive experiences in their life (Tavares et al., 2005). This "externalizing problem" appears to be motivated by several internal- and external-mediated variables (e.g., tension reduction, depression, poor family life) that are negatively reinforced. Individuals categorized as pathological gamblers also lack the requisite skills to contend with daily stressors and may tend to actually overreact. As identified in neuroimaging and neuropsychological studies, problem-solving ability can be limited and worsened by perseverative tendencies, with individuals unable to immediately recognize the negative consequences of their behavior.

C. Treatment of Pathological Gambling

We have categorized PG as a reward-seeking behavior, with individuals also exhibiting deficits in stress management. In targeting these two problems, individuals with PG require guidance in the identification of healthy alternatives to reward seeking and stress management. A majority of psychosocial treatment programs for individuals with PG are modeled after addiction programs and include self-help groups, inpatient treatment, and rehabilitation programs. However, programs such as Gamblers Anonymous (GA) have not demonstrated significant efficacy in the treatment of this problem, in isolation. Dropout rates from GA have ranged from 75–90% (Moody, 1990), with 8% reporting gambling abstinence at 1-year follow-up (Brown, 1985).

Cognitive behavioral methods, such as cognitive restructuring, have demonstrated some benefit in decreasing the frequency of gambling and irrational verbalizations associated with gambling (Hodgins and el-Guebaly, 2004). Others (Russo, Taber, McCormick et al., 1984; Taber, McCormick, Russo, et al., 1987) have suggested that professionally guided, multimodal treatment programs, provided alone or in combination with GA, may be more effective than GA alone. Self-help programs have reported some benefit (Hodgins, Currie, el-Gurbaly, and Peden, 2004). Hodgins and colleagues (2004) randomly assigned subjects (N = 67) to self-help workbook only or workbook and two motivational telephone interventions. At 1 year follow-up, 60% of the subjects in the motivational phone intervention group did not meet criteria for PG. The motivational interviewing appears to have had an effect on individuals inhibiting the urge to gamble and in developing healthy alternatives to gambling.

Pharmacological treatment may also offer significant promise in treating PG. Although the use of SSRIs, such as paroxetine, fluvoxamine, and sertraline for PG, has produced mixed findings (Grant and Potenza, 2004), they may be particularly beneficial for stress reduction in gamblers. Other randomized, placebo-controlled studies have demonstrated possible benefit from opioid antagonists (Grant et al., 2006; Kim et al., 2002) and lithium (Hollander, Pallanti, Allen, Sood, and Rossi, 2005). These medications may be better targeted to reduce reward-seeking behavior in gamblers. Studies of medication treatment, while providing short-term reduction of PG symptoms, have not demonstrated long-term benefits. The majority of the pharmacological studies, like the psychological studies, have failed to include co-occurring disorders and therefore the results may not generalize to the larger population of individuals with PG.

Future controlled-treatment studies for PG are needed in order to explore strategies (pharmacological and psychosocial)

that effect long-term change. We have discussed individuals with this impulse control problem experiencing an urge to engage in the problem behaviors, as seen in SUD, which can be mediated by internal and external stressors and/or triggers. Of concern, as reported by Tavares and colleagues (2005), is the fact that individuals with PG report significantly greater cravings compared to individuals with SUD. One possible treatment approach to be explored is cue exposure, which has been used successfully to treat other anxiety disorders (Barlow, 1993). The core idea in CE is that prolonged presentations of the conditioned cues (e.g., sights, sounds, and smells of gambling) in the absence of the naturally evocative experience (e.g., gambling behavior) will eliminate or substantially weaken (i.e., "extinguish" or "habituate") the pathological conditioned reactions (e.g., urge to gamble) that these cues produce (Foa and Kozak, 1986). In terms of CE treatment for PG, Symes and Nicki (1997) reported two cases of PG successfully treated with CE. McConaghy, Blaszczynski, and Frankova, (1991) (also see McConaghy, Armstrong, Blaszczynski, and Allock, 1983) reported one of the only randomized controlled trials of CE for PG. They found that CE procedures resulted in a greater percentage of PG cases that demonstrated "controlled" or "ceased" gambling at follow-up than did a control group undergoing relaxation training only. However, the control group actually had a higher proportion of participants that were actually abstinent from gambling at the follow-up. Future controlled studies are needed to determine the efficacy of CE for PG.

Additional risks for relapse in individuals with PG include unstructured time, boredom, and a lack of positive experiences in their lives (Hodgins and el-Guelby, 2004; Tavares et al., 2005). A multimodal approach to this problem would therefore consider training in healthy alternative coping skills that would include immediate and more enduring rewards, as experienced in gambling.

IV. HABIT BEHAVIOR: TRICHOTILLOMANIA (TTM)

Some impulse control disorders may be better conceptualized as habitual behaviors (for example, trichotillomania, skin picking, and nail biting) given that many individuals with trichotillomania (TTM) often report performing the behaviors without a clear driving force or a lack of premeditation (Whiteside and Lynam, 2001). Habits by definition are considered automatic processes and in the case of TTM, a maladaptive coping strategy to manage negative affect (depression) and serving to reduce tension.

CASE VIGNETTE

S.A. is a 16-year-old female who sought outpatient therapy for treatment of her hair pulling. She reported a depressed mood and significant hair loss. Her problem developed at age 10 when she would pull hair when upset about her parents fighting and when feeling sad, lonely, or bored. She reported that she usually pulled her hair "without thinking" or when under stress related to school, family, and relationship problems. Sometimes, however, she reported a significant urge to pull, with some relief (tension reduction) when she engaged in the behavior. At those times she found the hair pulling enjoyable.

As noted in this case vignette, individuals with TTM can experience a significant urge to engage in the hair-pulling behavior, and the behavior can become conditioned in the sense that it becomes an automatic response to stressors.

A. Tension Reduction

As defined in the *DSM-IV* (American Psychiatric Association, 2000), individuals with TTM experience an increased state of tension prior to pulling hair and a sense of relief when pulling. Azrin and Nunn (1973) characterize TTM as a nervous habit, starting as a normal reaction and becoming a strongly established habit. Rothbaum (1992) described hair pulling as occurring, increasing, and reappearing in conjunction with stress, leading to the conclusion that individuals with this problem would benefit from stress reduction training. Additional research has challenged the *DSM-IV* criteria requiring tension increase and reduction as overly restrictive (Christenson, Makenzie, and Mitchell, 1991). Christenson and colleagues (1991) reported that 17–23% of a sample of individuals diagnosed with TTM did not experience a sense of tension immediately before or while trying to resist hair pulling, or feelings of pleasure, gratification, or relief following hair pulling. Of interest in this study was the finding that each individual's experience of tension increase and subsequent relief was unique to the location of the hair pulled and type of hair pulled (e.g., scalp hair, gray hairs).

There have also been differences noted in the experience of tension and relief, with children and adolescents at times reporting none (Hanna, 1997) in comparison to adults. Hanna (1997) reported the differences in symptom endorsement could be attributed to the cognitive development of the different age groups, with younger children having less awareness of internal states.

The impact of heightened levels of stress on the psychosocial functioning of individuals struggling with TTM has also been examined. Diefenbach, Tolin, Hannan, Crocetto, and Workhunsky (2005) compared a psychiatric control group to individuals diagnosed with TTM and found the TTM group reported lower life satisfaction, higher levels of distress, and lower levels of self-esteem. The lower levels of self-esteem were related to concerns about appearance, feelings of embarrassment, and frustration with the inability to control the impulse to pull hair. In addition, the majority of the sample (96.4%) reported current problems with negative affect/negative self-evaluations. In terms of life functioning, the TTM group reported lifetime and current problems with grooming, physical health, social interaction, recreational activities, and work productivity (Diefenbach et al., 2005). In this study, the severity of hair loss was the most significant predictor of self-esteem.

B. TTM and SUD

Studies have reported upwards of 80% of individuals with TTM have comorbid *DSM-IV-TR* axis I disorders, with 20% reporting current or past SUDs and/or eating disorders (Christenson et al., 1991). Among alcohol-dependent patients (N = 79), 38% were diagnosed with impulse control disorders, with only one patient being diagnosed with TTM (Lejoyeux et al., 1999). Individuals with TTM do share similar characteristics with other impulse control disorders, but there appears to be less prevalence in having comorbid SUD. Nonetheless, individuals with TTM commonly experience mood and affective disorders, which are commonly reported as highly comorbid in SUD populations. The literature does not, however, reflect high comorbid SUD rates with TTM when TTM is studied independent of mood and affective disorders. As a result, there will not be as many comparisons between individuals with SUD and TTM in the following section.

C. Affective Regulation

Individuals with TTM frequently endorse comorbid *DSM-IV* Axis I disorders, with as

much as 82% of an adult clinical sample with TTM (N = 60) meeting criteria (Christenson et al., 1991). Lifetime prevalence rates of this adult sample included 65% for mood disorders, 57% for anxiety disorders, 22% for substance abuse disorders, 20% for eating disorders, and 42% for personality disorders. The presence of co-occurring mood disorders may suggest an association between TTM and impaired affective regulation. Mansueto, Stemberger, Thomas, and Golomb (1997) in construction of a behavioral model of TTM reported the affective experience as an important motivator for hair pulling, serving as both a stimulus cue and a reinforcer of the behavior. An additional variable in studying this problem is the behavioral sequence of the problem and associated emotional states. Stanley, Borden, Mouton, and Breckenridge (1995) found that hair pulling was associated with decreases in tension, boredom, sadness, and anger. Diefenbach, Mouton-Odum, and Stanley (2002) further investigated changes in emotional states across the hair-pulling cycle (pre to during to post), finding significant decreases in boredom across the entire cycle. The identified emotional states were found to act as both stimulus cues and reinforcers for hair pulling (Diefenbach et al., 2002). Additional emotional state changes included significant increases in sadness, guilt, and anger after hair pulling was completed.

Townsley-Stemberger, Mansueto, and Gardner-Carter (2000) found in a group of treatment seeking (N = 67) patients with TTM, marked, day-to-day distress and social impairment due to hair pulling. This treatment-seeking group reported avoidance of interpersonal activities, significant depressed mood, irritability, and relationship problems (Townsley-Stemberger et al., 2000). Simeon and colleagues (1997) surveyed 71 female hair-pullers for self-injurious behaviors. Two TTM groups with and without comorbid self-injurious behaviors were surveyed, with the former reporting more significant history of depression, suicide attempts, and thoughts of death during self-injurious acts. Of the comorbid self-injurious behaviors, nail biting and skin picking were most related to TTM. In regard to affective cues for hair pulling, the TTM-only group reported more anxiety, diminished motivation, and depression. These findings, however, are from a survey of a national magazine predominantly for women, and the diagnosis of TTM could not be verified using a structured clinical interview. Despite the limitations, Simeon and colleagues' (1997) findings were consistent with previous studies' (Christenson, Ristvedt, and MacKenzie, 1993) finding that subgroups of TTM patient behaviors were cued by negative affect. Christenson and colleagues (1993) found that negative affect and sedentary/contemplative states served as hair-pulling cues. Of interest to this discussion, the negative affective cues included feeling terms (e.g., feeling angry, hurt) and situations associated with negative self-evaluation (e.g., weighing oneself, interpersonal conflicts) (Christenson et al., 1993).

One hypothesis is that hair pulling develops as a habit to cope with stress, and then ironically the behavior results in negative intra- and interpersonal distress. Distress results from having to avoid certain activities due to hair loss, such as public activities, sexual intimacy, and athletic endeavors (Stemberger, Thomas, Mansueto, et al., 2000). Distress also results from the individual's inability to control the hair pulling resulting in lowered self-esteem (Casti, Toner, and Yu, 2000; Stemberger et al., 2000). Once this impulse control habit has developed into TTM, the negative self-evaluative thoughts and negative affect can serve to perpetuate this problem by prompting additional pulling episodes (Franklin, Tolin, and Diefenbach, In press).

D. Treatment of Trichotillomania

The experience of stress or distress in association with TTM has been identified at different stages of the hair-pulling process and is also associated with comorbid mood and affective disorders. We categorized TTM as a problem of habit, or maladaptive habit developed to deal with affective states and stress. Treatment therefore would need to target healthy stress reduction strategies with more enduring tension reduction effects. While tension reduction appears to be a motivating factor in TTM, negative affective states and the experience of "boredom" serve to perpetuate this problem. Behavioral strategies utilized with this problem have been found to be most successful with symptom reduction. Manseuto and colleagues (1997) proposed that functional analysis of the hair-pulling process and accompanying affective states could assist in identification of the most appropriate treatment options. Individuals who experience reductions in boredom as a result of hair pulling may benefit from activity planning or "competing behavioral response" training. In contrast, relaxation skills may be more relevant for individuals who experience tension and anxiety reduction while pulling hair. Individuals who experience negative affective states (e.g., guilt) as a result of hair pulling could benefit from cognitive restructuring and relapse prevention in order to reframe negative cognitions associated with the behavior. In a review of behavioral treatment strategies, Friman, Finney, and Christophersen (1984) reported additional components of successful treatment programs for individuals with TTM, to include hair collection and self-monitoring with therapist, self-imposed consequences, token reinforcement, and self-denial of privileges.

Habit reversal has been identified as the most successful strategy (Azrin, Nunn, and Frantz, 1980) with symptom improvements of 90% in the short term. This strategy includes practicing motor responses that compete with the habit, habit inconvenience review, solicitation of social support, and self-monitoring. Considering the tension reduction component of TTM, Rothbaum

(1992) added the use of deep muscle relaxation to habit-reversal training, as well as thought stopping, cognitive restructuring, and stimulus control (e.g., identification of high-risk situations). Controlled studies to date have reported short-term benefits of cognitive behavioral therapy (CBT; Ninan, Rothbaum, Marsteller, Knight, and Eccard, 2000; van Minnen, Hoogduin, Keijsers, Hellenbrand, and Jan Hendriks, 2003) compared to medication (clomipramine and fluoxetine). Unfortunately, the short-term CBT benefits for TTM have not been maintained in follow-up periods. Lerner, Franklin, Meadows et al. (1998) reported that only 4 of 13 subjects maintained their initial gains at 3.9 years post-treatment from CBT. Similarly, Mouton and Stanley (1996) found that two patients out of six maintained clinically significant gains at 6-month follow-up after participation in habit-reversal training.

Additional study is needed in the use of medications combined with CBT to further evaluate the efficacy of this combined approach. There are few studies examining medications other than serotonin reuptake inhibitors. Naltrexone, an opioid-blocking compound thought to decrease positive reinforcement by preventing the binding of endogenous opiates to relevant receptor sites in the brain, may offer some benefit beyond the antidepressants (Carrion, 1995; Christenson, Crow, and MacKenzie, 1994). Christenson and colleagues (1994) reported significant effects on decreasing TTM symptoms when comparing naltrexone to placebo. In an uncontrolled case study, Carrion (1995) reported the combination of fluoxetine and naltrexone decreased the duration and intensity of hair-pulling episodes, with the individual reporting "little pleasure" from the hair-pulling episodes. The early gains in this case study were maintained during 8 subsequent weeks of treatment and at a 4-month follow-up. The use of naltrexone necessitates further evaluation with larger controlled studies, combined with and compared to the behavioral treatments discussed. The benefit observed from these preliminary naltrexone studies may be related, in part, to individuals with TTM experiencing altered pain sensitivity at the site of pulling (Christenson et al., 1994). For those individuals with TTM that do experience pain, the pain itself could be reinforcing, because of the distraction from negative emotional or physiological states (Christenson and Mansueto, 1999). Ultimately, the goal for individuals with TTM is to learn healthy strategies for regulating negative affect and thereby inhibit the urge to pull.

Future directions in the treatment of TTM may include a combination of pharmacological and psychosocial treatments, as well as the components of CBT proven to be most effective in symptom reduction. Although there is a short-term benefit to CBT approaches, such as habit reversal, there is limited evidence of the long-term benefits. This problem of habit appears to require a multimodal approach to address the different components of TTM, including the pleasure-seeking aspects, need for tension reduction and affective regulation, and the psychosocial deficits (e.g., avoidance of social activities due to hair loss). Future treatment studies for TTM may also focus on the addition of mindfulness/acceptance strategies to traditional CBT approaches (Franklin, Tolin, and Diefenbach, In press) and in comparison to use of hypnosis (Robiner, Edwards, and Christensen, 1999).

V. LACK OF PREMEDITATION: INTERMITTENT EXPLOSIVE DISORDER (IED)

The final subtype of impulse control disorders is behavior characterized by its lack of premeditation. Intermittent explosive disorder (IED) is defined by recurrent, significant outbursts of aggression, often leading to assaultive acts against people or property, which are disproportionate to outside stressors and no better explained by another psychiatric diagnosis (American Psychiatric Association, 2000). Individuals with IED are prone to aggressive outbursts when under stress. They may perceive the stress as threat, frustration, insult, vulnerability, or any combination of the above. The person is often upset, guilt-laden, and remorseful after the rage-filled episode even though there may be a sense of relief after the aggressive outburst. A defining characteristic of IED is the complete lack of premeditation preceding the behavior, with individuals requiring only a subtle slight to feel provoked (Coccaro and Danehy, 2005).

CASE VIGNETTE

Jake is a 27-year-old male reporting for outpatient treatment for the first time due to his inability to manage his anger and outbursts. He reports a long-standing history of easily losing his temper in spite of illogical provocation. For example, Jake describes how, after getting cut off in traffic, he chased the car and crashed into it. He then approached the vehicle, was verbally aggressive to the driver, and pounded the driver's car window until it cracked. The police came and he was given a citation. After he calmed down, he was extremely embarrassed and remorseful of his actions. He describes anger episodes as "uncontrollable rages" which are never planned but instead "just happen." He reports a type of amnesic dissociative state during the outbursts with only partial memory of the particular details. Due to these outbursts, Jake has had numerous legal problems, and his finances and relationships are quite strained. He is on probation currently and is required to receive treatment.

Coccaro, Schmidt, Samuals, and Nestadt (2004) reported on prevalence rates of

individuals with IED in a community-based sample. In addition to *DSM-IV* criteria, Coccaro et al. added the following research criteria: verbal or physical aggression toward people, animals, or property; aggressive acts occurring twice weekly, on average, for 1 month or three episodes involving physical assault over a year; and the aggressive act was not premeditated and was not committed in order to achieve some tangible objective. Coccaro and colleagues (2004) reported 28 (11.07%) of 253 subjects met inclusion criteria for lifetime IED by either *DSM-IV* or research criteria. Of the individuals meeting criteria for IED, 81.3% reported significant psychosocial impairment, and 50% reported personal distress associated with their aggressive behavior. In addition, impairment was reported in association with aggression-related problems in relationships in 62.5% of subjects or psychosocial impairment with the law (50%). Despite the external consequences of their aggressive acts, individuals with IED perceive a limited capacity to resist the urge to engage in the behavior, as they tend to experience a tension build-up and are compelled to follow through with the aggressive act.

A. IED and SUD

Lifetime prevalence studies (McElroy, Soutullo, Beckman, Taylor, and Keck, 1998) of individuals with comorbid IED and SUD include 44% for alcohol, 33% for drug, and 48% for any substance use disorder. Subjects with IED have reported alcohol worsening or reducing symptoms, and cannabis use reducing symptoms (McElroy et al., 1998). Approximately 57% of a community sample of aggressive drivers (N = 30) reported current or past alcohol abuse or dependence (Galovski, Blanchard, and Veaszey, 2002). Of the individuals that were diagnosed with IED (N = 10), 70% reported current or past SUD. Individuals with IED are also likely to have comorbid personality disorders, including borderline personality disorder and antisocial personality disorder, which place individuals at a greater risk for SUD (Galovski et al., 2002). We will integrate discussion of SUD in the following section of the mediating factors contributing to IED.

B. Tension Reduction

As we have discussed with other impulse control problems, individuals can experience an urge to engage in the behavior, and it may be rewarding as in the case of PG, or develop out of habit, as seen with TTM. Most individuals with IED, however, do not appear to obtain similar benefits (e.g., reward) from acting on their impulsive tendencies, but rather, experience tension reduction alone (McElroy et al., 1998). McElroy and colleagues (1998) reported that all subjects (N = 27) with IED in a case series experienced an irresistible impulse to be aggressive prior to the aggressive acts. For subjects in this small case study, aggressive impulses were associated with a build-up in tension (88%), the aggressive acts were associated with a relief of tension (75%), and in a smaller percentage of cases (48%), individuals experienced pleasure following the aggressive acts. Impulsiveness and aggression, which are prominent symptoms among individuals with IED, are also strong predictors of craving substances in SUD (Zilberman, Taveres, and el-Guebaly, 2003). In addition, individuals with SUD reporting high levels of aggression have been found to endorse more situations that trigger use of substances (McCormick and Smith, 1995). Individuals with IED misinterpret benign environmental cues to be aggressive and are more likely to act on the aggressive impulse when disinhibited following substance use. Alcohol expectancies, or what benefit an individual expects from using drugs or alcohol, are strongly influenced by levels of impulsivity. Alcohol use and impulsivity were studied in a sample of

alcohol-dependent subjects with comorbid conduct disorder (Finn, Bobova, Wehner, Fargo, and Rickert, 2005). Finn and colleagues (2005) found that individuals considered high in impulsivity were more likely than nonimpulsive subjects to be accurate in their proximal (immediate) alcohol expectancies (e.g., expect negative outcomes), and despite their accuracy, they continue to engage in abusive substance use. However, negative distal (next day) alcohol expectancies in impulsive subjects could potentially act as a deterrent from successive heavy drinking episodes. This concept will be further discussed in treatment section for IED.

Biological models may offer a greater understanding of changes in tension in IED. Impulsive aggression has been correlated with reduced central serotonin function (Linnoila, Virkkunen, Scheinin, et al. 1983; Virkkunen, Rawlings, Tokola, et al. 1994). Human (Coccaro, Kavoussi, Hauger, Cooper, and Ferris, 1998) and animal (Ferris and Deville, 1994) studies suggest that central vasopressin and aggression are inversely related to serotonin. However, the inverse relationship between serotonin and aggression is not present when, for example, norepinephrine system function is diminished (Wetzler, Kahn, Asnis, et al., 1991). Brain imaging studies (Soloff, Meltzer, Greer, et al., 2000) of impulsive aggression in other populations such as borderline personality disorder have found an association between aggression and decreased serotonin uptake in the medial and orbital regions of the right, prefrontal cortex. Gerald and Higley (2002) proposed that one of the mediating factors that place subjects with low CNS serotonin functioning at an increased risk for alcohol dependence is impulsivity. Serotonin dysfunction, however, is not specific to IED and has been found in many psychiatric disorders (alcohol abuse and dependence) known to have impulse control deficits (Cloninger, 1987), as well as deficits in regulating negative affect.

C. Affective Regulation

Individuals with IED commonly have comorbid *DSM-IV* Axis I and II disorders. In their study, McElroy and colleagues (1998) reported 89% and 93% of IED subjects met criteria for a current and lifetime mood disorder, respectively. Additionally, IED subjects suffer from high rates of lifetime anxiety (48%) and substance use (48–57%) disorders (Coccaro et al., 2004; Galovski et al., 2002). These high rates of co-occurring mood, anxiety, and SUD suggest possible impairment in stress management skills, particularly the ability to tolerate negative emotion. McElroy and colleagues (1998) found that IED subjects commonly reported affective or manic-like symptoms, such as irritability and rage during their aggressive acts, and a rapid onset of depressed mood and fatigue after the acts. Subjects were excluded from this study if their aggressive acts were better accounted for by bipolar disorder, alcohol abuse, or antisocial personality disorders. The subjects with IED and comorbid bipolar disorder that were retained in the study (52%) reported that the mood and energy changes during aggressive acts were qualitatively similar, but much briefer than those associated with hypomanic or manic episodes (McElroy et al., 1998). Despite the limitations of this study, the findings are consistent with other research (McElroy, Pope, Keck, et al., 1996) reporting subjects with IED commonly having mood-related problems, and that IED is in fact comorbid, rather than secondary to mood, affective, or personality disorders (Coccaro, Posternak, and Zimmerman, In press). Treatment of individuals with IED should therefore consider addressing deficits in affective regulation as well as the maladaptive response to daily stressors.

D. Treatment of IED

IED was defined as a problem related to a lack of premeditation. Treatment efforts may therefore be aimed at increasing the person's ability to consider the consequences of his/her behavior, inhibiting aggressive urges, and developing alternative tension reduction strategies using a combination or individualized psychosocial and pharmacological interventions. A maladaptive coping strategy in which individuals with IED are likely to engage in is alcohol and substance use, which can lead to the development of SUD. As discussed throughout this section, individuals with IED share the common traits of impulsivity and aggression with individuals with SUD. Aggression is also considered a strong predictor for a strong urge to use substances and therefore is an added challenge for individuals with high levels of impulsivity. One strategy suggested by Finn and colleagues (2005) is to address negative alcohol expectancies in individuals high in impulsivity with comorbid SUD. A parallel that may be drawn between the comorbid disorders relates to delaying or inhibiting the impulse to act. Instructing individuals with comorbid IED and SUD to focus on the negative consequences of successive substance use episodes as well as aggressive acts in the context of the triggering situation may act to facilitate inhibition. Unfortunately, there is limited research in the area of psychotherapy specifically developed for individuals with IED, and this may reflect the reluctance of individuals with IED to acknowledge a need for or seek treatment. Coccaro and colleagues (2004) reported that only 2 of 28 subjects diagnosed with IED pursued help for their aggressive behaviors, and only 50% reported distress from their aggressive behaviors. Of those with IED that do seek treatment, the motivation is typically some externally related consequence, such as aggressive driving or other legal problems stemming from impulsive behaviors.

Although there are no published controlled psychological studies for IED, Grodnitsky and Tafrate (2000) found in a nonrandomized pilot study of adult outpatients that participated in imaginal exposure therapy for anger habituated to anger-provoking scenarios, while Deffenbacher et al. (2002) reported diminished anger for self-identified angry drivers following participation in relaxation training and cognitive therapy. In this study, individuals benefited equally from relaxation only and relaxation plus cognitive therapy. Anger and emotional regulation can also be addressed by dialectical behavior therapy (DBT; Linehan, Tutek, Heard, et al., 1994). Studies have demonstrated improvements in impulsivity and anger in individuals with borderline personality disorder following participation in DBT (Linehan et al., 1994).

Data concerning pharmacological treatment for IED is equally limited. The use of fluoxetine (Coccaro and Kavoussi, 1997) has resulted in diminished impulsive aggression in a double-blind, placebo-controlled study of individuals (N = 40) with personality disorders and current histories of impulsive aggression and irritability, and no current history of major depression, bipolar disorder, or schizophrenia. One randomized, placebo-controlled study of divalproex in impulsivity and aggression included subjects with IED as well as subjects with and without a Cluster B personality disorder (Hollander, Tracy, Swann, et al., 2003; Kavoussi and Coccaro, 1998). In that study divalproex was effective in reducing the aggression of subjects with borderline personality disorder, but no similar benefit was reported for subjects with IED. As noted by McElroy (1999) in an open-label study of patients with IED and comorbid manic or mixed bipolar symptoms, aggressive outbursts have been shown to decrease by greater than 50% using valproate (6 of 8 subjects) and lithium (1 of 2 subjects).

The preliminary treatment findings for individuals with IED require further validation with well-controlled studies to assess the use of various treatment combinations (e.g., pharmacological and psychosocial interventions). Cognitive, relaxation, and exposure therapies have demonstrated some benefit in treating individuals with aggressive behaviors. For example, components of programs such as DBT for individuals with borderline personality disorder may prove efficacious for individuals with IED. Individuals with IED have deficits in the ability to recognize and be mindful of behavioral consequences, necessitating training in self-control in order to inhibit stress responses to benign environmental cues. One additional component of treating anger and the lack of premeditation characteristic of individuals with IED is mindfulness training. A case study (Singh, Wahler, Adkins, and Myers, 2003) of an individual with comorbid psychiatric diagnosis and mental retardation demonstrated self-control over anger using a specific mindfulness strategy. A mindfulness strategy may involve learning a meditation technique that requires an individual to shift awareness and attention from the anger-producing situation to a neutral situation or a neutral part of the body (soles of the feet), as used in Singh and colleagues' pilot investigation. Other areas of research to be explored may include the accuracy of individuals with IED perception of emotion (Silver, Goodman, Knoll, Isakov, and Modai, 2005) as studied in individuals with schizophrenia, and more specifically, misperception of facial expressions (Eastwood and Smilek, 2004). As noted by Eastwood and Smilek, a rapid physiological response to an "unconsciously perceived" facial expression prepares us to react in an adaptive manner to the presence of a threatening individual. However, this adaptive function as mediated by the amygdala (Davidson and Irwin, 1999) may not function as well in individuals with IED in terms of who and what they perceive as threatening.

VI. CONCLUSIONS

In our review of the three categories of impulse control problems, reward, habit, and lack of premeditation, we came to understand the influence and impact of stress or stressors. Individuals with impulse control problems are understood to have deficits in the ability to regulate emotion, reduce tension, and engage in maladaptive sensation or reward-seeking behaviors. There is a characteristic experience of tension or stress throughout the process of engaging in the various impulsive behaviors, with some experiencing a complete lack of tension, as in TTM. There are many similarities between the impulse control problems and SUD. Individuals with PG problems were found to most closely resemble alcohol and substance dependence, with similar reward pathways and urge intensities, for example. Aggression and impulsivity were found to be mediating factors in IED as well as SUD and personality disorders such as antisocial personality disorder and borderline personality disorder. Individuals found to have higher levels of impulsivity and aggression are considered a higher risk for developing SUD, which is an argument for developing integrated treatment approaches to address inhibitory control for the comorbid problems. A review of the current literature on impulse control problems is limited in the areas of controlled treatment studies, especially with IED. Each of the impulse control problems would appear to benefit from a multimodal treatment approach including psychosocial and pharmacological interventions. CBT programs and specific medications have been utilized with moderate success in treating these problems, having short-term but not long-term benefits with TTM, for example. Future research can evaluate the most effective components of CBT and compare to other treatment approaches such as mindfulness training and self-hypnosis. In dealing with various stressors, individuals with different impulse control problems are not necessarily aware of the problem behavior while they are engaging in it, and the consequences, no matter how severe, don't necessarily deter them from engaging in the behavior. It is important for us to understand the motivations (e.g., reward, sensation seeking, tension release) behind these behaviors

and to recognize the strength of the craving or urge (as in PG) to engage in the behavior. Finally, there are numerous negative consequences as a result of engaging in the problem behaviors. Individuals with TTM avoid relationships and certain social activities, individuals with PG can experience severe financial consequences, and individuals with IED can endanger themselves and others by their behavior. Treating these complex impulse control problems requires increasing the individuals' awareness of the problem and positive/negative consequences, diminishing the urge to engage in the behaviors, implementing healthy alternative coping skills (e.g., affective regulation, tension reduction), and providing long-term support and maintenance plans.

REFERENCES

American Psychiatric Association. (2000). *Diagnostic and statistical manual of mental disorders* (4th ed., text rev.) Washington, D.C.: Author.

Azrin, N. H., and Nunn, R. G., (1973). Habit reversal: A method of eliminating nervous habits and tics. *Behavior Research and Therapy, 11*, 619–628.

Azrin, N. H., Nunn, R. G., and Frantz, S. E. (1980). Treatment of hair pulling (trichotillomania): A comparative study of habit reversal and negative practice training. *Behavior Therapy and Experimental Psychiatry, 11*, 13–20.

Barlow, D. H. (Ed.). (1993). *Clinical handbook of psychological disorders: A step-by-step treatment manual* (2nd ed.). New York: Guilford Press.

Blanchard, E. B., Wulfert, E., Freidenberg, B. M., and Malta, L. S. (2000). Psychophysiological assessment of compulsive gamblers' arousal to gambling cues: A pilot study. *Applied Psychophysiological Biofeedback, 25*, 155–165.

Brown, R. I. (1985). The effectiveness of gamblers anonymous. In W. R. Eadington (Ed.), *The gambling studies: proceedings of the 6th National Conference on Gambling and Risk Taking*. Reno, NV: University of Nevada.

Brown, S. L., Rodda, S., and Phillips, J. G. (2004). Differences between problem and non-problem gamblers in subjective arousal and affective valence amongst electronic gaming machine players. *Addictive Behaviors, 29*, 1863–1867.

Carrion, V. G. (1995). Naltrexone for the treatment of trichotillomania: A case report. Journal of Clinical *Psychopharmacology, 15*(6), 444–446.

Carrol, D., and Huxley, J. A. A. (1994). Cognitive, dispositional, and psychophysiological correlates of dependent slot machine gambling in young people. *Journal of Applied Social Psychology, 24*, 1070–1083.

Castellani, B., and Rugle, L. (1995). A comparison of pathological gamblers to alcoholics and cocaine misusers on impulsivity, sensation seeking, and craving. *International Journal of Addiction, 30*, 275–289.

Casti, J., Toner, B. B., and Yu, B. (2000). Psychosocial issues for women with trichotillomania. *Comprehensive Psychiatry, 41*, 344–351.

Christenson, G. A., Crow, S. J., and MacKenzie, T. B. (1994, May). A placebo controlled double blind study of naltrexone for trichotillomania. Paper presented at the 147th annual meeting of the American Psychiatric Association, Philadelphia, PA.

Christenson, G. A., MacKenzie, T. B., and Mitchell, J. E. (1991). Characteristics of 60 adult chronic hair pullers. *American Journal of Psychiatry, 148*(3), 365–370.

Christenson, G. A., and Manseuto, C. S. (1999). Trichotillomania: Descriptive characteristics and phenomenology. In D. G. Stein, G. A. Christenson, E. Hollander (Eds.), *Trichotillomania* (pp. 1–41). Washington, DC: American Psychiatric Press.

Christenson, G. A., Ristvedt, S. L., MacKenzie, T. B. (1993). Identification of trichotillomania cue profiles. Behavioral Research and Therapy, *31*, 315–320.

Clarke, D. (2004). Impulsiveness, locus of control, motivation, and problem gambling. *Journal of Gambling Studies, 20*(4), 319–345.

Cloninger, C. R. (1987). Neurogenetic adaptive mechanisms in alcoholism. *Science, 236*, 410–416.

Coccaro, E. F., and Danehy, M. (2005). Intermittent explosive disorder. In E. Hollander and D. J. Stein (Eds.), *Clinical manual of impulse-control disorders* (pp. 19–37). Arlington, VA: American Psychiatric Publishing Inc.

Coccaro, E. F., and Kavoussi, R. J. (1997). Fluoxetine and impulsive aggressive behavior and personality disordered subjects. *Archives of General Psychiatry, 54*(12), 1081–1088.

Coccaro, E. F., Kavoussi, R. J., Hauger, R. L., Cooper T. B., and Ferris, C. F. (1998). Cerebrospinal fluid vasopressin: Correlates with aggression and serotonin function in personality disordered subjects. *Archives of General Psychiatry, 55*, 708–714.

Coccaro, E. F., Posternak, M. A., and Zimmerman, M. (In press). Prevalence and features of intermittent explosive disorder in a clinical setting. *Journal of Clinical Psychiatry*.

Coccaro, E. F., Schmidt, C. A., Samuals, J. F., and Nestadt, G. (2004). Lifetime and 1-month prevalence rates of intermittent explosive disorder in a community sample. *Journal of Clinical Psychiatry, 65*(6), 820–824.

Cunningham-Williams, R. M., Cottler, L. B., Compton, W. M., and Spitznagel, E. L. (1998). Taking chances: Problem gamblers and mental health disorders. Results from the St. Louis Epidemiological Catchment Area study. *American Journal of Public Health, 88*, 1093–1096.

Cunningham-Williams, R. M., Gruzca, R. A., Cottler, L. B., Womack, W. B., Books, S. J., Rrzybeck, T. R., Spitznagel, E. L., and Cloninger, C. R. (2005). Prevalence and predictors of pathological gambling: Results from the St. Louis Personality, Health, and Lifestyle study (SLPHL). *Journal of Psychiatric Research, 39*, 377–390.

Davidson, R. J., and Irwin, W. (1999). The functional neuroanatomy of emotion and affective style. *Trends in Cognitive Sciences, 3*(1), 11–21.

Deffenbacher, J. L., Filetti, L. B., Lynch, R. S. Lynch, R. S., Dahlen, E. R., and Oetting, E. R. (2002). Cognitive behavioral treatment of high anger drivers. *Behavioral Research and Therapy, 40*, 895–910.

Diefenbach, G. J., Mouton-Odom, S., and Stanley, M. A. (2002). Affective correlates of trichotillomania. *Behavioral Research and Therapy, 40*, 1305–1315.

Diefenbach, G. J., Tolin, D. F., Hannan, S., Crocetto, J., and Worhunsky, P. (2005). Trichotillomania: Impact on psychological functioning and quality of life. *Behaviour Research and Therapy, 43*, 869–884.

Dom, G., Hulstijn, W., and Sabbe, B. (2006). Differences in impulsivity and sensation seeking between early and late-onset alcoholics. *Addictive Behaviors, 31*, 298–308.

Eastwood, J. D., and Smilek, D. (2005). Functional consequences of perceiving facial expressions of emotion without awareness. *Consciousness and Cognition, 14*, 565–584.

Ferris, C. F., and Delville, Y. (1994). Vasopressin and serotonin interactions in the control of agonistic behavior. *Psychoendocrinology, 19*, 593–601.

Finn, P. R., Bobova, B., Wehner, E., Fargo, S., and Rickert, M. E. (2005). Alcohol expectancies, conduct disorder and early-onset alcoholism: Negative alcohol expectancies are associated with less drinking in non-impulsive versus impulsive subjects. *Addiction, 100*, 953–962.

Foa, E. B., and Kozak, M. J. (1986). Emotional processing of fear: Exposure to corrective information. *Psychological Bulletin, 99*, 20–35.

Franklin, M. E., Tolin, D. F., and Diefenbach, G. J. (In press). Trichotillomania. In E. Hollander and D. J. Stein (Eds.), *Clinical manual of impulse-control disorders* (pp. 149 173). Arlington, VA: American Psychiatric Publishing Inc.

Friman, P. C., Finney, J. W., and Christopherson, E. R. (1984). Behavioral treatment of trichotillomania: An evaluative review. *Behavior Therapy, 15*, 249–265.

Galovski, T., Blanchard, E. B., and Veazey, C. (2002). Intermittent explosive disorder and other psychiatric comorbidity among court-referred and self-referred aggressive drivers. *Behaviour Research and Therapy, 40*, 641–651.

Gerald, M. S., and Higley, J. D. (2002). Evolutionary underpinnings of excessive alcohol consumption. *Addiction, 97*, 415–425.

Goldstein, L., and Carlton, P. L. (1988). Hemispheric EEG correlates of compulsive behavior: The case of pathological gamblers. *Research in Community Psychology and Psychological Behaviors, 13,* 103–111.

Goudriaan, A. E., Oosterlaan, J., de Beurs, E., and Van de Brink, W. (2004). Pathological gambling: A comprehensive review of biobehavioral findings. *Neuroscience and Biobehavioral Reviews, 28,* 123–141.

Grant, J. E., Kushner, M. G., and Kim, S. W. (2002). Pathological gambling and alcohol use disorder. *Alcohol Research and Health, 26*(2), 143–150.

Grant, J. E., and Potenza, M. N. (2004). Impulse control disorders: Clinical characteristics and pharmacological management. *Annals of Clinical Psychiatry, 16*(1), 27–34.

Grant, J. E., Potenza, M. N., Hollander, E., Cunningham-Williams, R., Nurminen, T., Smits, G., and Kallio, A. (2006). A multicenter investigation of the opioid antagonist nalmefene in the treatment of pathological gambling. *American Journal of Psychiatry, 163,* 303–312.

Grodnitzky, G. R., and Tafrate, R. C. (2000). Imaginal exposure for anger reduction in adult outpatients: A pilot study. *Journal of Behavioral Therapy and Experimental Psychiatry, 31,* 259–279.

Hanna, G. L. (1997). Trichotillomania and related disorders in children and adolescents. *Child Psychiatry and Human Development, 27,* 255–268.

Hardoon, K. K., Gupta, R., and Derevensky, J. L. (2004). Psychosocial variables associated with adolescent gambling. *Psychology of Addictive Behaviors, 18*(2), 170–179.

Hodgins, D. C., Currie, S., el-Guebaly, N., and Peden, N. (2004). Brief motivational treatment for problem gambling: A 24-month follow-up. *Psychology of Addictive Behaviors, 18*(3), 293–296.

Hodgins, D. C., and el-Guebaly, N. (2004). Retrospective and prospective reports of precipitants to relapse in pathological gambling. *Journal of Consulting and Clinical Psychology, 72,* 72–80.

Hollander, E., Pallanti, S., Allen, A., Sood, E., and Rossi, N. B. (2005). Does sustained-release lithium reduce impulsive gambling and affective instability versus placebo in pathological gamblers with bipolar spectrum disorders? *American Journal of Psychiatry, 162,* 137–145.

Hollander, E., Tracy, K. A., Swann, A. C., et al. (2003). Divalproex in the treatment of impulsive aggression: Efficacy in cluster B personality disorders. *Neuropsychopharmacology, 28,* 1186–1197.

Kavoussi, R. K., and Coccaro, E. F. (1998). Divalproex sodium for impulsive aggressive behavior in patients with personality disorder. *Journal of Clinical Psychiatry, 59,* 676–680.

Kim, S. W., Grant, J. E., and Adson, D. E. (2002). Double-blind placebo-controlled study in the treatment of pathological gambling. *Biological Psychiatry, 63,* 501–507.

Kreek, M. J., Nielsen, D. A., Butelman, E. R., and LaForge, K. S. (2005). Genetic influences on impulsivity and vulnerability to drug abuse and addiction. *Nature Neuroscience, 8*(11)1450–1457.

Lejoyeux, M., Feuche, N., Loi, S., Solomon, J., and Ades, J. (1999). Study of impulse control disorders among alcohol dependent patients. *Journal of Clinical Psychiatry, 60*(5), 302–305.

Lerner, J., Franklin, M. E., Meadows, E. A., et al. (1998). Effectiveness of a cognitive behavioral treatment program for trichotillomania: An uncontrolled evaluation. *Behavior Therapy, 29,* 157–171.

Linden, R. D., Pope, H. G., and Jonas, J. M. (1986). Pathological gambling and major affective disorders: Preliminary findings. *Journal of Clinical Psychiatry, 47,* 201–203.

Linehan, M. M., Tutek, D. A., Heard, H. L., et al. (1994). Interpersonal outcome of cognitive behavioral treatment for chronically suicidal borderline patients. *American Journal of Psychiatry, 151,* 1771–1776.

Linnoila, M., Virkkunen, M., Scheinin, M., et al. (1983). Low cerebral spinal fluid 5-hydroxyindoleacetic acid concentration differentiates impulsive from non-impulsive violent behavior. *Life Science, 33,* 2609–2614.

Mansueto, C. S., Stemberger, R. M. T., Thomas, A. M., and Golomb, R. G. (1997). Trichotillomania: A comprehensive behavioral model. *Clinical Psychology Review, 17,* 567–577.

Martins, S. S., Taveres, H., de Sliva Lobo, D.S., Galetti, A. M., and Gentil, V. (2004). Pathological gambling, gender, and risk-taking behaviors. *Addictive Behaviors, 29,* 1231–1235.

McConaghy, N., Armstong, M., Blaszczynski, A., and Allock, C. (1983). Controlled comparison of aversive therapy and imaginal desensitization in compulsive gambling addictions. *British Journal of Psychiatry, 142,* 366–372.

McConaghy, N., Blaszczynski, A., and Frankova, A. (1991). Comparison of imaginal desensitization with other behavioral treatments of pathological gambling: A two- to nine-year follow-up. *British Journal of Psychiatry, 159,* 390–393.

McCormick, R. A., Russo, A. M., Ramirez, L. F., et al. (1984). Affective disorders among pathological gamblers seeking treatment. *American Journal of Psychiatry, 141,* 215–218.

McCormick, R. A., and Smith, M. (1995). Aggression and hostility in substance abusers: The relationship to abuse patterns, coping styles, and relapse triggers. *Addictive Behaviors, 20*(5), 555–562.

McElroy, S. L. (1999). Recognition and treatment of DSM-IV intermittent explosive disorder. *Journal of Clinical Psychiatry,* 60(Suppl 15), 12–16.

McElroy, S. L., Pope, H. G., Keck, P. E., et al. (1996). Are impulse control disorders related to bipolar disorder. *Comprehensive Psychiatry, 37,* 229–240.

McElroy, S. L., Soutullo, C. A., Beckman, D. A., Taylor, P., and Keck, P. E. (1998). DSM-IV intermittent explosive disorder: A report of 27 cases. *Journal of Clinical Psychiatry, 59*(4), 203–210.

Moeller, F. G., Barratt, E. S., Dougherty, D. M., Schmitz, J. M., and Swann, A. C. (2001). Psychiatric aspects of impulsivity. *American Journal of Psychiatry, 158,* 1783–1793.

Moody, G. (1990). Quit compulsive gambling. London: Thorsons.

Mouton, S. G., and Stanley, M. A. (1996). Habit reversal training for trichotillomania: A group approach. *Cognitive and Behavioral Practice, 3,* 159–182.

Ninan, P. T., Rothbaum, B. O., Marstellar, F. A., Knight, B. T., and Eccard, M. B. (2000). A placebo-controlled trial of cognitive behavioral therapy and clomipramine in trichotillomania. *Journal of Clinical Psychiatry, 61*(1), 47–50.

Petry, N. M., Stinson, F. S., and Grant, B. F. (2005). Comorbidity of DSM-IV pathological gambling and other psychiatric disorders: Results from the national epidemiological survey on alcohol and related conditions. *Journal of Clinical Psychiatry, 66,* 564–574.

Potenza, M. N., Fiellin, D. A., Heninger, G. R., Rounsaville, B. J., and Mazure, C. M. (2002). Gambling: An addictive behavior with health and primary care implications. *Journal of General Internal Medicine, 17,* 721–732.

Potenza, M. N., Steinberg, M. A., Skudlarski, P., Fulbright, R. K., Lacadie, C. M., Wiber, M. K., Rounsaville, B. J., Gore, J. C., and Wexler, B. E. (2003). Gambling urges in pathological gambling: A functional magnetic resonance imaging study. *Archives of General Psychiatry, 60,* 828–836.

Robiner, W. N., Edwards, P. E., and Chistenson, G. A. (1999). Hypnosis in the treatment of trichotillomania. In D. J. Stein, G. A. Christenson, and E. Hollander (Eds.), *Trichotillomania* (pp. 176–199). Washington, DC: American Psychiatric Association.

Rothbaum, B. O. (1992). The behavioral treatment of trichotillomania. *Behavioral Psychotherapy, 20,* 85–90.

Roy, A., Adinoff, B., Roehrich, L., et al. (1988). Pathological gambling: A psychobiological study. *Archives of General Psychiatry, 45,* 369–373.

Russo, A. M., Taber, J. I., McCormick, R. A., et al. (1984). An outcome study of an inpatient treatment program for pathological gambling. *Hospital and Community Psychiatry, 35,* 823–827.

Schmitt, L. H., Harrison, G. A., and Spargo, R. M. (1998). Variation in epinephrine and cortisol excretion rates associated with behavior in Australian Aboriginal community. *American Journal of Physiological Anthropology, 106,* 249–253.

Sharpe, L., Tarrier, N., Schotte, D., and Spence, S. H. (1995). The role of autonomic arousal in problem gambling. *Addiction, 90,* 1529–1540.

Shinohara, K., Yanagisawa, A., Kagota, Y., et al. (1999). Physiological changes in pachinko players: Beta-endorphin, catecholamines, immune system substances and heart rate. *Journal of Physiological Anthropology and Applied Human Science, 18,* 37–42.

Silver, H., Goodman, C., Knoll, G., Isakov, V., and Modai, I. (2005). Schizophrenia patients with history of severe violence differ from nonviolent schizophrenia patients in perception of emotions but not cognitive function. *Journal of Clinical Psychiatry, 66*(3), 300–308.

Simeon, D., Cohen, L. J., Stein, D. J., Schmeidler, J., Spadaccinni, E., and Hollander, E. (1997). Comorbid self-injurious behaviors in 71 female hair-pullers: A survey study [Brief reports]. *The Journal of Nervous and Mental Disease, 185*(2), 117–119.

Singh, N. N., Wahler, R. G., Adkins, A., and Myers, R. E. (2003). Soles of the feet: A mindfulness-based self-control intervention for aggression by an individual with mild mental retardation and mental illness. *Research in Developmental Disabilities, 24,* 158–169.

Soloff, P. H., Meltzer, C. C., Greer, P. J., et al. (2000). A fenfluramine-activated FDG-PET study of borderline personality disorder. *Biological Psychiatry, 47,* 540–547.

Stanley, M. A., Borden, J. W., Mouton, S. G., and Breckenridge, J. K. (1995). Non-clinical hair-pulling: Affective correlates and comparison with clinical samples. *Behavior Research and Therapy, 33,* 179–186.

Stemberger, R. M. T., Thomas, A. M., Mansueto, C. S., et al. (2000). Personal toll of trichotillomania: Behavioral and interpersonal sequalae. *Journal of Anxiety Disorders, 14,* 97–104.

Stojanov, W., Karayanidis, F., Johnston, P., Bailey, A., Carr, V., and Schall, U. (2003). Disrupted sensory gating in pathological gambling. *Biological Psychiatry, 54,* 474–484.

Symes, B. A., and Nicki, R. M. (1997). A preliminary consideration of cue-exposure, response prevention treatment for pathological gambling behavior: Two case studies. *Journal of Gambling Studies, 13*(2), 145–157.

Taber, J. I., McCormick, R. A., Russo, A. M., et al. (1987). Follow-up of pathological gamblers after treatment. *American Journal of Psychiatry, 144,* 757–761.

Taveres, H., Zilberman, M. L., Beites, F. J., and Gentil, V. (2001). Gender differences in gambling progression. *Journal of Gambling Studies, 17,* 151–160.

Taveres, H., Zilberman, M. L., Hodgins, D. C., and el-Guebaly, N. (2005). Comparison of craving between pathological gamblers and alcoholics. *Alcoholism: Clinical and Experimental Research, 29*(8), 1427–1431.

Townsley-Stemberger, R. M., Mansueto, C. S., and Gardner-Carter, J. (2000). Personal toll of trichotillomania: Behavioral and interpersonal sequelae. *Journal of Anxiety Disorders, 14*(1), 97–104.

van Minnen, A., Hoogduin, K. A. L., Keijsers, G. P. J., Hellebrand, I., and Jan Hendricks, G. (2003). Treatment of trichotillomania with behavioral therapy or fluoxetine. *Archives of General Psychiatry, 60*, 517–522.

Virkkunen, M., Rawlings, R., Tokola, R., et al. (1994). CSF: Biochemistries, glucose metabolism, and diurnal activity rhythms in alcoholics, violent offenders, fire setters, and healthy volunteers. *Archives of General Psychiatry, 51*, 20–27.

Wetzler, S., Kahn, R. S., Asnis, G. M., et al. (1991). Serotonin receptor sensitivity and aggression. *Psychiatry Research, 37*, 271–279.

Whiteside, S. P., and Lynam, D. R. (2001). The five factor model and impulsivity: Using a structural model of personality to understand impulsivity. *Personality of Individual Differences, 30*, 669–689.

Zilberman, M. L., Tavares, H., and el-Guebaly, N. (2003). Relationship between craving and personality in treatment-seeking women with substance-related disorders. *BMC Psychiatry, 3*(1).

10

Psychosocial Determinants of the Stress Response

ANDREW STEPTOE AND MARK HAMER

Psychosocial factors relevant to health and addiction include sociodemographic characteristics such as socioeconomic status and ethnicity, adverse life experiences like acute life events and chronic stress, and social factors (social networks and support). This chapter outlines how these factors impact upon the pattern, magnitude, and duration of biobehavioral stress responses, and their relevance to addictive processes. We discuss the influence of psychosocial factors as investigated in epidemiological surveys, naturalistic everyday life monitoring studies, and laboratory psychophysiological stress testing. There is substantial evidence that lower socioeconomic status is associated with cardiovascular and neuroendocrine activation over the day, impaired recovery from acute stressors, and risk of addictive behaviors. Ethnicity has complex associations with psychobiological stress responses. Various adverse life experiences such as chronic work stress, caregiving, marital conflict, and childhood adversity are related to altered cardiovascular and neuroendocrine function during ambulatory monitoring and acute psychophysiological stress testing, while also influencing smoking, alcohol abuse, and drug dependence. Social support buffers acute physiological stress activation and addictive behavioral responses, while social isolation and loneliness are related to impaired psychobiological function. The chapter emphasizes the methodological difficulties of studying these relationships, but concludes that psychosocial factors are important determinants of stress responsivity and addictive behaviors.

I. INTRODUCTION

There is wide variation between people in the pattern, magnitude, duration, and rate of recovery of biobehavioral stress responses. These variations are not distributed randomly, but are systematically affected by a range of factors. These factors include genetic determinants, early life experiences, and psychological individual differences, as discussed in other chapters of this book. The present chapter focuses on psychosocial determinants of stress responses and their relevance to stress and addiction.

Psychosocial is the term used to describe a variety of social, demographic, and psychological factors that are relevant to health. Psychosocial factors include broad

Stress and Addiction: Biological and Psychological Mechanisms
Edited by **Mustafa al'Absi, Ph.D.**

sociodemographic concepts like socioeconomic status (SES) and ethnicity; adverse life experiences such as acute and chronic life stress; and social factors like social ties, social support, and social conflict. Psychological factors such as depression and hostility are often included within the umbrella of psychosocial factors, but will not be addressed in detail here, since individual differences are the topic of Chapter 11. The present chapter is therefore concerned with three sets of psychosocial factors: sociodemographic factors, life-stress exposure, and aspects of the social environment. The aim is to describe the extent to which stress responses are influenced by these factors. Our emphasis is on stress responses that are potentially relevant to addictions, so include both behavioral responses (smoking, alcohol consumption, etc.), and biological responses such as changes in cardiovascular, neuroendocrine, inflammatory, and immune function. Psychosocial factors are associated with physical and mental health outcomes and with problems of addiction. A theme that will emerge in the chapter is that psychosocial factors are related to stress responses in similar ways as they are to health outcomes; the evidence therefore suggests that stress processes in part mediate influences on health and addictive behavior.

Three basic research strategies have been used to evaluate the impact of psychosocial factors on biobehavioral stress responses (Steptoe, 2005). The first is to carry out epidemiological studies of associations between psychosocial factors and biobehavioral responses including smoking, alcohol consumption, blood pressure, heart rate variability, and neuroendocrine activity. The epidemiological approach is characterized by large samples, careful population sampling, measurement of potential confounders, and multivariate statistical techniques. Many epidemiological studies have longitudinal designs so that associations between psychosocial factors and health outcomes and mortality can

be investigated prospectively. A limitation is that it is not always clear whether the association between a biobehavioral variable and psychosocial factor is due to stress. For example, a relationship between chronic work stress and elevated blood pressure could be due not only to sympathoadrenal stress response, but also to selection factors related to choice of occupation, or concurrent lifestyle variables such as physical inactivity or excessive calorie intake. It is therefore necessary to complement epidemiological approaches with more dynamic methods of investigation.

A second strategy is naturalistic monitoring of behavioral and biological functioning in everyday life, using ambulatory physiological monitoring and behavioral diaries. This technique allows the relationship between psychosocial factors, daily activities, and emotional and biobehavioral responses to be evaluated. The most common biological responses assessed in this way are ambulatory blood pressure, heart rate, heart rate variability, and salivary cortisol. The method has ecological validity in that biological responses are measured in real life rather than in the artificial conditions of the laboratory clinic. Unfortunately, the range of biological markers that can be assessed is relatively small compared with the more sophisticated possibilities available in the laboratory.

The third strategy is laboratory psychophysiological stress testing, measuring biobehavioral responses to standardized challenges. This technique allows responses to be measured under controlled conditions from which other sources of variation are eliminated. Laboratory testing is being increasingly used to evaluate the impact of psychosocial factors in human health research, and important insights into the diversity of biological stress responses have emerged over recent years (Steptoe, In press). Laboratory methods can have problems of ecological validity and generalizability. An additional issue relevant to psychosocial investigations is that study samples need to be much larger than are typical in psychophysiological experiments, so that broad factors such as ethnicity or SES can be examined. Careful stratified sampling from defined populations is necessary.

All three methods are discussed in this chapter, but the full impact of psychosocial factors ultimately depends on the integration of findings from different research paradigms, and not on any single methodological approach.

II. SOCIODEMOGRAPHIC FACTORS AND STRESS RESPONSES

The sociodemographic factors that have been investigated most thoroughly in relation to biobehavioral stress responses are SES and ethnicity. Gender and age are sometimes placed in this category, but it could be argued that these are primarily biological rather than social factors.

A. Socioeconomic Status

There are wide socioeconomic disparities in many of the most common health problems in the modern world, including coronary heart disease, depression, type II diabetes, hypertension, lung disease, and many cancers (Marmot and Wilkinson, 2005). Effects are apparent with several different markers of SES including income, educational attainment, and occupational status or prestige; in each case, lower status individuals are at higher risk. For most diseases, there is an SES gradient and not just a difference between high and low SES groups, with people of intermediate status having an intermediate risk. Thus the crucial determinant is not poverty or serious deprivation, but relative deprivation and factors distributed throughout the population. There is also a marked SES gradient in behaviors such as smoking, alcohol abuse, and drug dependency.

Several factors might underlie the SES gradient in health and risk behavior, starting with childhood socioeconomic experiences. For example, one study of middle-aged men in Scotland showed a marked gradient in death from coronary heart disease, stroke, lung and stomach cancer related to the occupational status of participants' fathers (Davey Smith et al., 1998). After the participants' own SES was taken into account statistically, an influence of childhood SES persisted for stroke and stomach cancer mortality. Another important factor in some health systems is variation in access to primary care services and prioritization in secondary hospital care.

Stress processes are also related to SES. A number of laboratory studies have measured psychophysiological responses but have shown inconsistent relationships between SES and stress reactivity except in children, where lower SES groups appear to be more reactive (Steptoe and Marmot, 2002). One reason for these inconsistencies may be that emphasis has been placed on stress reactivity rather than recovery. In the Whitehall psychobiological study, our group compared white collar workers sampled from higher, intermediate, and lower occupational grades. Occupational grade was closely related both to income and educational attainment. We found that SES groups did not differ markedly in cardiovascular stress reactivity. However, post-stress recovery of systolic blood pressure, diastolic pressure, and heart rate variability was impaired in lower SES groups (Steptoe et al., 2002). These effects were substantial. For example, compared with the higher SES group, the odds of incomplete diastolic blood pressure recovery 45 minutes post-stress in lower SES participants were 3.85 (95% C.I. 1.48–10.0) after adjustment for age, gender, baseline blood pressure, and task reactivity. We also found that lower SES groups had slower recovery in factors related to blood clotting such as plasma viscosity and larger stress responses of the inflammatory cytokine interleukin (IL)-6 (Brydon et al., 2004).

Naturalistic monitoring studies have shown that salivary cortisol is slightly elevated over the day in lower than higher SES individuals (Cohen et al., 2006). Heart rate variability is reduced in lower SES groups, indicative of reduced vagal stimulation and autonomic imbalance (Lampert et al., 2005). There is also some evidence that variation in systemic biological function may be coupled with differences in central neurotransmitter activity. Matthews et al. (2000) studied central nervous system serotonergic activity by measuring the rise in prolactin following administration of the serotonin agonist fenfluramine. Lower SES participants showed blunted serotonin responsivity, and this may be related to depression and risk of substance abuse. More recently, it has been found that people living in lower SES communities defined by income, educational disadvantage, and housing costs also had reduced brain serotonergic responsivity, even after individual SES characteristics had been taken into account (Manuck et al., 2005).

The SES gradient in health-related behaviors such as smoking, binge drinking, physical activity, and fruit and vegetable intake is well established, and may be responsible in part for SES differences in health outcomes. For example, about a third of the educational difference in mortality in a longitudinal study from the Netherlands was accounted for by variations in smoking and physical inactivity across social groups (van Oort et al., 2004). But people of lower SES also tend to experience other adverse psychosocial factors including greater financial strain, lower control at work, chronic neighborhood and domestic stresses, and more limited social networks. SES differences in health-related behavior are due in part to the presence of these other psychosocial factors. For instance, in one large cohort study, the strong association between lower SES and excessive alcohol consumption was due in part to chronic financial strain and low social support (Droomers et al., 1998). Thus the impact of SES cannot be divorced

from the psychosocial factors discussed later in this chapter.

B. Ethnicity

There are substantial differences between ethnic groups in the prevalence of addictive behaviors and stress-related health outcomes. However, studying ethnic variations in stress responsivity is complicated by four factors. First, ethnic groups differ in levels of function in some biological processes as well as in psychosocial experience, and these factors may underlie stress responsivity. They include vascular differences and variations in genetic polymorphisms that regulate immune and neuroendocrine responses. Second, minority ethnic status is often confounded with SES, since many minority groups have low incomes and occupational status. Differences in stress response may therefore be due to socioeconomic rather than ethnic factors. Third, hypotheses about the stressful impact of ethnic minority status (due to discrimination and racism) must explain why not all minority groups are disadvantaged in health outcomes. Alcohol dependence, for example, is higher in African Americans than Caucasians, very low in Asians, but high in Native Americans. Hypertension by contrast is more common in African Americans than Caucasians. Fourth, few laboratory studies of stress responsivity have taken account of differences in task appraisal. It is well established that biological responses to behavioral tasks are strongly determined by task involvement and engagement; individuals who engage actively with the situation show heightened responsivity independently of any underlying variation in psychobiological processes. The experience of physiological monitoring and laboratory task performance may be very different in ethnic minority groups, and this needs to be properly assessed. It is also unfortunate that many studies of stress responsivity and ethnicity have been small, involving fewer than 50 people to represent each ethnic group, so have low statistical power.

The most substantial evidence on ethnicity concerns African Americans (Anderson et al., 1991). African Americans tend to have greater blood pressure and heart rate stress responsivity than Caucasians, and these responses are typically associated with larger vascular (peripheral resistance) changes. It has been argued that these differences contribute to the high prevalence of hypertension in African Americans, and relate to historical and genetic factors that were advantageous in hot, dry countries (such as sodium retention). African Americans show lower heart rate variability than Caucasians, with Hispanic people displaying an intermediate pattern (Lampert et al., 2005). By contrast, few differences have been observed in neuroendocrine function, including levels of cortisol, epinephrine, and norepinephrine (Masi et al., 2004). Other ethnic comparisons are sparse, but there is some evidence for differences in the response patterns of Asian Indians and people of Chinese origin.

An important issue is whether the impact of ethnic minority status on stress reactivity is due to racism and discrimination. A number of studies of blood pressure have been carried out, but results have been equivocal, though perceived racism has also been related to higher ambulatory blood pressure (Steffen et al., 2003). Troxel et al. (2003) demonstrated that African American women who experienced more chronic stress arising from unfair treatment and discrimination had higher carotid atherosclerosis. Evidence for direct effects of discrimination on psychological well-being, smoking, alcohol consumption, and self-reported physical health is stronger than for these physical health outcomes (Williams et al., 2003).

III. LIFE STRESS EXPOSURE

Life stress can be conveniently divided into three categories: acute life events such as divorce or a car crash which can be pinpointed in time; chronic stresses related to work, family conflict, financial strain, or other factors; and minor life events or daily hassles. Useful though such divisions are in theory, the distinctions between categories are blurred in practice. Exposure to life stress is of course the principal factor underlying most stress research. But in addition to the direct effects of adversity on biobehavioral stress responses, there may be indirect effects. People who experience chronic life stress may show either augmentation or diminution of biobehavioral stress responses to acute challenges, and these processes can be assessed using naturalistic monitoring and psychophysiological stress testing.

Acute life events are significant for many addictive behaviors and health outcomes, but their impact on biobehavioral stress responses tends to be transient unless they are transformed into sources of chronic strain. For example, the classic studies of the aftermath of the Three Mile Island nuclear accident showed enduring changes in blood pressure, catecholamine, and cortisol levels in local residents, but these changes were sustained by persistent intrusive thoughts and fears engendering chronic stress (Baum et al., 1993). The World Trade Center attacks stimulated mental and physical health symptoms, together with cardiovascular and neuroendocrine responses, some of which endured for several months in vulnerable individuals (Gerin et al., 2005).

A variety of enduring adverse life circumstances promote chronic stress, including factors related to work, domestic activity, financial life, spousal caregiving, and early life experiences. Work has been studied extensively since many people are exposed to their work environments for many years of their adult lives. The two models of work stress that have received the most attention are the "effort-reward imbalance" model developed by Johannes Siegrist and the "job strain" model formulated by Robert Karasek. The effort-reward imbalance model provides a framework for understanding the process of coping under conditions of limited control and hypothesizes that a lack of reciprocity between costs and gains leads to a state of emotional distress. Thus having a demanding but unstable job and achieving at a high level without any prospects of promotion are situations in which effort-reward imbalance will be high. The second model postulates that high job demands coupled with low job latitude or control induces a state of job strain. This is particularly common in jobs involving repetitive tasks with limited control over routines and a lack of creative outlet. Life stress from domestic sources includes family and marital conflict, and may also encompass financial strain and informal caregiving. Relevant early life experiences include adverse events such parental loss or separation, together with more subtle variations in affection and expressiveness in the family. In the following sections, we summarize the evidence linking life stress exposure with biological measures assessed in everyday life, acute psychobiological stress responsivity, and with addictive and health behaviors.

A. Effects on Naturalistic Stress Measures

Ambulatory blood pressure, cortisol, and catecholamine excretion are gener-ally higher when measured at work compared with the home environment. For example, the cortisol response to awakening, a sensitive psychobiological stress indicator, is greater on working days compared with the weekend. Figure 10-1 illustrates results from a study in which the cortisol awakening response was assessed on work and weekend days in 196 middle-aged men and women (Kunz-Ebrecht et al., 2004a). Salivary cortisol levels did not differ on waking on the 2 days, but the increase over the next 30 minutes was substantially larger on the working day. These findings suggest that anticipation of the working day is associated with greater physiological activation. Interestingly, the difference between days is more marked among women than men, probably because on working days, women often have greater domestic responsibilities than men.

Individual differences in the experience of chronic job stress influence these patterns. High effort-reward imbalance is correlated with reduced vagal tone over the day and evening (Vrijkotte et al., 2000), while overcommitment (a component of

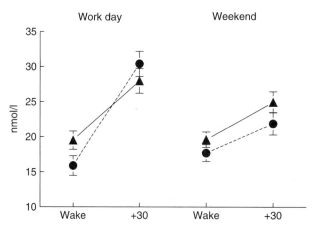

FIGURE 10-1   Mean levels of salivary free cortisol on waking and 30 minutes later on work and weekend days in women (dashed lines) and men (solid lines). Error bars are standard errors of the mean. From Kunz-Ebrecht et al., 2004a.

the effort-reward imbalance model) in men is associated with a heightened cortisol response to awakening and greater levels of cortisol and systolic blood pressure over the working day (Steptoe et al., 2004a). Job strain, and especially low job control, is accompanied by elevated daytime ambulatory blood pressure and raised salivary cortisol levels (Kunz-Ebrecht et al., 2004b; Schnall et al., 1994). In a longitudinal study of workers in New York City, high job strain was consistently associated with greater 24-hour ambulatory blood pressure, and those individuals who reduced their job strain over the 3-year study showed reductions in blood pressure both at work and home (Schnall et al., 1998).

Chronic work stressors do not act in isolation, but are modified by family experience. In a sample of Canadian white collar workers, the combination of large family responsibilities and high job strain had adverse effects on ambulatory blood pressure in women but not men (Brisson et al., 1999). In another Canadian sample, high job strain was associated with lower 24-hour systolic blood pressure in participants reporting high marital cohesion (Tobe et al., 2005).

Marital conflict has also been shown to be related to psychobiological stress indicators (Kiecolt-Glaser and Newton, 2001). In one study of middle-aged men and women, marital role concerns were associated with greater self-reported stress throughout the day, an attenuated cortisol response to awakening, a flatter cortisol slope over the day, and elevated ambulatory blood pressure over the middle of the working day (Barnett et al., 2005). Other chronic stressors are relevant as well. For example, financial strain, a potent source of marital conflict and chronic distress, is related to heightened neuroendocrine and cardiovascular activation during the day. Interestingly, improvements in financial strain may lead to a reduction in these psychobiological responses, suggesting that chronic adversity is driving the pattern of physiological change (Steptoe et al., 2005). This pattern is shown in Figure 10-2, which compares the ambulatory systolic and diastolic blood pressure of men and women who reported an improvement in financial strain over 3 years with those who had a deterioration or no change in their financial situation. Blood pressure levels were lower in participants who had improved financial strain. The values are adjusted statistically for initial levels of blood pressure in the two groups.

Family caregivers experience a high degree of enduring stress. A number of studies have shown disturbances in hypothalamic-pituitary-adrenocortical (HPA) axis function in informal caregivers of dementing relatives, including elevated cortisol levels early in the day (Vedhara et al., 1999). However, biological effects have not all been consistent. In a meta-analysis of the literature, Vitaliano et al. (2003) concluded that the evidence was strong for differences in neuroendocrine function and antibody levels, but less consistent for cardiovascular or metabolic variables.

An enduring effect on adult stress responsivity is a legacy of poor and disrupted childhood family relationships (Luecken and Lemery, 2004). For example, elevated cortisol in middle age is found in people who lost a parent through death early in their lives (Nicolson, 2004). Other psychosocial factors (e.g., depression, anxiety, hostility, social isolation) and cognitive-affective pathways such as coping may mediate the effects of childhood family experiences on psychobiological indicators (Luecken and Lemery, 2004).

B. Effects on Acute Stress Responsivity

The literature relating background levels of psychosocial stress with acute responses to laboratory challenges shows different patterns for different types of exposure. Recent negative life events have been associated with both increased and reduced acute

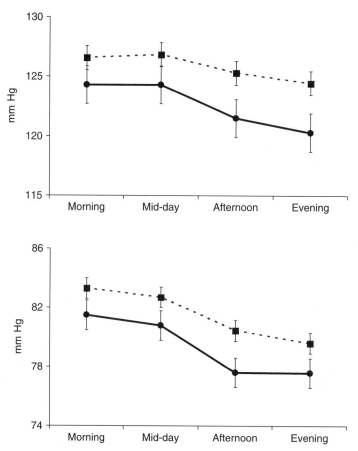

FIGURE 10-2 Systolic (upper panel) and diastolic (lower panel) blood pressure in middle-aged participants who reported improved financial strain (solid lines) or worse/no change in financial strain (dashed line) over a 3-year period. Values are adjusted for blood pressure 3 years earlier, and for age, gender, grade of employment, body mass, smoking status, and baseline financial strain. From Steptoe et al., 2005.

cardiovascular reactivity (Musante et al., 2000; Roy et al., 1998). Gump and Matthews (1999) reviewed the evidence for the influence of background acute and chronic life stressors on stress reactivity and found that six studies reported a positive association between ongoing stressors and reactivity, while four reported a negative association. One possible reason for the variation may be that some acute stressors are not of long enough duration to permit the effects of background stress to emerge and that physiological monitoring did not continue into the post-stress recovery period. Indeed, the studies that continued to measure physiological responses during recovery show

that greater background stress is related to slower blood pressure recovery.

The evidence relating background levels of chronic work stress with acute reactivity is also inconsistent. Our group found that chronic work stress conceptualized with the job strain model predicted increased acute blood pressure responses to uncontrollable tasks (Steptoe et al., 1993), but an inverse relationship between effort-reward imbalance and cardiovascular activation to public speech and mirror tracing stressors has been described (Hamer et al., 2006). In contrast, effort-reward imbalance is positively associated with acute responses in markers of inflammation such as C-reactive

protein and von Willebrand Factor antigen. Either the various facets of work stress
operate through different pathways, or they
have varying effects depending on duration
of exposure. It is possible, for example, that
high effort-reward imbalance is initially
associated with heightened cardiovascular reactivity, but that this is reversed after
many years of unrewarded effort.

There is a growing literature relating
marital/partner relationship strain with
acute physiological stress responses
(Kiecolt-Glaser and Newton, 2001). The
most robust results have emerged from
studies involving discussion of conten-
tious issues by the couple, a method that
reliably induces substantial cardiovascular,
endocrine, and immunological reactivity.
Individuals reporting marital dissatisfaction or conflict show heightened blood pressure, catecholamine, and cortisol reactivity,
responses that are strongly associated with
displays of hostile affect.

Few investigations have been carried
out of the impact of caregiver status on
responsivity to acute stressors. Redwine
et al. (2004) compared spousal caregivers
for Alzheimer's disease with controls in
responses to standardized laboratory tasks.
There were no differences between groups in
blood pressure, heart rate, or catecholamine
responses, but the caregiver group showed
reduced lymphocyte chemotaxis, suggesting alterations in the release of immune
cells into the circulation. Some work has
also been conducted on stress responses in
adult life of individuals who experienced
childhood adversity. Heim et al. (2000)
found that women with a history of childhood abuse had increased cortisol, adrenocorticotropic hormone (ACTH), and heart
rate stress responsivity compared with
nonabused controls, indicating persistent
disturbances of stress-related regulatory
processes.

An important aspect of psychosocial
influence on acute responsivity is the nature
of the acute stress demands. As noted earlier, job strain (high demands and low con-

trol) is associated with heightened reactivity
to controllable but not uncontrollable tasks,
and physiological response differences related to marital conflict are particularly
prominent when acute tasks involve marital interaction. This suggests that a match
between acute demands and the nature of
the underlying chronic stress exposure may
stimulate heightened responsivity. In general, neuroendocrine stress responses tend
to be greater when people are confronted
with uncontrollable and social-evaluative
tasks (Dickerson and Kemeny, 2004), so it
is plausible that acute stress reactivity will
be preferentially enhanced in people who
experience chronic social stress in their
lives.

C. Effects on Health and Addictive Behaviors

Research on brain neurocircuitry has
demonstrated how stress can impact on
reward systems regulating addictive behaviors, and on the central processes governing peripheral physiological activation
(Koob and Le Moal, 2001). Unfortunately,
causal relationships between life stress
and addictive behaviors are often difficult to tease out, since stress and negative
affect have reciprocal relationships with
all stages of addictive behaviors from initiation to maintenance and relapse (e.g.,
Kassel et al., 2003). Associations between
life stress and health behaviors such as
smoking, alcohol consumption, and eating
habits have been documented in epidemiological studies. In one of the largest cross-
sectional studies to date, with over 40,000
Finnish men and women working in the
public sector, high job strain and effort-
reward imbalance were associated with
smoking and reduced physical activity
but not with heavy drinking after adjustment for occupational position, education,
marital status, and other demographic factors (Kouvonen et al., 2005a; 2005b). In a
smaller cohort of Japanese rural workers,
high job strain was associated with lower

prevalence of smoking but greater alcohol consumption (Tsutsumi et al., 2003), while British civil servants experiencing high effort-reward imbalance were at increased risk of alcohol dependence after adjustment for employment grade and other risk factors (Head et al., 2004). These cross-sectional findings are corroborated in longitudinal studies. For example, Crum et al. (1995) found that men with high strain jobs were more than 20 times more likely to develop alcohol dependence over a 1-year period than were matched controls. In a 6-year prospective study of Danish nurses who were all smokers at baseline, high job control among other factors predicted smoking cessation at follow-up (Sanderson et al., 2005).

Loss of paid employment can have profound effects on addictive behaviors. Catalano et al. (1993) showed how job loss increased risk of alcohol abuse independently of alcohol history, SES, gender, and other risk factors in an analysis of the Epidemiologic Catchment Area project. Interestingly, these effects may be reversible, with favorable changes in employment leading to reduced alcohol abuse (Dooley and Prause, 1997). A cross-sectional association between financial strain and smoking has been shown in household panel data that were independent of education, income, and socioeconomic disadvantage, suggesting an additional effect of this source of chronic stress (Siahpush et al., 2003). Financial strain is also related to alcohol abuse, although effects are mediated by negative affect and motives for drinking (Peirce et al., 1994).

There has been relatively little research on the impact of informal caregiving on behaviors such as smoking and alcohol consumption, so it is difficult to draw general conclusions (Connell et al., 2001; Polen and Green, 2001). Other forms of chronic stress such as marital conflict appear to have a reciprocal relationship with health behaviors. For example, marital conflict can be both a precursor and a consequence of

alcohol and drug abuse (Kiecolt-Glaser and Newton, 2001).

The literature on acute stress and health behavior has been dominated by topics such as dietary restraint in relation to eating disorders (Greeno and Wing, 1994), the supposed stress-dampening effects of alcohol (Sayette, 1999), and the effects of nicotine on performance. These issues are detailed in other chapters and will not therefore be discussed here.

IV. PROTECTIVE PSYCHOSOCIAL FACTORS

Social relationships are fundamental to psychobiological function and may help to buffer the impact of psychosocial stress. One of the most extensively researched topics is social support, which can be defined as both structural and functional. Structural measures of support examine the number, density, and reciprocity of relationships (with measures of social ties or networks), whereas functional measures of support assess the particular roles that social relationships play (e.g., emotional, informational, or material support). An extensive review of this research indicated that social support is reliably related to lower levels of autonomic activity (assessed with ambulatory monitoring and psychophysiological stress testing), better immunosurveillance (aspects of both cellular and humoral immune responses), and lower levels of stress hormones such as catecholamines, while effects on cortisol are less consistent (Uchino et al., 1996). High levels of social support have also been associated with healthier lifestyles (e.g., Allgower et al., 2001).

Social support may also buffer acute stress responses. This outcome has been documented in laboratory studies in which volunteers were exposed to behavioral challenges in the presence of others, or else in isolation. Many variations have been tested, including whether or not the supportive other was a

TABLE 10-1 Summary of Psychosocial Influences on Biological Responses

	Naturalistic Monitoring	Responsivity to Acute Stressors
Low socioeconomic status	Increased blood pressure and cortisol over the day Inconsistent effect on cortisol awakening response Reduced heart rate variability	Inconsistent blood pressure and heart rate reactivity effects Increased inflammatory cytokine response Slow recovery of blood pressure, heart rate variability, and hemostatic variables
Recent life events and chronic environmental threats	Increased blood pressure, catecholamines and cortisol Altered hemostatic function	Inconsistent blood pressure and heart rate reactivity effects Slow blood pressure recovery
Job strain (demand/control)	Increased blood pressure and cortisol over the day Reduced heart rate variability	Increased blood pressure reactivity
Effort/reward imbalance	Increased blood pressure and cortisol awakening response Reduced heart rate variability	Reduced blood pressure and heart rate reactivity Increased inflammatory responses
Marital conflict	Increased blood pressure Reduced cortisol awakening response Flat cortisol profile over the day	Increased blood pressure, catecholamine, immune, and cortisol reactivity
Caregiving	Disrupted cortisol profile, lower immune antibody responses Inconsistent effect on cardiovascular and metabolic function	Reduced immune responses
Financial strain	Increased blood pressure and cortisol awakening response	Increased cortisol, ACTH, and heart rate reactivity
Childhood adversity	Increased cortisol, catecholamines, blood pressure	Increased cardiovascular reactivity
Low social support	Increased blood pressure and catecholamines Impaired immune function Inconsistent effects on cortisol	
Loneliness	Increased peripheral resistance, reduced cardiac output Impaired immune function Increased cortisol awakening response	Increased diastolic blood pressure, peripheral resistance, and fibrinogen reactivity

friend, touched the participant, made supportive comments, and so on (Lepore, 1998). There is even evidence that pets promote a diminution in cardiovascular stress reactions (Allen et al., 2001). The relevance of these effects (which involve the actual presence of a supportive individual) to stress responsivity in everyday life has not been evaluated extensively. However, one ambulatory monitoring study assessed subjective stress concurrently with blood pressure measures every 20 minutes over a working day (Steptoe, 2000). Systolic pressure was modestly increased during periods of high versus low subjective stress, after controlling for physical activity. Interestingly, this response was attenuated in people reporting high social support, suggesting a stress buffering effect on physiological function in real life as well as the laboratory. The buffering effects of social support have been demonstrated for addictive behaviors as well, with the impact of financial strain on alcohol problems being reduced in individuals who enjoyed high levels of material support (Peirce et al., 1996).

The psychological correlate of social isolation and low perceived intimacy is loneliness, and this has also been linked with stress reactivity. In one series of studies, lonely individuals were characterized by increased peripheral resistance and lower cardiac output during ambulatory monitoring and acute psychophysiological testing (Hawkley and Cacioppo, 2003). Loneliness is also associated with larger cortisol awakening responses, heightened acute inflammatory stress reactions, and diminished cellular immune function (Steptoe et al., 2004b). At present, however, there is little evidence to suggest that it has a marked impact on smoking, alcohol use, or exercise habits (Hawkley and Cacioppo, 2003).

V. CONCLUSIONS

Psychosocial factors are important determinants of stress responses. Table 10-1 summarizes the findings that have been outlined in this chapter. It is evident that background characteristics such as SES and ethnicity, recent and early life adversity, and features of the social environment all influence the magnitude of biobehavioral stress reactions and patterns of post-stress recovery, and have an impact on physiological function in naturalistic as well as laboratory settings. Yet despite some uniformity emerging in this field, much of the literature is inconsistent. The reason for this is partly that all too often, studies of psychosocial factors have involved small convenience samples. A population-based stratified approach to selection of participants is required for the investigation of psychosocial factors, with power calculations to determine appropriate sample size. As this literature evolves, it is likely that the role of psychosocial factors in determining stress reactivity and addictive behaviors will be increasingly appreciated.

REFERENCES

Allen, K., Shykoff, B. E., and Izzo, J. L., Jr. (2001). Pet ownership, but not ace inhibitor therapy, blunts home blood pressure responses to mental stress. *Hypertension, 38*, 815–820.

Allgower, A., Wardle, J., and Steptoe, A. (2001). Depressive symptoms, social support, and personal health behaviors in young men and women. *Health Psychol, 20*, 223–227.

Anderson, N. B., McNeilly, M., and Myers, H. (1991). Autonomic reactivity and hypertension in blacks: A review and proposed model. *Ethn Dis, 1*, 154–170.

Barnett, R. C., Steptoe, A., and Gareis, K. C. (2005). Marital-role quality and stress-related psychobiological indicators. *Ann Behav Med, 30*, 36–43.

Baum, A., Cohen, L., and Hall, M. (1993). Control and intrusive memories as possible determinants of chronic stress. *Psychosom Med, 55*, 274–286.

Brisson, C., Laflamme, N., Moisan, J., Milot, A., Masse, B., and Vezina, M. (1999). Effect of family responsibilities and job strain on ambulatory blood pressure among white-collar women. *Psychosom Med, 61*, 205–213.

Brydon, L., Edwards, S., Mohamed-Ali, V., and Steptoe, A. (2004). Socioeconomic status and stress-induced increases in interleukin-6. *Brain Behav Immun, 18*, 281–290.

Catalano, R., Dooley, D., Wilson, G., and Hough, R. (1993). Job loss and alcohol abuse: A test using data from the Epidemiologic Catchment Area project. *J Health Soc Behav, 34*, 215–225.

Cohen, S., Schwartz, J. E., Epel, E., Kirschbaum, C., Sidney, S., and Seeman, T. (2006). Socioeconomic status, race, and diurnal cortisol decline in the Coronary Artery Risk Development in Young Adults (CARDIA) Study. *Psychosom Med, 68*, 41–50.

Connell, C. M., Janevic, M. R., and Gallant, M. P. (2001). The costs of caring: Impact of dementia on family caregivers. *J Geriatr Psychiatry Neurol, 14*, 179–187.

Crum, R. M., Muntaner, C., Eaton, W. W., and Anthony, J. C. (1995). Occupational stress and the risk of alcohol abuse and dependence. *Alc, Clin Exp Res, 19*, 647–655.

Davey Smith, G., Hart, C., Blane, D., and Hole, D. (1998). Adverse socioeconomic conditions in childhood and cause specific adult mortality: Prospective observational study. *Br Med J, 316*, 1631–1635.

Dickerson, S. S., and Kemeny, M. E. (2004). Acute stressors and cortisol responses: A theoretical integration and synthesis of laboratory research. *Psychol Bull, 130*, 355–391.

Dooley, D., and Prause, J. (1997). Effect of favorable employment change on alcohol abuse: One- and five-year follow-ups in the National Longitudinal Survey of Youth. *Am J Community Psychol, 25*, 787–807.

Droomers, M., Schrijvers, C. T., van de Mheen, H., and Mackenbach, J. P. (1998). Educational differences in leisure-time physical inactivity: A descriptive and explanatory study. *Soc Sci Med, 47*, 1665–1676.

Gerin, W., Chaplin, W., Schwartz, J. E., Holland, J., Alter, R., Wheeler, R., Duong, D., and Pickering, T. G. (2005). Sustained blood pressure increase after an acute stressor: The effects of the 11 September 2001 attack on the New York City World Trade Center. *J Hypertens, 23*, 279–284.

Greeno, C. G., and Wing, R. R. (1994). Stress-induced eating. *Psychol Bull, 115*, 444–464.

Gump, B. B., and Matthews, K. (1999). Do background stressors influence reactivity to and recovery from acute stressors? *J Appl Soc Psychol, 29*, 469–494.

Hamer, M., Williams, M., Vuononvirta, R., Giacobazzi, P., Gibson, E. L., and Steptoe, A. (2006). The effects of effort-reward imbalance on inflammatory and cardiovascular responses to mental stress. *Psychosom Med, 68*, 408–415.

Hawkley, L. C., and Cacioppo, J. T. (2003). Loneliness and pathways to disease. *Brain Behav Immun, 17*, 98–105.

Head, J., Stansfeld, S. A., and Siegrist, J. (2004). The psychosocial work environment and alcohol dependence: A prospective study. *Occup Environ Med, 61*, 219–224.

Heim, C., Newport, D. J., Heit, S., Graham, Y. P., Wilcox, M., Bonsall, R., Miller, A. H., and Nemeroff, C. B. (2000). Pituitary-adrenal and autonomic responses to stress in women after sexual and physical abuse in childhood. *JAMA, 284*, 592–597.

Kassel, J. D., Stroud, L. R., and Paronis, C. A. (2003). Smoking, stress, and negative affect: Correlation, causation, and context across stages of smoking. *Psychol Bull, 129*, 270–304.

Kiecolt-Glaser, J. K., and Newton, T. L. (2001). Marriage and health: His and hers. *Psychol Bull, 127*, 472–503.

Koob, G. F., and Le Moal, M. (2001). Drug addiction, dysregulation of reward, and allostasis. *Neuropsychopharmacology, 24*, 97–129.

Kouvonen, A., Kivimaki, M., Cox, S. J., Poikolainen, K., Cox, T., and Vahtera, J. (2005a). Job strain, effort-reward imbalance, and heavy drinking: A study in 40,851 employees. *J Occup Environ Med, 47*, 503–513.

Kouvonen, A., Kivimaki, M., Virtanen, M., Pentti, J., and Vahtera, J. (2005b). Work stress, smoking status, and smoking intensity: An observational study of 46,190 employees. *J Epidemiol Community Health, 59*, 63–69.

Kunz-Ebrecht, S. R., Kirschbaum, C., Marmot, M., and Steptoe, A. (2004a). Differences in cortisol awakening response on work days and weekends in women and men from the Whitehall II cohort. *Psychoneuroendocrinology, 29*, 516–528.

Kunz-Ebrecht, S. R., Kirschbaum, C., and Steptoe, A. (2004b). Work stress, socioeconomic status and neuroendocrine activation over the working day. *Soc Sci Med, 58*, 1523–1530.

Lampert, R., Ickovics, J., Horwitz, R., and Lee, F. (2005). Depressed autonomic nervous system function in African Americans and individuals of lower social class: A potential mechanism of race- and class-related disparities in health outcomes. *Am Heart J, 150*, 153–160.

Lepore, S. J. (1998). Problems and prospects for the social support-reactivity hypothesis. *Ann Behav Med, 20*, 257–269.

Luecken, L. J., and Lemery, K. S. (2004). Early caregiving and physiological stress responses. *Clin Psychol Rev, 24*, 171–191.

Manuck, S. B., Bleil, M. E., Petersen, K. L., Flory, J. D., Mann, J. J., Ferrell, R. E., and Muldoon, M. F. (2005). The socio-economic status of communities predicts variation in brain serotonergic responsivity. *Psychol Med, 35*, 519–528.

Marmot, M., and Wilkinson, R. G. (Eds.). (2005). *Social determinants of health* (2nd ed.). Oxford: Oxford University Press.

Masi, C. M., Rickett, E. M., Hawkley, L. C., and Cacioppo, J. T. (2004). Gender and ethnic differences in urinary stress hormones: The population-based Chicago Health, Aging, and Social Relations Study. *J Appl Physiol, 97*, 941–947.

Matthews, K. A., Flory, J. D., Muldoon, M. F., and Manuck, S. B. (2000). Does socioeconomic status relate to central serotonergic responsivity in healthy adults? *Psychosom Med, 62*, 231–237.

Musante, L., Treiber, F. A., Kapuku, G., Moore, D., Davis, H., and Strong, W. B. (2000). The effects of life events on cardiovascular reactivity to behavioral stressors as a function of socioeconomic status, ethnicity, and sex. *Psychosom Med, 62*, 760–767.

Nicolson, N. A. (2004). Childhood parental loss and cortisol levels in adult men. *Psychoneuroendocrinology, 29*, 1012–1018.

Peirce, R. S., Frone, M. R., Russell, M., and Cooper, M. L. (1994). Relationship of financial strain and psychosocial resources to alcohol use and abuse: The mediating role of negative affect and drinking motives. *J Health Soc Behav, 35*, 291–308.

Peirce, R. S., Frone, M. R., Russell, M., and Cooper, M. L. (1996). Financial stress, social support, and alcohol involvement: A longitudinal test of the buffering hypothesis in a general population survey. *Health Psychol, 15*, 38–47.

Polen, M. R., and Green, C. A. (2001). Caregiving, alcohol use, and mental health symptoms among HMO members. *J Community Health, 26*, 285–301.

Redwine, L., Mills, P. J., Sada, M., Dimsdale, J., Patterson, T., and Grant, I. (2004). Differential immune cell chemotaxis responses to acute psychological stress in Alzheimer caregivers compared to non-caregiver controls. *Psychosom Med, 66*, 770–775.

Roy, M. P., Steptoe, A., and Kirschbaum, C. (1998). Life events and social support as moderators of individual differences in cardiovascular and cortisol reactivity. *J Pers Soc Psychol, 75*, 1273–1281.

Sanderson, D. M., Ekholm, O., Hundrup, Y. A., and Rasmussen, N. K. (2005). Influence of lifestyle, health, and work environment on smoking cessation among Danish nurses followed over 6 years. *Prev Med, 41*, 757–760.

Sayette, M. A. (1999). Does drinking reduce stress? *Alcohol Res Health, 23*, 250–255.

Schnall, P. L., Landsbergis, P. A., and Baker, D. (1994). Job strain and cardiovascular disease. *Annu Rev Public Health, 15*, 381–411.

Schnall, P. L., Schwartz, J. E., Landsbergis, P. A., Warren, K., and Pickering, T. G. (1998). A longitudinal study of job strain and ambulatory blood pressure: Results from a three-year follow-up. *Psychosom Med, 60*, 697–706.

Siahpush, M., Borland, R., and Scollo, M. (2003). Smoking and financial stress. *Tob Control, 12*, 60–66.

Steffen, P. R., McNeilly, M., Anderson, N., and Sherwood, A. (2003). Effects of perceived racism and anger inhibition on ambulatory blood pressure in African Americans. *Psychosom Med, 65*, 746–750.

Steptoe, A. (2000). Stress, social support and cardiovascular activity over the working day. *Int J Psychophysiol, 37*, 299–308.

Steptoe, A. (2005). Tools of psychosocial biology in health care research. In A. Bowling and S. Ebrahim, Eds. *Handbook of health research methods* (pp. 471–493). Maidenhead: Open University Press.

Steptoe, A. (In press). Psychophysiological contributions to behavioral medicine and psychosomatics. In J. T. Cacioppo, L. G. Tassinary, and G. Bernston, Eds. *The Handbook of Psychophysiology* (3rd ed.). New York: Cambridge University Press.

Steptoe, A., Brydon, L., and Kunz-Ebrecht, S. (2005). Changes in financial strain over three years, ambulatory blood pressure, and cortisol responses to awakening. *Psychosom Med, 67*, 281–287.

Steptoe, A., Feldman, P. M., Kunz, S., Owen, N., Willemsen, G., and Marmot, M. (2002). Stress responsivity and socioeconomic status: A mechanism for increased cardiovascular disease risk? *Euro Heart J, 23*, 1757–1763.

Steptoe, A., Fieldman, G., Evans, O., and Perry, L. (1993). Control over work pace, job strain and cardiovascular responses in middle-aged men. *J Hypertension, 11*, 751–759.

Steptoe, A., and Marmot, M. (2002). The role of psychobiological pathways in socio-economic inequalities in cardiovascular disease risk. *Euro Heart J, 23*, 13–25.

Steptoe, A., Siegrist, J., Kirschbaum, C., and Marmot, M. (2004a). Effort-reward imbalance, overcommitment, and measures of cortisol and blood pressure over the working day. *Psychosom Med, 66*, 323–329.

Steptoe, A., Owen, N., Kunz-Ebrecht, S., and Brydon, L. (2004b). Loneliness and neuroendocrine, cardiovascular, and inflammatory stress responses in middle-aged men and women. *Psychoneuroendocrinology, 29*, 593–611.

Tobe, S. W., Kiss, A., Szalai, J. P., Perkins, N., Tsigoulis, M., and Baker, B. (2005). Impact of job and marital strain on ambulatory blood pressure results from the double exposure study. *Am J Hypertens, 18*, 1046–1051.

Troxel, W. M., Matthews, K. A., Bromberger, J. T., and Sutton-Tyrrell, K. (2003). Chronic stress burden, discrimination, and subclinical carotid artery disease in African American and Caucasian women. *Health Psychol, 22*, 300–309.

Tsutsumi, A., Kayaba, K., Yoshimura, M., Sawada, M., Ishikawa, S., Sakai, K., Gotoh, T., and Nago, N. (2003). Association between job characteristics and health behaviors in Japanese rural workers. *Int J Behav Med, 10*, 125–142.

Uchino, B. N., Cacioppo, J. T., and Kiecolt-Glaser, J. K. (1996). The relationship between social support and physiological processes: A review with emphasis on underlying mechanisms and implications for health. *Psychol Bull, 119*, 488–531.

van Oort, F. V., van Lenthe, F. J., and Mackenbach, J. P. (2004). Cooccurrence of lifestyle risk factors and the explanation of education inequalities in mortality: Results from the GLOBE study. *Prev Med, 39*, 1126–1134.

Vedhara, K., Cox, N. K. M., Wilcock, G. K., Perks, P., Hunt, M., Anderson, S., Lightman, S. L., and Shanks,

N. M. (1999). Chronic stress in elderly carers of dementia patients and antibody response to influenza vaccination. *Lancet, 353*, 627–631.

Vitaliano, P. P., Zhang, J., and Scanlan, J. M. (2003). Is caregiving hazardous to one's physical health? A meta-analysis. *Psychol Bull, 129*, 946–972.

Vrijkotte, T. G., van Doornen, L. J., and de Geus, E. J. (2000). Effects of work stress on ambulatory blood pressure, heart rate, and heart rate variability. *Hypertension, 35*, 880–886.

Williams, D. R., Neighbors, H. W., and Jackson, J. S. (2003). Racial/ethnic discrimination and health: Findings from community studies. *Am J Public Health, 93*, 200–208.

11

Individual Differences in Response to Stress and Risk for Addiction

WILLIAM R. LOVALLO

Addiction to alcohol and other drugs follows a trajectory of increasingly frequent and heavy intake leading to a dependence on the substance to maintain normal mood regulation. The gradual acquisition of dependence indicates that mechanisms of neural plasticity may underlie the addiction trajectory. Studies in animal models indicate that the limbic system is central to this process. This chapter explores individual differences in response to stress, in particular altered hypothalamic-pituitary-adrenocortical reactivity, in relation to familial vulnerability to addiction. Addictions are more common in persons with a family history of substance use disorders (FH+), suggesting an inherited disposition. FH+ persons also have a tendency toward behavioral undercontrol, characterized by antisocial behaviors, excitement seeking, impulsivity, and poor mood regulation. FH+ have a blunted stress cortisol response, but they respond positively to pharmacological challenge with opioid receptor blockers. These findings are consistent with a hypothesis that FH+ have a chronically enhanced central opioid activation. The $val^{158}met$ polymor-

phism of the catechol-O-methyltransferase gene may underlie these risk-associated characteristics. Persons who have the val/val homozygous form also have high levels of central opioid activity, behavioral disinhibition, and low stress responsiveness. The polymorphism is more common among patients with substance use disorders than in healthy controls. This evidence converges on a possible FH+ genotype with altered central opioid function that may render affected individuals vulnerable to severe stress and predispose them toward risky experimentation with alcohol and drugs of abuse, thereby contributing to addiction.

I. INTRODUCTION

Addictions are chronic disorders that carry negative social and medical consequences for the individual. A propensity toward substance-use disorders may have biological roots, as suggested by studies of family inheritance patterns (Cloninger, Bohman, and Sigvardsson, 1981). Addictions evolve over time as the person consumes alcohol or other drugs more frequently, in increasing amounts, at inappropriate times, and with increasingly severe consequences. This trajectory is captured by the American Psychiatric Association's diagnostic criteria for abuse and dependence on alcohol and psychoactive substances (American Psychiatric Association, 1994). The compulsive character of the progression and maintenance of addictions suggests that the brain's motivational systems are critically involved in the addiction trajectory (Koob, 2003). These motivational systems include the limbic system and its interactions with the prefrontal cortex and their joint regulation of attention and control over endocrine, autonomic, and skeletal motor behavior (Lovallo, 2005). It is noteworthy that these motivational systems overlap fully with brain systems that respond during stress and also in learning and motivation of behavior.

Alcoholism is known to run in families, raising the question of genetic contributions and the person's susceptibility to environmental factors, including life stress. This chapter presents selected data on persons with a family history of alcohol or drug abuse (FH+) and discusses altered limbic system function and response to stress that may underlie their propensity toward addiction. In such persons, the limbic system and prefrontal cortex are seen to undergo neural plasticity during times of emotional distress and also in response to drug intake, and these processes are therefore seen as having a common impact on the vulnerable individual.

II. STRESS AND THE BRAIN'S MOTIVATIONAL SYSTEMS

Survival calls for an organism to approach and obtain what is needed to sustain life and to avoid what is life threatening. These basic approach and avoid-

ance tendencies represent the fundamental descriptive framework for all behavior and are a useful departure for a brief overview of brain systems involved in motivated behavior, stress reactivity, and inherited risk for addictions.

A. Brain Systems Involved in Motivated Behavior

The limbic system and cerebral cortex work together in regulating behavior. The limbic system includes the amygdala, stria terminalis, bed nuclei of the stria terminalis (BNST), nucleus accumbens, and related ventral forebrain nuclei. They interact with overlying areas of the cerebral cortex, including the medial temporal gyrus, the cingulate gyrus, and the ventromedial prefrontal cortex (Iversen, Kupfermann, and Kandel, 2000). These structures function to orient attention to behaviorally significant events, motivate approach and avoidance behaviors, and shape bodily responses to support the requisite behaviors (Rolls, 2000a). The amygdala, located bilaterally in the medial temporal lobes, is crucial for generating the initial response to significant events, increasing the likelihood that such inputs will be evaluated accurately and that appropriate approach or avoidance behaviors will occur (Bechara, Damasio, and Damasio, 2003). At such times, the amygdala engages medial forebrain structures, including the BNST, the ventromedial prefrontal cortex, and anterior cingulate gyrus to aid in evaluation of behavioral options and to shape behavioral choices (Bechara, Damasio, Damasio, and Lee, 1999; Ridderinkhof, Ullsperger, Crone, and Nieuwenhuis, 2004). The interactions between the limbic system and prefrontal cortex are significant in shaping behavioral choices, and they collectively determine autonomic and endocrine responses during states of stress (Davis, 2000). In addition to its role in short-term behavioral regulation, the amygdala is essential for the formation of Pavlovian-conditioned associations that underlie long-term regulation of motivated behaviors. Finally, the amygdala interacts with the hippocampus in the formation of declarative memories (Cahill, Babinsky, Markowitsch, and McGaugh, 1995; Rolls and Stringer, 2001).

B. Brain Systems Altered in the Addictions and in Inherited Risk for Addictions

The coming together of limbic structures, subcortical nuclei, and the cingulate gyrus and ventromedial prefrontal cortex forms what we will call a frontal-limbic convergence (Damasio, 1994). This convergence is essential to the process of decision making and behavioral regulation and is therefore a focal point for the study of individual differences in addiction potential. This frontal-limbic region receives dopaminergic (DA), serotonergic, and noradrenergic projections from the brain stem that regulate the behavioral state of the organism (Swanson, 2000). DA is released at the nucleus accumbens in response to administration of abused drugs (Koob and Bloom, 1988). Although DA is often associated with hedonically positive events, a more general formulation is that it is secreted in this region when events depart from normal or expected patterns, thus allowing the system to adjust adaptively to changed environmental contingencies (Oswald et al., 2005; Tobler, Fiorillo, and Schultz, 2005). In this sense, DA release at the nucleus accumbens may operate with surrounding regions to support a behavioral and motivational set point (Koob and Le Moal, 1997). Modification of the DA-mediated set point by stress or drug exposure and withdrawal may move the individual to a less stable behavioral homeostasis, eventually requiring drug intake for normal function. Actions of DA, norepinephrine, and serotonin are accordingly targets of study for inherited differences that may underlie vulnerability to addiction.

C. Brain Systems Mediating the Stress Response and Individual Differences in Stress Reactivity

While these frontal-limbic systems guide behavior under normal circumstances, they are notably activated during periods of stress. A comprehensive discussion of the acute stress response and individual differences in stress reactivity is presented elsewhere (Lovallo, 2005). (See Clemens Kirschbaum's discussion in Chapter 1 of this volume and Andrew Steptoe's discussion of psychosocial determinants of stress responses in Chapter 10.) The central nervous system response to stress is integrated by a widespread system of neurons that release corticotropin-releasing factor (CRF) that leads the limbic system, cerebral cortex, and the hypothalamus and brain stem to produce an integrated fight-or-flight response (Petrusz and Merchenthaler, 1992; Swanson, Sawchenko, Rivier, and Vale, 1983). The central outcome of this response is the systemic release of the glucocorticoid hormone, cortisol (Selye, 1936). In a normal day, cortisol output is stimulated by the hypothalamus and restrained by negative feedback to maintain homeostasis (Czeisler and Klerman, 1999). This daily pattern of feedforward and feedback regulation is disrupted during periods of stress when the central CRF system stimulates high levels of cortisol release accompanied by a reduction in the effectiveness of cortisol's negative feedback (Reul and de Kloet, 1986).

D. Some Effects of Stress on the Brain

High levels of cortisol prevailing during times of stress may alter brain systems engaged in long-term regulation of behavior. The limbic system and temporal and prefrontal cortexes are extensively supplied with cortisol receptors (Sanchez, Young, Plotsky, and Insel, 2000). Cortisol may alter states of global activation (Buchanan, Brechtel, Sollers, and Lovallo, 2001), increase anxiety and stress responsivity

(Shepard, Barron, and Myers, 2003), and affect the formation of declarative memories and Pavlovian associations (Buchanan and Lovallo, 2001; Cahill, Babinsky, Markowitsch, and McGaugh, 1995; Okuda, Roozendaal, and McGaugh, 2004). Three examples illustrate these effects. (1) The hippocampus acts as the primary point of negative cortisol feedback (Sapolsky, Meaney, and McEwen, 1985). Prolonged and severe stress can leave the hippocampus vulnerable to excitatory neurotoxins leading to a loss of neurons, impairing its negative-feedback ability (Sapolsky, Krey, and McEwen, 1985). The loss of negative feedback regulation may contribute to a tonic upregulation of circulating cortisol and a loss of its diurnal cycle. (2) Formation of long-term memories for emotional events is enhanced by stress levels of circulating cortisol (Buchanan and Lovallo, 2001; Okuda, Roozendaal, and McGaugh, 2004), increasing responses to previously rewarded stimuli. (3) The amygdala is sensitized by exposure to stress levels of glucocorticoid (Shepard, Barron, and Myers, 2003), which causes an upregulation of amygdalar and forebrain CRF receptors, resulting in exaggerated anxiety and cortisol responses to subsequent stressors (Shepard, Barron, and Myers, 2000). Accordingly, extensive exposure to high levels of cortisol during periods of stress or drug withdrawal is likely to affect both memory formation and behavioral tendencies, possibly including decision making. Evidence reviewed below suggests that regulation of these structures by brain stem neuronal systems may be altered in FH+ persons.

III. HEDONIC HOMEOSTASIS IN ADDICTION RISK

The region of frontal-limbic convergence, essential for making behavioral choices and generating stress responses, is also affected by drug intake and withdrawal and is therefore seen as being centrally involved in the development of addictions. (1) All

drugs of abuse evoke an acute release of DA in the shell of the nucleus accumbens and in nearby areas, including the anterior cingulate gyrus (Koob and Bloom, 1988). (2) Cortisol secretion increases acutely in response to drug intake and remains elevated during such times. As such, intake of alcohol and other drugs mimics the cortisol component of the stress response (Adinoff, Ruether, Krebaum, Iranmanesh, and Williams, 2003). (3) Stress increases drug craving (Ahmed and Koob, 1998; Breese et al., 2005; Sinha, Catapano, and O'Malley, 1999). (4) Drug withdrawal increases CRF activity and precipitates a stress-like level of cortisol secretion (Adinoff and Risher-Flowers, 1991; Rodriguez de Fonseca, Carrera, Navarro, Koob, and Weiss, 1997), again mimicking features of the cortisol response during stress. This stress mimicry leads us to view drug intake and severe stress as affecting overlapping brain structures and neurochemical processes.

George Koob has pointed to a systematic dysregulation of dopamine release in this region of frontal-limbic convergence as a central feature of the process of addiction, referring to this dysregulation as the "hijacking" of the brain's motivational systems (Koob, Rassnick, Heinrichs, and Weiss, 1994). Under his formulation, alcohol and other drugs would cause repeated pharmacologic stimulation of DA release at the nucleus accumbens, simultaneously activating attentional processes and motivating behavioral approach tendencies. This may result in the system detecting reduced DA activity between episodes of drug intake and stimulating a stress-like CRF response. This pattern may contribute to further intake, as seen in studies on animal models showing prior episodes of alcohol exposure followed by withdrawal and abstinence to lead to still higher levels of intake when alcohol again becomes available (Valdez et al., 2002). These effects are attenuated by CRF blockade (Valdez, Sabino, and Koob, 2004). Koob has hypothesized that over time, the hedonic set point of the system may move from its normal homeostatic center, resulting in biases in motivation and decision making to maintain hedonic homeostasis, ultimately through maladaptive or allostatic means (Koob, 2003). The stress levels of cortisol prevailing during drug intake and withdrawal may therefore contribute to this departure from the normal hedonic homeostasis. Others provide a similar depiction (Adinoff, 2004; de Jong and de Kloet, 2004).

The foregoing suggests that there should be some evidence for overlapping responses to stress and drug exposure and their impact on brain motivational systems. At an anecdotal and clinical level, persons with substance use disorders, including smokers, report more severe cravings during periods of acute stress. Persons with a history of traumatic stress exposure are likely to become heavy users of alcohol and drugs in an apparent attempt at self-medication (see Chapter 17 of this volume). Patients in treatment for substance use disorders are likely to report high rates of lifetime trauma exposure (Bernardy, King, Parsons, and Lovallo, 1996).

Recent animal work has shown that drug exposure and stress both have common effects on the brain's mesolimbic DA system (Saal, Dong, Bonci, and Malenka, 2003). Rats were exposed to single doses of morphine, nicotine, alcohol, cocaine, and amphetamine and were then killed and their brains subjected to electrophysiological study. Brain slices showed long-term potentiation in DA-neuron response to excitatory neurotransmitters, suggesting enhanced DA neuronal plasticity in response to all of the drugs tested. An acute swim stressor produced a nearly identical pattern of DA response change. The connection between stress and drug exposure was further indicated by the involvement in glucocorticoid mechanisms in the formation of the DA potentiation following stress. Brain tissue from animals exposed to the cold swim, but pretreated with the glucocorticoid receptor blocker, RU-486, did not show the facilita-

tion of the DA response. This indicates that the stress-induced potentiation acted specifically through actions of stress hormones on the central nervous system. Such work indicates that not only do stress and drugs of abuse act on the same brain systems, they also have similar effects on the midbrain DA system.

IV. AFFECTIVE REGULATION AND VULNERABILITY TO ADDICTION

The discussion of brain systems involved in addiction leads to the question of whether risk for addiction is inherited through vulnerabilities in these same systems. Do persons who are genetically at risk for addiction also have different patterns of stress response that may reflect inherited differences in these common brain systems? Do persons who are vulnerable to addiction have different responses to severe stress? Does severe stress in early life alter the brain regions that regulate motivated behavior and increase addiction vulnerability?

With regard to the first question, we may ask if persons at increased risk of future drug abuse have less stable behavioral and emotional regulation than their low-risk counterparts. In a longitudinal study from California, Block and colleagues performed detailed psychological and personality evaluations of children 5–7 years of age and reassessed them into early adulthood (Shedler and Block, 1990). In evaluating drug intake when the cohort was 17–18 years of age, the researchers had the subjects complete a drug use inventory, by which they were classified as having never used drugs or alcohol; experimenting at about the usual level for their peers; or as being regular users of tobacco, alcohol, and illicit drugs. Clinical psychologists, who were blind to the subjects' drug use patterns, assessed the groups using an adjective sorting procedure. The heavy users were described as being "undependable, irresponsible, unproductive, unable to delay gratification, rebellious, self-indulgent, and ethically inconsistent." During their childhood evaluations, clinicians rated these same future heavy users as "maladjusted, insecure, and emotionally distressed." Other workers have pointed to poor behavioral regulation, impulsivity, and deficient executive controls over behavior as characterizing those at high risk of future addictions (Tapert, Baratta, Abrantes, and Brown, 2002).

Studies of alcohol abuse etiology have characterized those with an early-onset of alcoholism as being more likely to show oppositional-defiant behavior as children and conduct disorder in adolescence (Babor et al., 1992; Johann, Bobbe, Putzhammer, and Wodarz, 2003). Twin-adoption data suggest a common pattern of inheritance of substance use disorders, antisocial tendencies, and diagnosis of antisocial personality disorder (Cloninger, 1987; Cloninger and Reich, 1983; Langbehn, Cadoret, Caspers, Troughton, and Yucuis, 2003). Increased risk for alcohol and drug abuse is associated with poor regulation of affect and behavior. A model of psychological and behavioral characteristics of FH+ indicates a combination of excitement seeking and antisocial behavior as contributing to excessive drinking and maladaptive patterns of intake (Figure 11-1) (Finn, 2002; Finn,

Mazas, Justus, and Steinmetz, 2002; Mazas, Finn, and Steinmetz, 2000), a pattern Sher has termed *behavioral undercontrol* (Sher, Walitzer, Wood, and Brent, 1991). Other evidence implicates differences in stress responsivity, particularly in cortisol secretion, that coincide with addiction and elevated risk for addiction.

V. ADDICTIONS AND ABNORMALITIES OF HPAC REGULATION OF CORTISOL SECRETION

Studies of substance abusers and FH+ boys and young adults provide converging evidence that HPA regulation differs from that seen in nonaddicted controls and in FH–. The evidence discussed here shows consistently diminished cortisol response to stress and increased risk for addiction. Diminished stress cortisol reactivity is seen in (1) alcoholic patients, (2) FH+ preadolescent boys with no history of substance use, and (3) FH+ young adults with moderate to heavy social drinking histories; and diminished stress cortisol responses predict (4) which preadolescents will later begin early drug and alcohol experimentation, and (5) which smokers will fail in smoking cessation programs; and finally (6) studies showing that FH+ have differential responses to

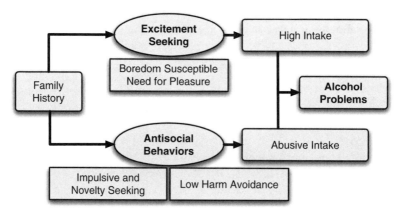

FIGURE 11-1   A structural model relating family history of alcoholism to behavioral dispositions and risk-related drinking patterns. Drawn from Finn (2002).

opioid receptor blockade. Further discussion of the HPAC and risk for addiction is provided in Chapter 2 of the present volume.

A. Studies in Alcoholism and Drug Abuse

In our initial studies, abstinent alcoholics had blunted HPAC responses to a range of physical and psychological stressors, including mental arithmetic plus a painful cold pressor, mental arithmetic plus isometric handgrip, and public speaking plus handgrip (Figure 11-2) (Bernardy, King, Parsons, and Lovallo, 1996; Errico, Parsons, King, and Lovallo, 1993). Blunting of the stress response was more pronounced in polysubstance abusers than in patients reporting only problems with alcohol, leading to the speculation that the polysubstance abusers may have had a

more severe level of addiction with more attenuation of cortisol reactivity. Cortisol secretion had the same slope over the waking hours in all three groups, allowing us to rule out fundamental disturbances in diurnal and metabolic regulation of HPA function in the patients. Work with abstinent users of "ecstasy" and opioids also found these groups to have deficient stress and affect-related cortisol responses as compared to nonabusing controls (Gerra, Baldaro et al., 2003; Gerra, Bassignana, et al., 2003). However, such findings cannot fully rule out exposure to high levels of alcohol and other substances as a cause of the patients' blunted stress cortisol responses.

B. Studies in Preadolescent FH+

The first studies to examine the impact of psychological stressors on offspring of

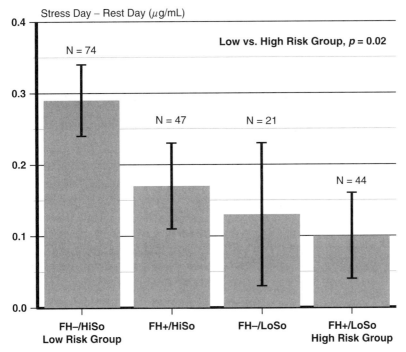

Cortisol Stress Response

FIGURE 11-2   Cortisol stress responses defined as the increase in the mean cortisol level during the stress period on a stress day from the corresponding time period on the rest day. Reprinted from Sorocco, Lovallo, Vincent, and Collins (2006).

substance abusers come from a longitudinal study by Ralph Tarter and colleagues of 10–12-year-old boys whose fathers had substance use disorders (Moss, Vanyukov, and Martin, 1995). These boys were brought to the hospital for an electroencephalographic procedure calling for attachment of scalp electrodes and exposure to an unfamiliar laboratory environment, considered anxiety provoking and mildly stressful. They provided saliva samples before and after this procedure for analysis of cortisol. The FH– had a significant elevation of cortisol in the first sample, indicating an anticipatory response to the impending novel experience, and they had a reduction afterward, indicating recovery. In contrast, the FH+ had low levels at both times, indicating an absence of anticipation or a reduced HPA activation in relation to the anticipation. Further analyses indicated that antisocial tendencies were a significant predictor of the reduced HPA response (Dawes et al., 1999).

C. Studies in Young-Adult FH+

Our work also suggests a diminished stress response in 18–30-year-old FH+, especially if antisocial tendencies are present (Sorocco, Lovallo, Vincent, and Collins, 2006). FH+ exposed to a public speaking and mental arithmetic stress had smaller cortisol responses than the FH– controls (Figure 11-2). The small cortisol responses in the FH+ group were due to the presence of many subjects with low scores on the Sociability scale of the California Personality Inventory (Gough, 1994), in agreement with the Moss findings that small cortisol responses in preadolescent boys were especially prominent among those with antisocial tendencies (Dawes et al., 1999). As in the case of our studies with alcoholics, the absence of FH group differences in cortisol on the resting control day indicates that basal HPA function is intact and normal across all of the FH and sociability subgroups. Other work with these same subjects showed that the FH+ who were low in sociability were

likely to have poor performance on the Stroop task, and the FH+ males were found to be strongly oriented to monetary gains in performing the Iowa Gambling task (Lovallo, Yechiam, Sorocco, Vincent, and Collins, 2006). Gianoulakis and colleagues also reported a numerically smaller cortisol response during mental arithmetic stress in 20 FH+ vs. that seen in 20 FH– males (Dai, Thavundayil, and Gianoulakis, 2002), although this difference did not achieve statistical significance.

Two studies have contradictory findings. Zimmermann tested cortisol responses in 29 paternal FH+ and 23 FH– controls in response to public speaking and mental arithmetic following alcohol versus placebo administration given in two sessions (Zimmermann et al., 2004). The 15 FH+ exposed to placebo and stress on their first session had larger cortisol responses than the 10 FH– controls in that condition. There were no differences between FH groups receiving placebo and stress on their second lab day, and no FH group differences overall. FH+ had greater stress cortisol reactivity than FH– in one study (Uhart, Oswald, McCaul, Chong, and Wand, 2006), as described by Wand in Chapter 4 of this volume.

D. Studies in Smoking Relapse

Studies of smoking cessation show that cigarette smokers who have the smallest stress cortisol responses are the ones most likely to relapse in the short term (al'Absi, 2006). Both relapsers and abstainers had significant histories of nicotine exposure, reducing the likelihood that attenuated cortisol responses were secondary to nicotine history. The data are broadly consistent with the idea that an attenuated HPA response is tied to likelihood of drug taking.

E. Studies Predicting Experimentation with Substance Nicotine and Marijuana in FH+

Predictive evidence for the tie between addiction-proneness and blunted HPA reactivity comes from the study cited above in which 10–12-year-old boys were tested for anticipatory stress cortisol responses (Moss, Vanyukov, and Martin, 1995). Although the FH+ boys had smaller cortisol responses than the FH–, a follow-up over 5 years showed that the strongest predictor of early experimentation with marijuana was a diminished cortisol response, regardless of FH status (Moss, Vanyukov, Yao, and Kirillova, 1999).

F. Opioid Blockade and HPA Response in FH+

Other investigators have examined opioid systems in persons addicted to alcohol and illicit drugs as part of studies on treatment for addiction (Kreek, 1996). In the process, workers examined the impact of opioid blockade on the secretion of cortisol in FH+ persons. Wand and colleagues have carried out systematic observations of naloxone's effects on acute changes in cortisol secretion in FH+ young adults and FH– controls, as reviewed in the present volume (Chapter 4). FH+ have a stress-like cortisol response to naloxone, in contrast to the FH– (Wand, McCaul, Gotjen, Reynolds, and Lee, 2001). The cortisol response occurs at lower doses, more promptly, and more persistently in the FH+. In a related study, King and colleagues administered naltrexone to FH+ and found the same response differential (King et al., 2002).

What might account for FH effects on cortisol response to opioid blockade? The fact that FH+ are more sensitive to blockade suggests some form of reliance on endogenous opioid actions for normal HPA function. To put this thought another way, it is possible that FH+ have a higher tonic level of central opioid function and that this restrains the central CRF system, causing diminished cortisol responses to stress and other provocations. The fact that basal cortisol secretion is not disturbed in the FH+ suggests that the system reacts normally to diurnal and metabolic signals, indicat-

ing intact HPA function, but this does not rule out differences in CRF actions at higher levels. Others have also argued that greater endogenous opioid activity is responsible for these differential effects of naloxone (Shoblock and Maidment, 2006).

Accordingly, the view advanced here is that alcoholics, FH+ young adults, and smokers have diminished stress cortisol responses due to a constitutionally based difference in central HPA regulation. The similarity of HPA function at rest suggests that the difference is confined to stress-responsive systems, implicating the limbic system and central CRF neurons above the hypothalamus (Lovallo, 2006). Studies reviewed in this section point to diminished stress cortisol responsivity as indicating increased addiction potential. Converging evidence is seen in the increased response of FH+ to opioid blockade. This paired set of findings provides circumstantial evidence that the altered frontal-limbic activity associated with risk for substance use disorders may be centrally involved with alterations of the central CRF system. These studies also indicate that HPA function is a useful system to probe for limbic system response differences in relation to individual differences in risk for the addictions. The first question that arises in this connection is how diminished stress reactivity and enhanced response to opioid blockade might fit into a consistent picture of increased risk for addiction.

VI. RISK FOR ADDICTION, CENTRAL OPIOID FUNCTION, AND REGIONAL BRAIN FUNCTION

We have seen that the brain systems responsible for motivation of adaptive behavior are the same ones that are involved in responses to stress and acute administration of psychoactive substances. Koob has argued that these stress-responsive systems may be fundamentally altered during repeated administration of drugs, as occurs in the development of addictions (Koob, 2003). He has indicated that repeated use of drugs destabilizes the ability of this system to maintain hedonic homeostasis, driving it to maintain a hedonic balance through allostatic processes, including repeated use of a drug.

The hypothesis advanced here follows the premise that loss of hedonic homeostasis and the altered response of the HPA to stress are both vulnerabilities to addiction that derive from the same inherited alteration in central opioid function.

HYPOTHESIS

FH+ persons inherit an active central opioid system. This high-level of opioid function is a tonic restraint on the central CRF system. Increased central opioid regulation of CRF systems may fulfill requirements of Koob's postulated vulnerability to hedonic dysregulation in response to stress and drug intake.

This restraint has four consequences:

(1) The HPA of the FH+ individual is adapted to a high level of opioid regulation in its basal state.
(2) Acute removal of opioid restraint by blockade causes increased CRF activity leading to a stress-like cortisol response.
(3) Persons with higher levels of opioid control of CRF function may experience lower than normal levels of anxiety and may consequently lack an aversion to risky behaviors, such as binge drinking and experimentation with illicit drugs.
(4) This heightened opioid regulation may affect how the HPA reacts to repeated cycles of drug intake and withdrawal.

A useful point of departure for considering this hypothesis is a model developed by Gary Wand that focuses on three points in the central nervous system where opioid neurons regulate brain structures crucial for determining HPA reactivity to stress. The model is illustrated in Figure 11-3 (Wand, Mangold, El Deiry, McCaul, and Hoover, 1998). The key points of opioid neuron interactions are at the locus coeruleus (LC) in the brain stem, the PVN of the hypothalamus, and the nucleus accumbens of the septal region. Collectively, these three points of opioidergic regulation have the potential to greatly alter the reactivity of the HPA.

A. Brain Stem Mechanisms

The LC is responsible for the ability of the CNS to mount global activational responses to homeostatic challenges (Aston–Jones, 1986). It contains 85% of the norepinephrine containing cell bodies in the CNS; and the axons extend upward to the amygdala, hypothalamus, and the cerebral cortex; and they also extend downward through all levels of the spinal cord (Grant and Redmond, 1981). The LC responds to homeostatic challenges arising internally or externally, and in the latter case these arise from the amygdala via the BNST. During both types of challenges, LC fibers activate the central CRF system (Petrusz and Merchenthaler, 1992; Valentino, Page, Van Bockstaele, and Aston–Jones, 1992) and initiate a stress cortisol response. The Wand model indicates that the LC is under tonic inhibitory control by brain stem opioid neurons. Administration of opioid-blocking agents would remove this tonic regulation, reducing the restraint over LC neuronal firing (Grant, Huang, and Redmond, 1988). Increased firing by norepinephrine neurons would contribute to increased activation of the limbic system, including the amygdala, and extrahypothalamic CRF neurons.

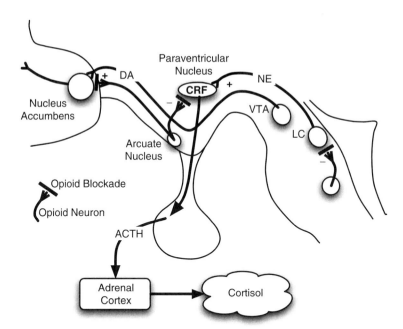

FIGURE 11-3   Effects of opioid blockade on cortisol secretion. Opioid blockade acts in the brain to increase cortisol secretion and alter mood. (1) Opioid neurons from the arcuate nucleus of the hypothalamus normally inhibit CRF output by neurons of the PVN, reducing CRF secretion at the pituitary gland and thereby reducing ACTH release and cortisol production. Opioid blockade releases the PVN from this inhibitory influence, allowing cortisol production to increase. (2) The LC contains about 85% of the NE cell bodies in the central nervous system, and it is largely responsible for the amount of global activation in the brain. Opioid neurons in the brain stem normally inhibit the NE-producing cells of the LC. Opioid blockade releases the LC from this inhibitory influence, allowing NE to activate the CRF-neurons of the PVN, resulting in increased cortisol production. (3) The nucleus accumbens is a site of DA release in response to all drugs of abuse. This nucleus is in extensive two-way communication with the prefrontal cortex. Opioid neurons from the arcuate nucleus normally activate DA release at the nucleus accumbens. Opioid blockade inhibits this effect, reducing DA release by the nucleus accumbens at the prefrontal cortex. This may alter hedonic states and attention to reward cues. Cortisol feedback to the central nervous system is capable of altering the excitability of dopamine neurons as discussed in the text. ACTH = adrenocorticotropic hormone; CNS = central nervous system; CRF = corticotropin-releasing factor; DA = dopamine; LC = locus coeruleus; NE = norepinephrine; VTA = ventral tegmental area. Adapted with permission of the author (Wand et al., 1998).

B. Hypothalamic PVN

The second component of the model is the regulation of the PVN of the hypothalamus by opioidergic neurons branching from the arcuate nucleus of the hypothalamus. These opioidergic neurons inhibit activity of CRF neurons within the PVN (Hellbach et al., 1998). PVN CRF neurosecretory neurons are directly responsible for HPA activation as they stimulate ACTH output from the pituitary during states of distress, including periods of drug withdrawal (Milanes,

Laorden, Chapleur-Chateau, and Burlet, 1998). Opioid blockade would therefore leave the PVN more readily activated by any stress-related input and by activational signals arising from the LC. Accordingly, opioid blockade may increase HPA activation by way of noradrenergic inputs from the LC and by reduced restraint from the arcuate nucleus. In a person with normally high levels of opioid regulation, opioid blockade would stimulate the PVN to initiate a stress-like cortisol response.

C. Nucleus Accumbens and Prefrontal Cortex

The third point of opioid interaction with the stress response is at the nucleus accumbens, a subcortical structure located in the region of frontal-limbic convergence, and a point where opioid variations could affect how DA influences the prefrontal cortex (Herkenham, Edley, and Stuart, 1984). Some writers have described this region, along with the orbitofrontal cortex, as one where the reward value of stimulus inputs is processed as part of a cognitive stream of information arriving from more dorsal and parietal regions of the cortex (Damasio, 1994; LaBar, Crupain, Voyvodic, and McCarthy, 2003; Rolls, 2000b). Accordingly, this area is one that is potentially highly reactive to DA release during periods of acute drug intake and also to the reduced DA release during periods of withdrawal.

The effects of drug exposure and withdrawal on DA function in this motivationally critical brain region may have implications for motivation to engage in further experimentation and drug intake. Exposure to cues that may signal reward is associated with approach behaviors accompanied by DA release in the shell of the nucleus accumbens (Nicola, Taha, Kim, and Fields, 2005; Yun, Wakabayashi, Fields, and Nicola, 2004). Disruption of DA function in these areas appears to diminish the hedonic value of drugs of abuse (Carr, Kutchukhidze, and Park, 1999; Koob, Vaccarino, Amalric, and Bloom, 1986; Lyons and Porrino, 1997). Alterations in the character of these frontal-limbic interactions may therefore change the person's affective state, with consequences for approach and avoidance tendencies. The timing and magnitude of DA release at the nucleus accumbens may therefore affect decision making (Shidara and Richmond, 2002) and alter the evaluation of risks and benefits between response alternatives (Ridderinkhof, Ullsperger, Crone, and Nieuwenhuis, 2004) when choosing to consume alcohol or other drugs. Opioid interactions at the nucleus accumbens may therefore affect attention to environmental cues, evaluation of the hedonic value of those cues, decision making, motivation of approach behaviors, and reward mechanisms. A connection with cortisol secretion is seen in the finding that increases in negative affect contribute to cortisol response during stress (al'Absi et al., 1997). The sensitivity of FH+ persons to opioid blockade suggests that an inherited alteration in opioid function could account for some of the behavioral and psychophysiological characteristics of these persons.

VII. THE VAL[158]MET POLYMORPHISM AND OPIOID FUNCTION

Research on genetic contributions to substance use disorders has been reviewed extensively by others (Dick and Foroud, 2003; Goldman, Oroszi, and Ducci, 2005; Kreek, Bart, Lilly, LaForge, and Nielsen, 2005; Kreek, Nielsen, Butelman, and LaForge, 2005) and in Chapter 6 of this volume. The discussion here is confined to work on variants of the gene that codes for expression of catechol-O-methyltransferase (COMT). Gene variations that determine differing levels of COMT activity have implications for understanding differences in central opioidergic function and differing HPA responses to opioid blockade.

COMT is an enzyme that degrades norepinephrine, serotonin, and DA in the extracellular environment when the transmitter fails to be transported back into the presynaptic neuron. In such cases, a deficit of COMT activity would tend to leave neurotransmitter active in the synaptic cleft, prolonging activity of the postsynaptic neuron, in turn leading to downregulation of postsynaptic receptors. Because the transmitters that are subject to COMT degradation affect many brain systems and behaviors, a single polymorphism has the potential to exert a range of effects on behavioral dispositions. A common polymorphism has been described that codes for two forms of the COMT molecule, one that is a relatively stable molecular configuration (High Activity) and one that is less stable (Low Activity; Ishiguro, Haruo Shibuya, Toru, Saito, and Arinami, 1999). These COMT variants derive from a single-nucleotide polymorphism at codon 158 of the COMT gene, in which case the amino acid valine (val) may substitute for methionine (met). The *val*^{158}*met* polymorphism is inherited from both parents and accordingly, the offspring may be typed as val/val, val/met, or met/met.

The val/val genotype codes for a stable, High Activity, pool of the molecule, the met/met pool is the least stable, considered Low Activity, while the val/met pool is intermediate in stability and activity. Among Euro-American populations, 25% are estimated to be val/val homozygous (Li et al., 1997). The functional consequences of inheriting these polymorphisms are laid out in Table 11-1. A person with the val/val genotype and High Activity COMT will have rapid synaptic inactivation of DA and norepinephrine. This results in reduced DA activity in the prefrontal cortex and other brain regions, and it has implications for activity of the central opioid system. Low levels of DA activity in frontal-limbic regions may result in a greater DA response to drug intake in view of a relatively low endogenous or baseline level of activity, and it would similarly cause a larger decline in DA activity during acute withdrawal as the effect of a single dose declines. This would be consistent with Koob's model of vulnerability to loss of hedonic homeostasis. On the opioid side, animal models having low DA function tend to have high levels of endogenous opioids in presynaptic

storage vesicles. The postsynaptic neurons therefore tend to downregulate their receptor populations in response to the active opioid transmission. This appears to result in more efficient opioidergic activity and highly effective opioidergic regulation of other neuron populations. The met/met genotype may be seen as the mirror opposite, in which lower levels of central opioid function result in less effective opioid regulation of other systems. The val/val pattern of low DA activity and high opioidergic function raises the question of whether that combination could account for FH-group differences in HPA response to stress and opioid blockade, as well as behavioral disinhibition, risky behavioral choices, and experimentation with drugs.

A. Behavioral and Affective Characteristics of the val/val Genotype

Given the above considerations, we hypothesize that differences in central CRF regulation may derive from differences in central opioid function resulting from different levels of COMT activity. Studies on the val/val and met/met genotypes indicate that they differ in stress-proneness, impulsiveness, and behavioral restraint (Lipsky et al., 2005; Smolka et al., 2005). In a study of response to prolonged muscle pain, val/val subjects required greater application of the pain stimulus to reach a preset subjective pain level, while the met/met counterparts required the least, and intermediate responses were seen in the val/met subjects, consistent with the proposed functional opioid differences (Zubieta et al., 2003). Ratings of negative affect paralleled these group differences, with the val/val group experiencing the least distress and the met/met the most, even though actual pain ratings were equalized by design. Central opioid activity in these groups was estimated by positron emission tomographic (PET) measures of cerebral uptake of an opioid ligand. The greatest endogenous opioid activity was seen in the val/val group

TABLE 11-1 Characteristics of Persons with Three Variant Polymorphism combinations of the Gene for Catechol-O-methyltransferase

val158met Allele	COMT Activity	CNS DA Activity	μ-Opioid in Terminals	Opioid Receptors	Opioid Activity	Addiction Proneness	% with Allele in lo/med/hi Risk	Impulsive
				WARRIORS				
VAL/VAL	HIGH	LOW	HIGH	FEW	HIGH	HIGH	18 31 39	HIGH
VAL/MET	MED	MED	MED	MED	MED	MED	31 24 29	MED
				WORRIERS				
MET/MET	LOW	HIGH	LOW	MANY	LOW	LOW	51 45 32	LOW

Note: Frequency of alleles in three risk groups based on data from Vandenburgh et al. (1997) on 122 community controls (low risk), 185 heavy substance users (medium risk), and 41 patients meeting DSM-IIIR criteria for substance use disorders (high risk). Description of characteristics of Warriors and Worriers from Goldman et al. (2005).

and lowest in the met/met group. Brain areas showing the greatest opioid activity were the thalamus, nucleus accumbens and surrounding structures, and the amygdala, consistent with our focus on this frontal-limbic convergence zone. In Goldman's shorthand terminology, the val/val group may be considered stress-resistant "Warriors" and the met/met group, stress-prone "Worriers."

Other evidence implicates COMT polymorphisms in regulation of affect and behavioral propensities. The val/val genotype has been linked to psychiatric disorders, including schizophrenia (Shifman et al., 2002). Behavioral studies indicate that the val/val genotype may confer impairments of executive function, as seen in perseverative errors on the Wisconsin Card Sorting Task (Lipsky et al., 2005). Consistent with a predicted lower response to aversive stimuli, exposure to unpleasant visual stimuli led to lower activation of the right amygdala and selected prefrontal regions in val/val subjects than in the met/met group, although no such difference was seen to pleasant stimuli (Smolka et al., 2005). Other evidence implicates the val/val genotype in risk for addiction. The frequency of the val/val allele is low in community controls (18%) but higher in persons who report heavy drinking and drug use (31%) and higher still in persons meeting criteria for substance abuse or dependence (39%; Table 11-1) (Vandenbergh, Rodriguez, Miller, Uhl, and Lachman, 1997). These proportions were opposite for the met/met group. This evidence of association with addiction potential is complimented by a haplotype analysis of the COMT gene implicated in nicotine addiction (Beuten, Payne, Ma, and Li, 2006).

In summary, persons possessing the val/val genotype have high levels of central opioid activity, display differences in frontal regulation of behavior, have differential limbic system responses to aversive visual stimuli, and display higher pain tolerance.

The val/val genotype is more prevalent among drug abusers than among controls, and persons possessing it share phenotypic characteristics with FH+ persons. Like the val/val Warriors, FH+ also display reduced responses to stress, greater responses to opioid blockade, and greater potential for addiction.

VIII. ADDICTION, RESPONSE TO STRESS, AND HEDONIC DYSREGULATION

Are the val/val Warriors vulnerable to hedonic dysregulation of the sort postulated by George Koob to underlie addictions, and can stress contribute to this process? Under Koob's model, frontal–limbic interactions are crucial to regulating approach and avoidance behaviors and their accompanying affective states. At one extreme are persons with a more active fear-related system with attendant higher levels of acute fear and anxiety responses (akin to Goldman's Worriers) and at the other extreme is a low-fear group with deficient limbic system activation to aversive threats and events (like Goldman's Warriors). Optimal interactions between limbic inputs and prefrontal function, deriving from a normal neurochemical environment, also imply a normal, homeostatic, hedonic balance associated with a midrange regulation of approach-avoidance and affective tendencies. Persons who are at genetic risk for substance abuse appear to have an inborn vulnerability in this system, indicated by poorly regulated approach-avoidance tendencies, exemplified by risk-taking, norm violations, and impulsivity. These tendencies may account for a greater willingness to initiate experimentation with alcohol and other drugs and for a greater response to that early experimentation. Enhanced experimentation then has the potential to initiate a shift in hedonic regulation, as called for in Koob's model, but the risk may be exaggerated by other characteristics of FH+.

A contributor to increased risk of addiction is a postulated lower endogenous activity in prefrontal DA systems. As indicated in Table 11-1, increased COMT activity suggests lowered DA function in the basal state. If so, compared to Worriers, the Warriors may experience a greater relative increase in DA concentration in the ventral striatum in response to alcohol and other drugs. For example, in humans, the extent of DA release in the nucleus accumbens following amphetamine intake correlates positively with the intensity of self-rated feelings of euphoria (Drevets et al., 2001). As a result, greater euphoria and reward could increase the tendency of Warriors to engage in further drug intake. Correspondingly, their return to a basal state could be experienced as more unpleasant. Cocaine abusers exposed to drug cues in the abstinent state experience the event as a stressor and also produce an HPA response to those events (Sinha et al., 2003). The common pattern of cyclical use and acute withdrawal could therefore begin to move the person toward more frequent consumption of larger amounts of alcohol or other drugs (Ahmed and Koob, 1998; Koob, 2003). The long-term effect is that an initially vulnerable, but homeostatic, hedonic state becomes an increasingly allostatic one. That is, the return to a normal subjective level of hedonic balance would be achieved at a greater cost of system resources and would be more easily disturbed by future perturbations (Sterling and Eyer, 1988).

Studies showing the Warrior type to be low in anxiety and high in central opioid function indicate a resistance to mild stresses (Zubieta et al., 2003). We speculate that resistance to mild stress need not rule out an impact of long-term or severe stress in such persons. Their neurochemical characteristics may render them vulnerable to severe stress in three ways: (1) Risk taking may result in increased total lifetime stress exposure with consequent effects on central CRF systems. (2) Cortisol's negative feedback is essential for normal modulation of the feedforward portion of the stress response, and deleterious consequences of unchecked feedforward processes are well known in humans and animals that are deficient in adrenal steroids (Selye, 1936). During periods of stress, a blunted cortisol response in Warriors would result in poorer counterregulation by cortisol feedback to critical CRF systems that generate the initial response, including the amygdala and BNST. (3) A willingness to engage in drug and alcohol intake may induce limbic system adaptations as described above (Saal, Dong, Bonci, and Malenka, 2003; Shepard, Barron, and Myers, 2000). Drug intake and withdrawal are both accompanied by cortisol release (Adinoff and Risher-Flowers, 1991), which may sensitize limbic system structures to future stress episodes and induce long-term potentiation in frontal-limbic structures.

A difficulty in rigorously addressing the addiction trajectory in val/val Warriors is a current absence of prospective data to examine the hypothesis, although the limited data on antisocial FH+ boys with low cortisol reactivity is suggestive (Moss, Vanyukov, and Martin, 1995). In addition, at least some evidence from animal models makes a plausible case that stress exposure can have long-term effects on brain motivational systems in ways that may fulfill some of the criteria of Koob's homeostatic dysregulation. This somewhat general formulation is refined by work by Rainnie and colleagues (2004) who have shown that central CRF activity affects neuronal plasticity at the amygdala, and that this may alter the response of the limbic system in the development of emotional disorders. The influence of early stress on brain systems underlying addictions is presented in Chapter 5 of this volume, and the effect of stress on DA pathways is presented in Chapter 3.

IX. LIFE EVENTS, BEHAVIORAL DISPOSITIONS, AND ADDICTION RISK

The evidence reviewed above has focused on differences in acute stress reactivity in FH+ and persons with substance use disorders. Koob's model of homeostatic dysregulation specifies that alcohol and other drug exposure gradually alters the hedonic homeostasis of the abuser such that the person comes to use drugs to maintain that homeostasis at an allostatic level. A corollary to that argument is that such persons may be vulnerable to stress as well. Unfortunately, the state of knowledge on inherited vulnerabilities to addiction does not allow us to make strong statements about the interplay of genes and life events that may help explain stress vulnerabilities in FH+. Work on the $val^{158}met$ polymorphism was presented here because the val/val Warrior type appears to have several characteristics in common with FH+ persons, including a tendency to be risk-taking, initially stress resistant, and to have altered opioid function.

Do FH+ persons differ in how they experience the consequences of severe stress relative to FH–? There are consistent reports of increased amounts of life stress in persons addicted to alcohol and other drugs, and this differential is greater among women than men. Up to 70% of female alcoholics report experiencing severe physical or sexual abuse during childhood and adolescence. This creates at least a presumption that severe stress is a contributing cause, but it does not prove this to be the case. Significant numbers of persons begin to escalate their alcohol and drug intake in response to prolonged stress exposure. Persons with post-traumatic stress disorder have markedly higher rates of alcoholism and drug abuse than the general population (see Chapter 17 of the present volume). For the most part this sort of evidence suggests that there may be stress vulnerabilities in relation to risk for substance abuse operating in humans. Such vulnerabilities are likely to have a genetic basis.

Connections between central CRF activity and addiction proneness are seen in rat strains that are readily trained to self-administer alcohol: (1) Notably the Lewis rat readily learns to consume alcohol and also has reduced HPA reactivity and a paucity of PVN CRF neurons (Baird and Lewis, 1964; Da Silva, Ramos, and Takahashi, 2004); (2) strains that readily self-administer alcohol are also more tolerant of noxious stimulation (Knapp, Kampov-Polevoy, Overstreet, Breese, and Rezvani, 1997). (3) Manipulation of the brain's stress response systems also increases and decreases self-administration (Barone and Roberts, 1996; Valdez, Zorrilla, Roberts, and Koob, 2003).

New work on a longitudinal cohort in Duneden, New Zealand, indicates the occurrence of well-documented gene-environment interactions that may render vulnerable persons susceptible to untoward outcomes in the presence of stress during early life (Moffitt, Caspi, and Rutter, 2006). In one report, males who had a specific variant of the promoter region of the gene for the enzyme, monoamine oxidase-a, were shown to be violence-prone as young adults, but only if abused as children (Caspi et al., 2002). In a second paper on this cohort, young adults with a variant allele for the serotonin transporter molecule were vulnerable to depression, but again only if they had had more than the usual amount of adversity as a child (Caspi et al., 2003). In both cases, persons with the contrasting alleles were resistant to the effects of early adversity. In an adoption study, persons with a genetic background of antisocial personality disorder were more likely to develop conduct disorder and antisocial personality disorder if they were exposed to adversity in their adoptive homes (Cadoret, Yates, Troughton, Woodworth, and Stewart, 1995).

X. CONCLUSIONS

Evidence suggests a connection between stress cortisol responsiveness and risk for addiction. Studies on FH+ persons show a reduction in stress reactivity that is enhanced in relation to behavioral undercontrol. Such persons also display diminished working memory and a propensity toward risky decision making. Persons with the greatest blunting of cortisol responsiveness to stress appear to be most vulnerable to early drug experimentation and to relapse during smoking cessation. Studies on a the $val^{158}met$ polymorphism that studying activity of the COMT molecule has the potential to explain these relationships among FH, risks-taking, reduced stress responsivity, and risk for addiction. In particular, persons possessing the val/val genotype have higher levels of central opioid activity that may reduce their aversion to risky behaviors and also diminish their acute stress reactivity. The work on altered HPA reactivity and addiction proneness may fulfill some of the conditions of Koob's model of hedonic homeostasis; both stress and drugs of abuse interact with neuronal plasticity in the mesolimbic DA system, perhaps biasing the organism to increased drug intake. This work tends to reinforce the connections between individual differences in stress reactivity and addiction proneness. Studies of familial risk for addiction, life stress, and long-term stress vulnerability in relation to outcomes will provide further insights into these processes.

ACKNOWLEDGMENTS

Preparation of this chapter was made possible by the Medical Research Service of the United States Department of Veterans Affairs, Washington, D.C., and by grants AA 12207 and RR-14467 from the National Institutes of Health, Bethesda, MD. We thank Gary Wand for generously allowing us to redraw his diagram of opioid interactions with stress-related brain systems. We similarly acknowledge the use of information from David Goldman's characterization of individuals possessing the val/val polymorphism of the gene for catechol-O-methyltransferase.

REFERENCES

Adinoff, B. (2004). Neurobiologic processes in drug reward and addiction. *Harvard Review of Psychiatry, 12*, 305–320.

Adinoff, B., and Risher-Flowers, D. (1991). Disturbances of hypothalamic-pituitary-adrenal axis functioning during ethanol withdrawal in six men. *American Journal of Psychiatry, 148*, 1023–1025.

Adinoff, B., Ruether, K., Krebaum, S., Iranmanesh, A., and Williams, M. J. (2003). Increased salivary cortisol concentrations during chronic alcohol intoxication in a naturalistic clinical sample of men. *Alcoholism, Clinical and Experimental Research, 27*, 1420–1427.

Ahmed, S. H., and Koob, G. F. (1998). Transition from moderate to excessive drug intake: Change in hedonic set point. *Science, 282*, 298–300.

al'Absi, M. (2006). Hypothalamic-pituitary-adrenocortical responses to psychological stress and risk for smoking relapse. *International Journal of Psychophysiology, 59*, 218–227.

al'Absi, M., Bongard, S., Buchanan, T., Pincomb, G. A., Licinio, J., and Lovallo, W. R. (1997). Cardiovascular and neuroendocrine adjustment to public speaking and mental arithmetic stressors. *Psychophysiology, 34*, 266–275.

American Psychiatric Association. (1994). *Diagnostic and statistical manual of mental disorders*. Washington, D.C.: Author.

Aston–Jones, G., Ennis, M., Pieribone, R. A., Nickell, W. T., and Shipley, M. T. (1986). The brain nucleus locus coeruleus: Restricted afferent control of a broad efferent network. *Science, 234*, 734–737.

Babor, T. F., Hofmann, M., DelBoca, F. K., Hesselbrock, V., Meyer, R. E., Dolinsky, Z. S., et al. (1992). Types of alcoholics, I. Evidence for an empirically derived typology based on indicators of vulnerability and severity. *Archives of General Psychiatry, 49*, 599–608.

Baird, J. R., and Lewis, J. J. (1964). The effects of cocaine, amphetamine and some amphetamine-like compounds on the in vivo levels of noradrenaline and dopamine in the rat brain. *Biochemical Pharmacology, 13*, 1475–1482.

Barone, J. J., and Roberts, H. R., (1996). Caffeine consumption. *Food and Chemical Toxicology, 34*, 119–129.

Bechara, A., Damasio, H., and Damasio, A. R. (2003). Role of the amygdala in decision-making. *Annals of the New York Academy of Sciences, 985*, 356–369.

Bechara, A., Damasio, H., Damasio, A. R., and Lee, G. P. (1999). Different contributions of the human amygdala and ventromedial prefrontal cortex to decision-making. *Journal of Neuroscience, 19*, 5473–5481.

Bernardy, N. C., King, A. C., Parsons, O. A., and Lovallo, W. R. (1996). Altered cortisol response in sober alcoholics: An examination of contributing factors. *Alcohol, 13*, 493–498.

Beuten, J., Payne, T. J., Ma, J. Z., and Li, M. D. (2006). Significant association of catechol-O-methyltransferase (COMT) haplotypes with nicotine dependence in male and female smokers of two ethnic populations. *Neuropsychopharmacology, 31*, 675–684.

Breese, G. R., Chu, K., Dayas, C. V., Funk, D., Knapp, D. J., Koob, G. F., et al. (2005). Stress enhancement of craving during sobriety: A risk for relapse. *Alcoholism, Clinical and Experimental Research, 29*, 185–195.

Buchanan, T. W., Brechtel, A., Sollers, J. J., and Lovallo, W. R. (2001). Exogenous cortisol exerts effects on the startle reflex independent of emotional modulation. *Pharmacology, Biochemistry, and Behavior, 68*, 203–210.

Buchanan, T. W., and Lovallo, W. R. (2001). Enhanced memory for emotional material following stress-level cortisol treatment in humans. *Psychoneuroendocrinology, 26*, 307–317.

Cadoret, R. J., Yates, W. R., Troughton, E., Woodworth, G., and Stewart, M. A. (1995). Adoption study demonstrating two genetic pathways to drug abuse. *Archives of General Psychiatry, 52*, 42–52.

Cahill, L., Babinsky, R., Markowitsch, H. J., and McGaugh, J. L. (1995). The amygdala and emotional memory. *Nature, 377*, 295–296.

Carr, K. D., Kutchukhidze, N., and Park, T. H. (1999). Differential effects of mu and kappa opioid antagonists on Fos-like immunoreactivity in extended amygdala. *Brain Research, 822*, 34–42.

Caspi, A., McClay, J., Moffitt, T. E., Mill, J., Martin, J., Craig, I. W., et al. (2002). Role of genotype in the cycle of violence in maltreated children. *Science, 297*, 851–854.

Caspi, A., Sugden, K., Moffitt, T. E., Taylor, A., Craig, I. W., Harrington, H., et al. (2003). Influence of life stress on depression: Moderation by a polymorphism in the 5-HTT gene. *Science, 301*, 386–389.

Cloninger, C. R. (1987). Neurogenetic adaptive mechanisms in alcoholism. *Science, 236*, 410–416.

Cloninger, C. R., Bohman, M., and Sigvardsson, S. (1981). Inheritance of alcohol abuse: Cross fostering analysis of adopted men. *Archives of General Psychiatry, 38*, 861–868.

Cloninger, C. R., and Reich, T. (1983). Genetic heterogeneity in alcoholism and sociopathy. *Research Publication of the Association for Research in Nervous and Mental Disease, 60*, 145–166.

Czeisler, C. A., and Klerman, E. B. (1999). Circadian and sleep-dependent regulation of hormone release in humans. *Recent Progress in Hormone Research, 54*, 97–130; discussion 130–132.

Dai, X., Thavundayil, J., and Gianoulakis, C. (2002). Response of the hypothalamic-pituitary-adrenal axis to stress in the absence and presence of ethanol in subjects at high and low risk of alcoholism. *Neuropsychopharmacology, 27*, 442–452.

Damasio, A. R. (1994). *Descartes' error: Emotion, reason, and the human brain.* New York, NY: G.P. Putnam's Sons.

Da Silva, G. E., Ramos, A., and Takahashi, R. N. (2004). Comparison of voluntary ethanol intake by two pairs of rat lines used as genetic models of anxiety. *Brazilian Journal of Medical and Biological Research, 37*, 1511–1517.

Davis, M. (2000). The role of the amygdala in conditioned and unconditioned fear and anxiety. In J. P. Aggleton (Ed.), *The amygdala: A functional analysis* (pp. 213–287). Oxford, England: Oxford University Press.

Dawes, M. A., Dorn, L. D., Moss, H. B., Yao, J. K., Kirisci, L., Ammerman, R. T., et al. (1999). Hormonal and behavioral homeostasis in boys at risk for substance abuse. *Drug and Alcohol Dependence, 55*, 165–176.

de Jong, I. E., and de Kloet, E. R. (2004). Glucocorticoids and vulnerability to psychostimulant drugs: Toward substrate and mechanism. *Annals of the New York Academy of Sciences, 1018*, 192–198.

Dick, D. M., and Foroud, T. (2003). Candidate genes for alcohol dependence: A review of genetic evidence from human studies. *Alcoholism, Clinical and Experimental Research, 27*, 868–879.

Drevets, W. C., Gautier, C., Price, J. C., Kupfer, D. J., Kinahan, P. E., Grace, A. A., et al. (2001). Amphetamine-induced dopamine release in human ventral striatum correlates with euphoria. *Biological Psychiatry, 49*, 81–96.

Errico, A. L., Parsons, O. A., King, A. C., and Lovallo, W. R. (1993). Attenuated cortisol response to biobehavioral stressors in sober alcoholics. *Journal of Studies on Alcohol, 54*, 393–398.

Finn, P. R. (2002). Motivation, working memory, and decision making: A cognitive-motivational theory of personality vulnerability to alcoholism. *Behavioral and Cognitive Neuroscience Reviews, 1*, 183–205.

Finn, P. R., Mazas, C. A., Justus, A. N., and Steinmetz, J. (2002). Early-onset alcoholism with conduct disorder: Go/no go learning deficits, working memory capacity, and personality. *Alcoholism, Clinical and Experimental Research, 26*, 186–206.

Gerra, G., Baldaro, B., Zaimovic, A., Moi, G., Bussandri, M., Raggi, M. A., et al. (2003). Neuroendocrine responses to experimentally-induced emotions among abstinent opioid-dependent subjects. *Drug and Alcohol Dependence, 71*, 25–35.

Gerra, G., Bassignana, S., Zaimovic, A., Moi, G., Bussandri, M., Caccavari, R., et al. (2003). Hypothalamic-pituitary-adrenal axis responses to stress in subjects with 3,4-methylenedioxy-methamphetamine ('ecstasy') use history: Correlation with dopamine receptor sensitivity. *Psychiatry Research, 120*, 115–124.

Goldman, D., Oroszi, G., and Ducci, F. (2005). The genetics of addictions: Uncovering the genes. *Nature Reviews. Genetics, 6*, 521–532.

Gough, H. (1994). Theory, development, and interpretation of the CPI socialization scale. *Psychological Reports, 75*, 651–700.

Grant, S. J., Huang, Y. H., and Redmond, D. E., Jr. (1988). Behavior of monkeys during opiate withdrawal and locus coeruleus stimulation. *Pharmacology, Biochemistry, and Behavior, 30*, 13–19.

Grant, S. J., and Redmond, D. E., Jr. (1981). The neuroanatomy and pharmacology of the nucleus locus coeruleus. *Progress in Clinical Biological Research, 71*, 5–27.

Hellbach, S., Gartner, P., Deicke, J., Fischer, D., Hassan, A. H., and Almeida, O. F. (1998). Inherent glucocorticoid response potential of isolated hypothalamic neuroendocrine neurons. *The FASEB Journal, 12*, 199–207.

Herkenham, M., Edley, S. M., and Stuart, J. (1984). Cell clusters in the nucleus accumbens of the rat, and the mosaic relationship of opiate receptors, acetylcholinesterase and subcortical afferent terminations. *Neuroscience, 11*, 561–593.

Ishiguro, H., Haruo Shibuya, T., Toru, M., Saito, T., and Arinami, T. (1999). Association study between high and low activity polymorphism of catechol-O-methyltransferase gene and alcoholism. *Psychiatric Genetics, 9*, 135–138.

Iversen, S., Kupfermann, I., and Kandel, E. R. (2000). Emotional states and feelings. In E. R. Kandel, Schwartz, J. H. and T. M. Jessell (Eds.), *Priniciples of Neural Science* (4th ed., pp. 982–997). New York: McGraw-Hill.

Johann, M., Bobbe, G., Putzhammer, A., and Wodarz, N. (2003). Comorbidity of alcohol dependence with attention-deficit hyperactivity disorder: Differences in phenotype with increased severity of the substance disorder, but not in genotype (serotonin transporter and 5-hydroxytryptamine-2c receptor). *Alcoholism, Clinical and Experimental Research, 27*, 1527–1534.

King, A. C., Schluger, J., Gunduz, M., Borg, L., Perret, G., Ho, A., et al. (2002). Hypothalamic-pituitary-adrenocortical (HPA) axis response and biotransformation of oral naltrexone: Preliminary examination of relationship to family history of alcoholism. *Neuropsychopharmacology, 26*, 778–788.

Knapp, D. J., Kampov-Polevoy, A. B., Overstreet, D. H., Breese, G. R., and Rezvani, A. H. (1997). Ultrasonic vocalization behavior differs between lines of ethanol-preferring and nonpreferring rats. *Alcoholism, Clinical and Experimental Research, 21*, 1232–1240.

Koob, G. F. (2003). Alcoholism: Allostasis and beyond. *Alcoholism, Clinical and Experimental Research, 27*, 232–243.

Koob, G. F., and Bloom, F. E. (1988). Cellular and molecular mechanisms of drug dependence. *Science, 242*, 715–723.

Koob, G. F., and Le Moal, M. (1997). Drug abuse: Hedonic homeostatic dysregulation. *Science, 278*, 52–58.

Koob, G. F., Rassnick, S., Heinrichs, S., and Weiss, F. (1994). Alcohol, the reward system and dependence. *EXS, 71*, 103–114.

Koob, G. F., Vaccarino, F. J., Amalric, M., and Bloom, F. E. (1986). Neurochemical substrates for opiate reinforcement. *NIDA Research Monographs, 71*, 146–164.

Kreek, M. J. (1996). Opiates, opioids and addiction. *Molecular Psychiatry, 1*, 232–254.

Kreek, M. J., Bart, G., Lilly, C., LaForge, K. S., and Nielsen, D. A. (2005). Pharmacogenetics and human molecular genetics of opiate and cocaine addictions and their treatments. *Pharmacological Reviews, 57*, 1–26.

Kreek, M. J., Nielsen, D. A., Butelman, E. R., and LaForge, K. S. (2005). Genetic influences on impulsivity, risk taking, stress responsivity and vulnerability to drug abuse and addiction. *Nature Neuroscience, 8*, 1450–1457.

LaBar, K. S., Crupain, M. J., Voyvodic, J. T., and McCarthy, G. (2003). Dynamic perception of facial affect and identity in the human brain. *Cerebral Cortex, 13*, 1023–1033.

Langbehn, D. R., Cadoret, R. J., Caspers, K., Troughton, E. P., and Yucuis, R. (2003). Genetic and environmental risk factors for the onset of drug use and problems in adoptees. *Drug and Alcohol Dependence, 69*, 151–167.

Li, T., Vallada, H., Curtis, D., Arranz, M., Xu, K., Cai, G., et al. (1997). Catechol-O-methyltransferase Val158Met polymorphism: Frequency analysis in Han Chinese subjects and allelic association of the low activity allele with bipolar affective disorder. *Pharmacogenetics, 7*, 349–353.

Lipsky, R. H., Sparling, M. B., Ryan, L. M., Xu, K., Salazar, A. M., Goldman, D., et al. (2005). Association of COMT Val158Met genotype with executive functioning following traumatic brain injury. *Journal of Neuropsychiatry and Clinical Neurosciences, 17*, 465–471.

Lovallo, W. R. (2005). *Stress and health: Biological and psychological interactions* (2nd ed.). Thousand Oaks, CA: Sage Publications.

Lovallo, W. R. (2006). Cortisol secretion patterns in addiction and addiction risk. *International Journal of Psychophysiology, 59*, 195–202.

Lovallo, W. R., Yechiam, E., Sorocco, K. H., Vincent, A. S., and Collins, F. L. (2006). Working memory and decision-making biases in young adults with a family history of alcoholism: Studies from the Oklahoma Family Health Patterns Project. *Alcoholism, Clinical and Experimental Research, 30.* 763–773.

Lyons, D., and Porrino, L. J. (1997). Dopamine depletion in the rostral nucleus accumbens alters the cerebral metabolic response to cocaine in the rat. *Brain Research, 753,* 69–79.

Mazas, C. A., Finn, P. R., and Steinmetz, J. E. (2000). Decision-making biases, antisocial personality, and early-onset alcoholism. *Alcoholism, Clinical and Experimental Research, 24,* 1036–1040.

Milanes, M. V., Laorden, M. L., Chapleur-Chateau, M., and Burlet, A. (1998). Alterations in corticotropin-releasing factor and vasopressin content in rat brain during morphine withdrawal: Correlation with hypothalamic noradrenergic activity and pituitary-adrenal response. *Journal of Pharmacology and Experimental Therapeutics, 285,* 700–706.

Moffitt, T. E., Caspi, A., and Rutter, M. (2006). Measured gene-environment interactions in psychopathology. *Perspectives in Psychological Science, 1,* 5–27.

Moss, H. B., Vanyukov, M., Yao, J. K., and Kirillova, G. P. (1999). Salivary cortisol responses in prepubertal boys: The effects of parental substance abuse and association with drug use behavior during adolescence. *Biological Psychiatry, 45,* 1293–1299.

Moss, H. B., Vanyukov, M. M., and Martin, C. S. (1995). Salivary cortisol responses and the risk for substance abuse in prepubertal boys. *Biological Psychiatry, 38,* 547–555.

Nicola, S. M., Taha, S. A., Kim, S. W., and Fields, H. L. (2005). Nucleus accumbens dopamine release is necessary and sufficient to promote the behavioral response to reward-predictive cues. *Neuroscience, 135,* 1025–1033.

Okuda, S., Roozendaal, B., and McGaugh, J. L. (2004). Glucocorticoid effects on object recognition memory require training-associated emotional arousal. *Proceedings of the National Academy of Sciences of the United States of America, 101,* 853–858.

Oswald, L. M., Wong, D. F., McCaul, M., Zhou, Y., Kuwabara, H., Choi, L., et al. (2005). Relationships among ventral striatal dopamine release, cortisol secretion, and subjective responses to amphetamine. *Neuropsychopharmacology, 30,* 821–832.

Petrusz, P., and Merchenthaler, I. (1992). The corticotropin-releasing factor system. In C. B. Nemeroff (Ed.), *Neuroendocrinology* (1st ed., pp. 129–183). Boca Raton, FL: CRC Press.

Rainnie, D. G., Bergeron, R., Sajdyk, T. J., Patil, M., Gehlert, D. R., and Shekhar, A. (2004). Corticotropin releasing factor-induced synaptic plasticity in the amygdala translates stress into emotional disorders. *Journal of Neuroscience, 24,* 3471–3479.

Reul, J. M., and de Kloet, E. R. (1986). Anatomical resolution of two types of corticosterone receptor sites in rat brain with in vitro autoradiography and comput-

erized image analysis. *Journal of Steroid Biochemistry, 24,* 269–272.

Ridderinkhof, K. R., Ullsperger, M., Crone, E. A., and Nieuwenhuis, S. (2004). The role of the medial frontal cortex in cognitive control. *Science, 306,* 443–447.

Rodriguez de Fonseca, F., Carrera, M. R., Navarro, M., Koob, G. F., and Weiss, F. (1997). Activation of corticotropin-releasing factor in the limbic system during cannabinoid withdrawal. *Science, 276,* 2050–2054.

Rolls, E. T. (2000a). Precis of the brain and emotion. *The Behavioral and Brain Sciences, 23,* 177–191; discussion 192–233.

Rolls, E. T. (2000b). The orbitofrontal cortex and reward. *Cerebral Cortex, 10,* 284–294.

Rolls, E. T., and Stringer, S. M. (2001). A model of the interaction between mood and memory. *Network, 12,* 89–109.

Saal, D., Dong, Y., Bonci, A., and Malenka, R. C. (2003). Drugs of abuse and stress trigger a common synaptic adaptation in dopamine neurons. *Neuron, 37,* 577–582.

Sanchez, M. M., Young, L. J., Plotsky, P. M., and Insel, T. R. (2000). Distribution of corticosteroid receptors in the rhesus brain: Relative absence of glucocorticoid receptors in the hippocampal formation. *Journal of Neuroscience, 20,* 4657–4668.

Sapolsky, R. M., Krey, L. C., and McEwen, B. S. (1985). Prolonged glucocorticoid exposure reduces hippocampal neuron number: Implications for aging. *Journal of Neuroscience, 5,* 1222–1227.

Sapolsky, R. M., Meaney, M. J., and McEwen, B. S. (1985). The development of the glucocorticoid receptor system in the rat limbic brain. III. Negative-feedback regulation. *Brain Research, 350,* 169–173.

Selye, H. (1936). Thymus and adrenals in the response of the organism to injuries and intoxications. *British Journal of Experimental Pathology, 17,* 234–248.

Shedler, J., and Block, J. (1990). Adolescent drug use and psychological health. *American Psychologist, 45,* 612–630.

Shepard, J. D., Barron, K. W., and Myers, D. A. (2000). Corticosterone delivery to the amygdala increases corticotropin-releasing factor mRNA in the central amygdaloid nucleus and anxiety-like behavior. *Brain Research, 861,* 288–295.

Shepard, J. D., Barron, K. W., and Myers, D. A. (2003). Stereotaxic localization of corticosterone to the amygdala enhances hypothalamo-pituitary-adrenal responses to behavioral stress. *Brain Research, 963,* 203–213.

Sher, K. J., Walitzer, K. S., Wood, P. K., and Brent, E. E. (1991). Characteristics of children of alcoholics: Putative risk factors, substance use and abuse, and psychopathology. *Journal of Abnormal Psychology, 100,* 427–448.

Shidara, M., and Richmond, B. J. (2002). Anterior cingulate: Single neuronal signals related to degree of reward expectancy. *Science, 296,* 1709–1711.

Shifman, S., Bronstein, M., Sternfeld, M., Pisante-Shalom, A., Lev-Lehman, E., Weizman, A., et al. (2002). A highly significant association between a COMT haplotype and schizophrenia. *American Journal of Human Genetics, 71*, 1296–1302.

Shoblock, J. R., and Maidment, N. T. (2006). Constitutively active mu opioid receptors mediate the enhanced conditioned aversive effect of naloxone in morphine-dependent mice. *Neuropsychopharmacology, 31*, 171–177.

Sinha, R., Catapano, D., and O'Malley, S. (1999). Stress induced craving and stress response in cocaine dependent individuals. *Psychopharmacology, 142*, 343–351.

Sinha, R., Talih, M., Malison, R., Cooney, N., Anderson, G. M., and Kreek, M. J. (2003). Hypothalamic-pituitary-adrenal axis and sympatho-adreno-medullary responses during stress-induced and drug cue-induced cocaine craving states. *Psychopharmacology, 170*, 62–72.

Smolka, M. N., Schumann, G., Wrase, J., Grusser, S. M., Flor, H., Mann, K., et al. (2005). Catechol-O-methyltransferase val158met genotype affects processing of emotional stimuli in the amygdala and prefrontal cortex. *Journal of Neuroscience, 25*, 836–842.

Sorocco, K. H., Lovallo, W. R., Vincent, A. S., and Collins, F. L. (2006). Blunted hypothalamic-pituitary-adrenocortical axis responsivity to stress in persons with a family history of alcoholism. *International Journal of Psychophysiology, 58*, 210–217.

Sterling, P., and Eyer, J. (1988). Allostasis: A new paradigm to explain arousal pathology. In S. Fisher, Reason, J. (Eds.), *Handbook of life stress, cognition, and health* (pp. 629–649). New York: John Wiley and Sons, Ltd.

Swanson, L. W. (2000). Cerebral hemisphere regulation of motivated behavior. *Brain Research, 886*, 113–164.

Swanson, L. W., Sawchenko, P. E., Rivier, J., and Vale, W. W. (1983). Organization of ovine corticotropin-releasing factor immunoreactive cells and fibers in the rat brain: An immunohistochemical study. *Neuroendocrinology, 36*, 165–186.

Tapert, S. F., Baratta, M. V., Abrantes, A. M., and Brown, S. A. (2002). Attention dysfunction predicts substance involvement in community youths. *Journal of the American Academy of Child and Adolescent Psychiatry, 41*, 680–686.

Tobler, P. N., Fiorillo, C. D., and Schultz, W. (2005). Adaptive coding of reward value by dopamine neurons. *Science, 307*, 1642–1645.

Uhart, M., Oswald, L. M., McCaul, M., Chong, R., and Wand, G. S. (2006). Hormonal responses to psychological stress and family history of alcoholism. *Neurospychopharmacology*. (In Press). 1–9.

Valdez, G. R., Roberts, A. J., Chan, K., Davis, H., Brennan, M., Zorrilla, E. P., et al. (2002). Increased ethanol self-administration and anxiety-like behavior during acute ethanol withdrawal and protracted abstinence: Regulation by corticotropin-releasing factor. *Alcoholism, Clinical and Experimental Research, 26*, 1494–1501.

Valdez, G. R., Sabino, V., and Koob, G. F. (2004). Increased anxiety-like behavior and ethanol self-administration in dependent rats: Reversal via corticotropin-releasing factor-2 receptor activation. *Alcoholism, Clinical and Experimental Research, 28*, 865–872.

Valdez, G. R., Zorrilla, E. P., Roberts, A. J., and Koob, G. F. (2003). Antagonism of corticotropin-releasing factor attenuates the enhanced responsiveness to stress observed during protracted ethanol abstinence. *Alcohol, 29*, 55–60.

Valentino, R. J., Page, M., Van Bockstaele, E., and Aston-Jones, G. (1992). Corticotropin-releasing factor innervation of the locus coeruleus region: Distribution of fibers and sources of input. *Neuroscience, 48*, 689–705.

Vandenbergh, D. J., Rodriguez, L. A., Miller, I. T., Uhl, G. R., and Lachman, H. M. (1997). High-activity catechol-O-methyltransferase allele is more prevalent in polysubstance abusers. *American Journal of Medical Genetics, 74*, 439–442.

Wand, G. S., Mangold, D., El Deiry, S., McCaul, M. E., and Hoover, D. (1998). Family history of alcoholism and hypothalamic opioidergic activity. *Archives of General Psychiatry, 55*, 1114–1119.

Wand, G. S., McCaul, M. E., Gotjen, D., Reynolds, J., and Lee, S. (2001). Confirmation that offspring from families with alcohol-dependent individuals have greater hypothalamic-pituitary-adrenal axis activation induced by naloxone compared with offspring without a family history of alcohol dependence. *Alcoholism, Clinical and Experimental Research, 25*, 1134–1139.

Yun, I. A., Wakabayashi, K. T., Fields, H. L., and Nicola, S. M. (2004). The ventral tegmental area is required for the behavioral and nucleus accumbens neuronal firing responses to incentive cues. *Journal of Neuroscience, 24*, 2923–2933.

Zimmermann, U., Spring, K., Kunz-Ebrecht, S. R., Uhr, M., Wittchen, H. U., and Holsboer, F. (2004). Effect of ethanol on hypothalamic-pituitary-adrenal system response to psychosocial stress in sons of alcohol-dependent fathers. *Neuropsychopharmacology, 29*, 1156–1165.

Zubieta, J. K., Heitzeg, M. M., Smith, Y. R., Bueller, J. A., Xu, K., Xu, Y., et al. (2003). COMT val158met genotype affects mu-opioid neurotransmitter responses to a pain stressor. *Science, 299*, 1240–1243.

12

Addiction and Stress in Adolescents

SUSAN R. TATE, KATHERINE A. PATTERSON, BONNIE J. NAGEL,
KRISTEN G. ANDERSON, AND SANDRA A. BROWN

We briefly summarize the unique biological, cognitive, emotional, and psychosocial developmental transitions occurring throughout these years. With this essential foundation for understanding adolescent interpretation and management of life challenges, we discuss assessment and evaluation of prevalent stressors during this developmental period and the interplay of stress and alcohol and drug use behaviors of youth. Adolescent-specific stressors, gender considerations, and consequences of life stress for substance involvement and later development are presented. We highlight empirical findings that clarify the bidirectional relations of stress and the initiation, progression, and escalation of substance use in youth. Risk and protective factors, moderating influences, and cumulative developmental consequences are considered.

I. INTRODUCTION

Adolescence is a period characterized by significant developmental changes spanning multiple domains of functioning: biological, cognitive, emotional, and psychosocial. To the extent that stress is conceptualized in terms of change and adjustment, adolescence is clearly a stressful time. In addition to stress inherently associated with adolescent development, external stressors (e.g., family conflicts, health problems, financial stress) also contribute to the stress load during these years. There is ample evidence to support this view of high stress during the teen years from both adolescent self-reports and the reports of adults interacting with them (Buchanan and Holmbeck, 1998; Gest et al., 1999; Offer et al., 1981). Although research has not always supported the characterization of adolescence as inevitably stressful (Eccles et al., 1993; Offer and Schonert-Reichl, 1992), findings have consistently documented adolescence as "the period when storm and stress is *more likely* to occur than at other ages" (Arnett, 1999).

The relationship between developmental shifts in functioning and the emergence of adolescent substance involvement is reciprocal and synergistic. Similarly, life stress has a bidirectional relationship with changes in functioning across these major areas. The influence of normal developmental change on adolescent substance use must be considered within the context of their complex interaction with environmental stressors and preexisting characteristics of the individual.

We first summarize the developmental transitions occurring in adolescence and then describe stress-related issues specific to the adolescent years. With this foundation, we proceed to present findings on life stress in relation to addiction in adolescence followed by recommendations for clinical and research work with this age group.

II. ADOLESCENT DEVELOPMENT

Perhaps the most salient event associated with early adolescence is the onset of puberty. During puberty, there is triggering of the biological systems responsible for adrenal and gonadal hormone secretion. Research has demonstrated that fluctuations in hormone levels impact levels of emotional arousal, sensation seeking, and motivation (Buchanan et al., 1992; Halpern et al., 1998; Martin et al., 2002), which ultimately drive changes in adolescent behavior.

Further complicating hormone-related changes, there is evidence to suggest that adolescents experience greater psychophysiological response to stressful environmental stimuli (Miller and Shields, 1980). Elevated exposure to stress can activate the hypothalamic-pituitary-adrenal (HPA) axis, increasing glucocorticoid release, and by way of triggering the release of gonadal steroids, ultimately may lead to the early onset of puberty (Walker et al., 2004). It has been demonstrated that, while later pubertal maturation is associated with higher levels of psychopathology in boys (Graber et al., 1997), early pubertal onset is particularly stressful for girls (Tremblay and Frigon, 2005). The hormonal perturbations of puberty, in concert with the increase in psychosocial stress during adolescence, appear to play a role in modulating development of the neurocognitive systems that

underlie the regulation of emotion (for review, see Cameron, 2004). The perception and processing of social or emotional stimuli may further exacerbate responses to stress during adolescence, as social relationships are rapidly changing, and peer relationships emerge as more central (Steinberg and Morris, 2001). With greater levels of stress and emotional responsiveness, the need to be able to regulate affect and behavior becomes increasingly important. However, many of the biomaturational changes that heighten a teen's emotional arousal and motivation occur prior to the neuromaturation and development of cognitive functions that allow more sophisticated cognition and regulation of behavior.

In addition to early hormone-related biological processes, a number of continuing neuromaturational processes occur throughout adolescence. Recently, attention has been given to the developing prefrontal cortex, a region that undergoes both progressive and regressive change throughout adolescence and into adulthood. Specifically, there are increases in prefrontal white matter volume and density (Giedd et al., 1999; Paus et al., 1999), which are thought to reflect a greater degree of axonal myelination allowing for more efficient communication and connectivity with other brain regions. Concomitantly, there are decreases in prefrontal gray matter and density across adolescence (Giedd et al., 1999; Gogtay et al., 2004) reflecting synaptic pruning, needed for more efficient processing. There is some degree of gender specificity for the timing of these changes, with females typically maturing earlier than males in most brain regions (Durston et al., 2001; Giedd et al., 1999). The prefrontal cortex is most known for the role that it plays in higher level abstract cognition and in the control and modulation of cognitive processes such as inhibition, cognitive monitoring, and affective control (Fuster, 2002). Each of these cognitive functions improves across the adolescent age-range

(Luciana et al., 2005). Further, maturation of the circuitry between frontal and emotion-processing limbic systems allows for greater affective control and modulation of emotional responsiveness and affective functioning (Chambers et al., 2003; Nelson et al., 2005). As mentioned earlier, the pubertal heightening of emotional responsiveness to stress precedes the development of these higher-level cognitive functions that allow the teen to regulate, inhibit, and contextually process information.

Subserved by the many biological and neuromaturational alterations that occur during adolescence, a number of changes in cognitive processing impact a teen's ability to regulate both behavior and emotion. In addition to the likely contribution of hormonal changes, role transitions, and environmental stressors to the emotional volatility in the teen years, self-regulation skills for managing emotional states are also less mature for adolescents than adults (Cauffman and Steinberg, 2000; Gross et al., 1997). The neuromaturational processes occurring throughout adolescence allow for greater executive control over one's ability to inhibit, control, and modulate behavior. Improvements in these cognitive functions enhance one's ability to more accurately perceive, process, and cope with stressful and emotional stimuli.

Accompanying the biological and cognitive developmental changes, adolescence is a period marked by changes in emotionality. Negative affect is higher during adolescence than at any other developmental stage (Buchanan et al., 1992; Petersen et al., 1993), including frequently reported feelings of depression, embarrassment, awkwardness, loneliness, and nervousness. Findings of one review suggested that more than one-third of adolescents experience significant levels of depressed mood at any given time (Petersen et al., 1993). Adolescents also report more intense or extreme emotional reactions than do other age groups (Larson and Richards, 1994). Accompanying this

increase in the intensity and negativity of mood states are notable declines in positive emotional states (e.g., happy, proud, in control; Larson and Richards, 1994). Thus, adolescents face the challenge of managing significant emotional lability at a time when assistance in regulating and soothing affective distress previously provided by adults is declining.

Marked psychosocial challenges are salient throughout adolescence. Although the family environment remains important, peer influences become a central focus. In addition to the increased significance placed on peer relations, there are qualitative changes within the teen's social sphere, including the introduction of dating and intimate relations. Adolescents must navigate increasingly complex social relationships, without the adult guidance provided during childhood. Additionally, teens must learn to adeptly transition from one context (home, school, peers) to another, and in adolescence above any other developmental period, the behavioral expectations are markedly different across these contexts.

Across these changing social contexts, adolescents continue the process of exploring and defining a cohesive self-identity. In Erikson's influential social stages framework, successful adolescent development is conceptualized as a time of identity formation (Erikson, 1959). Shifts in self-identity, coupled with increased autonomy and perceptions of invulnerability, are associated with experimentation with new behaviors, some of which may have serious implications for the future. Teens can evidence a clear lack of future orientation, exhibiting high levels of risk taking behaviors with the potential for negative long-term or even lifelong consequences. Risk-taking behaviors common in adolescence include dangerous driving, risky sexual activity, and substance misuse (Fergusson and Lynskey, 1996; Halpern-Felsher et al., 1996; Jonah, 1990; Spear, 2002). Substance use may additionally elevate sexual risk taking and other risky behaviors in adolescence (Aarons et al., 2003; Tapert et al., 2001).

III. LIFE STRESS IN ADOLESCENCE

A. Assessment

One critical challenge associated with life stress research is the task of clearly defining the construct of interest. Consequently, inconsistencies in measurement are pervasive in both the adult and adolescent stress literature. With a focus on adolescent development, Grant and colleagues (2003) defined stressors as "environmental events or chronic conditions that objectively threaten the physical and/or psychological health or well-being of individuals of a particular age in a particular society." This expanded objective definition acknowledges that stressors in adolescence differ in their impact from other periods during the life span. Objective definitions for life stressors have been advocated in both the adult and adolescent literature to avoid confounds associated with subjective cognitive influences, subjective perceptions of stress related to personality and temperament, and personal meaning attributed to stressors post hoc based on subsequent consequences (Brown and Harris, 1989; Grant et al., 2003; O'Doherty and Davies, 1987). Of particular importance in relation to addiction is the distinction between life stressors which occur independent of substance use and those stressors occurring as a result of substance involvement (O'Doherty and Davies, 1987; Vik and Brown, 1998).

The impact of a stressor may be influenced by its severity and chronicity. Severity of stressful life events during adolescence can range from minor daily hassles such as completing schoolwork to major losses and traumas. Stressors also vary by chronicity, some being ongoing stressful experiences (e.g., persistent conflict within the family, financial problems) and others being acute

events with a discrete occurrence (e.g., romantic break-up, automobile accident). During adolescence, stressors can also be classified in terms of their prevalence, ranging from universal (e.g., transition through puberty, academic tasks) to common (e.g., occasional conflict with siblings or parents) to rare (e.g., death of a parent, being injured in a gang fight).

As with adults, adolescent stress is typically assessed through the use of self-report checklists and structured interviews. Progress has been made in developing life stress assessments specifically for adolescent samples, with at least 11 general stressor checklists available (see Grant et al., 2004). Checklists vary widely and range from general measures, covering a broad range of potential stressors, to specialized instruments for specific populations of adolescents (e.g., teens belonging to a particular ethnic minority) or a specific domain of stressors (e.g., catastrophic events). The popularity of checklists is due, in large part, to their ease of administration relative to interview assessments. Criticisms of such checklists include the limitation on items available for endorsement, lack of information regarding temporal sequencing, and confounds related to the independence of stressors from a respondent's actions (Grant et al., 2004). Checklists can also result in duplicate endorsement of stressors under multiple items, and checklists seldom distinguish between acute and chronic stressors that have shown distinct relationships to substance involvement (Tate et al., 2005).

Stressor interviews offer an alternative method for identifying stressors that include consideration of contextual background and chronology. Despite being less cost effective due to increased time required for the adolescent, interviewer, and evaluating procedures, research with adults has generally supported the interviewing method as preferable to checklists (Gorman, 1993; Katschnig, 1986; McQuaid et al., 2000). However, one extensive review of child and adolescent life stress evaluation noted that less than 2% of the 500 studies utilized interview-based assessments, noting the substantially decreased time and financial cost associated with checklist measures (Grant et al., 2004).

B. Adolescent and Gender-Specific Stressors

As previously noted, teens frequently report high levels of life stress. Adolescents commonly endorse stress related to autonomy, emotional distress, and sexual issues and frequently report stressors associated with family problems, relocation, and accidents/illness (Brown, 1989). Ethnic minority adolescents may experience added challenge, given that many of these youth report experiencing racial discrimination perceived as highly stressful (Fisher et al., 2000; Outlaw, 1993). Universally experienced developmental changes can also be markedly stressful for adolescents when they occur out of the normal developmental sequence or time frame. For example, accelerated or delayed puberty/maturation may trigger adverse social consequences (Ellis, 2004), demonstrating the importance of the timing of specific life events. As in other developmental stages, the family environment and peer social networks can serve as both a source of support and a source of stress in relation to developmental changes. In adolescence, family disruption and parental substance use or other parental problems may lead to a cascade of stressful experiences (Brown, 1989). Figure 12-1 depicts a few examples of adolescent life stressors occurring in the context of background characteristics, environmental factors, and developmental considerations.

Gender is an important consideration in understanding the relations between stress and addiction during adolescence. Adolescent girls report experiencing more stressors than do adolescent boys (Ames, et al., 2005; Bruns and Geist, 1984; Compas and Phares, 1991; Jose and Ratcliffe, 2004). Further, there are gender differences in

perceptions of severity of stressful experiences, with adolescent girls showing greater stressor sensitivity than boys (Jose and Ratcliffe, 2004; Silberg et al., 1999; Wagner and Compas, 1990). Compas and Phares (1991) found that interpersonal stressors were viewed as more stressful by girls during early adolescence compared to boys of the same age. In a recently developed measure for minor stress experienced by youth, faking good and faking bad adjustment scales were included (Ames et al., 2005). Consistent with prior findings, girls reported more stress than boys, but girls did not differ on the faking bad scale, suggesting that girls are not merely exaggerating stress experiences. However, gender differences were observed in the faking good scale, with boys having significantly higher values. Thus, underreporting by boys, consistent with male gender roles, may result in minimization in reports of psychological distress and emotional expression during this developmental stage.

Gender-specific patterns in response to stressors have also been demonstrated among youth. Girls are more likely than boys to respond with internalizing reactions to severe life stress such as sexual abuse (Chandy et al., 1996; Jose and Ratcliffe, 2004), whereas boys have been shown to exhibit greater externalizing reactions to severe stressors (Chandy et al., 1996; Garnefski and Arends, 1998). Additionally, there appear to be gender-linked reactions to specific types of stressors. For example, physical abuse, but not sexual abuse, was related to depression and general distress among boys. However, for girls, sexual abuse, but not physical abuse, was related to depression and general distress (Meyerson et al., 2002). These stress response differences have implications for identification of youth in need of mental health services.

C. Consequences of Life Stress for Later Development

Stressful life experiences increase the risk for a variety of negative outcomes

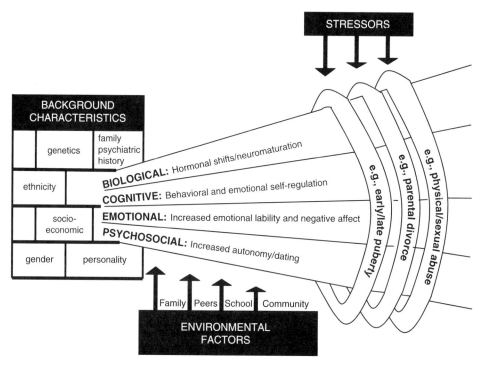

FIGURE 12-1   Adolescent life stress in the context of development.

during adolescence and later development. For example, life stress has been shown to contribute to early initiation of sexual intercourse (Waller and DuBois, 2004), and adolescents who exhibit early transition into puberty are also more likely to be sexually active compared to peers (Flannery et al., 1993). In turn, developmentally premature initiation of sexual intercourse during the adolescent years is associated with increased risk for sexually transmitted disease and pregnancy (CDC, 2000; Crockett et al., 1996).

Similarly, research documents a relationship between stressors in adolescence and risk for the development of psychopathology. In one review, 88% of studies supported a relationship between life stressors and child/adolescent psychopathology (Grant et al., 2004). The predictive value of specific types of stressors for later maladjustment may vary throughout the course of adolescence. For example, Wagner and Compas (1990) found that for young adolescents,

family stressors were significant predictors of psychopathology; for middle adolescents, peer stressors were more significant predictors; and for older adolescents, academic stressors were the strongest predictors of maladjustment. Experiencing severe stressors (physical/sexual assault, witnessing violence, severe neglect) increases the risk for substance use disorders during adolescence (Kilpatrick et al., 2000). Clearly, the relationship between stressors and psychopathology in adolescence is reciprocal, and there is the potential for this bidirectional relationship established in adolescence to evolve into a self-perpetuating cycle of stress and psychopathology that persists into adulthood.

IV. ADOLESCENT STRESS AND ADDICTIVE BEHAVIORS

The body of research on stress and addictive behaviors in adolescence has grown considerably in recent years. Adolescent drug use has been associated with retrospective reports of stress (Bruns and Geist, 1984), and concurrently, stressful life events have been associated with both alcohol and other drug use (Byrne and Mazanor, 1999; D'Elio et al., 1996; Windle, 1992). While some direct effects have been shown across time (Wills, 1986; Wills et al., 2002), cross-sectional and prospective studies have identified a number of moderating (Bates and Pandina, 1989; D'Elio et al., 1996; Nash et al., 2005; Wills et al., 2002) and mediating (Colder and Chassin, 1993; Newcomb and Harlow, 1986; Wills et al., 2004) influences on the youth stress-substance involvement relation. These mediating and moderating factors include individual characteristics (e.g., family history of substance use, self-control, coping skills) and environment factors (e.g., economic resources, family support, peer behavior). These findings suggest a complex interplay of risk and protective factors influencing stress and substance involvement over the course of adolescence (Dawes et al., 2000; Vik and Brown, 1998).

As mentioned above, life stress and life events are not equivalent over the course of human development. While transitions in parental influence and accelerations in peer influences are a hallmark of adolescence, the family environment is a stable influence for most individuals throughout childhood and adolescence. The family environment can exert both positive and negative influences on life stress experiences and substance involvement of youth. More positive family environment characteristics have been shown to predict less stress among high school students, and correspondingly, lower alcohol use (particularly for youth with high perceived parental disapproval for use; Nash et al., 2005). In addition to positive and negative influences, familial interactions differ along multiple dimensions (e.g., degree of support, level of conflict, cohesion) related to teen substance use. For example, in the

initial years following addiction treatment, families of abstaining teens experienced gradual steady increases in cohesiveness (commitment and support) and expressiveness (open communication), as well as decreases in familial conflict compared to families of teens who continued to drink or use heavily (Stewart and Brown, 1993). Both positive and negative life events have been implicated in a causal chain connecting the protective influence of parental support on adolescent substance use (Wills et al., 2004).

Most commonly, the focus of research has been on how risk factors within the family system, parental psychopathology in particular, lead to adolescent substance use. In a review of etiological factors, Zucker and Gomberg (1986) noted that parents of individuals who later developed alcohol disorders were more likely to be alcoholic, antisocial, or sexually deviant. Parental substance use, and subsequent family disruption, has been associated with stress and substance involvement in adolescence. Parental alcohol and drug abuse has been associated with greater stress among offspring (Brown, 1989; Johnson and Pandina, 1991) and lower parental attachment in adolescence (Johnson and Pandina, 1991). As suggested above, many of the effects of parental substance use and abuse unfold indirectly for youth. Some research suggests that stress from family conflict might mediate the relation between parental psychopathology, including alcoholism, and adolescent adjustment (i.e., adolescent substance use, negative affect, and associations with drug-using peers; Pillow et al., 1998). A retrospective study of adult women with alcoholic parents suggests that the experience of low family cohesion, more so than child and adolescent life stress, predicted adult alcohol problems (Griffin et al., 2005). In addition, the relations between life stress in children of alcoholics (ages 10–16) and youth drinking also are influenced by temperamental and other personal characteristics such as negative affect (Colder and Chassin, 1993).

While disruptions to the family system can be a function of parental substance use, divorce and youth substance use also serve to stress the family network. A number of forms of parental conflict and family disruption have been associated with greater teen drinking and development of alcohol disorders (Zucker and Gomberg, 1986). For example, among 7th and 10th grade students, youth from divorced families have been shown to have greater quantity and frequency of drinking than counterparts from nondivorced families (Burnside et al., 1986). Prospective investigation has demonstrated that across a 5-year period following parental divorce, boys increased their alcohol and drug use compared to girls and age-matched peers (Doherty and Needle, 1991). In general, children of divorced parents have been shown to have higher levels of life stress, less problem-focused coping, and more substance using friends and family members than children from intact marriages (Short, 1998). These family and personal factors were associated with greater substance use, aggressive behavior, and depression among youth ages 9–12 years.

The impact of substance use in the family environment is not one sided; youth substance involvement creates stress for the family system. Substance use disordered adolescents experience more life stress than their nondisordered peers, and greater inconsistency between parental use patterns and adolescent use patterns seems to exacerbate stress (Brown, 1987, 1989). Adolescent substance use and subsequent substance-related problems can tax family resources and cause disruption (Vik and Brown, 1998). A longitudinal study demonstrates that even among those youth who stop their abuse or dependence, extended abstinence is required before family relations return to normal (Stewart and Brown, 1993).

While families continue to influence adolescent behavior, major contextual changes unfold, particularly those involving peers, and become more salient across this period of development. Peer use and peer support have been consistently identified as mediators of the life stress-substance use relation for youth. In conjunction with their findings regarding parental support, Wills et al. (2004) found that peer support can have both risk and protective effects on adolescent drinking through influences on self-control to positive and negative life events. Associating with heavy-using peers can expose youth to higher levels of substance-related problems, greater access to substances, and environments supportive of risky and deviant behaviors (Brown et al., 1989). These problems, both within and external to the family, can lead to increased stress on the adolescent and the family system.

Individual factors, such as self-regulation and coping, have been implicated in the adolescent stress-substance use relation. Wills and colleagues (2002) found that the negative impact of adolescent life events on substance use was significantly higher for youth with poor self-control. Youth with less developed self-regulation skills may also react more strongly to life stress, making them prone to use substance use as a coping strategy (Wills et al., 1999). Coping strategies are important predictors of both adolescent substance use and treatment outcomes (Myers et al., 1993; Vaccaro and Wills 1998). In school-based samples of young adolescents, both life stress and coping influence the level of substance use and rate of change in use across time (Wills et al., 2001). Among community youth, life stress and coping by disengagement serve as risks for substance use, whereas behavioral coping efforts decrease substance use. Life stress pertaining to exposure to gangs and violence in conjunction with avoidance and withdrawal coping, peer use, and availability of substances were found to predict teen alcohol use

(Allison et al., 1997). For marijuana use, this type of stress, positive action coping, peer use, and pressure to use were also associated among high school students. In addition, coping and life stress have been shown to interact in predicting substance use outcomes for substance use disordered youth after treatment such that the ability to cope with the temptation to use in social situations reduced the rates of substance use 6 months after treatment for youth with higher levels of life stress (Anderson et al., In press).

V. IMPLICATIONS FOR ADOLESCENT ADDICTION INTERVENTIONS

A. Prevention

Many prevention programs incorporate adolescent interest and competence with computers. Findings from a CD-ROM drug prevention intervention with junior high school students indicated improvements in pro-drug attitudes, normative impressions of peer and adult substance use, anxiety reduction skills, and relaxation skills knowledge (Williams et al., 2005). CD-ROM and web-based prevention interventions are quite promising, given their relatively low cost and accessibility across multiple settings (e.g., home, school, library; Skinner et al., 2001).

Schools also provide an ideal opportunity for reaching a "captive" adolescent audience. As a result, many prevention efforts are school-based. Advantages of school-based interventions include limited reliance on parents to provide transportation or funding for services. When high school students were provided a choice of selecting a group, individual, or web-based format for an alcohol intervention, the majority of teens selected a group format (Project Options; D'Amico et al., under review). However, 17% of participating students selected the individual or web-based

formats, and minority youth disproportionately sought these more private types of services (D'Amico et al., under review). Thus, providing multiple choices is important to reaching larger numbers of teens.

We have previously reported research evidence documenting a stress-substance use relationship in adolescence. One possibility for preventing escalation of alcohol and drug use is through provision of alternative skills for managing life stress. Although most stress management interventions have focused on adults, preliminary findings suggest that similar stress reduction interventions may prove beneficial for adolescents coping with stressors (Hains and Szyjakowski, 1990).

B. Treatment

Youth who have already begun abusing alcohol report they would be less likely than their nonabusing peers to take advantage of alcohol-related resources (i.e., websites, helplines, counselors, groups, school programs, and community 12-step meetings; D'Amico et al., 2004). Strategies that are successful with alcohol-abusing adolescents also differ from those that work with adults. Alcohol and drug treatment services traditionally employed with adults do not respond to youth preferences and the critical cognitive, emotional, and social transitions that occur during adolescence (Brown, 1993; Brown and D'Amico, 2001). Interventions that are shorter in length, with adolescent group formats, and incentives (e.g., free food) were endorsed as facilitating participation (D'Amico et al., 2004).

Adolescents seldom identify themselves as having alcohol or drug-related problems and thus rarely self-present for traditional treatments. Because teens are commonly mandated to addiction treatment by juvenile legal authorities, school officials, or parents, internal motivation is likely to be low. Therefore, motivational interviewing techniques that target ambivalence, resistance, and motivational factors may be particularly beneficial. Motivational strategies have been developed with specific adjustments for working with adolescents (Baer and Peterson, 2002) and those coerced into treatment (Ginsburg et al., 2002).

In addition to intervention strategies focused on motivation, some stressful experiences may provide a window of opportunity to engage teens in treatment. For example, one brief motivational intervention was developed for adolescents receiving emergency room treatment for alcohol-related injuries, resulting in subsequent reductions in drinking and drinking-related behaviors (Monti et al., 2002). Another study targeted the frequently stressful transition to college life, providing an intervention to incoming college freshmen who reported drinking heavily in high school. The study intervention resulted in decreased drinking and negative consequences (Marlatt et al., 1998). Thus, some salient stressors may provide unique circumstances for engaging teens in reevaluating consequences of alcohol and drug use.

The increasing influence of peers during teen years is also an important treatment consideration. Twelve-step programs (Alcoholics Anonymous, Narcotics Anonymous) are routinely recommended for adults with substance use disorders, and although youth in general report much less satisfaction with AA/NA, a limited body of research documents the benefit of these community-based programs for teens as well (Kelly et al., 2002). Adolescents attend more frequently and place more value on aftercare and AA/NA meetings when other group members are approximately the same age (Kelly et al., 2005) or perceived as similar to the teens (Vik et al., 1992), highlighting the importance of peer influences.

In addition to peers, the family continues to exert a strong influence. Interventions that incorporate the family, such as MultiSystemic Therapy (MST; Henggeler

et al., 1998), have proven effective in reducing teen substance use (Henggeler et al., 2002). Departing from usual services provided to adults, MST typically includes delivery of services in the home at times convenient for the family and incorporates family, peer, school, and community-related risk factors and coping strategies.

As we have previously noted, life stress is associated with adolescent psychopathology including, but not limited to, alcohol and drug use disorders. Comorbid psychiatric disorders among substance-abusing teens commonly include mood, anxiety, conduct, and attention-deficit/hyperactivity disorders (e.g., Lewinsohn et al., 1995). Screening, and additional assessment if indicated, to identify and treat comorbid disorders is recommended to enhance addiction treatment efforts (Myers et al., 2002).

Finally, it is important to acknowledge increased sources of stress following addiction treatment. Major stressors facing newly abstaining teens include dealing with family conflicts, establishing a new group of friends, making changes in activities, and resolving academic problems. Different strategies may prove successful for teens depending on environmental and developmental factors. Younger teens from families with no drug use and modest or no alcohol use view the family as helpful in the recovery process and utilize the family for support. A second pattern, more commonly observed among older teens with parental alcohol and drug abuse, involves the adolescent becoming more involved in school, recreational activities, and work rather than relying on the family for support for reducing alcohol use (Brown, 1993).

VI. SUMMARY

Clearly, the relation between stress and addiction during adolescence is a complex interplay of personal factors and the changing environment, in the midst of adolescent development. While many relations between these factors are understood, few studies have examined biological, environmental, and personal characteristics of youth and their families in concert. Such research is necessary to truly understand ways in which development drives both the nature and fluctuations in stress and youth ability to successfully respond to these challenges. Further, such multilevel research can aid in directing prevention and early intervention efforts to arrest the adverse consequences of both stress and youth addiction.

REFERENCES

Aarons, G. A., Ziegenhorn, L. A., and Brown, S. A. (2003). Adolescent conduct disorder, substance use, and traumatic injury. *Journal of Child and Adolescent Substance Abuse, 12*, 1–18.

Allison, K. R., Adlaf, E. M., and Mates, D. (1997). Life strain, coping, and substance use among high school students. *Addiction Research, 5*, 251–272.

Ames, S. C., Offord, K. P., Nirelli, L. M., Patten, C. A., Friedrich, W. N., Decker, P. A., and Hurt, R. D. (2005). Initial development of a new measure of minor stress for adolescents: The Adolescent Minor Stress Inventory. *Journal of Youth and Adolescence, 34*, 207–219.

Anderson, K. G., Ramo, D. E., and Brown, S. A. (In press). Life stress, coping and comorbid youth: An examination of the stress-vulnerability model for substance use. *Journal of Psychoactive Drugs.*

Arnett, J. J. (1999). Adolescent storm and stress, reconsidered. *American Psychologist, 54*, 317–326.

Baer, J. S., and Peterson, P. G. (2002). Motivational interviewing with adolescents. In W. R. Miller and S. Rollnick, Eds. *Motivational interviewing: Preparing people for change* (2nd ed., pp. 320–332). New York: Guilford Press.

Bates, M. E., and Pandina, R. J. (1989). Individual differences in the stability of personality needs: Relations to stress and substance use during adolescence. *Personality and Individual Differences, 10*, 1151–1157.

Brown, G., and Harris, T. O. (1989). Depression. In G. W. Brown and T. O. Harris, Eds. *Life events and illness* (pp. 49–93). New York: Guilford Press.

Brown, S. A. (1987). Alcohol use and type of life events experienced during adolescence. *Psychology of Addictive Behaviors, 1*, 104–107.

Brown, S. A. (1989). Life events of adolescents in relation to personal and parental substance abuse. *American Journal of Psychiatry, 146*, 484–489.

Brown, S. A. (1993). Recovery patterns in adolescent substance abuse. In R. J. McMahon, Ed. *Addictive behaviors across the life span* (pp. 161–183). Beverly Hills, CA: Sage Publications, Inc.

Brown, S. A., and D'Amico, E. J. (2001). Outcomes of alcohol treatment for adolescents. In M. Galanter, Ed. *Recent developments in alcoholism: Volume XV: Services research in the era of managed care* (pp. 307–327). New York: Kluwer Academic/Plenum Publishers.

Brown, S. A., Vik, P. W., and Creamer, V. A. (1989). Characteristics of relapse following adolescent substance abuse treatment. *Addictive Behaviors, 14*, 291–300.

Bruns, C., and Geist, C. S. (1984). Stressful life events and drug use among adolescents. *Journal of Human Stress, 10*, 135–139.

Buchanan, C. M., Eccles, J., and Becker, J. (1992). Are adolescents the victims of raging hormones? Evidence for activational effects of hormones on mood and behavior at adolescence. *Psychological Bulletin, 111*, 62–107.

Buchanan, C. M., and Holmbeck, G. N. (1998). Measuring beliefs about adolescent personality and behavior. *Journal of Youth and Adolescence, 27*, 609–629.

Burnside, M. A., Baer, P. E., McLaughlin, R. J., and Pokarny, A. D. (1986). Alcohol use by adolescents in disrupted families. *Alcoholism: Experimental and Clinical Research, 10*, 274–278.

Byrne, D. G., and Mazanov, J. (1999). Sources of adolescent stress, smoking and the use of other drugs. *Stress Medicine, 15*, 215–227.

Cauffman, E., and Steinberg, L. (2000). (Im)maturity in judgment in adolescence: Why adolescents may be less culpable than adults. *Behavioral Sciences and the Law, 18*, 741–760.

Cameron, J. L. (2004). Interrelationships between hormones, behavior, and affect during adolescence: Complex relationships exist between reproductive hormones, stress-related hormones, and the activity of neural systems that regulate behavioral affect. Comments on part III. *Annals of the New York Academy of Sciences, 1021*, 134–142.

Centers for Disease Control and Prevention. (2000). *Youth risk behavior surveillance—United States, 1999.* Report No. 49 SS03, pp. 1–96. Atlanta, GA: U.S. Department of Health and Human Services.

Chambers, R. A., Taylor, J. R., and Potenza, M. N. (2003). Developmental neurocircuitry of motivation in adolescence: A critical period of addiction vulnerability. *American Journal of Psychiatry, 160*, 1041–1052.

Chandy, J. M., Blum, R. W., and Resnick, M. D. (1996). Gender-specific outcomes for sexually abused adolescents. *Child Abuse and Neglect, 20*, 1219–1231.

Compas, B. E., and Phares, V. (1991). Stress during childhood and adolescence: Sources of risk and vulnerability. In E. M. Cummings, A. L. Greene, and

K. H. Karraker, Eds. *Life-span developmental psychology: Perspectives on stress and coping* (pp. 111–129). New Jersey: LEA.

Colder, C. R., and Chassin, L. (1993). The stress and negative affect model of adolescent alcohol use and the moderating effects of behavioral undercontrol. *Journal of Studies on Alcohol, 54,* 326–333.

Crockett, L. J., Bingham, C. R., Chopak, J. S., and Vicary, J. R. (1996). Timing of first sexual intercourse: The role of social control, social learning, and problem behavior. *Journal of Youth and Adolescence, 25,* 89–112.

D'Amico, E. J., Anderson, K. G., Metrik, J., Frissell, K. C., Ellingstad, T., and Brown, S. A. (Under review). Adolescent self-selection of service formats: Implications for secondary interventions targeting alcohol use.

D'Amico, E. J., McCarthy, D. M., Metrik, J., and Brown, S. A. (2004). Alcohol-related services: Prevention, secondary intervention, and treatment preferences of adolescents. *Journal of Child and Adolescent Substance Abuse, 14*(2), 61–80.

Dawes, M. A., Antelman, S. M., Vanyukov, M. M., Giancola, P., Tarter, R. E., Susman, E. J., et al. (2000). Developmental sources of variation in liability to adolescent substance use disorders. *Drug and Alcohol Dependence, 61,* 3–14.

D'Elio, M. A., O'Brien, R. W., Iannotti, R. J., Bush, P. J., and Galper, D. I. (1996). Early adolescents' substance use and life stress: Concurrent and prospective relationships. *Substance Use and Misuse, 31,* 873–894.

Doherty, W. J., and Needle, R. H. (1991). Psychological adjustment among adolescents before and after a parental divorce. *Child Development, 62,* 328–337.

Durston, S., Hulshoff Pol, H. E., Casey, B. J., Giedd, J. N., Buitelaar, J. K., and Van Engeland, H. (2001). Anatomical MRI of the developing human brain: What have we learned? *Journal of the American Academy of Child and Adolescent Psychiatry, 40,* 1012–1020.

Eccles, J. S., Midgely, C., Wigfield, A., Buchanan, C. M., Reuman, D., Flanagan, C., and MacIver, D. (1993). Development during adolescence: The impact of stage-environmental fit on young adolescents' experiences in schools and in families. *American Psychologist, 48,* 90–101.

Ellis, B. J. (2004). Timing of pubertal maturation in girls: An integrated life history approach. *Psychological Bulletin, 130,* 920–958.

Erikson, E. H. (1959). Identity and the life cycle. *Psychological Issues, 1,* Monograph 1.

Fergusson, D. M., and Lynskey, M. T. (1996). Alcohol misuse and adolescent sexual behaviors and risk taking. *Pediatrics 98,* 91–96.

Fisher, C. B., Wallace, S. A., and Fenton, R. E. (2000). Discrimination distress during adolescence. *Journal of Youth and Adolescence, 29,* 679–695.

Flannery, D. J., Rowe, D. C., and Gulley, B. L. (1993). Impact of pubertal status, timing, and age on adolescent sexual experience and delinquency. *Journal of Adolescent Research, 8,* 21–40.

Fuster, J. M. (2002). Frontal lobe and cognitive development. *Journal of Neurocytology, 31,* 373–385.

Garnefski, N., and Arends, E. (1998). Sexual abuse and adolescent maladjustment: Differences between male and female victims. *Journal of Adolescence, 21,* 99–107.

Gest, S. D., Reed, M. G., and Masten, A. S. (1999). Measuring developmental changes in exposure to adversity: A life chart and rating scale approach. *Development and Psychopathology, 11,* 171–192.

Giedd, J. N., Blumenthal, J., Jeffries, N. O., Castellanos, F. X., Liu, H., Zijdenbos, A., et al. (1999). Brain development during childhood and adolescence: A longitudinal MRI study. *Nature Neuroscience, 2,* 861–863.

Ginsburg, J. I. D., Mann, R. E., Rotgers, F., and Weekes, J. R. (2002). Motivational interviewing with criminal justic populations. In W. R. Miller and S. Rollnick, Eds. *Motivational interviewing: Preparing people for change* (2nd ed., pp. 333–346). New York: Guilford Press.

Gogtay, N., Giedd, J. N., Lusk, L., Hayashi, K. M., Greenstein, D., Vaituzis, A. C., et al. (2004). Dynamic mapping of human cortical development during childhood through early adulthood. *Proceedings of the National Academy of Sciences of the United States of America, 17,* 17.

Gorman, D. M. (1993). A review of studies comparing checklist and interview methods of data collection in life event research. *Behavioral Medicine, 19,* 66–73.

Graber, J. A., Lewinsohn, P. M., Seeley, J. R., and Brooks-Gunn, J. (1997). Is psychopathology associated with the timing of pubertal development? *Journal of the American Academy of Child and Adolescent Psychiatry, 36,* 1768–1776.

Grant, K. E., Compas, B. E., Stuhlmacher, A., Thurm, A. E., McMahon, S., and Halpert, J. (2003). Stressors and child/adolescent psychopathology: Moving from markers to mechanisms of risk. *Psychological Bulletin, 129,* 447–466.

Grant, K. E., Compas, B. E., Thurm, A. E., McMahon, S. D., and Gipson, P. Y. (2004). Stressors and child and adolescent psychopathology: Measurement issues and prospective effects. *Journal of Clinical Child and Adolescent Psychology, 33,* 412–425.

Griffin, M. L., Amodeo, M., Fassler, I., Ellis, M. A., and Clay, C. (2005). Mediating factors for the long-term effects of parental alcoholism in women: The contribution of other childhood stresses and resources. *The American Journal on Addictions, 14,* 18–34.

Gross, J. J., Carstensen, L. L., Pasupathi, M., Tsai, J., Goetestam, S., and Hsu, A. (1997). Emotion and aging: Experience, expression, and control. *Psychology and Aging, 12,* 590–599.

Hains, A. A., and Szyjakowski, M. (1990). A cognitive stress-reduction intervention program for adolescents. *Journal of Counseling Psychology, 37,* 79–84.

Halpern, C. T., Udry, J. R., and Suchindran, C. (1998). Monthly measures of salivary testosterone predict sexual activity in adolescent males. *Archives of Sexual Behavior, 27*, 445–465.

Halpern-Felsher, B. L., Millstein, S. G., and Ellen, J. M. (1996). Relationship of alcohol use and risky sexual behavior: A review and analysis of findings. *Journal of Adolescent Health, 19*, 331–336.

Henggeler, S. W., Clingempeel, W. G., Brondino, M. J., and Pickrel, S. G. (2002). Four-year follow-up of multisystemic therapy with substance abusing and dependent juvenile offenders. *Journal of the American Academy of Child and Adolescent Psychiatry, 41*, 868–874.

Henggeler, S. W., Schoenwald, S. K., Borduin, C. M., Rowland, M. D., and Cunningham, P. B. (1998). *Multisystemic treatment of antisocial behavior in children and adolescents*. New York: Guilford Press.

Johnson, V., and Pandina, R. J. (1991). Familial and personal drinking histories and measures of competence in youth. *Addictive Behaviors, 16*, 453–465.

Jonah, B. (1990). Age differences in risky driving. *Health Education Research, 5*, 139–149.

Jose, P. E., and Ratcliffe, V. (2004). Stressor frequency and perceived intensity as predictors of internalizing symptoms: Gender and age differences in adolescence. *New Zealand Journal of Psychology, 33*, 145–154.

Katschnig, H. (1986). Measuring life stress—a comparison of the checklist and the panel technique. In H. Katschnig, Ed., *Life events and psychiatric disorders: Controversial issues* (pp. 74–106). England: Cambridge University Press.

Kelly, J. F., Myers, M. G., and Brown, S. A. (2002). Do adolescents affiliate with 12-step groups? A multivariate process of model effects. *Journal of Studies on Alcohol, 63*(3), 293–304.

Kelly, J. F., Myers, M. G., and Brown, S. A. (2005). The effects of age composition of 12-step groups on adolescent 12-step participation and substance use outcome. *Journal of Child and Adolescent Substance Abuse, 15*(1), 63–72.

Kilpatrick, D. G., Acierno, R., Saunders, B., Resnick, H. S., Best, C. L., and Schnurr, P. P. (2000). Risk factors for adolescent substance abuse and dependence: Data from a national sample. *Journal of Consulting and Clinical Psychology, 68*, 19–30.

Larson, R., and Richards, M. H. (1994). *Divergent realities: The emotional lives of mothers, fathers, and adolescents*. New York: Basic Books.

Lewinsohn, P. M., Rhode, P., and Seeley, J. R. (1995). Adolescent psychopathology: The clinical consequences of comorbidity. *Journal of the American Academy of Child and Adolescent Psychiatry, 34*(4), 510–519.

Luciana, M., Conklin, H. M., Hooper, C. J., and Yarger, R. S. (2005). The development of nonverbal working memory and executive control processes in adolescents. *Child Development, 76*, 697–712.

Marlatt, G. A., Baer, J. S., Kivlahan, D. R., Dimeff, L. A., Larimer, M. E., and Quigley, L. A. (1998). Screening and brief intervention for high-risk college student drinkers: Results from a 2-year follow-up assessment. *Journal of Consulting and Clinical Psychology, 66*, 604–615.

Martin, C. A., Kelly, T. H., Rayens, M. K., Brogli, B. R., Brenzel, A., Smith, W. J., et al. (2002). Sensation seeking, puberty, and nicotine, alcohol, and marijuana use in adolescence. *Journal of the American Academy of Child and Adolescent Psychiatry, 41*, 1495–1502.

McQuaid, J. R., Monroe, S. M., Roberts, J. E., Kupfer, D. J., and Frank, E. (2000). A comparison of two life stress assessment approaches: Prospective prediction of treatment outcome in recurrent depression. *Journal of Abnormal Psychology, 109*, 787–791.

Meyerson, L. A., Long, P. J., Miranda, Jr., R., and Marx, B. P. (2002). The influence of childhood sexual abuse, physical abuse, family environment, and gender on the psychological adjustment of adolescents. *Child Abuse and Neglect, 26*, 387–405.

Miller, E. M., and Shields, S. A. (1980). Skin conductance response as a measure of adolescents' emotional reactivity. *Psychological Reports, 46*, 587–590.

Monti, P. M., Barnett, N. P., O'Leary, T. A., and Colby, S. M. (2002). Motivational enhancement for alcohol-involved adolescents. In P. M. Monti, S. M. Colby, and T. A. O'Leary, Eds. *Adolescents, alcohol, and substance abuse: Reaching teens through brief interventions* (pp. 145–182). New York: Guilford Press.

Myers, M. G., Brown, S. A., and Mott, M. A. (1993). Coping as a predictor of adolescent substance abuse treatment outcome. *Journal of Substance Abuse, 5*, 15–29.

Myers, M. G., Brown, S. A., Tate, S., Abrantes, A., and Tomlinson, K. (2002). Toward brief interventions for adolescents with substance abuse and comorbid psychiatric problems. In P. M. Monti, S. M. Colby, and T. A. O'Leary, Eds. *Adolescents, alcohol, and substance abuse: Reaching teens through brief interventions*, (pp. 275–296). New York: Guilford Press.

Nash, S. G., McQueen, A., and Bray, J. H. (2005). Pathways to adolescent alcohol use: Family environment, peer influence, and parental expectations. *Journal of Adolescent Health, 37*, 19–28.

Nelson, E. E., Leibenluft, E., McClure, E. B., and Pine, D. S. (2005). The social re-orientation of adolescence: A neuroscience perspective on the process and its relation to psychopathology. *Psychological Medicine, 35*, 163–174.

Newcomb, M. D., and Harlow, L. L. (1986). Life events and substance use among adolescents: Mediating effects of perceived loss of control and meaninglessness in life. *Journal of Personality and Social Psychology, 51*, 564–577.

O'Doherty, F., and Davies, J. B. (1987). Life events and addiction: A critical review. *British Journal of Addiction, 82*, 127–137.

Offer, D., Ostrov, E., and Howard, K. I. (1981). The mental health professional's concept of the normal adolescent. *Archives of General Psychiatry, 38*, 149–153.

Offer, D., and Schonert-Reichl, K. A. (1992). Debunking the myths of adolescence: Findings from recent research. *Journal of the American Academy of Child and Adolescent Psychiatry, 31*, 1003–1014.

Outlaw, F. H. (1993). Stress and coping: The influence of racism on the cognitive appraisal processing of African Americans. *Issues in Mental Health Nursing, 14*, 399–409.

Paus, T., Zijdenbos, A., Worsley, K., Collins, D. L., Blumenthal, J., Giedd, J. N., et al. (1999). Structural maturation of neural pathways in children and adolescents: In vivo study. *Science, 283*, 1908–1911.

Petersen, A. C., Compass, B. E., Brooks-Gunn, J., Stemmler, M., Ey, S., and Grant, K. E. (1993). Depression in adolescence. *American Psychologist, 48*, 155–168.

Pillow, D. R., Barrera, M., Jr., and Chassin, L. (1998). Using cluster analysis to assess the effects of stressful life events: Probing the impact of parental alcoholism on child stress and substance use. *Journal of Community Psychology, 26*, 361–380.

Short, J. L. (1998). Predictors of substance use and mental health of children of divorce: A prospective analysis. *Journal of Divorce and Remarriage, 29*, 147–166.

Silberg, J., Pickles, A., Rutter, M., Hewitt, J., Simonoff, E., Maes, H., et al. (1999). The influence of genetic factors and life stress on depression among adolescent girls. *Archives of General Psychiatry, 56*, 225–232.

Skinner, H., Maley, O., Smith, L., Chirrey, S., and Morrison, M. (2001). New frontiers: Using the Internet to engage teens in substance abuse prevention and treatment. In P. M. Monti, S. M. Colby, and T. A. O'Leary, Eds. *Adolescents, alcohol, and substance abuse: Reaching teens through brief interventions* (pp. 297–318). New York: Guilford Press.

Spear, L. (2002). The adolescent brain and the college drinker: Biological basis of propensity to use and misuse alcohol. *Journal of Studies on Alcohol. Special Issue: College drinking, what it is, and what to do about it: Review of the state of the science, 14*, 71–81.

Steinberg, L., and Morris, A. S. (2001). Adolescent development. *Annual Reviews of Psychology, 52*, 83–110.

Stewart, M. A., and Brown, S. A. (1993). Family functioning following adolescent substance abuse treatment. *Journal of Substance Abuse, 5*, 327–339.

Tapert, S. F., Aarons, G. A., Sedlar, G. R., and Brown, S. A. (2001). Adolescent substance use and sexual risk-taking behavior. *Journal of Adolescent Health, 28*, 181–189.

Tate, S. R., McQuaid, J. R., and Brown, S. A. (2005). Characteristics of life stressors predictive of substance treatment outcomes. *Journal of Substance Abuse Treatment, 29*, 107–115.

Tremblay, L., and Frigon, J. Y. (2005). Precocious puberty in adolescent girls: A biomarker of later psychosocial adjustment problems. *Child Psychiatry and Human Development, 36*, 73–94.

Vaccaro, D., and Wills, T. A. (1998). Stress-coping factors in adolescent substance use: Test of ethnic and gender differences in samples of urban adolescents. *Journal of Drug Education, 28*, 257–282.

Vik, P. W., and Brown, S. A. (1998). Life events and substance abuse during adolescence. In T. W. Miller, Ed. *Children of trauma: Stressful life events and their effect on adolescents* (pp. 179–205). International University Press, Inc. Madison, CT

Vik, P. W., Grizzle, K. L., and Brown, S. A. (1992). Social resource characteristics and adolescent substance abuse relapse. *Journal of Adolescent Chemical Dependency, 2*(2), 59–74.

Wagner, B. M., and Compas, B. E. (1990). Gender, instrumentality, and expressivity: Moderators of the relation between stress and psychological symptoms during adolescence. *American Journal of Community Psychology, 18*, 383–406.

Walker, E. F., Sabuwalla, Z., and Huot, R. (2004). Pubertal neuromaturation, stress sensitivity, and psychopathology. *Developmental Psychopathology, 16*, 807–824.

Waller, E. M., and DuBois, D. L. (2004). Investigation of stressful experiences, self-evaluations, and self-standards as predictors of sexual activity during early adolescence. *Journal of Early Adolescence, 24*, 431–459.

Williams, C., Griffin, K. W., Macaulay, A. P., West, T. L., and Gronewold, E. (2005). Efficacy of a drug prevention CD-ROM intervention for adolescents. *Substance Use and Misuse, 40*, 869–878.

Wills, T. A. (1986). Stress and coping in early adolescence: Relationships to substance use in urban school samples. *Health Psychology, 5*, 503–529.

Wills, T. A., Resko, J. A., Ainette, M. G., and Mendoza, D. (2004). Role of parent support and peer support in adolescent substance use: A test of mediated effects. *Psychology of Addictive Behaviors, 18*, 122–134.

Wills, T. A., Sandy, J. M., Shinar, O., and Yaeger, A. M. (1999). Contributions of positive and negative affect to adolescent substance use: Test of a bidimensional model in a longitudinal study. *Psychology of Addictive Behaviors, 13*, 327–338.

Wills, T. A., Sandy, J. M., and Yaeger, A. M. (2002). Moderators of the relation between substance use level and problems: Test of a self-regulation model in middle adolescence. *Journal of Abnormal Psychology, 111*, 3–21.

Wills, T. A., Sandy, J. M., Yaeger, A. M., Cleary, S. D., and Shinar, O. (2001). Coping dimensions, life stress, and adolescent substance use: A latent growth analysis. *Journal of Abnormal Psychology, 110*, 309–323.

Windle, M. (1992). A longitudinal study of stress buffering for adolescent problem behaviors. *Developmental Psychology, 28*, 52.

Zucker, R. A., and Gomberg, E. S. L. (1986). Etiology of alcoholism reconsidered: The case for a biopsychosocial process. *American Psychologist, 41*, 783–793.

CLINICAL IMPLICATIONS: ASSESSMENT AND INTERVENTION

Assessment of Stress in Research and Clinical Settings

GARY L. DAVIS, MUSTAFA AL'ABSI, AND JANE HOVLAND

The assessment of stress is an exciting and dynamic area of research. Assessment measures range from the macroscopic to the microscopic, from the obvious to the subtle. This chapter reviews the measurement of stress and begins with questionnaire and interview measures and concludes with biological measures. The measures range in complexity and difficulty from interviews that take hours to administer and score, to those as simple as a blood pressure taken in a matter of seconds. Included in this review are life events scales, semistructured interviews, self-report scales, hormonal measures, catecholamine levels, cardiovascular measures, and immune system parameters. The chapter is not exhaustive in its review but is selective of those measures that are commonly used and have substantial literature to support their reliability and validity. Recent, innovative, and promising measures are also included such as the Adverse Childhood Experience Scale, the "D" Personality Scale, and various hormonal and immunological measures. Principles to consider in selecting specific measures of stress are discussed.

I. INTRODUCTION

The relationship of stress to a wide range of human conditions has been the subject of intense interest and research for many decades. Stress has been implicated in the development of substance abuse and dependence, psychopathologies, cancer, cardiovascular diseases, and autoimmune diseases, to mention a few. A fundamental and vexing question in the investigation of the relationship between stress and these various conditions is how to measure stress. The assessment of stress has taken many forms in an attempt to answer this question. These forms have included the use of simple questionnaires asking about symptoms of stress or the occurrence of stressful life experiences, semistructured interviews probing the contextual elements of stressful events, questionnaires tailored to specific situations such as trauma-related stress or stress from work environments, scales that measure the effects of stress indirectly (e.g., depression and anxiety scales), and the assessment of biological markers of stress. As a consequence of the use of such diverse and multifaceted instruments, the stress research literature is one that is rich in results, complicated in nature, and contradictory in part.

This chapter is an introductory overview of many of the common approaches to the measurement of stress. The chapter begins with the assessment approaches that are more external and global in nature, the use of semistructured interviews to measure stressful life events, and concludes with those assessment approaches that are more internal and microscopic in nature, the measurement of immune response parameters. The chapter is divided into two major sections. The first section reviews the interviews, checklists, and self-report questionnaires to measure stress; the second section reviews the biological measures of stress. Major methodological issues are discussed, and the advantages and disadvantages of the various approaches to measurement are reviewed. The measures selected are those that are commonly used and have a substantial body of evidence to support their utility, or in some cases, those that show promise for future research. As with any overview, the authors intend to give the reader a feel for the "lay of the land" and point the way for the stimulated reader to pursue his/her specific interest through additional reading and research.

II. THE ASSESSMENT OF STRESSFUL LIFE EVENTS

A. Methodological Issues

Even casual readers of the stress literature are familiar with the classic research of Holmes and Rahe (1967) and their checklist approach to the assessment of stressful life events exemplified by the Social Readjustment Rating Questionnaire (SRRQ). This seminal publication spawned decades of research examining the relationship of stressful life events to human problems. Although the SRRQ was a major contribution to the literature, numerous investigators have identified significant methodological problems with the checklist approach (Brown and Harris, 1989;

Dohrenwend et al., 1987; McQuaid et al., 2000). Among the most important of these problems is that the subject is left to interpret the significance of an event in his/her own life and the event's relationship to an item on the checklist. Each subject uses idiosyncratic and personal criteria to determine whether or not a life event matches the item on the scale, thereby introducing error variance into the measurement process. Other methodological concerns with the checklist approach are the weighting of the items on the checklist, the confounding of mental and physical symptoms with life events, the effects of personal characteristics and behaviors on the occurrence of life events, the over-reporting of minor events, and the distortion of events in the negative direction or selective memory of negative events by subjects who are depressed or anxious. Collectively, these concerns coalesce around the issue of whether the subject or the researcher should define or identify stressful events.

In order to reduce the error variance or bias introduced by the checklist approach, semistructured interviews to assess life events have been developed. Three of these will be briefly discussed, and they are the ones most frequently used by researchers. They are the Interview for Recent Life Events (IRLE; Paykel, 1997), Structured Event Probe and Narrative Rating Method (SEPRATE; Dohrenwend et al., 1993), and the Bedford College Life Events and Difficulties Scale (LEDS; Brown and Harris, 1978). Table 13-1 contains all of the assessment approaches reviewed in this section on interviews and checklists.

B. Semistructured Interview Methods

The Bedford College LEDS (Brown, 1974; Brown and Harris, 1978) was the first widely published attempt to improve upon life events checklists through the use of a semistructured interview. The LEDS interview solicits information about events and life difficulties in 10 areas: education,

TABLE 13-1   Life Events Measures

Semistructured interviews
  Bedford College Life Events and Difficulties Scale (Brown and Harris, 1978)
  Structured Event Probe and Narrative Rating Method (Dohrenwend et al., 1993)
  Interview for Recent Life Events (Paykel, 1997)
Life events scales
  Social Readjustment Rating Scale (Holmes and Rahe, 1967)
  Psychiatric Epidemiology Research Interview Life Events Scale (Dohrenwend et al., 1978)
  Adverse Childhood Events Scale (Felitti et al., 1998)
  Hassles and Uplifts Scales (Lazarus and Folkman, 1989)

work, reproduction, financial, housing, legal, health, romantic relationships, other social/family relationships, and miscellaneous. The interviews are tape-recorded, and judges rate the interviews on a number of dimensions while listening to the tapes. The judges are required to assess the meaning of an event by taking into account the subject's history and current circumstances, described as the context of the event. The ratings are intended to be normative in nature, reflecting what an average person in the same circumstances with the same history would experience. Life events (those of short duration) and difficulties (those lasting 4 weeks or more) are rated for severity independent of the subjects' reported reactions. The raters are guided by a dictionary of events compiled by the Bedford College group. Events are also rated for their independence from the subjects' psychological disorders. Stress researchers generally use only those events rated as independent or possibly independent in the investigations into the relationship of life events to health outcomes. The interviews can take several hours to complete, and interviewers and judges must undergo rather extensive training in the LEDS system. High inter-rater reliabilities have been reported for the LEDS and generally have been in the .80–.90 range. The LEDS has been studied in relation to a wide range of psychological problems including addictions (O'Doherty and Davies, 1987), bipolar disorder (Malkoff-Schwartz et al., 1998),

major depression (Leskala et al., 2004), schizophrenia (Day et al., 1987), eating disorders (Schmidt et al., 1997), and adolescent depression (Williamson et al., 1998).

Paykel created the first version of the Interview for Recent Life Events in the late 1960s as a measure of depression. He intended the IRLE to reduce the methodological concerns that had been raised about life events checklists (Paykel, 1983). The IRLE underwent modifications and expansion over the years and currently exists as a semistructured interview of 64 life events (Paykel, 1997). A guiding principle in the development of the IRLE was that the events were to be independent of psychological disorder and its potential outcomes, such as hospitalization. The events in the IRLE can be traced to specific dates and reflect changes in the external environment. The events are grouped into 10 categories: work, education, finance, health, bereavement, migration, dating and cohabitation, legal, family and social relationships, and marital. The events that are reported are probed by the interviewer to determine their natures and circumstances. For each event, the month of occurrence is noted, and the event is scored for independence from psychological disorder and objective negative impact. Independence is scored from one (almost certainly independent) to five (almost certainly dependent). Objective negative impact is scored from one (severe negative impact) to five (no negative impact). The rater is asked to "evaluate the degree of unpleasant impact, stress, or threat the event would be expected to bear when its full nature and circumstances are taken into account" (Paykel, 1997). The interview takes up to 2 hours to complete and varies in length according to the number of life events reported. Interrater reliabilities were reported that ranged from .58–.96, with most results in the .80s and .90s. The IRLE has been used with alcohol- and drug-abusing populations (Cooke and Allan, 1984; Turrina et al., 1993).

The Structured Event Probe and Narrative Rating Method (Dohrenwend et al., 1993) was developed, like the IRLE, as a semistructured interview designed to reduce measurement error inherent in the checklist approach to assessing stressful life events. Event checklists have been found to have low correlations to health outcomes, and measurement error variance has been suspected to be an explanation for the low correlation. SEPRATE was intended to reduce intracategory variability by taking a more "normative" approach to rating events. The SEPRATE inquires about 74 events grouped into 10 categories: schooling, work, love and marriage, having children, family matters, living situation, crime and legal matters, financial matters, social life and recreation, and miscellaneous matters. Subjects are asked which of the events occurred to themselves or their spouses/mates. Events that are reported are then probed by the interviewer with a predetermined set of questions to elicit factually detailed accounts of the events. Subjects are explicitly asked not to report personal feelings or an evaluation of what happened. The event descriptions are stripped of personal information prior to being rated. The interview data are reviewed by two or more judges who rate each event occurrence on five factors: the event's negative valence, the event's fatefulness, the extent to which the event may be life-threatening, the amount of change in daily activities that would be expected for an average person, and whether the event is likely to be physically exhausting. The interview takes 2 hours or more, and the rating process is also quite time consuming. Research conducted by the SEPRATE authors found that the interview method reduced intracategory variability and produced high interrater reliabilities (Dohrenwend et al., 1990; Shrout et al., 1989).

C. Life Events Scales

Stress responses are significantly associated with life events, and in general, life event scales represent gradations of increasingly stressful events. These gradations are established using sorting techniques, with subsequent validation by larger samples.

The most widely cited scale associated with life events is the Social Readjustment Rating Scale (SRRS) developed by Holmes and Rahe (1967). The SRRS reflects an understanding of the biological, psychological, and sociological implications of stress, and acknowledges that positive and negative, as well as unexpected or expected, events require an adaptive response. Two primary categories of items comprise the scale: those related to the lifestyle of the individual and those related to possible positive or negative events. In the SRRS, events are ranked based on the intensity of the stress event as well as the length of time necessary to adapt to the stress. Statistical transformation of the ratings of the events on the scale resulted in a ratio scale associated with each of the 43 rank-ordered items. Correlation coefficients between discrete groups in the original sample range from 0.82 to 0.97 (Holmes and Rahe, 1967). Although developed over 40 years ago, the instrument's rank ordering of stressors appears to have maintained its robustness, with only minor changes suggested by a recent reevaluation of its psychometrics (Scully et al., 2000). Most of the rank order changes involve events requiring moderate to low adjustment, and an upward shift in financial stressors. Scully et al. (2000) reported correlation coefficients between the original SRRS and the re-ranked version of 0.8.

The Psychiatric Epidemiology Research Interview (PERI) Life Events Scale (Dohrenwend et al., 1978) was developed to address several of the criticisms of the SRRS, particularly whether weighting events is better than simply tallying the number of events, and if weighted, should the reference point for the weightings be based on the individuals' perceptions or those of a referenced group. Items in the SRRS were based on events that roughly coincided with the onset of illness. Dohrenwend et al. (1978) noted that illness onset is subtle and generally gradual; therefore, correlating stressors with illness onset is difficult, if not impossible, in etiological research. Additionally, the SRRS does not address many of the confounding states individuals experience at the time they are also dealing with a stressor, nor are the effects of ethnic backgrounds or urban living considered on the perception of the stressful events. To address these issues as well as other related methodological issues, Dohrenwend's group generated a list of 101 events that were then rated by judges on a number of variables: universal versus limited event, desirability, whether the event happened to the respondent or another, whether the event involved psychological or physical health states, and whether or not the event could be viewed as under the control of the respondent. The result was a set of group-specific rank orderings for respondents based on race, gender, and socioeconomic status that allowed for more meaningful comparison of events within subjects and between groups. The construction of the PERI is described in detail (Dohrenwend et al., 1978). Initial reliability and validity procedures were based on achieving inter-rater agreement of at least 0.90. Later analyses factored in probabilities for type 2 errors with the goal of eliminating bias in the scale. Those items preserved had coefficients of 0.8 or better.

The Adverse Childhood Events Scale (ACEs) (Felitti et al., 1998) is a retrospective scale created from a number of instruments, primarily the Conflict Tactic Scale (Straus and Gelles, 1990), designed to measure exposure to parental and family dysfunction in childhood. Seven categories of childhood exposures are identified: psychological abuse, physical abuse, contact sexual abuse, substance abuse by an adult in the home, mental illness in an adult in the home, criminal behavior by an adult in the home, and maltreatment of a parent. Positive responses to a total of 17 yes-no questions are tallied, and based on these, a categorical score of 0 to 7 is obtained. Scores on this scale have been correlated with health-risk behavioral assessments (Anda et al., 1999; Felitti, 2002). Test-retest scores (using the kappa coefficient) range from .41 to .86 for individual dichotomously scored items, and .64 for the total ACEs score (Dube et al., 2004). The ACEs instrument is currently being refined as a semistructured interview by our group to improve its psychometric sensitivity and specificity.

The Hassles and Uplifts Scales represent a much different approach to the study of stress. Rather than examining major events, the scales rate the cumulative effects of minor stressors—the kinds individuals face in everyday life (Kanner et al., 1981; Lazarus and Folkman, 1989). This instrument has also found wide use in a number of settings, including use with occupational groups and may be a better predictor of ongoing psychological symptoms. Test-retest correlations have been reported as .79 (for frequency of hassles), .48 (for intensity of hassles), .72 (for uplifts frequency), and .60 (for uplifts intensity) at a 30-day interval (Kanner et al., 1981).

III. THE ASSESSMENT OF SELF-REPORTED STRESS

A. Methodological Issues

The life events assessment approach, as we have seen, has been characterized by efforts to depersonalize and objectify stress measurement. By contrast, other stress researchers have taken the polar opposite approach and asserted that stress is a perceptual experience and that events are only stressful when they are appraised or judged to be so by the person. This theoretical position is most closely identified with Richard Lazarus and Susan Folkman in their classic work on stress, appraisal, and coping (Lazarus and Folkman, 1984). The interaction between the event and the person is seen as a dynamic transaction in which the person actively shapes the nature of the event. Events are only stressful when they are judged to be threatening or to represent loss, and when the coping resources available are judged to be inadequate to cope with the event. A stressful event to one person may be a nonevent to another. A fuller discussion of these theoretical issues is beyond the scope of this chapter and has been done well elsewhere (Cohen et al., 1995; Lovallo, 2004; Monroe and Kelley, 1995).

Many scales have been developed to assess stress from a subjective frame of reference. These range from scales designed to globally assess stress, e.g., Perceived Stress Scale (PSS; Cohen et al., 1983) to scales created for a specific situation such as occupational stress, e.g., Nursing Stress Inventory (Numeroff and Abrams, 1984) or trauma, e.g., Mississippi Scale for Combat-related PTSD (Keane et al., 1988). Table 13-2 contains the self-report stress scales reviewed in this section. All of the subjective self-report scales are vulnerable to the same inherent problem. Items on the scale may duplicate or be highly similar to symptoms of a psychological disorder that the subject is experiencing leading to a misattribution of the symptom to stressful events. For example, on the 14-item version of the PSS, an item reads, "In the last month how

TABLE 13-2   Self-Report Stress Scales

Clinician Administered PTSD Scale (Foa et al., 1993)

Expanded Nursing Stress Scale (French et al., 2000)

Impact of Events Scales (Horowitz, Wilner, and Alvarez, 1979)

Impact of Events Scales-Revised (Weiss and Marmar, 1997)

Job Diagnostics Survey (Hackman and Lawler, 1971)

Job Stress Survey (Vagg and Spielberger, 1998)

Mississippi Scale (Keane, Malloy, and Fairbank, 1984)

Nursing Stress Inventory (Numeroff and Abrams, 1984)

Occupational Stress Inventory (Osipow and Spokane, 1981)

Occupational Stress Indicator (Cooper, Sloan, and Williams, 1988)

Perceived Stress Scale (Cohen, Kamarck, and Mermelstein, 1983)

Work Environment Scale (Insel and Moos, 1974)

Self-Report Stress-Related Scales

Beck Depression Inventory-II (Beck, Steer, and Brown, 1998)

Center for Epidemiological Studies Depression Scale (Radloff, 1977)

State-Trait Anxiety Inventory (Spielberger and Gorsuch, 1983)

Positive and Negative Affect Schedule (Watson, Clark, and Tellegen, 1988)

Profile of Mood States (McNair, Lorr, and Droppleman, 1992)

Distress Scale 14 (Denollet, 2005)

often have you felt nervous and 'stressed'?" A subject who feels nervous due to an anxiety disorder is quite likely to respond "fairly often" or "very often," resulting in an elevation of the stress score. Self-report scales are also vulnerable to the cumulative effects of stress from sources other than discrete events. Work-related pressures, worry about upcoming deadlines or events, and concern about problems that friends and family members may be experiencing are just a few examples of circumstances that may raise stress scores on self-report scales. Scales designed to measure stress from a specific source are especially prone to this type of error variance as subjects are likely to misattribute general life stress to a specific stressor (Cohen et al., 1983).

B. Self-Report Stress Scales

1. Global Stress Measure

The most widely used instrument as a measure of globally perceived stress is the Perceived Stress Scale (PSS; Cohen et al., 1983). The PSS grew out of Lazarus' work (Lazarus and Folkman, 1984) on stress appraisal. The most reliable version of the PSS (Cohen and Williamson, 1988) contains 10 items that ask subjects about the extent of unpredictability, uncontrollability, and overloading they experience in their lives. Subjects respond to each item on a five-point Likert-type scale from "never" to "almost always." The PSS has been reported to have good internal consistency, alpha = .78 (Cohen and Williamson, 1988). The PSS is significantly correlated to a wide range of health behaviors and outcomes. The reader is referred to Cohen and Williamson (1988) for a comprehensive review of this literature.

2. Post-Traumatic Stress

PTSD as a diagnosis has only recently been included in the *Diagnostic and Statistical Manual of Mental Disorders* (*DSM-IV*) American Psychiatric Association (1994), although long-lasting responses to trauma

have been described for centuries. Based on the expansion of research and scholarship in the area, the psychometric properties of assessment scales for PTSD must be emphasized. Only a few examples of PTSD-related scales are included in this discussion, and the reader is referred to Brewin (2005) for a more complete review.

The Impact of Events Scale (IES; Horowitz et al., 1979) is a 15-item self-report tool developed to measure an individual's subjective distress after experiencing trauma, using indicators of intrusiveness and avoidance associated with the trauma. The IES was constructed before PTSD was established as a mental disorder, yet the instrument has been shown to discriminate between those who meet PTSD diagnostic criteria and those who do not (Bryant and Harvey, 1996). Cronback's alpha is reported as .86 for the entire IES, .78 for intrusion, and .82 for avoidance (Joseph, 2000). Critics have cited content validity as a primary problem with the IES. The scale does not sample all PTSD diagnostic symptom categories (e.g., hypervigilence), nor does it encompass many of the symptoms currently described in the *DSM-IV* (e.g., detachment and a foreshortened future). In addition to not being a specific PTSD measure, the IES has been criticized for being easy to fake, thus portraying psychopathology where none actually exists. Additional psychometric problems are explored by Joseph (2000) in a review of the psychometric properties of the scale.

A revised IES (IES-R) was designed to parallel the *DSM-IV* criteria for PTSD (Weiss and Marmar, 1997). The IES-R contains the 15 items of the IES, an additional 6 items to assess hypervigilence/hyperarousal, and 1 item to assess reexperiencing the trauma through flashbacks. Cronbach's alpha for the full scale is reported as .94, with subscale measures ranging from .77 to .85. Test-retest correlations at 2 weeks are .91. Issues of faking have still not been addressed in this revised version.

The psychometric properties of the MMPI-2 (Butcher et al., 1989), with its emphasis on detecting faking, lying, or malingering make it a valuable instrument in stress-related research, particularly in PTSD. The MMPI-2 incorporates Keane's original PTSD scale (Keane et al., 1984). Refinements in norming and scaling now demonstrate that the diagnosis of PTSD can be reliably established in general populations of subjects (Lyons and Wheeler-Cox, 1999) using the MMPI-2.

Foa et al. (1993) reported on a comparison of the Clinician Administered PTSD Scale (CAPS), the PTSD Symptom Scale-Interview Version (PSS-I), and a 17-item self-report inventory, the PSS-SR with rape victims. They concluded that the self-report PSS-SR is somewhat more "conservative" in its ability to identify PTSD; however, since the CAPS and the PSS-I require significant interviewer time to administer, the PSS-SR may be an acceptable alternative. Alpha coefficients for the PSS-SR and PSS-I instruments are similar (.65–.86 and .71–.88, respectively). Validity coefficients range from .73 to .83.

3. Occupational Stress Scales

Work-related stress exacts a toll on worker productivity and safety. Assessing occupational stress can involve general instruments or those designed specifically for an occupation. In the case of general assessment, several instruments are widely used, including the Job Diagnostics Survey (Hackman and Lawler, 1971), the Work Environment Scale (Insel and Moos, 1974), the Occupational Stress Inventory (Osipow and Spokane, 1981), and the Occupational Stress Indicator (Cooper et al., 1988). Use of these particular scales depends on theoretical orientation, particularly from a management perspective. A more job-neutral instrument is the Job Stress Survey (JSS; Vagg and Spielberger, 1998). The JSS measures perceptions of severity and frequency of 30 job-related events, such as being assigned new duties and working with those who are not motivated. It has applicability of use in white- and blue-collar situations as well as with men and women.

It incorporates information on job pressures as well as degree of support a worker feels in the work environment.

Assessment of high stress work conditions for specific occupational groups has occurred in many settings, including teaching, air traffic control, medicine, and the petrochemical industry. Most of these studies have involved assessment of the mental and physical consequences of stress rather than worker-occupation interaction. Examples of worker-occupation interaction tools involve several instruments designed to measure stress of nursing personnel. The Nursing Stress Inventory (NSI; Numeroff and Abrams, 1984) focuses on stressors experienced in the six areas: organizational, work demands, affective demands, death issues, lack of administrative support, and the role of the supervisor. The Expanded Nursing Stress Scale (ENSS; French et al., 2000) incorporates some of the same categories and adds job discrimination and peer conflict. Internal consistency coefficients for these scales are reported between .75 and .89.

C. Stress-Related Scales

Up to this point, we have reviewed measurement approaches that are designed to directly measure stress. However, in the stress research literature, many studies exist that use less direct measures of stress. Examples of these are scales measuring depression, anxiety, and other negative mood states. A comprehensive review of these scales is well beyond the scope of this chapter, and the interested reader will find that excellent literature reviews are available (McDowell and Newell, 1996). We have selected a few for brief mention, and they are listed in Table 13-2.

The Beck Depression Inventory-II (BDI-II; Beck et al., 1996) is one of the most widely used and best-researched instruments for measuring depression. The BDI-II has high reliability (coefficient alpha = .92) and is easy to administer. The Center for Epidemiological Studies Depression

Scale (CES-D; Radloff, 1977) has been used extensively in research, especially community-based survey research. The test is composed of 20 items that were taken from other measures of depression. Alpha coefficients are reported in the .85–.91 range (Hann et al., 1999; Himmelfarb and Murrell, 1983). The State-Trait Anxiety Inventory (Spielberger and Gorsuch, 1983) is the most often used measure of anxiety in research studies, and is used frequently in clinical settings as well. An extensive review of psychometric data on the STAI (Barnes et al., 2002) reported that the mean internal consistency coefficient for the State scale was .91, and the mean stability (test-retest) coefficient was .70. For the Trait scale the internal consistency mean was .89, and the stability was .88. The Positive and Negative Affect Schedule (PANAS; Watson et al., 1988) was developed to measure the two dominant dimensions of affective structure from factor analyses of self-rated mood studies. Alpha coefficients are high for both scales and range from .86 to .90 for positive affect and .84 to .87 for negative affect. Stability coefficients are .47 to .68 for positive affect and .39 to .71 for negative affect. The Profile of Mood States (POMS; McNair et al., 1992) is also widely used in stress research, and a recent bibliography (McNair et al., 2003) listed more than 2,900 publications related to the POMS. The alpha coefficients reported for the six subscales range from .63 to .96, and stability coefficients exceed .75 (Gibson, 1997).

The Distress Scale (DS16; Denollet, 1998) was designed to be a measure of negative affectivity and social inhibition or the Type D personality. DS16 was later revised to the DS14 and is a 14-item questionnaire (Denollet, 2005). Denollet (1998; Denollet and De Vries, 2006; Denollet and Van Heck, 2001) demonstrated that Type D is a significant risk factor for morbidity and mortality in coronary heart disease as well as other poor outcomes. DS14 has seven items that assess social inhibition (SI) or a tendency to inhibit self-expression from others, and seven items that assess negative affectivity (NA) or the tendency to experience negative emotions. Alpha coefficients were reported to be .88 for NA and .86 for SI. Stability or test-retest reliabilities were reported to be .72 for NA and .82 for SI after 3 months (Denollet, 2005). The DS14 is self-administered and takes 5–10 minutes to complete.

IV. BIOLOGICAL AND PHYSIOLOGICAL ASSESSMENT

There has been a significant growth of methods and procedures to examine the effects of acute and chronic stress on various biological and physiological functions. These methods have demonstrated the utility and benefits of using these measures to gain a better understanding of how stress may affect peripheral and central processes. To that end, research over many decades has identified multiple systems that are involved in manifesting the physiological response to stress. These systems include the hypothalamic-pituitary-adrenocortical (HPA) axis and the sympatho-adreno-medullary (SAM) system. In the following sections we briefly describe measures used to assess the effects of stress on these systems. These biological measures are listed in Table 13-3.

V. HYPOTHALAMIC-PITUITARY-ADRENOCORTICAL (HPA) MEASURES

The HPA system involves three brain and peripheral structures: the hypothalamus, the pituitary, and the cortex of the adrenal gland. The activity of this system is triggered by the release of corticotropin-releasing factor (CRF) from neuronal cell bodies of the paraventricular nucleus (PVN). CRF travels from the median eminence of the hypothalamus through the portal circulation system to the anterior part of the pituitary gland.

TABLE 13-3   Biological and Physiological Measures
of Stress

Hypothalamic-pituitary-adrenocortical (HPA)
Measures
    Cortisol
    Adrenocorticotropic hormone (ACTH)
    Corticotropin-releasing factor (CRF)
Sympatho-adreno-medullary Measures
    Catecholamines
        Epinephrine
        Norepinephrine
    Cardiovascular
        Blood pressure
        Heart rate
        Stroke volume
Immune Response
    Cellular
        T cells
        NK cells
    Humoral
        Immunoglobulins (IgG)
    Cytokines
        Tumor necrosis factor
        Interleukin-1
        Interleukin-6

There it acts on the corticotrope cells stimulating the synthesis of proopiomelanocortin leading to the subsequent release of adrenocorticotropic hormone (ACTH) and beta-endorphin into systemic circulation.

Vasopressin (AVP) is also synthesized and secreted in the PVN. AVP participates in stimulating ACTH release. Although AVP is a weak secretagogue at ACTH-producing cells, when it is combined with CRF, it markedly potentiates ACTH secretion. ACTH travels through the peripheral circulation to reach the adrenal cortex where it leads to the synthesis and release of corticosteroids—most notably in humans, cortisol (Dallman, 1993). About 95% of cortisol is bound to corticosteroid-binding globulin (CBG). The remaining free cortisol enters cells to affect their metabolic activity. The liver is the main site for cortisol metabolism, and free cortisol (40–100 µg/day) is excreted in urine.

A. Assessment of Cortisol and ACTH

Both cortisol and ACTH have been used frequently to assess the biological effects of acute stress. These measures can also be used as an indicator of dysregulation in the system, such as that might result from exposure to chronic stress. While cortisol can be measured in saliva and plasma, ACTH can be measured only in plasma. Cortisol can also be measured in urine over an extended period of time. This modality is less widely used currently due to the additional information that can be obtained using more frequent sampling, such as that obtained from saliva or plasma. Due to the low quantities of CRF in peripheral circulation, it is not possible at this time to assess CRF from plasma, but it can be assessed in cerebrospinal fluid, which requires invasive procedures.

Several acute laboratory challenges have been found to be effective in probing the HPA response, including tasks that are socially salient and are characterized by uncertainty, distress, and lack of control. Examples of the stressors that have been successfully used to challenge the HPA system are public speaking, extended mental arithmetic, and pain-induction procedures (al'Absi et al., 1997; 2000).

One method to assess the integrity of the HPA axis is to assess response to waking up. Cortisol increase upon awakening is considered a promising marker of adrenocortical functional status (Born et al., 1999; Edwards et al., 2001; Pruessner et al., 1999). This increase may reach 50–100%, and peaks approximately 30 minutes after awakening in healthy subjects (Pruessner et al., 1999). The sharp rise to a morning wake-up challenge followed by a clear short-term decline suggests a well-regulated system, while a lower rise or a delayed decline may indicate a dysfunctional state of the system. For example, in a chronically stressed population the decline may be less steep, indicating continued HPA overstimulation (Born et al., 1999; Edwards et al., 2001).

1. Assessment Considerations

When measuring cortisol, the choice of what sampling procedure to use, saliva or plasma, depends on the question at hand. Salivary cortisol reflects the free portion of cortisol (unbound), while plasma cortisol measurement reflects total available cortisol (bound and unbound). Because of the ease in measuring cortisol in saliva, there has been a growing use of this method. Salivary cortisol assessment can also be conducted ambulatory over 24-hour periods.

An important factor to consider is the diurnal pattern of HPA activity. For example, cortisol production has a clear diurnal variation (Bailey and Heitkemper, 1991; Weitzman et al., 1971) with the peak activity of cortisol occurring at about 8:00 a.m. in the normal sleeper, followed by a steady decline until noon. The lowest activity occurs around 8:00 p.m. It is therefore important to collect frequent samples, especially in the morning, to assess this pattern and to assess response to awakening, if that is a desired measure.

Methods used for handling data obtained from such assessment vary depending on the population and the questions being addressed. For example, measures of area-under-the-curve (total cortisol concentration over a period of time) may be better when working with healthy, normal populations, while assessment of diurnal changes and identifying rhythm profiles may be helpful when examining effects of certain diseases or disorders that may affect HPA activity.

When collecting samples in ambulatory settings, it is important to provide specific instructions on collection methods and handling of samples. For the morning sample period, participants should be instructed not to brush their teeth before completing saliva sampling to avoid contamination of saliva with blood caused by microinjuries in the oral cavity from brushing. They should also be asked to refrain from food, beverages, and cigarettes during the awakening sampling period.

A primary concern in the ambulatory assessment of cortisol is compliance with the timing of sample collections. Researchers are advised to explore the use of devices or certain prompts to promote compliance. Different types of technologies may increase adherence. For example, a personal digital assistant or alarm watch may be effective in providing reminders. The Electronic Drug Exposure Monitor (eDEM, Aardex Ltd., Switzerland) used to document sampling times can be useful. The saliva-sampling swabs used for saliva collection (e.g., Salivette™ tubes, Sarstedt, Rommelsdorf, Germany) can be placed in the eDEM. When a swab is removed from the container, the time is recorded (Kudielka et al., 2003). Although it is preferable to store samples in a freezer, the integrity of salivary cortisol samples does not seem to be compromised by storage at room temperature for up to 24 hours (Kirschbaum and Hellhammer, 1994).

Several commercially available kits that utilize immunoassays can be used in the assay of HPA hormones. Kits that assay for salivary cortisol differ from those used to assay cortisol in plasma in various technical ways. Technical details about these assays are beyond the scope of this chapter.

VI. THE SYMPATHO-ADRENO-MEDULLARY (SAM) SYSTEM

The sympathetic nervous system, in concert with the parasympathetic nervous system, plays an essential role in the body's adjustments to normal demands, and is essential for the integration and expression of the fight-flight response during times of stress (Cannon, 1914). The sympathetic nervous system controls the activity of smooth muscles or cardiac muscles by secreting norepinephrine at specialized synaptic junctions. Norepinephrine (NE) enhances the rate and force of contraction of the innervated smooth muscles. Thus, the sympathetic nervous system generally increases the activation and function of the organs it innervates.

A. Catecholamine Measures

One important element of the SAM is the sympathetic innervation of the medulla of the adrenal gland. The adrenal medulla receives sympathetic preganglionic fibers directly from the spinal cord. These fibers secrete acetylcholine causing the adrenal medulla to release epinephrine and norepinephrine into the systemic circulation where epinephrine acts as an endocrine messenger. Norepinephrine is secreted at the same time as epinephrine, but its effect on tissues via circulation is limited (Lovallo, 2004). The outcome of this cascade of actions is the mobilization of energy to the muscles and the heart, and reduction of blood flow to the internal organs and the gastrointestinal system.

In the assessment of stress, several SAM measures can be collected. The two biochemical measures, epinephrine and norepinephrine, can be obtained from blood (plasma) or in urine. The source of circulating epinephrine is primarily the adrenal medulla, but most of the circulating norepinephrine is produced by sympathetic nerve endings. There are data that indicate a positive relationship between urinary and plasma catecholamines (Akerstedt et al., 1983; Steptoe, 1985).

The choice of the type of samples to be used for the assessment of epinephrine and norepinephrine depends on the purpose for the assessment. For example, plasma levels are better suited to assess short-term effects of acute stress, while urinary levels provide integrated measurements of these catecholamines over extended periods of time (e.g., 12 hours). Assessing catecholamines in urine is more appropriate than in plasma when examining the effects of chronic stress or the effects of ongoing psychosocial factors (Baum et al., 1985).

Relative to blood sampling, collection of urine samples is logistically easier, involves no discomfort, and may not interfere with the subject's normal habits and environment. On the other hand, plasma levels can be useful to identify the effects of a specific stressor, but can be unpleasant and susceptible to multiple sources of error. Plasma also requires careful attention to the timing of when samples are collected because of the short half-life of catecholamines. While collection of blood samples requires experienced staff (e.g., a nurse), urinary collection is usually conducted by the participant. Specific instructions are provided to participants when collecting urinary samples, emphasizing that the participant should empty his/her bladder completely into the containers provided during the entire observation period.

The amount of catecholamines excreted in urine sample collected during a specific period is usually multiplied by the total urine volume, or by relating the concentration to creatinine excretion, used as a reference. The most widely used method to assay catecholamines is the high-performance liquid chromatography with electrochemical detection (Hjemdahl et al., 1989; Lundberg et al., 1988).

1. Assessment Considerations

Several methodological issues have to be considered when assaying catecholamine response to stress. Catecholamine levels are influenced by diurnal variations. The levels peak in the middle of the day and reach their lowest levels during night sleep (Akerstedt, 1979). Changes in the sleep pattern may significantly influence the circadian rhythm of the catecholamine production. In addition to sleep, other factors may influence catecholamine levels such as caffeine intake, alcohol use, smoking, heavy physical exercise, and taking certain medications that influence sympathetic activity.

In addition to these sources of variance, there may also be significant individual differences in baseline concentrations of these measures that influence the magnitude of the stress response (Forsman and Lundberg, 1982). A method to reduce the influence of circadian rhythms and individual differences in baseline levels is to calculate response measures, by subtracting baseline level obtained during relaxation from measures obtained during stress.

B. Cardiovascular Measures

Several noninvasive physiological measures can also be used to assess response to stress. These measures can be collected in a repeated fashion. Baseline measures are obtained while the person is resting; then exposure to specific behavioral or psychological stressors takes place. The difference between baseline and measures obtained during the stressor reflect the stress response. These measures include blood pressure and heart rate. Some laboratories also collect additional hemodynamic measures, including stroke volume that is used to calculate the cardiac output and total peripheral resistance. Stroke volume can be estimated in behavioral studies of humans using impedance cardiography, based on the principle that a conductor, such as the blood moving in an alternating current field, produces impedance changes that are proportional to the volume of blood. In this manner a pulsatile signal can be produced whose characteristics reflect the volume of blood ejected from the heart on each beat. The accurate estimation of stroke volume with this technique involves a number of considerations in the design of the apparatus and in the specific application to humans. More details on this technique have been published before (see Sherwood et al., 1990).

VII. THE IMMUNE RESPONSE

In addition to the HPA and SAM measures of stress, other indices of the biological response to stress involve the immune system. This system provides essential protection for the body from various invasive agents. It includes a cellular component (e.g., T cells), a humoral component (e.g., immunoglobulins), and a cytokine component (e.g., interleukins). Over the last 2 decades, a growing literature has demonstrated the value of assessing various immune measures to document individual difference in response to acute stress and to identify a propensity for negative effects of chronic stress (Kelly et al., 1997).

There are two major classes of immune system cells: phagocytes and lymphocytes. The phagocytes consist of macrophages, neutrophils, and eosinophils. Phagocytes ingest and destroy antigen. The lymphocytes consist of T cells, B cells, and natural killer (NK) cells that help in mounting a defense response. The activity of immune system cells is coordinated by a set of messengers known as cytokines. Cytokines stimulate immune cell replication and division, and because of their signaling activity, they are essential for understanding the effects of stress on immune functions.

Research has demonstrated that psychological stressors activate the production of the multiple pro-inflammatory cytokines (Dunn, 1989), and this activation seems to be mediated by cortisol production (Dobbs et al., 1996). Studies have shown that tumor necrosis factor, interleukin-1, and interleukin-6 stimulate the production of glucocorticoids (Glaser et al., 1990), while glucocorticoids have a negative-feedback effect on these cytokines. Also, B cell lymphocytes can be stimulated by corticotropin-releasing hormone and inhibited by cortisol (Reichlin, 1993).

A. Immune Response Measures

Evaluation of the immune response to stress may focus on enumerating immune cells in whole blood or measuring the level of circulating substances. Relying on measures of cell counts, however, may be limited due to the fact that cell counts are influenced by multiple biological processes, and therefore likely to produce inconsistent results. Serum immunoglobulin concentrations may be helpful in assessing effects of unhealthy lifestyles. For example, some research shows increased IgG concentrations in individuals with high job strain among those with low social support (Theorell et al., 1990).

Functional response measures may provide more information than using enumeration measures, due to the sensitivity of these measures to the competence of the immune system. They may include the assessment of antibody response to vaccines, such as the response to hepatitis B vaccine. Stress may influence our response to these vaccines, and may also decrease our control over viruses that we carry in a latent state (Kelly et al., 1997). There are also indications that certain lymphocyte measures may be used as biological markers of the effects of stress on immune function. These measures include T cell and natural killer (NK) cell activity assessed *in vitro*.

One important aspect of the assessment of immune functions in response to stress is to measure cytokine activity. Evidence has demonstrated a close interaction between immune functions and the stress response, and cytokines seem to be an essential component of this communication. The immune system signals the central nervous system with cytokines, and the central nervous system regulates the immune response through the HPA axis. Immune system cells have receptors for epinephrine, and organs of the immune system are innervated by both sympathetic and parasympathetic systems (Felten and Felten, 1991). The interactions between the immune system and the two primary stressor biological systems provide a framework for how stress may affect immune functions.

1. Assessment Considerations

Blood sampling is required to assess immune functions. There are, however, important issues that need to be considered,

including the rapid changes that occur in the numbers and types of circulating immune cells due to the circulation of the cell around the body. In order to maintain the viability of the sample for the assessment of lymphocyte proliferation and natural killer cell activity, cells must be kept alive. This limits the feasibility of using such measures in large-scale investigations or in ambulatory settings. In addition, a relatively large volume of blood is required for this assessment. By contrast, the assessment of viral antibodies and immunoglobins may be accomplished readily in such studies because assessment of antigenic response does not require blood sampling; however, multiple visits may be required by the participant over an extended period to ascertain the effects of the test. Assay techniques to measure various immune response variables are widely available and well established, and there are many suppliers of reliable kits used in these assays. Many laboratories with advanced technical expertise and equipment are usually available to conduct these assays.

VIII. CONCLUSIONS

In this chapter we briefly described a variety of assessment methods useful in the measurement of stress in research and clinical settings. These methods were selected from an almost bewildering array of assessment methods available in the literature. We conclude this chapter by discussing criteria that can guide the selection of methods that are appropriate for use in a specific research or clinical setting. These criteria are psychometric properties, "goodness of fit" to the specific setting or research question, practical considerations, comprehensiveness, multimethod or single-method assessment, and the availability of relevant measures.

A. Psychometric Properties

Reliability, generally measured with Cronbach's alpha and test-retest correlations, is important information in judging an assessment method. The reliability of a method is fundamental to being able to make meaningful sense of the results. Clinical settings require an even higher standard since one person at a time is being tested rather than large groups. The assessment methods discussed in this chapter generally have reliabilities in the .75–.90 range. Similarly, the validity of the method is crucial information in the selection process. Has the method been used in longitudinal research with established outcomes and appropriate populations? Has it been found to be valid with clinical populations similar to the ones in which it is being considered to be used? Does it correlate well to related constructs and correlate poorly to dissimilar constructs? Validity is generally established over time, with multiple investigators, and varied populations. Consequently, most of the methods we discussed were developed 10 to 30 years ago and were used in many studies with good results.

B. "Goodness of Fit"

How well does the method fit the specific research question being asked or the clinical setting in which it is being used? While seemingly simplistic, this question is too often overlooked in selecting a method. For example, one might be enamored with the MMPI-2 and decide to use it in an addiction treatment setting as a measure of stress and depression, only to find later that the BDI-II is much shorter, cheaper, and user-friendly. Similarly, one would not use the LEDS as a measure of stress in a clinical setting because of the inordinate amount of time it takes to administer and rate, as well as the tangential nature of much of the information acquired to clinical questions. Researchers looking for a biological measure of stress to relate to a paper/pencil measure of stress would probably be well advised to select a cardiovascular measure, such as blood pressure, rather than an immunological measure, whose relationship to perceived stress is less transparent.

C. Practical Considerations

Although practical considerations are the least scientific of the criteria, they often determine the final choice. Is the method likely to be accepted by the subject or patient? Is the method too invasive, unnecessarily probing, or too wide ranging in content? Can you afford the time, space, and staff required? Do you have the financial resources to use the method? Are laboratory facilities adequate and available to do the necessary analyses? Are the results easily scored and amenable to manipulation in a database? Will the clinic administration find the method acceptable and support its use? Is the method commonly used in addiction treatment facilities? These are the types of practical considerations that need to be considered in selecting a method. The method that is the soundest from a scientific point of view may not be the most practical.

D. Comprehensiveness

Brief questionnaires are tempting from an economic frame of reference. They are generally well accepted by patients and subjects, easy to score, simple to administer, and inexpensive. Their simplicity may also be their liability. By their very nature, brief questionnaires cannot sample the relevant universe of events or experiences. Important gaps occur in the assessment process that lead to inadequate results and incomplete findings. On the other hand, the most comprehensive method may be overkill and yield too much information for the question of interest.

E. Multimethod or Single-Method Measurement

When possible, the use of multiple methods of assessment is always preferable to the use of a single method. All methods have their shortcomings and sources of error. The use of multiple methods is compensatory for this error. In clinical settings, one is tempted to use a single measure because of considerations of economy. But even there, multiple measures are preferable if feasible. In research, results are generally more compelling if multiple questionnaire and biological measures are used. One set of measures amplifies the other, producing a much richer results section and more meaningful findings.

F. Availability of Relevant Measures

If measures exist that meet the preceding criteria, use them. The world probably does not need another paper/pencil measure of depression, for example. In the literature can be found thousands of measures of mental and physical health status, most of which have very little evidence, if any, attesting to their psychometric soundness. Fortunately, the literature also contains measures with excellent psychometric properties that have been used in many studies and clinical settings. If you have a research problem or a clinical question, almost certainly an assessment method exists to help you.

REFERENCES

Akerstedt, T. (1979). Altered sleep/wake patterns and circadian rhythms. Laboratory and field studies of sympathomedullary and related variables. *Acta Physiologica Scandinavica, Supplement 469*.

Akerstedt, T., Gillberg, M., Hjemdahl, P., Sigurdson, K., Gustavsson, I., Daleskog, M., and Pollare, T. (1983). Comparison of urinary and plasma catecholamine responses to mental stress. *Acta Physiologica Scandinavica, 117*, 19–26.

al'Absi, M., Petersen, K., & Wittmer, L. (2000). Blood pressure and not parental history for hypertension predicts pain perception in women. *Pain, 88*, 61–68.

al'Absi, M., Bongard S., Buchanan, T., Pincomb, G., Licinio, J., and Lovallo, W. R. (1997). Neuroendocrine and hemodynamic responses to extended mental and interpersonal stressors. *Psychophysiology, 34*, 266–275.

American Psychatric Association (1994). *Diagnostic and Statisticol Manual of Mental Disorders (DSM-IV)*. Washington, D.C. American Psychiatric Association.

Anda, R. F., Croft, J. B., Felitti, V. J., Nordenberg, D., Giles, W. F., Williamson, D. F., and Giovino, G. A. (1999). Adverse childhood experiences and smok-

ing during adolescence and adulthood. *Journal of the American Medical Association, 282*(17), 1652–1658.

Bailey, S. L., and Heitkemper, M. M. (1991). Morningness-eveningness and early-morning salivary cortisol levels. *Biological Psychology, 32*, 181–192.

Barnes, L. L. B., Harp, D., and Jung, W. S. (2002). Reliability generalization of scores on the Spielberger State-Trait Anxiety Inventory. *Educational and Psychological Measurement, 62*(4), 603–618.

Baum, A., Lundberg, U., Grunberg, N., Singer, J., and Gatchel, R. (1985). Urinary catecholamines in behavioral research in stress. In C. R. Lake and M. G. Ziegler (Eds.), *The catecholamines in psychiatric and neurologic disorders* (pp. 55–72). Ann Arbor: Butterworths.

Beck, A. T., Steer, R. A., and Brown, G. K. (1996). *The Beck Depression Inventory Second Edition (BDI-II)*. San Antonio, TX: Harcourt Assessment.

Born, J., Hansen, K., Marshall, L., Molle, M., and Fehm, H. L. (1999). Timing the end of nocturnal sleep. *Nature, 397*, 29–30.

Brewin, C. R. (2005). Systematic review of screening instruments for adults at risk of PTSD. *Journal of Traumatic Stress, 18*(1), 53–62.

Brown, G. W. (1974). Meaning, measurement and stress of life events. In B. S. Dohrenwend and B. P. Dohrenwend (Eds.), *Stressful life events: Their nature and effects* (pp. 217–244). New York: John Wiley.

Brown, G. W., and Harris, T. O. (1978). *Social origins of depression: A study of psychiatric disorders in women*. London: Tavistock.

Brown, G. W., and Harris, T. O. (1989). *Life events and illness*. New York: Guilford Press.

Bryant, R., and Harvey, A. (1996). Visual imagery in posttraumatic stress disorder. *Journal of Traumatic Stress, 9*, 613–619.

Butcher, J. N., Dahlstrom, W. G., Graham, J. R., Tellegen, A., and Kaemmer, B. (1989). *Minnesota Multiphasic Personality Inventory (MMPI-2). Manual for administration and scoring*. Minneapolis: University of Minnesota Press.

Cannon, W. B. (1914). The emergent function of the adrenal medulla in pain and the major emotions. *American Journal of Physiology, 33*, 356–372.

Cohen, S., Kamarck, T., and Mermelstein, R. (1983). A global measure of perceived stress. *Journal of Health and Social Behavior, 24*, 385–396.

Cohen, S., Kessler, R. C., and Gordon, L. U. (1995). *Measuring stress: A guide for health and social scientists*. New York: Oxford University Press.

Cohen, S., and Williamson, G. M. (1988). Perceived stress in a probability sample of the United States. In S. Spacapan and S. Oskamp (Eds.), *The social psychology of health*. Newbury Park, CA: Sage.

Cooke, D. J., and Allan, C. A. (1984). Stressful life events and alcohol abuse in women: A general population study. *British Journal of Addiction, 79*(4), 425–430.

Cooper, C., Sloan, S., and Williams, S. (1988). *The Occupational Stress Indicator: Management guide*. Windsor, England: NFER-Nelson.

Dallman, M. (1993). Stress update: Adaptation of the hypothalamic-pituitary-adrenal axis to chronic stress. *Trends in Endocrinology and Metabolism, 4,* 62–69.

Day, R., Nielsen, J. A., Korten, A., Ernberg, G., Dube, K. C., Gebhart, J., Jablensky, A., Leon, C., Marsella, A., Olatawura, M., Sartorius, N., Stromgren, E., Takahashi, R., Wig, N., and Wynne, L. C. (1987). Stressful life events preceding the acute onset of schizophrenia: A cross-national study from the world health organization. *Culture, Medicine and Psychiatry, 11*(2), 123–205.

Denollet, J. (1998). Personality and coronary heart disease: The Type-D Scale-16. *Annals of Behavioral Medicine, 20*(3), 209–215.

Denollet, J. (2005). DS14: Standard assessment of negative affectivity, social inhibition, and Type D personality. *Psychosomatic Medicine, 67,* 89–97.

Denollet, J., and De Vries, J. (2006). Positive and negative affect within the realm of depression, stress and fatigue: The two factor distress model of the global mood scale (GMS). *Journal of Affective Disorders, 12.*

Denollet, J., and Van Heck, G. (2001). Psychological risk factors in heart disease: What Type D personality is (not) about. *Journal of Psychosomatic Research, 51,* 465–468.

Dobbs, C. M., Feg, N., Beck, F. M., and Sheridan, J. F. (1996). Neuroendocrine regulation of cytokine production during experimental influenza viral infection. *Journal of Immunology, 157,* 1870–1877.

Dohrenwend, B. P., Link, B., Kern, G., Shrout, P., and Markowitz, J. (1987). *Measuring life events: The problem of variability within event categories.* London: Croom Helm.

Dohrenwend, B. P., Link, B. G., Kern, R., Shrout, P., and Markowitz, J. (1990). Measuring life events: The problem of variability within event categories. *Stress Medicine, 6*(3), 179–187.

Dohrenwend, B. P., Raphael, K. G., Schwartz, S., Stueve, A., and Skodol, A. (1993). The structural event probe and narrative rating method for measuring stressful life events. In L. Goldberger and S. Breznitz (Eds.), *Handbook of stress. Theoretical and clinical aspects* (2nd ed., pp. 174–196). New York: The Free Press.

Dohrenwend, B. S., Krasnoff, L., Askensay, A. R., and Dohrenwend, B. P. (1978). Exemplification of a method for scaling life events. The PERI Life Events scale. *Journal of Health and Social Behavior, 19,* 205–229.

Dube, S., Williamson, D., Thompson, T., Felitti, V. J., and Anda, R. (2004). Assessing the reliability of retrospective reports of adverse childhood experiences among adult HMO members attending a primary care clinic. *Child Abuse and Neglect 28,* 729–737.

Dunn, A. J. (1989). Psychoneuroimmunology for the psychoneuroendocrinologist: A review of animal studies of nervous system immune system interactions. *Psychoneuroendocrinology, 14,* 251.

Edwards, S., Evans, P., Hucklebridge, F., and Clow, A. (2001). Association between time of awakening and diurnal cortisol secretory activity. *Psychoneuroendocrinology, 26,* 613–622.

Felitti, V. J. (2002). The relation between adverse childhood experiences and adult health: Turning gold into lead. *The Permanente Journal, 6*(1), 44–47.

Felitti, V. J., Anda, R. F., Nordenberg, D., Williamson, D. F., Spitz, A. M., Edwards, V., et al. (1998). Relationship of childhood abuse and household dysfunction to many of the leading causes of death in adults. *American Journal of Preventive Medicine, 14*(4), 245–258.

Felten, S., and Felten, D. (1991). Innervation of lymphoid tissue. In R. Ader, D. L. Felten, and S. Cohen (Eds.), *Psychoneuroimmunology* (2nd ed., pp. 27–69). San Diego, CA: Academic Press.

Foa, E. B., Riggs, D. S., Dancu, B. O., and Rothbaum, B. (1993). Reliability and validity of a brief instrument for assessing post-traumatic stress disorder. *Journal of Traumatic Stress, 6*(4), 459–473.

Forsman, L., and Lundberg, U. (1982). Consistency in catecholamine and cortisol excretion in males and females. *Pharmacology, Biochemistry and Behavior, 17,* 555–562.

French, S., Lenton, R., Walters, V., and Eyles, J. (2000). An empirical evaluation of an expanded nursing stress scale. *Journal of Nursing Measurement, 8*(2), 161–178.

Gibson, S. J. (1997). The measurement of mood states in older adults. *Journals of Gerontology Series B, 52*(4), 167–174.

Glaser, R., Kennedy, S., Lafuse, W. P., Bonneau, R. H., Speicher, C., Hillhouse, J., and Kielcolt-Glaser, J. K. (1990). Psychological stress-induced modulation of interleukin 2 receptor gene expression and interleukin 2 production in peripheral blood leukocytes. *Archives of General Psychiatry, 47,* 707–712.

Hackman, J., and Lawler, E. (1971). Employee reactions to job characteristics. *Journal of Applied Psychology, 55,* 259–285.

Hann, D., Winter, K., and Jacobsen, P. (1999). Measurement of depressive symptoms in cancer patients: Evaluation of the Center for Epidemiological Studies Depression scale (CES-D). *Journal of Psychosomatic Research, 46*(5), 437–443.

Himmelfarb, S., and Murrell, S. A. (1983). Reliability and validity of five mental health scales in older persons. *Journal of Gerontology, 38*(3), 333–339.

Hjemdahl, P., Larsson, P. T., Bradley, T., Akerstedt, T., Anderzén, I., Sigurdson, K., Gillberg, M., and Lundberg, U. (1989). Catecholamine measurements in urine with high-performance liquid chromatography with amperometric detection-comparison with an autoanalyser fluorescence method. *Journal of Chromatography, 494,* 53–66.

Holmes, T. H., and Rahe, T. H. (1967). The social readjustment rating scale. *Journal of Psychosomatic Research, 11,* 213–218.

Horowitz, M., Wilner, N., and Alvarez, W. (1979). Impact of Event Scale: A measure of subjective stress. *Psychosomatic Medicine, 41*, 209–218.

Insel, P., and Moos, R. (1974). *Work Environment Scale.* Palo Alto: CA: Consulting Psychologists Press.

Joseph, S. (2000). Psychometric evaluation of Horowitz's Impact of Event Scale: A review. *Journal of Traumatic Stress, 13*, 101–113.

Kanner, A., Coyne, J., Schaefer, C., and Lazarus, R. (1981). Comparison of two models of stress measurement: Daily hassles and uplifts versus major life events. *Journal of Behavioral Medicine, 4*, 1–39.

Keane, T. M., Caddell, J. M., and Taylor, K. L. (1988). Mississippi scale for combat-related post traumatic stress disorder: Three studies in reliability and validity. *Journal of Consulting and Clinical Psychology, 56*(1), 85–90.

Keane, T. M., Malloy, P. E., and Fairbank, J. A. (1984). Empirical development of an MMPI subscale for the assessment of combat-related posttraumatic stress. *Journal of Consulting and Clinical Psychology, 52*(5), 888–891.

Kelly, S., Hertzman, C., and Daniels, M. (1997). Searching for the biological pathways between stress and health. *Annual Review of Public Health, 18*, 437–462.

Kirschbaum, C., and Hellhammer, D. H. (1994). Salivary cortisol in psychoneuroendocrine research: Recent developments and applications. *Psychoneuroendocrinology, 19*, 313–333.

Kudielka, B. M., Broderick, J. E., and Kirschbaum, C. (2003). Compliance with saliva sample protocols: Electronic monitoring reveals invalid cortisol daytime profile in noncompliant subjects. *Psychosomatic Medicine, 65*, 313–319.

Lazarus, R. S., and Folkman, S. (1984). *Stress, appraisal, and coping.* New York: Springer Publishing Company.

Lazarus, R. S., and Folkman, S. (1989). *Manual: Hassles and uplifts scales.* Redwood City, CA: Mind Garden.

Leskala, U. S., Melartin, T. K., Lestela-Mielonen, P. S., Rytsala, H. J., Sokero, T. P., Heikkinen, M. E., et al. (2004). Life events, social support, and onset of major depressive episode in Finnish patients. *Journal of Nervous and Mental Disease, 192*(5), 373–381.

Lovallo, W. R. (2004). *Stress and health: Biological and psychological interactions.* Thousand Oaks, CA: Sage.

Lundberg, U., Holmberg, L., and Frankenhaeuser, M. (1988). Urinary catecholamines: Comparison between HPLC with electrochemical detection and fluorophotometric assay. *Pharmacology, Biochemistry and Behavior, 31*, 287–290.

Lyons, J. A., and Wheeler-Cox, T. (1999). MMPI, MMPI-2, and PTSD: Overview of scores, scales, and profiles. *Journal of Traumatic Stress, 12*(1), 175–183.

Malkoff-Schwartz, S., Frank, E., Anderson, B., Sherrill, J. T., Siegel, L., Patterson, D., and Kupfer, D. (1998). Stressful life events and social rhythm disruption in the onset of manic and depressive bipolar episodes:

A preliminary investigation. *Archives of General Psychiatry, 55*(8), 702–707.

McDowell, I., and Newell, C. (1996). *Measuring health: A guide to rating scales and questionnaires.* New York: Oxford University Press.

McNair, D. M., Heuchert, J., and Shilony, E. (2003). *Profile of mood states.* North Tonawanda, NY: Multi-Health Systems, Inc.

McNair, D. M., Lorr, M., and Droppleman, L. (1992). *POMS: Profile of mood states.* San Diego: Educational and Industrial Testing Service.

McQuaid, J. R., Monroe, S. M., Roberts, J. E., Kupfer, D. J., and Frank, E. (2000). A comparison of two life stress approaches: Prospective prediction of treatment outcome in recurrent depression. *Journal of Abnormal Psychology, 109*(4), 787–791.

Monroe, S. M., and Kelley, J. M. (1995). Measurement of stress appraisal. In S. Cohen, R. C. Kessler, and L. U. Gordon (Eds.), *Measuring stress: A guide for health and social scientists.* New York: Oxford University Press.

Numeroff, R., and Abrams, M. (1984). Sources of stress among nurses: An empirical investigation. *Journal of Human Stress, 10*, 88–100.

O'Doherty, F., and Davies, J. B. (1987). Life events and addiction: A critical review. *British Journal of Addiction, 82*, 127–137.

Osipow, S., and Spokane, A. (1981). *Occupational Stress Inventory: Research guide.* Odessa, FL: Psychological Resources.

Paykel, E. S. (1983). Methodological aspects of life events research. *Journal of Psychosomatic Research, 27*(5), 342–351.

Paykel, E. S. (1997). The interview for recent life events. *Psychological Medicine, 27*, 301–310.

Pruessner, J. C., Hellhammer, D. H., and Kirschbaum, C. (1999). Burnout, perceived stress, and cortisol responses to awakening. *Psychosomatic Medicine, 61*, 197–204.

Radloff, L. (1977). The CES-D scale—a self report depression scale for research in the general population. *Applied Psychological Measurement, 1*, 385–401.

Reichlin, S. (1993). Neuroendocrine-immune interactions. *New England Journal of Medicine, 329*, 1246–1253.

Schmidt, U., Tiller, J., Andrews, B., Blanchard, M., and Treasure, J. (1997). Is there a specific trauma precipitating onset of an eating disorder? *Psychological Medicine, 27*, 523–530.

Scully, J. A., Tosi, H., and Banning, K. (2000). Life events checklists: Revisiting the social readjustment rating scale after 30 years. *Educational and Psychological Measurement, 60*(6), 864–876.

Sherwood, A., Dolan, C. A., and Light, K. C. (1990). Hemodynamics of blood pressure responses during active and passive coping. *Psychophysiology, 27*, 656–668.

Shrout, P. E., Link, B. G., Dohrenwend, B. P., Skodol, A. E., Stueve, A., and Mirotznik, J. (1989). Characterizing life events as risk factors for depression:

The role of fateful loss events. *Journal of Abnormal Psychology, 98,* 460–467.

Spielberger, C. D. (1989). *State Trait Anxiety Inventory: A comprehensive bibliography.* Palo Alto, CA: Mind Garden.

Spielberger, C. D., and Gorsuch, R. L. (1983). *Manual for the State-Trait Anxiety Inventory (STAI).* Palo Alto: Mind Garden.

Steptoe, A. (1985). The assessment of sympathetic nervous function in human stress research. *Journal of Psychosomatic Research, 31,* 141–152.

Straus, M., and Gelles, R. (1990). *Physical violence in American families: Risk factors and adaptations to violence in 8,145 families.* New Brunswick, NJ: Transaction Press.

Theorell, T., Orth-Gomer, K., and Eneroth, P. (1990). Slow-reacting immunoglobulin in relation to social support and changes in job strain: A preliminary note. *Psychosomatic Medicine, 52,* 511–516.

Turrina, C., Zimmerman-Tansella, C., Micciolo, R., and Siciliani, O. (1993). A community survey of psychotropic drug consumption in South Verona: Prevalence and associated variables. *Social Psychiatry and Psychiatric Epidemiology, 28*(1), 40–44.

Vagg, P., and Spielberger, C. (1998). Occupational stress: Measuring job pressure and organizational support in the workplace. *Journal of Occupational Health Psychology, 3,* 294–305.

Watson, D., Clark, L., and Tellegen, A. (1988). Development and validation of brief measures of positive and negative affect: The PANAS scales. *Journal of Personality and Social Psychology, 54,* 1063–1070.

Weiss, D., and Marmar, C. (1997). Impact of Event Scale-Revised. In J. Wilson and T. Keane (Eds.), *Assessing psychological trauma and PTSD.* New York: Guilford Press.

Weitzman, E. D., Fukushima, D., Nogeire, C., Roffwarg, H., Gallagher, T. F., and Hellman, L. (1971). Twenty-four hour pattern of the episodic secretion of cortisol in normal subjects. *Journal of Clinical Endocrinology, 33,* 14–21.

Williamson, D. E., Birmaher, B., Frank, E., Anderson, B., Matty, M., and Kupfer, D. (1998). Nature of life events and difficulties in depressed adolescents. *Journal of the American Academy of Child and Adolescent Psychiatry, 37*(10), 1049–1057.

14

Assessment of Addictions in Clinical and Research Settings

MICHAEL ELLERY AND SHERRY H. STEWART

People who are suffering from stress-related illness are at risk for the development of an addiction (Stewart, 1996), and stress often precedes relapse among people in recovery from an addiction (Marlatt and Gordon, 1985). In both research and therapeutic intervention, accurate assessment is essential for the development of effective case formulations, planning treatments, and evaluating outcomes. To these ends, important areas to assess include problem severity, relapse risk, substance use expectancies, motivations to engage in addictive behavior, and treatment readiness. When one is selecting appropriate assessment instruments, it is important to consider factors such as acceptability of the instrument to clients, the availability of population norms, the time required to administer the measure, clinician training required for administration, and the psychometric properties of the measure. Instruments have been developed for such purposes as to screen for possible addiction, diagnose addictive disorders, measure the quantity and frequency of addictive behaviors, assess symptom severity, and plan treatment. Instruments should be selected in accordance with the purpose

for which they have been developed. This chapter reviews the purposes and psychometric properties of a number of addiction measures.

I. INTRODUCTION

Whether one is conducting research or doing clinical work, accurate assessment is necessary for effective case formulation, treatment planning, intervention, and outcome evaluation. In addition to data gathered by means of less formal clinical interviewing, and data gathered from collateral sources (e.g., review of medical charts, legal records, etc.), the information acquired by using more formal assessment instruments is often extremely useful.

When one is selecting a measure, or a battery of measures, a number of considerations are important including the measure's psychometric properties, the population on which it was normed, clinician training requirements, administration time, and the purpose of the assessment. One of the most important considerations in test selection is reviewing the measure's

Stress and Addiction: Biological and Psychological Mechanisms
Edited by **Mustafa al'Absi, Ph.D.**

psychometric properties. In general, standards of test reliability and validity are rigorous for clinical use and somewhat less so for research purposes. Moreover, it is important to be aware of whether a measure has been normed for the population with whom it is being considered for use. Also to be considered when selecting an instrument are clinician training requirements, time required for administration, scoring and interpretation, the acceptability of the measure to clients, and general ease of use. Because addictive behavior instruments can be used for a number of purposes, including screening, diagnosis, measurement of addiction-related behavior, treatment planning, assessment of treatment process, and outcome evaluation (Allen and Wilson, 2003), an appropriate instrument should be selected with its specific purpose in mind. An instrument designed for one purpose should not be used for another. For instance, the purpose of an addiction screen is to detect the possible presence of an addictive problem for further inquiry. As such, screens are often designed to be more sensitive than specific. Thus, the use of a screen for diagnosis would frequently result in a number of false positives and, consequently, overdiagnosis of the addictive disorder. A positive score on a screen warrants a more thorough assessment, which may include diagnostic measures. The topics of a thorough assessment might include the current presentation of the problem, coming to a diagnosis (including the duration and severity of the problem), description of the patient's strengths and social supports, measurement of the patient's readiness for treatment, determination of the patient's needs with respect to treatment, and treatment planning. Obviously, considerable resources are required to conduct a thorough assessment. While not diagnostic, the utility of screens becomes apparent when attempting to appropriately allocate limited assessment resources.

There are a number of other important factors to evaluate when conducting assessments in addiction (Negrete, 2005). One is the severity of substance use levels and problems, which is useful clinically when matching treatment options to the problems being experienced. Knowledge of the severity of the addictive problem can also be useful in the research context (e.g., to homogenize severity in the selected sample in order to minimize confounds in research). Several instruments that are useful in this regard are the Quantity-Frequency Index, the Alcohol Dependence Scale (ADS; Skinner and Allen, 1982), the Timeline Follow-Back method (TLFB; Sobell and Sobell, 1973), the Fagerstrom Tolerance Questionnaire (FTQ; Fagerstrom, 1978), and the Fagerstrom Test for Nicotine Dependence (FTND; Heatherton, Kozlowski, Frecker, and Fagerstrom, 1991). Another important construct to assess is individual vulnerability to relapse across specific high-risk situations. Useful instruments to measure this construct include the Inventory of Drinking Situations (IDS; Annis, Graham, and Davis, 1987), the Inventory of Drug Taking Situations (IDTS; Turner, Annis, and Sklar, 1997), the Inventory of Gambling Situations (IGS; Turner and Littman-Sharp, 2001), and the Situational Confidence Questionnaire (SCQ; Annis and Graham, 1988). Substance use expectancies are also important to assess when developing cognitive strategies to treat addiction. Useful instruments to measure outcome expectancies in the alcohol research area include the Alcohol Expectancy Questionnaire (AEQ; Brown, Goldman, Inn, and Anderson, 1980), the expectancy subscales of the Alcohol Craving Questionnaire (ACQ; Singleton, Tiffany, and Henningfield, 1994), and the Comprehensive Effects of Alcohol (CEOA; Fromme, Stroot, and Kaplan, 1993) scale. Like expectancies, it is helpful to understand the motivation to use substances when planning treatment. Measures to assess substance use motives include the Drinking Motives Questionnaire (DMQ; Cooper, Russell, Skinner, and Windle, 1992), the Marijuana Motives Measure (Simons, Correia, and Carey, 2000), and the Reasons for Smoking Test (RFS; Ikard, Green, and Horn, 1969). Readiness to engage in treatment is another important construct to tap in assessment. One instrument to measure this factor is the Stages of Change Readiness and Treatment Eagerness Scale (SOCRATES; Miller and Tonigan, 1996). The psychometrics of each of these instruments, along with several addiction screens and a diagnostic instrument (i.e., the Structured Clinical Interview for DSM [SCID]; Spitzer, Williams, Gibbon, and First, 1992), are reviewed in this chapter. See Table 14-1.

II. ADDICTION SCREENS

A. Michigan Alcoholism Screening Test (MAST; Selzer, 1971)

The MAST was initially devised as an instrument that could accurately detect alcoholism and that could be administered quickly by both professionals and nonprofessionals (Selzer, 1971). Since its development over 30 years ago, it has undergone numerous evaluations and reviews (e.g., Martin, Liepman, and Young, 1990; Storgaard, Nielson, and Gluud, 1994; Tulevski, 1989). The original MAST contained 25 dichotomous (i.e., "Yes" or "No") items, which were scored zero or one, two, or five, depending on the item (Selzer, 1971). The MAST has high internal consistency (alpha = .83–.95; Hedlund and Vieweg, 1984). Estimates of the MAST's sensitivity and specificity have both ranged widely (from .36 to nearly 1.00; Storgaard et al., 1994). The MAST demonstrates acceptable validity against clinicians' diagnoses (Magruder-Habib, Fraker, and Peterson, 1983) and biochemical alcoholic markers (Bell and Steensland, 1987). Criticisms of the MAST include its inability to discriminate between active alcoholism and alcoholism in remission (Rounsaville, Weissman, Wilber, and Kleber, 1983; Toland and Moss, 1989), the ability of alcoholics

to deliberately misrepresent themselves and go undetected (Otto and Hall, 1988), and its tendency to overidentify alcoholism (Gibbs, 1983), particularly among young people (Brady, Foulks, Childress, and Pertshuk, 1982; Martin et al., 1990). The latter issue has been shown to be corrected by elevation of the MAST's usual cutoff score (Martin et al., 1990). The MAST is frequently administered as a 10-item instrument, with similar psychometric properties (Brief MAST; Pokorny, Miller, and Kaplan, 1972). It is also available as a 13-item Short MAST (SMAST; Selzer, Vinokur, and van Rooijen, 1975) or a 9-item instrument called the Malmo modified MAST (Mm-MAST; Kristenson and Trell, 1982). The MAST demonstrates adequate psychometric properties as an alcoholism screen, as long as the subpopulation on which it is used remains a consideration. It should not be used with clients whom the clinician suspects may be motivated to go undetected.

B. Drug Abuse Screening Test (DAST; Skinner, 1982)

The 28 self-report items of the original DAST were modified from the MAST. It was initially developed to quantify problems with drugs other than alcohol (Skinner, 1982). Skinner (1982) recommended a 20-item version of the DAST which has very similar psychometric properties to the original and is shorter to administer. A 10-item version has also been developed (Bohn, Babor, and Kranzler, 1991), also with similar psychometric properties to the original. The DAST items are scored dichotomously (i.e., "Yes" or "No"), with cutoff scores that balance the sensitivity and specificity of the instrument set around five or six for the 20- and 28-item versions (Cocco and Carey, 1998; Gavin, Ross, and Skinner, 1989; Skinner, 1982; Staley and el-Guebaly, 1990) and three or four for the 10-item version (Bohn et al., 1991; Cocco and Carey, 1998). The DAST is unifactorial (Skinner, 1982; Staley and el-Guebaly, 1990), with

TABLE 14-1   Addiction Measures and Their Uses

Measure	Use				
	Screening	Diagnosis	Symptom Severity	Behavioral Measure	Treatment Planning
Alcohol Craving Questionnaire (ACQ)					X
Alcohol Dependence Scale (ADS)			X		
Alcohol Expectancy Questionnaire (AEQ; AEQ-III)					X
Alcohol Use Inventory (AUI)			X		
Brief Michigan Alcoholism Screening Test (Brief MAST)	X				
Canadian Problem Gambling Index (CPGI)	X				
Comprehensive Effects of Alcohol (CEOA)					X
Decisional Balance Scale (DBS)					X
Drinking Motives Questionnaire (DMQ; DMQ-R)					X
Drug Abuse Screening Test (DAST)	X				
Fagerstrom Test for Nicotine Dependence (FTND)			X		
Fagerstrom Tolerance Questionnaire (FTQ)			X		
Inventory of Drinking Situations (IDS)					X

Screen	
Inventory of Drug Taking Situations (IDTS)	
Inventory of Gambling Situations (IGS)	X
Malmo modified Michigan Alcoholism Screening Test (Mm-MAST)	X
Marijuana Motives Measure (MM)	
Michigan Alcoholism Screening Test (MAST)	X
Quantity-Frequency Index (QFI)	X
Reasons for Smoking Test (RFS)	X
Short Michigan Alcoholism Screening Test (SMAST)	X
Situational Confidence Questionnaire (SCQ)	X
South Oaks Gambling Screen (SOGS)	X
Stages of Change Readiness and Treatment Eagerness Scale (SOCRATES)	
Structured Clinical Interview for DSM (SCID)	X
Timeline Follow-Back method (TLFB)	X

Note: Adapted from Allen and Wilson (2003).

excellent internal consistency (alphas = .92–.94; Cocco and Carey, 1998; Skinner, 1982; Staley and el-Guebaly, 1990). Two week test-retest reliability is good (20-item version = .78; 10-item version = .71; Cocco and Carey, 1998).

C. South Oaks Gambling Screen (SOGS; Lesieur and Blume, 1987)

The SOGS was developed to provide a structured instrument for detecting pathological gambling that could be easily administered by both professionals and nonprofessionals (Lesieur and Blume, 1987). Its content was derived from the third version of the *Diagnostic and Statistical Manual of Mental Disorders* (*DSM-III*; American Psychiatric Association [APA], 1980) criteria, the 20 questions of Gamblers Anonymous (GA), and also from the expert opinion of counselors working in the area of pathological gambling. Subsequently, the instrument was cross-validated against *DSM-III-R* (APA, 1987) criteria, using scores obtained from three populations: GA members, university students, and hospital employees (Lesieur and Blume, 1987). Validated against the *DSM-III-R* criteria, the SOGS appears to be both sensitive and specific (Lesieur and Blume, 1987). False positives range from 0.7% to 1.4%, and false negatives range from 0.0% to 3.4% (Lesieur and Blume, 1987). Internal consistency is high (alpha = .97), and retest reliability is adequate (r = .71; Lesieur and Blume, 1987).

The SOGS has become a widely used clinical and epidemiological screen (Lesieur and Blume, 1993; Volberg and Banks, 1990). Until recently, the SOGS was the "gold standard" for the clinical screening of probable pathological gamblers (Volberg and Banks, 1990). However, newer instruments such as the Canadian Problem Gambling Index (CPGI; Ferris and Wynne, 2001), which was developed using *DSM-IV* (APA, 1994) criteria for pathological gambling, have begun to compete with the SOGS for this status.

III. DIAGNOSTIC MEASURES

A. The Structured Clinical Interview for DSM (SCID; Spitzer et al., 1992)

Structured clinical interviews play a very important role in the diagnosis of addictive disorders. They operationalize the criteria for making a given diagnosis as outlined in existing diagnostic systems such as the current version of the *DSM* (APA, 1994). They also ensure that interviewers ask questions in a standardized manner to enhance inter-rater agreement. The SCID is one such structured psychiatric interview that can be used to assist in making diagnoses of substance use disorders. It was originally developed as a semistructured interview for making diagnoses for various Axis I disorders according to the criteria outlined in the *DSM-III-R* (APA, 1987). It has since been revised for use with the *DSM-IV* (APA, 1994)—i.e., the SCID-IV. The SCID was specifically designed to be administered by trained clinicians rather than by lay interviewers to allow for the benefit of the clinicians' wealth of experience in assisting the diagnostic interview process.

Various editions have been developed specifically for use with particular populations such as psychiatric patients (SCID-P) and nonpatient samples (SCID-NP; Spitzer et al., 1992). Both of these versions include a module assessing psychoactive substance use disorders: alcohol; sedatives, hypnotics, and anxiolytics; cannabis; stimulants; opioids; cocaine; hallucinogens/PCP; polysubstance; and other substances. In addition to making each of these diagnoses, the SCID is also used to obtain additional information such as age at onset and time since last symptoms (if the disorder is not current; Spitzer et al., 1992).

Structured interviews are intended to improve inter-rater reliability of diagnoses. The reliability of the SCID was tested in a multisite study (Williams et al., 1992): Two clinicians independently interviewed and rated each participant, and rate of diagnostic agreement was examined. Kappa values above .70 indicate good agreement. In the total sample of 390 psychiatric patients, kappas for lifetime and current alcohol use disorder and other drug use disorder were all good (range = .73–.85). In the sample of 202 nonpatients, kappas for lifetime alcohol use disorder and other drug use disorder were similarly good (kappas = .76 and .85, respectively). Agreement was variable across specific classes of drug dependence, however, ranging from a low kappa of .22 for current cannabis dependence, to a high of .95 for lifetime opioid dependence. Since the sample on which these data were based was very small (n = 50), additional information is needed on the reliability of specific drug dependence diagnoses in future research.

This same study also compared interrater agreement with the SCID to that obtained with other established structured interviews. The SCID performed as well or better than several other interviews across a variety of substance use disorder diagnoses for both the patient and nonpatient samples (Williams et al., 1992). Overall, these findings support the use of the SCID Psychoactive Substance Use Disorders module for making diagnoses of addictive disorders, at least when administered by appropriately trained clinicians.

IV. SYMPTOM SEVERITY MEASURES

A. Alcohol Use Inventory (AUI; Horn, Wanberg, and Foster, 1990) and Alcohol Dependence Scale (ADS; Skinner and Allen, 1982)

Based on early factor analytic studies of self-reports completed by people seeking treatment for alcohol problems, Wanberg and Horn (1983) theorized that alcohol abuse is actually composed of a wide range of dimensions (i.e., alcohol use, background,

current situation, personality, immediate response to treatment, and long-term outcome), rather than a unitary construct. The AUI (Horn et al., 1990) was developed to assess the domain of alcohol use. The 25-item ADS (Skinner and Allen, 1982; Skinner and Horn, 1984) is derived from one of the subscales of the original AUI. The ADS is well validated, and a user's manual and normative data are available on this self-report measure of dependence severity. A conservative cutoff for "alcohol dependence" is an ADS score of 21 (the 50th percentile in the normative sample). Respondents scoring below this cutoff have rarely experienced severe alcohol withdrawal symptoms such as hallucinations, seizures, or delirium tremens (Skinner and Horn, 1984). Unlike many available measures of alcohol dependence severity, the ADS is sensitive at lower levels of dependence (Skinner and Allen, 1982; Sobell and Sobell, 1993). It is quick to administer and has adequate psychometric properties (Sobell and Sobell, 1993).

B. Fagerstrom Tolerance Questionnaire (FTQ; Fagerstrom, 1978) and the Fagerstrom Test for Nicotine Dependence (FTND; Heatherton et al., 1991)

The FTQ and later the FTND were both designed to quantify smokers' level of physical dependence on nicotine. The FTND is embedded within the original FTQ and is now used more commonly than the original. A sample item includes: "Do you find it difficult to refrain from smoking in places where it is forbidden such as church, the library, or movie theatres?" Heatherton et al. (1991) provided scoring details for the FTND. The FTND score can also be used to classify smokers into one of five levels of smoking dependence: very low, low, moderate, high, and very high (Fagerstrom, Heatherton, and Kozlowski, 1990). The FTND has shown good reliability in terms of both internal consistency and test-retest stability coefficients, and has demonstrated validity in terms of positive relations with key smoking variables such as saliva cotinine (Heatherton et al., 1991; Payne, Smith, McCracken, McSherry, and Antony, 1994; Pomerleau, Carton, Lutzke, Flessland, and Pomerleau, 1994).

V. BEHAVIORAL MEASURES

A. Quantity-Frequency Index (QFI)

The assessment of drinking levels is common in alcohol research either because drinking level is the focus of the research or simply to provide descriptive information on the drinking behavior of the sample in question. It is also a critical feature of any treatment for alcohol use problems (Sobell and Sobell, 1993). One method of assessing drinking levels is via the QFI self-report method (e.g., Stewart, Peterson, and Pihl, 1995; Stewart, Angelopoulos, Baker, and Boland, 2000). For frequency, respondents are asked to report on the number of occasions per week on which they usually consume alcohol. Options are normally given for respondents to provide monthly or yearly drinking frequency if they typically drink less often than once a week. For quantity, respondents are asked to indicate the average number of alcoholic beverages they usually consume per drinking occasion. They are normally provided a definition of what constitutes one standard drink. Sometimes these two indices are multiplied to yield a composite "drinks per week" variable (e.g., Stewart et al., 1995). However, it has been noted that valuable information can be lost when the composite is used rather than examining quantity and frequency separately. For example, quantity is more associated with alcohol problems than drinking frequency (see Stewart et al., 2000). Although much research indicates that people are generally quite accurate when self-reporting drinking levels (Sobell and Sobell, 1990), several

recommended procedures for enhancing self-report accuracy should be employed when using QFI measures (e.g., drinking questions should be presented in an open-ended as opposed to forced-choice format to minimize socially desirable responding; confidentiality should be assured; assessment should be conducted when respondent is in a drug-free state; drinking measures should be embedded within other questions to reduce their salience; Sobell and Sobell, 1990).

One of the main problems with the QFI method is that heavy drinking episodes tend to be missed if they are not the part of the typical or average pattern (Conrod, Stewart, and Pihl, 1998). Another problem is that the QFI method forces respondents to impose a pattern on their drinking behavior when in fact their drinking may be far from patterned (Sobell and Sobell, 1993). For these reasons, some have recommended against the QFI for use in clinical settings (Room, 1990; Sobell and Sobell, 1992). An alternative to the QFI for self-report assessment of drinking levels is described next.

B. Timeline Follow-Back (TLFB; Sobell and Sobell, 1973)

The TLFB method was developed over 30 years ago as a treatment outcome instrument. The TLFB method overcomes the limitations noted for the QFI, reviewed above, by having respondents recall all of their drinking within a specified interval. The method involves having the respondents reconstruct their drinking using a blank calendar, and recalling, as well as possible, their drinking behavior on each day. They are asked to indicate the number of standard drinks consumed on each day. The intervals over which clients recall their drinking have varied from 90 days prior to the assessment (commonly used in clinical practice) to 1 year prior to the assessment (typically used for research purposes) (Sobell and Sobell, 1993). This method provides additional information to the QFI by assessing drinking pattern and degree of variability, in addition to quantity and frequency.

Several aids are used to help improve respondents' accuracy on this retrospective memory task, such as the use of "anchor dates." Specifically, respondents are asked to identify the dates of significant events during the reporting period (e.g., New Year's Eve; their spouse's birthday), and to write these out on the calendar to help facilitate recall of drinking levels around those times.

A substantial body of research shows that people can provide reliable and valid retrospective estimates of their drinking behavior with the TLFB method. With respect to reliability, reports over the same interval have been shown to be stable over time. With respect to validity, TLFB estimates by treatment-seeking clients have been shown to correspond well with reports of significant others, and to correlate with official records of alcohol-related consequences (Babor, Stephens, and Marlatt, 1987; Sobell and Sobell, 1992; Sobell, Sobell, and Riley, 1988). The TLFB is used not only in the assessment of drinking behavior, but also in the assessment of other addictive behaviors like drug use.

VI. TREATMENT PLANNING

A. Inventory of Drinking Situations (IDS; Annis et al., 1987)

The IDS is a 100-item self-report questionnaire that was originally developed for research purposes that many now use for treatment planning (e.g., Sobell and Sobell, 1993). The IDS is designed to assess relative frequency of heavy drinking across the situations specified in Marlatt and Gordon's (1985) model of high-risk situations for alcoholic relapse. Thus, the scale is used clinically to assess the types of situations in which the client is most likely to relapse to heavy drinking, and to target therapy

accordingly to best prepare the client for managing these specific types of situations in order to prevent relapse.

The IDS contains subscales tapping relative frequency of heavy alcohol use in eight distinct types of drinking situations (e.g., Physical Discomfort). Respondents rate their frequency of heavy drinking over the year prior to being interviewed in each situation on a scale from 1 (never drank heavily in that situation) to 4 (always drank heavily in that situation). The IDS is proposed to possess a hierarchical structure with eight lower-order factors (the specific drinking situation subscales like Physical Discomfort) that are said to combine to form two higher-order classes of high-risk drinking situations—namely Personal States versus Situations Involving Other People (Annis et al., 1987). Factor analyses do support a hierarchical structure for the IDS with eight lower-order factors combining to form a smaller number of core higher-order factors. However, factor analyses suggest the presence of three (rather than two) higher-order high-risk drinking situations: negative (e.g., unpleasant emotions), positive (e.g., pleasant emotions), and temptation (e.g., urges and temptations; e.g., Stewart, Samoluk, Conrod, Pihl, and Dongier, 1999).

The IDS possesses good psychometric properties in both clinical (Annis et al., 1987; Cannon, Leeka, Patterson, and Baker, 1990; Isenhart, 1991; Stewart et al., 1999) and nonclinical (Carrigan, Samoluk, and Stewart, 1998) samples. They include adequate internal consistency of the eight subscales and three higher-order scales (e.g., Stewart et al., 1999) and good construct, concurrent, and predictive validity (Annis et al., 1987). For example, there is good concordance between the IDS subscale scores and the types of situations that clients identify as most problematic in their therapy homework (Sobell and Sobell, 1993). Two limitations of the IDS are the assumption that situations that trigger a relapse are the same as situations associated with regular heavy drinking prior to treatment—an issue that requires further investigation—and the absence of a definition of heavy drinking in the instructions to the measure (Sobell and Sobell, 1993). With respect to the latter problem, some have suggested asking clients to indicate the following at the end of the measure "By 'heavy drinking,' I mean drinking at least ____ standard drinks in any particular situation" (Sobell and Sobell, 1993). The IDS is also available as a much briefer instrument, the IDS-42, which retains most of the excellent psychometric properties of the original (Annis et al., 1987).

Measures similar to the IDS have been developed for the assessment of situational risk for other addictive behaviors—specifically, the Inventory of Drug Taking Situations (IDTS; Turner et al., 1997) for drugs other than alcohol, and the Inventory of Gambling Situations (IGS; Turner and Littman-Sharp, 2001) for gambling behavior. The IDTS uses the same eight situational subscales as the IDS and has been shown to have good psychometric properties (Turner et al., 1997). The IGS has 11 subscales assessing situational risk for heavy gambling: Negative Emotions, Conflict with Others, Urges and Temptations, Testing Personal Control, Pleasant Emotions, Social Pressure to Gamble, Need for Excitement, Worried about Debts, Winning and Chasing, Confidence in Skill, and Need to be in Control. Although a much more recently developed measure, the IGS has already demonstrated good psychometric properties (Turner and Littman-Sharp, 2001).

B. Situational Confidence Questionnaire (SCQ; Annis and Graham, 1988)

The SCQ is a parallel instrument to the IDS and is designed to assess the client's self-efficacy to abstain from heavy drinking/drug-taking/gambling in various situations. The SCQ contains the same items as the IDS. Respondents are asked to indicate on a six-point scale how confident they feel that they could resist the urge to engaging in heavy drinking/drug-taking/gam-

bling in that situation. The time frame for answering the items is at the present time. The scale for each item ranges from 0 to 100 in increments of 20 points. It is typical for scores on the SCQ to mirror scores on the IDS (i.e., when a client indicates he/she typically consumes heavily in a given situation, that situation is often also associated with poor self-efficacy about his/her ability to abstain or control use in that context). However, discrepancies can be informative for treatment planning. For example, if a client indicates on the IDS that most of his past year heavy drinking occurred in situations involving physical discomfort and those involving conflict with others, but indicates a high self-efficacy to refrain from heavy drinking in physical discomfort situations but a low self-efficacy to refrain from heavy drinking in conflict with others situations, then treatment should obviously focus on providing him with skills for dealing with interpersonal conflict in order to best prevent relapse. The SCQ has adequate psychometric properties (Annis and Graham, 1988).

C. Alcohol Expectancy Questionnaire (AEQ; Brown et al., 1980)

Alcohol outcome expectancies are learned beliefs about the mental, behavioral, and emotional consequences of drinking (Leigh, 1989; Marlatt and Gordon, 1985). They have been reliably found to serve as potent incentives for drinking behavior (Goldman, Del Boca, and Darkes, 1999). Assessment of expectancies can be useful in cognitive types of therapy to determine the kinds of beliefs about alcohol that are particularly important to challenge in treatment because they are maintaining problematic alcohol use.

The AEQ is the most widely used alcohol outcome expectancy measure. The AEQ was originally designed as a 90-item questionnaire that measured six positive alcohol outcome expectancy domains (i.e., beliefs regarding the positive consequences of drinking). However, Goldman, Greenbaum, and Darkes (1997) recommended that the original 90-item AEQ be reduced to a shorter 68-item version (the AEQ-III) which includes only those items that showed salient loadings on the six factors identified for the scale in exploratory factor analyses (Brown et al., 1980). The AEQ-III requires respondents to indicate whether they agree or disagree with a series of statements, based upon what they personally believe is true about the outcomes of drinking alcohol. Each item belongs to one of six subscales: global positive changes (24 items), sexual enhancement (7 items), social and physical pleasure (9 items), social assertiveness (10 items), relaxation/tension reduction (9 items), and arousal/aggression (9 items). Each endorsed statement is assigned a value of 1 point, and a total score for each subscale is tabulated.

The newer AEQ-III also shows adequate to excellent reliability (MacDonald and Stewart, 1999), good construct validity (Goldman et al., 1997; MacDonald and Stewart, 1999), and good predictive validity (Goldman et al., 1997). For example, Goldman et al. (1997) found that AEQ-III subscale scores accounted for about 49% of the variance in drinking levels measured 1 year after the initial expectancy assessment.

Despite these strong psychometric properties, the AEQ and its revisions have nonetheless been criticized on several grounds (e.g., Leigh, 1989). For example, on the AEQ, expectancies are measured in a global fashion where no specific drinking context is specified (Fromme et al., 1993; Goldman, Brown, Christiansen, and Smith, 1991). More recent research suggests that the specific alcohol expectancies activated and the strength of activation of various expectancies do indeed differ across contexts (e.g., Birch, Stewart, Wall, McKee, Eisnor, and Theakston, 2004; MacLatchy-Gaudet and Stewart, 2001). In response to this criticism of the AEQ, a measure called the Expectancy Context Questionnaire has been developed which allows assessment of expectancies in a variety of specific drinking contexts (e.g., at a bar with friends; on a romantic date; Levine, 1988; MacLatchy-Gaudet and Stewart, 2001). Similarly, the Alcohol Craving Questionnaire (Singleton et al., 1994) contains two expectancy subscales (i.e., emotional reward versus emotional relief expectancies) where expectancies are assessed as current states (see Birch et al., 2004). A further criticism of the AEQ is that it assesses only expectancies, but not the subjective valuations that respondents place on each outcome. For example, an individual might believe that alcohol has tension-reducing consequences, but he/she would be unlikely to drink as result of this belief unless he/she also highly valued the outcome of tension-reduction. Measures have also been developed to assess subjective valuations in addition to expectancies. For example, the Comprehensive Effects of Alcohol measure (Fromme et al., 1993) assesses subjective valuations of each outcome specified (i.e., is the outcome good or bad?), as well as expectancy strength.

D. Drinking Motives Questionnaire (DMQ; Cooper et al., 1992)

Motives are the underlying reasons that people engage in a given behavior such as drinking or drug use. Information on underlying motives for any addictive behavior can be very useful for treatment planning in clinical practice. For example, if a client reports drinking primarily to cope with negative emotions and deal with stress, then the intervention should include a focus on helping the client better manage stress and negative emotions without the use of alcohol. There are several substance use motives measures available in the literature. For example, there is a 25-item Marijuana Motives measure that taps use of marijuana for coping, conformity, social, enhancement, and expansion motives (Simons et al., 2000). There is also an 18-item smoking motives measure called the Reasons for Smoking Test (RFS; Ikard et al., 1969; see

Shiffman, 1993 for psychometric properties) that taps use of tobacco for a variety of reasons: Stimulation (e.g., "I smoke cigarettes to give me a lift"), Craving (e.g., "I get a real gnawing hunger for a cigarette when I haven't smoked for a while"), Crutch (e.g., "When I feel uncomfortable or upset about something, I light up a cigarette"), Pleasure (e.g., "I find cigarettes pleasurable"), Habit (e.g., "I light up a cigarette without realizing I still have one burning in the ashtray"), and Handling (e.g., "Handling a cigarette is part of the enjoyment of smoking it"), each of which is tapped by a specific subscale.

In the alcohol literature, two motivational measures have received a good deal of empirical attention: the DMQ (Cooper et al., 1992), and its revision for adolescents the DMQ-R (Cooper, 1994). The original 15-item DMQ contains three subscales of 5 items each. The Enhancement Motives subscale taps drinking for the positively reinforcing emotional consequences of drinking (e.g., "Because it makes you feel good"). The Coping Motives subscale taps drinking for the negatively reinforcing emotional consequences of drinking (e.g., "To forget your worries"). Finally, the Social Motives subscale taps drinking for reasons related to social affiliation (e.g., "To be sociable"). Respondents are first asked to indicate whether they have ever consumed alcohol; then those who indicate a history of alcohol consumption are asked to estimate the relative frequency of their alcohol use for each of the indicated reasons on a scale ranging from 1 (almost never/never) to 4 (almost always). Subscale scores are computed as the mean of the ratings for each of the 5 items on each subscale (Cooper et al., 1992). The adolescent DMQ-R includes a fourth 5-item subscale tapping Conformity Motives—drinking to reduce social censure (e.g., "To fit in"). Research has shown the original three-factor DMQ to display good structural validity in both young adults and community-recruited middle-aged adults (Cooper et al., 1992; Stewart, Zeitlin, and Samoluk, 1996). Similarly, the revised four-factor DMQ-R displays good structural validity in community-recruited adolescents (Cooper, 1994). In terms of construct validity, the drinking motives assessed by the DMQ and DMQ-R have been found to predict distinct patterns of alcohol use behavior and alcohol abuse symptoms (Cooper, 1994; Cooper et al., 1992).

Limitations of the DMQs are that they were developed for use in the general (nonclinical) population, and norms and validation data do not yet exist regarding the use of these measures in clinical samples. Thus, we recommend using these measures only in nonclinical samples at present. Another problem identified regarding the DMQs is their core assumption that people are aware of, and can accurately report on, the motivations underlying their behavior. Measures such as the IDS (Annis et al., 1987; reviewed above) avoid this problem by assessing motives more indirectly (i.e., by examining the situational contexts in which drinking typically occurs).

E. Stages of Change Readiness and Treatment Eagerness Scale (SOCRATES; Miller and Tonigan, 1996)

The transtheoretical model of change (Prochaska, DiClemente, and Norcross, 1992) posits that people pass through a number of stages in the process of initiating and maintaining changes in behavior. Ideally, knowing the stage in which a person currently rests with respect to a particular behavior change (i.e., whether he/she is in precontemplation, contemplation, preparation, action, or maintenance) would allow clinicians to tailor their interventions to help people move toward a beneficial change. The ability to assess stages of change would also permit clinicians to evaluate the effectiveness of their interventions at promoting movement through the stages toward change (Miller and Tonigan, 1996). The SOCRATES is one such measure (see Carey, Purnine, Maisto, and Carey, 1999, for a review of instruments measuring stages of change).

The SOCRATES consists of 19 items scored on a 5-point Likert scale ranging from "strongly disagree" to "strongly agree." The three factors of this instrument measure: (1) "Ambivalence" or degree of uncertainty about one's drinking (conceptually located in the contemplation stage), (2) "Recognition" or extent of identification that one may have an alcohol problem (conceptually located at the end of the contemplation stage, and in the preparation stage); and (3) "Taking Steps" or degree to which one is in the process of changing his/her drinking (conceptually located at the end of the preparation stage, and in the action stage) (Miller and Tonigan, 1996). The 8-item Taking Steps factor has very good internal consistency (alpha = .83–.96). Retest reliability over several days is also very good (intraclass correlation = .82–.91). The 7-item Recognition factor also has very good internal consistency (alpha = .85–.95). Retest reliability over several days is also excellent (intraclass correlation = .90–.94). The 4-item Ambivalence factor has marginal to good internal consistency (alpha = .60–.88). Retest reliability over several days is fair to good (intraclass correlation = .79–.82; Carey, Maisto, and Carey, 2001; Miller and Tonigan, 1996). The test developers demonstrated that Ambivalence was unrelated to either Recognition or Taking Steps (Miller and Tonigan, 1996). However, a more recent study found that Ambivalence was correlated with Recognition (r = .49; Carey et al., 2001). Recognition and Taking Steps are correlated (r = .33–.60; Carey et al., 2001; Miller and Tonigan, 1996). While no true gold standard currently exists for the assessment of stages of change (Hodgins, 2001), Carey and colleagues (2001) provided some evidence for the convergent validity of the SOCRATES with aspects of the Decisional Balance Scale (DBS; King and DiClemente, 1993), which assesses pros and cons of changing versus remaining the same. Their results support the position that the Recognition and Taking Steps subscales of the SOCRATES are reliable and tentatively valid, while the Ambivalence subscale may be too unreliable to be usefully valid (Carey et al., 1999). The SOCRATES has also been modified to assess readiness to change the use of drugs other than alcohol (Carey et al., 1999, 2001).

VII. CONCLUSIONS

The complexity of issues associated with conducting accurate assessment of addictive disorders in special populations is affirmed by the number of excellent resources that have been published on this issue (e.g., Allen and Wilson, 2003; Skinner, 2005). While the relationship between stress and substance use isn't always clear in nonclinical populations (e.g., Brennan, Schutte, and Moos, 1999), it has been clearly established that substance misuse is an enormous concern for people who are experiencing clinically relevant levels of stress (e.g., post-traumatic stress disorder; see Stewart, 1996, for a review) and that stress is a major predictor of relapse among people recovering from an addictive disorder (Brown, Vik, Patterson, Grant, and Schuckit, 1995). While advances have been made in the assessment of stress in addicted populations (e.g., McQuaid, Brown, and Aarons, 2000), there currently do not exist recommendations for the use of particular addiction measurement instruments for populations suffering from stress-related disorders. Future research would do well to examine the psychometric properties of an addiction assessment battery in populations of individuals suffering from stress-related illnesses.

ACKNOWLEDGMENTS

Dr. Stewart is supported through an Investigator Award from the Canadian Institutes of Health Research and by a Killam Research Professorship from the Faculty of Science at Dalhousie University.

REFERENCES

Allen, J., and Wilson, P. (Eds.) (2003). *Assessing alcohol problems: A guide for clinicians and researchers* (2nd ed.). Rockville, MD: National Institute on Alcohol Abuse and Alcoholism.

American Psychiatric Association. (1980). *Diagnostic and statistical manual of mental disorders* (3rd ed.). New York: Author.

American Psychiatric Association. (1987). *Diagnostic and statistical manual of mental disorders* (3rd ed., rev.) New York: Author.

American Psychiatric Association. (1994). *Diagnostic and statistical manual of mental disorders* (4th ed.). New York: Author.

Annis, H. M., and Graham, J. M. (1988). *Situational Confidence Questionnaire (SCQ-39) user's guide.* Toronto, Canada: Addiction Research Foundation.

Annis, H. M., Graham, J. M., and Davis, C. S. (1987). *Inventory of Drinking Situations (IDS) user's guide.* Toronto, Canada: Addiction Research Foundation.

Babor, T. F., Stephens, R. S., and Marlatt, G. A. (1987). Verbal report methods in clinical research on alcoholism: Response bias and its minimization. *Journal of Studies on Alcohol, 48,* 410–424.

Bell, H, and Steensland, H. (1987). Serum activity of gamma-glutamyltranspeptidase (GGT) in relation to estimated alcohol consumption and questionnaires in alcohol dependence syndrome. *British Journal of Addiction, 82,* 1021–1026.

Birch, C. D., Stewart, S. H., Wall, A.-M., McKee, S. A., Eisnor, S. J., and Theakston, J. A. (2004). Mood-induced increases in alcohol expectancy strength in internally motivated drinkers. *Psychology of Addictive Behaviors, 18,* 231–238.

Bohn, M. J., Babor, T. F., and Kranzler, H. R. (1991). Validity of the Drug Abuse Screening Test (DAST-10) in inpatient substance abusers. *Problems of Drug Dependence, 119,* 233–235.

Brady, J. P., Foulks, E. T., Childress, A. R., and Pertshuk, M. (1982). The Michigan Alcoholism Screening Test as a survey instrument. *Journal of Operational Psychiatry, 13,* 27–31.

Brennan, P. L., Schutte, K. K., and Moos, R. H. (1999). Reciprocal relations between stressors and drinking behavior: A three-wave panel study of late middle-aged and older women and men. *Addiction, 94,* 737–749.

Brown, S. A., Goldman, M., Inn, A., and Anderson, L. (1980). Expectations of reinforcement from alcohol: Their domain and relation to drinking patterns. *Journal of Consulting and Clinical Psychology, 43,* 419–426.

Brown, S. A., Vik, P. W., Patterson, T. L., Grant, I., and Schuckit, M. A. (1995). Stress, vulnerability, and adult alcohol relapse. *Journal of Studies on Alcohol, 56,* 528–545.

Cannon, D. S., Leeka, J. K., Patterson, E. T., and Baker, T. B. (1990). Principal components analysis of the Inventory of Drinking Situations: Empirical categories of drinking by alcoholics. *Addictive Behaviors, 15,* 265–269.

Carey, K. B., Maisto, S. A., and Carey, M. P. (2001). Measuring readiness-to-change substance misuse among psychiatric outpatients: I. Reliability and validity of self-report measures. *Journal of Studies on Alcohol, 62,* 79–88.

Carey, K. B., Purnine, D. M., Maisto, S. A., and Carey, M. P. (1999). Assessing readiness to change substance abuse: A critical review of the instruments. *Clinical Psychology: Science and Practice, 6,* 245–266.

Carrigan, G., Samoluk, S. B., and Stewart, S. H. (1998). Examination of the short form of the Inventory of Drinking Situations (IDS-42) in a young adult university student sample. *Behaviour Research and Therapy, 36,* 789–807.

Cocco, K. M., and Carey, K. B. (1998). Psychometric properties of the Drug Abuse Screening Test in psychiatric outpatients. *Psychological Assessment, 10,* 404–418.

Conrod, P. J., Stewart, S. H., and Pihl, R. O. (1998). Validation of a measure of excessive drinking: Frequency per year BAL exceeds 0.08%. *Substance Use and Misuse, 32,* 587–607.

Cooper, M. L. (1994). Motivations for alcohol use among adolescents: Development and validation of a four-factor model. *Psychological Assessment, 6,* 117–128.

Cooper, M. L., Russell, M., Skinner, J. B., and Windle, M. (1992). Development and validation of a three-dimensional measure of drinking motives. *Psychological Assessment, 4,* 123–132.

Fagerstrom, K. O. (1978). Measuring degree of physical dependence to tobacco smoking with reference to individualization of treatment. *Addictive Behaviors, 3,* 235–241.

Fagerstrom, K. O., Heatherton, T. F., and Kozlowski, L. T. (1990). Nicotine addiction and its assessment. *Ear, Nose, and Throat Journal, 69,* 763–765.

Ferris, J. and Wynne, H. (2001). *The Canadian problem gambling index.* Ottawa, ON: Canadian Centre on Substance Abuse.

Fromme, K., Stroot, E., and Kaplan, D. (1993). Comprehensive effects of alcohol: Development and psychometric assessment of a new expectancy questionnaire. *Psychological Assessment, 5,* 19–26.

Gavin, D. R., Ross, H. E., and Skinner, H. A. (1989). Diagnostic validity of the Drug Abuse Screening Test in the assessment of DSM-III drug disorders. *British Journal of Addiction, 84,* 301–307.

Gibbs, L. E. (1983). Validity and reliability of the Michigan Alcoholism Screening Test: A preview. *Drug and Alcohol Dependence, 12,* 279–285.

Goldman, M., Brown, S., Christiansen, B., and Smith, G. (1991). Alcoholism and memory: Broadening the scope of alcohol expectancy research. *Psychological Bulletin, 110,* 137–146.

Goldman, M., Del Boca, F., and Darkes, J. (1999). Alcohol expectancy theory: The application of cognitive neuroscience. In K. E. Leonard and H. T. Blane (Eds.), *Psychological theories of drinking and alcoholism* (2nd ed., pp. 203–246). New York: Guilford Press.

Goldman, M., Greenbaum, P., and Darkes, J. (1997). A confirmatory test of hierarchical expectancy structure and predictive power: Discriminant validation of the Alcohol Expectancy Questionnaire. *Psychological Assessment, 9,* 145–157.

Heatherton, T. F., Kozlowski, L. T., Frecker, R. C., and Fagerstrom, K-O. (1991). The Fagerstrom Test for Nicotine Dependence: A revision of the Fagerstrom Tolerance Questionnaire. *British Journal of Addiction, 86,* 1119–1127.

Hedlund, J. L., and Vieweg, B. W. (1984). The Michigan Alcoholism Screening Test (MAST): A comprehensive review. *Journal of Operational Psychology, 15,* 55–65.

Hodgins, D. C. (2001). Stages of change assessments in alcohol problems: Agreement across self- and clinician-reports. *Substance Abuse, 22,* 87–96.

Horn, J. L., Wanberg, K. W., and Foster, F. M. (1990). *Guide to the Alcohol Use Inventory (AUI).* Minneapolis, MN: National Computer Systems.

Ikard, F. F., Green, D. E., and Horn, D. (1969). A scale to differentiate between types of smoking related to the management of affect. *The International Journal of the Addictions, 4,* 649–659.

Isenhart, C. E. (1991). Factor structure of the Inventory of Drinking Situations. *Journal of Substance Abuse, 3,* 59–71.

King, T. K., and DiClemente, C. C. (1993). *A decisional balance measure for assessing and predicting drinking behavior.* Unpublished manuscript. Department of Psychology, University of Houston, Houston, Texas.

Kristenson, H., and Trell, E. (1982). Indicators of alcohol consumption: Comparisons between a questionnaire (Mm-MAST), interviews and serum γ-glutamyl transferase (GGT) in a health survey of middle-aged males. *British Journal of Addiction, 77,* 297–304.

Leigh, B. (1989). In search of the seven dwarves: Issues of measurement and meaning in alcohol expectancy research. *Psychological Bulletin, 105,* 361–373.

Lesieur, H. R., and Blume, S. B. (1987). The South Oaks Gambling Screen (SOGS): A new instrument for the identification of pathological gamblers. *American Journal of Psychiatry, 144,* 1184–1188.

Levine, B. (1988). *Situational variations in alcohol expectancies.* Unpublished master's thesis, University of South Florida, Tampa.

MacDonald, A. B., and Stewart, S. H. (1999, May). *Factor analytic investigation of the Alcohol Expectancy Questionnaire—3rd version in a university sample.* Presented at the Annual Convention of the Canadian Psychological Association, Halifax, NS, Canada.

MacLatchy-Gaudet, H. A., and Stewart, S. H. (2001). The context-specific positive alcohol outcome expectancies of university women. *Addictive Behaviors, 26,* 31–49.

Magruder-Habib, K., Fraker, G. G., and Peterson, G. L. (1983). Correspondence of clinicians judgments with the Michigan Alcoholism Screening Test in determining alcoholism in Veterans Administration outpatients. *Journal of Studies on Alcohol, 44,* 872–884.

Marlatt, G. A., and Gordon, J. R. (1985). *Relapse prevention: Maintenance strategies in the treatment of addictive behaviors.* New York: Guilford Press.

Martin, C. S., Liepman, M. R., and Young, C. M. (1990). The Michigan Alcoholism Screening Test: False positives in a college student sample. *Alcoholism: Clinical and Experimental Research, 14,* 853–855.

McQuaid, J. R., Brown, S. A., and Aarons, G. A. (2000). Correlates of life stress in an alcohol treatment sample. *Addictive Behaviors, 25,* 131–137.

Miller, W. R., and Tonigan, J. S. (1996). Assessing drinkers' motivation for change: The stages of change readiness and treatment eagerness scale (SOCRATES). *Psychology of Addictive Behaviors, 10,* 81–89.

Negrete, J.C. (2005). Screening and assessing for concurrent disorders. In W. J. W. Skinner (Ed.), *Treating concurrent disorders: A guide for counsellors* (pp. 29–76). Toronto, ON: Centre for Addiction and Mental Health.

Otto, R. K., and Hall, J. E. (1988). The utility of the Michigan Alcoholism Screening Test in the detection of alcoholics and problem drinkers. *Journal of Personality Assessment, 52,* 499–505.

Payne, T. J., Smith, P. O., McCracken, L. M., McSherry, W. C., and Antony, M. M. (1994). Assessing nicotine dependence: A comparison of the Fagerstrom Tolerance Questionnaire (FTQ) with the Fagerstrom Test for Nicotine Dependence (FTND) in a clinical sample. *Addictive Behaviors, 19,* 307–317.

Pokorny, A. D., Miller, B. A., and Kaplan, H. A. (1972). The brief MAST: A shortened version of the Michigan Alcoholism Screening Test. *American Journal of Psychiatry, 129,* 342–345.

Pomerleau, C. S., Carton, S. M., Lutzke, M. L., Flessland, K. A., and Pomerleau, O. F. (1994). Reliability of the Fagerstrom Tolerance Questionnaire and the Fagerstrom Test for Nicotine Dependence. *Addictive Behaviors, 19,* 33–39.

Prochaska, J. O., DiClemente, C. C., and Norcross, J. C. (1992). In search of how people change: Applications to addictive behaviors. *American Psychologist, 47,* 1102–1114.

Room, R. (1990). Measuring alcohol consumption in the United States: Methods and rationales. In L. T. Kozlowski, H. M. Annis, H. D. Cappell, F. B. Glaser, M. S. Goodstadt, Y. Israel et al. (Eds.), *Research advances in alcohol and drug problems* (vol. 10, pp. 39–80). New York: Plenum Press.

Rounsaville, B. J., Weissman, M. M., Wilber, C., and Kleber, H. (1983). Identifying alcoholism in treated opiate addicts. *American Journal of Psychiatry, 140,* 764–766.

Selzer, M. L. (1971). The Michigan Alcoholism Screening Test: The quest for a new diagnostic instrument. *American Journal of Psychiatry, 127,* 1653–1658.

Selzer, M. L., Vinokur, A., and van Rooijen, L. (1975). A self-administered Short Michigan Alcoholism Screening Test (SMAST). *Journal of Studies on Alcohol, 36,* 117–126.

Shiffman, S. (1993). Assessing smoking patterns and motives. *Journal of Consulting and Clinical Psychology, 5,* 732–742.

Simons, J., Correia, C. J., and Carey, K. B. (2000). A comparison of motives for marijuana and alcohol use among experienced users. *Addictive Behaviors, 25,* 153–160.

Singleton, E. G., Tiffany, S. R., and Henningfield, J. E. (1994). *The multidimensional aspects of craving for alcohol.* Unpublished research, Intramural Research Program, National Institute on Drug Abuse, National Institutes of Health, Baltimore.

Skinner, H. A. (1982). The drug abuse screening test. *Addictive Behaviors, 7,* 363–371.

Skinner, H. A., and Allen, B. A. (1982). Alcohol dependence syndrome: Measurement and validation. *Journal of Abnormal Psychology, 91,* 199–209.

Skinner, H. A., and Horn, J. L. (1984). *Alcohol Dependence Scale (ADS) user's guide.* Toronto: Addiction Research Foundation.

Skinner, W. J. W. (Ed.) (2005). *Treating concurrent disorders: A guide for counsellors.* Toronto, ON: Centre for Addiction and Mental Health.

Sobell, L. C., and Sobell, M. B. (1973). A self-feedback technique to monitor drinking behavior in alcoholics. *Behaviour Research and Therapy, 11,* 237–238.

Sobell, L. C., and Sobell, M. B. (1990). Self-report issues in alcohol abuse: State of the art and future directions. *Behavioral Assessment, 12,* 77–90.

Sobell, L. C., and Sobell, M. B. (1992). Timeline Follow-Back: A technique for assessing self-reported ethanol consumption. In J. Allen and R. Z. Litten (Eds.), *Measuring alcohol consumption: Psychosocial and biological methods* (pp. 41–72). Totowa, NJ: Humana Press.

Sobell, L. C., Sobell, M. B., and Riley, D. M. (1988). The reliability of alcohol abusers' self-reports of drinking and life events that occurred in the distant past. *Journal of Studies on Alcohol, 49,* 225–232.

Sobell, M. B., and Sobell, L. C. (1993). *Problem drinkers: Guided Self-Change Treatment.* New York: Guilford.

Spitzer, R. L., Williams, J. B. W., Gibbon, M., and First, M. B. (1992). The Structured Clinical Interview for DSM-III-T (SCID). I: History, rationale, and description. *Archives of General Psychiatry, 49,* 624–629.

Staley, D., and el-Guebaly, N. (1990). Psychometric properties of the Drug Abuse Screening Test in a psychiatric patient population. *Addictive Behaviors, 15,* 257–264.

Stewart, S. H. (1996). Alcohol abuse in individuals exposed to trauma: A critical review. *Psychological Bulletin, 120,* 83–112.

Stewart, S. H., Angelopoulos, M., Baker, J. M., and Boland, F. J. (2000). Relations between dietary restraint and patterns of alcohol use in young adult women. *Psychology of Addictive Behaviors, 14,* 77–82.

Stewart, S. H., Peterson, J. B., and Pihl, R. O. (1995). Anxiety sensitivity and self-reported alcohol consumption rates among university women. *Journal of Anxiety Disorders, 9,* 283–292.

Stewart, S. H., Samoluk, S. B., Conrod, P. J., Pihl, R. O., and Dongier, M. (1999). Psychometric evaluation of the short form Inventory of Drinking Situations (IDS-42) in a community-recruited sample of substance-abusing women. *Journal of Substance Abuse, 11,* 305–321.

Stewart, S. H., Zeitlin, S. B., and Samoluk, S. B. (1996). Examination of a three-dimensional drinking motives questionnaire in a young adult university student sample. *Behaviour Research and Therapy, 34,* 61–71.

Storgaard, H., Nielson, S. D., and Gluud, C. (1994). The validity of the Michigan Alcoholism Screening Test (MAST). *Alcohol and Alcoholism, 29,* 493–502.

Toland, A. M., and Moss, H. B. (1989). Identification of the alcoholic schizophrenic: Use of clinical laboratory tests and the MAST. *Journal of Studies on Alcohol, 30,* 49–53.

Tulevski, I. G. (1989). Michigan Alcoholism Screening Test (MAST)—Its possibilities and shortcomings as a screening device in a pre-selected non-clinical population. *Drug and Alcohol Dependence, 24,* 255–260.

Turner, N. E., Annis, H. M., and Sklar, S. M. (1997). Measurement of antecedents to drug and alcohol use: Psychometric properties of the Inventory of Drug-Taking Situations (IDTS). *Behaviour Research and Therapy, 35,* 465–483.

Turner, N. E., and Littman-Sharp, N. (2001). *Inventory of gambling situations user's guide.* Toronto, ON, Canada: Centre for Addictions and Mental Health.

Volberg, R. A., and Banks, S. M. (1990). A review of two measures of pathological gambling in the United States. *Journal of Gambling Studies, 6,* 153–163.

Wanberg, K. W., and Horn, J. L. (1983). Assessment of alcohol use with multidimensional concepts and measures. *American Psychologist, 38,* 1055–1069.

Williams, J. B. W., Gibbon, M., First, M. B., Spitzer, R. L., Davies, M., Borus, J., et al. (1992). The Structured Clinical Interview for DSM-III-R (SCID). II: Multisite test-retest reliability. *Archives of General Psychiatry, 49,* 630–636.

15

Stress, Anxiety, and Addiction: Intervention Strategies

CHRISTOPHER B. DONAHUE AND MATT G. KUSHNER

This chapter explores the relationship between anxiety symptoms, stress responding and substance use disorders (alcohol and drug). Special emphasis is given to treatment approaches. Having an anxiety disorder increases the probability of having substance use disorder (SUD) with research showing the short-term effects of alcohol and drug use dampening stress responding. Factors that can contribute to individuals developing SUD include stress reduction alcohol and drug outcome expectancies, and avoidant and impulsive personality styles. Individuals with an SUD are at an increased risk for relapse following standard substance abuse treatment. This observation provides the basis for developing treatment approaches that specifically target SUD. Different treatment approaches for dual diagnosis are discussed, including parallel, sequential, and hybrid strategies. We conclude that hybrid treatment approaches that focus on the interactive aspects of stress, anxiety, and substance use are the most promising approaches for future study.

I. INTRODUCTION

Stress and anxiety are ubiquitous human conditions. Anxiety disorders represent clinical-level manifestations of maladaptive stress responding and are among the most common psychiatric conditions found in the general community (Kessler et al., 1997). Because alcohol and drug problems are also very common, it is not surprising that stress and anxiety disorders are common among individuals with alcohol and drug problems. Beyond the likely coincidence of two pervasive problems, two core questions have emerged when considering this association: (1) Do stress and anxiety disorders occur more frequently among individuals with addictions than individuals without addictions? and (2) what are the best strategies for treating stress and anxiety disorders in individuals with addictions?

While anxiety disorders conform to highly specific criteria outlined in the *DSM IV-TR* (American Psychiatric Association, 2000), stress is variously defined. Not everyone who is exposed to stressful situations ("stressors") experiences problematic stress responses. On the other hand, some

Stress and Addiction: Biological and Psychological Mechanisms
Edited by **Mustafa al'Absi, Ph.D.**

individuals experience significant stress responses when confronting situations that others cope with well. According to Brady and Sonne (1999) stress can be defined as

> The reactions of the body to certain events or stimuli, which are defined as stressors, can be either physical (e.g., unusual environmental conditions or a physical attack) or psychological (e.g., occupational or familial difficulties) in nature. (p. 264)

Anisman and Merali (1999) provide further elaboration with a working definition of stress or a commonly used term "stressor," indicating

> A situation or event appraised as being aversive in that it elicits a stress response which taxes a person's physiological or psychological resources as well as possibly provoking a subjective state of physical or mental tension. (p. 241)

Individuals' response to stress or stressors can be characterized in a number of ways. First, if the individuals' response is in proportion to the circumstance, and if they have well-developed coping skills, they are more likely to be able to respond to stressors in a healthy and/or protective manner. However, individuals likely to experience a pathological response to stress are those who (a) are exposed to unusually high intensity stressors, (b) are psychologically prone to catastrophize (i.e., exaggerate) the seriousness of otherwise normal stressors, and/or (c) have deficits in their coping skills so that common stressors overwhelm their ability to cope. Such individuals could be at an increased risk for abusing drugs or alcohol as a makeshift coping strategy (e.g., abuse of drug or alcohol) (Lazarus and Folkman, 1984).

A. Distinguishing Anxiety Symptoms from Stress Responding

Because of the significant overlap and potential confusion in the meaning of anxiety symptoms and stress responding,

it is necessary to address this distinction for our present purposes. From a psychiatric perspective, anxiety symptoms are indicative of a psychopathological process. Inasmuch as psychiatric nosology is (for the time being) a descriptive enterprise, disorders associated with anxiety symptoms are identified primarily based on one's self-reported subjective feelings of relatively long-standing and chronic distress (e.g., panic attacks, worry, nervousness). This may be contrasted with stress responding, which refers to the subjective, physiological, and behavioral responses of an organism to an environmental challenge. The stress-response system in humans is well understood and involves the hypothalamic-pituitary-adrenal (HPA) axis (Tsigos and Chrousos, 2002). Chronic activation of these stress response symptoms is subjectively unpleasant and may have adverse health consequences (Chrousos and Gold, 1992). Among "at risk" individuals, chronic stress system activation might cause the onset of an anxiety or affective disorder. For our present purposes, we note that studies have shown that the acute effects of alcohol may dampen both anxiety symptoms and stress responding, thereby promoting escalating drinking via negative reinforcement.

Data reviewed in the chapter will show that abnormal stress responding and anxiety syndromes are linked to increased risk for co-occurring ("comorbid") alcohol or drug addictions. We also review theories and some data suggesting that the acute effects of alcohol can, under some circumstances, relieve stress and anxiety states, which, in turn, can promote problematic alcohol use. Further, we review data suggesting that stress and anxiety states are significantly associated with failed attempts at treating pathological drug and alcohol use (i.e., stress and anxiety promote relapse to alcohol use following treatment). Finally, we review and comment on the extent that literature focused on treatment approaches related to comorbid cases.

The majority of research in the area of stress-related substance use has focused on alcohol use and the possibility that stress-induced drinking ("self-medication") can lead to alcohol use disorders (Cooper, Russel, Skinner, Frone, and Mudar, 1992; Kushner, Abrams, and Borchardt, 2000; Sher, 1987). However, there is also evidence of high comorbid rates between anxiety states and other substance use disorders (e.g., Kessler et al., 1997), which can imply similar (e.g., self-medication) or different (e.g., cocaine use–induced panic attacks in susceptible individuals) mechanisms. In fact, individuals with anxiety disorders have been found to be at an increased risk for having both drug and alcohol dependence in the United States and other countries (e.g., Merikangas et al., 1998). For the purposes of this discussion, we will refer to alcohol and drug use disorders generically as substance use disorders (SUDs), unless otherwise identified in specific alcohol or drug use studies.

II. STRESS AND SUBSTANCE USE DISORDERS (SUDs)

It is well documented that, under limited circumstances, alcohol consumption can reduce the magnitude of an organism's response to stress—a phenomenon termed *stress response dampening* (SRD) by Levenson, Sher, Grossman, Neman, and Newlin (1980). The SRD effects appear to be moderated by dose (Sher and Walitzer, 1986), alcohol outcome expectancies (Kushner, Sher, Wood, and Wood, 1994) and other individual differences (Sher and Levenson, 1982). Regarding the latter, more pronounced SRD effects are produced in problem drinkers and those with personality characteristics such as impulsiveness, aggressiveness, or extroversion. Studies have consistently shown reduced heart rate following alcohol consumption (Levenson et al., 1980; Sher and Levenson, 1982; Wilson, Abrams, and Lipscomb, 1980) and a smaller number of

studies have shown that alcohol reduces clinical anxiety phenomena (e.g., "panic reactions") for individuals suffering from full-blown anxiety disorders (e.g., Kushner et al., 1996). However, the fact that alcohol can reduce such responses does not, in and of itself, provide evidence that individuals are inclined to drink alcohol for the purpose of stress management. It is to this question we turn next.

Not only does alcohol reduce anxiety and stress, lab investigations have found that both humans and animals tend to increase their alcohol use following exposure to stressful conditions (Abrams, Kushner, Lisdahl-Medina, and Voight, 2002; Liu and Weiss, 2002; McNally and Noel, 1996). This includes exposure to both acute and repeated stressors and even when the stress is experienced indirectly by observing others exposed to stress (Piazza and Le Moal, 1998). Further, Sinha and colleagues (1999) reported that brief exposure to distressing imagery in a controlled lab study was capable of inducing drug and alcohol cravings, as well as negative affect.

Work-related stressors and SUD have also been investigated. Frone (1999) suggested that a variety of factors determine whether stress will contribute to pathological alcohol use. For example, Vasse, Nijhuis, and Kok (1998) proposed a model that included a number of factors that contribute to SUD, such as high work demands and poor employee relations. Similarly, Martin, Roman, and Blum (1996) found that low job control related to higher levels of drinking to cope with negative affect. Employees experiencing stress in the context of poorly defined job roles are more likely to engage in heavy drinking (Frone and Windle, 1997). Frone, Yardley, and Markel (1997) also described work-family conflict in which individuals who use alcohol to cope with work-related stressors tend to have symptoms of anxiety and depression and mistaken beliefs (i.e., expectancies) that alcohol promotes lasting effects such as relaxation and allows the avoidance of negative emotions. In short, stress may lead to SUD only in a subset of vulnerable individuals.

III. ANXIETY DISORDERS AND SUBSTANCE USE DISORDERS (SUDs)

Anxiety disorders can be understood as an extreme form of stress response dysregulation and/or reactions to stressors for which a person's ability to cope is inadequate (Cooper et al., 1992). From this perspective, the association between SUD and psychiatric anxiety disorders is relevant to and may be indicative of the nexus of extreme stress with problematic alcohol and drug use. From this perspective, one would expect to see high rates of SUDs among individuals with anxiety disorders and vice versa.

Consistent with this prediction, epidemiological studies have found consistently a significant connection between the presence of anxiety disorders and SUDs. For example, the Epidemiologic Catchment Area study (ECA; Regier et al., 1990) and National Comorbidity Survey (NCS; Kessler et al., 1997) reported a two- to four-fold increase in the odds for either an anxiety disorder or SUD given the presence of the other. This association was found to be as strong or stronger in an international consortium in psychiatric epidemiology (Merikangas et al., 1998). The association between anxiety disorders and SUDs implies co-variation (i.e., correlation) but does not clarify the causal and maintaining mechanisms underlying the association. An understanding of these causal influences would be helpful for, if not necessary to develop, effective treatment options for comorbidity. In particular, we are interested in determining whether anxiety and stress promote pathological substance use as a means of coping.

Several studies and theories do offer support for the idea that drugs such as alcohol can, at least temporarily, ameliorate the symptoms of specific anxiety disorders. For example, Kushner and colleagues (1996) found the acute pharmacological effects of alcohol intoxication to include a dampening of panic attack susceptibility. Similar findings were reported for individuals with social phobia (Abrams, Kushner, Lisdahl-Medina, and Voight, 2001; Abrams et al., 2002). Animal work also links substance use to post-traumatic stress. Volpicelli, Balaraman, Hahn, Wallace, and Bux (1999) theorized that endorphin dysregulation following a trauma could result in increased emotional distress, and, in many cases, a desire for the analgesic effect that can be achieved by drug or alcohol intoxication. This effect has been observed in controlled animal studies (Volpicelli and Ulm, 1990). Rats exposed to inescapable shocks showed increasing alcohol preference one day later compared to controls. Such findings suggest that individuals might be at an increased risk for the development of alcohol use disorders when they self-administer alcohol in response to social anxiety. Also consistent with this conclusion, anxiety disorder tends to begin prior to comorbid SUDs (Kushner et al., 1990).

IV. MODERATORS OF THE ANXIETY AND SUD ASSOCIATION

While stress and anxiety increase the risk for SUD (above), it is important to consider that most stressed/anxious individuals do not develop substance use problems. This observation raises the important question of what distinguishes individuals who are prone to SUD from those who are not. In other words, what are the characteristics (or moderators) that mark those with stress for whom alcohol or drug use to cope is most likely? Answering this question may also provide important clues as to the most effective prevention and treatment approaches by allowing us to focus our energies on these risk factors.

In fact, a number of variables have been identified as contributing to the likelihood an individual might use alcohol or drugs to cope with stress and anxiety. They include alcohol outcome expectancies, personality variables, and gender (Cooper et al., 1992). Cooper and colleagues (1992) found that being male, holding strongly positive alcohol outcome expectancies (e.g., "alcohol will help manage my emotions"), and having an avoidant coping style all predicted stress-related alcohol use and abuse. Interestingly, Cooper and colleagues interpreted their data to suggest that a maladaptive or inadequate set of coping skills may have contributed more to the likelihood of using alcohol to cope than were the experience of unusually strong stressors per se. In other words, good coping skills were protective against SUD across a range of stressful situations.

Kushner et al. (1994) replicated Cooper et al. (1992) findings and controlled for a number of confounding variables not addressed by the earlier work. Kushner and colleagues reported that males with higher outcome expectancies for alcohol to reduce tension demonstrated a stronger association between measures of anxiety and alcohol consumption. As in the Cooper et al. (1992) study, Kushner and colleagues (1994) found no moderation effects for expectancies among females in their study. This finding led them to conclude that males and females appear to have a different interrelationship of stress/anxiety, alcohol consumption, and alcohol outcome expectancies (Kushner et al., 1994). Different relationships among these variables have also been found in individuals who develop PTSD and drug addictions (e.g., Montoya, Covarrubias, Patek, and Graves, 2003).

Such findings suggest that tension-reduction alcohol and drug expectancies and deficient alternative coping skills are important in considering treatment for this group. Consistent with this, individuals with SUD who do not receive an intervention to address mistaken alcohol or drug expectancies and increase coping skills are

at an increased relapse risk (Young and Longmore, 1987; Brown, Vik, Patterson, Grant, and Schuckitt, 1995). Beyond the expectancies and coping skills, reducing anxiety/stress response symptoms should also help to reduce the relapse risk.

V. TREATMENT OF COMORBID DISORDERS

Although prevention perspectives have received some attention (Kushner et al., 2000), interventions are typically reserved for individuals with full-blown drug and alcohol use disorders. Because of this, individuals with SUD are typically identified when they seek treatment for either anxiety (i.e., in psychiatry or primary care) or substance abuse. Further, those with both stress-related and substance use–related problems are even more likely to be found in treatment settings than in the community at large (Berkson, 1949). Further, the specific treatment venue impacts on the likelihood of finding individuals with co-occurring anxiety disorder and SUD. Kushner et al. (1990) reviewed literature showing that it was more likely that alcoholism treatment patients would have a co-occurring anxiety disorder than it was for anxiety disorder treatment patients to have co-occurring alcoholism. This may reflect referral and triage biases. For example, individuals with both SUD and a stress/anxiety disorder may routinely be referred for substance abuse (versus psychiatric) treatment.

The fact that patients with the dual problems are often found in substance abuse treatment raises the question of the optimal treatment protocol for such patients in these treatment settings. Is standard substance use treatment necessary and sufficient for such patients? For example, if the stress disorder was caused and/or maintained by ongoing substance abuse (e.g., Schuckit and Hesselbrock, 1994), then simply treating the SUD should also resolve the stress problem as well. However, if the stress/anxiety disorder exerts a maintaining influence on the SUD (as we argue above), then it would be critical to also specifically treat the stress anxiety disorder. This could be done serially (i.e., either SUD or anxiety treatment first and then the other) or in parallel (i.e., both SUD and anxiety treatment are given simultaneously). Regardless of whether serial or parallel, this approach uses conventional SUD and anxiety disorder treatment. However, we should not overlook the possibility that comorbidity requires the development of new hybrid treatments tailored to the unique needs of those with SUD.

One way to approach the basic question of whether treatment beyond standard substance abuse is necessary is to evaluate the relative course of stress/anxiety symptoms and relapse following standard treatment. Individuals reporting higher rates of "trait" anxiety at discharge from inpatient treatment have higher relapse rates (Brown, Irwin, Schuckit, 1991). Similarly, individuals with untreated anxiety disorders (e.g., panic disorder, social phobia) have been shown to relapse at much higher rates than noncomorbid individuals (Driessen et al., 2001; Kushner, 2005). Based on this, the view that untreated anxiety disorder contributes to relapse following SUD is compelling. These findings are also indirectly supportive of the idea that treating comorbid anxiety, in addition to SUD, would provide a better outcome for comorbid individuals.

VI. ANXIETY AND SUD TREATMENT PROGRAM CONCEPTS

Parallel and serial treatment programs employ SUD and psychiatric treatments as usual, while hybrid treatment programs employ novel techniques. The starting point for considering hybrid treatments is to identify the noxious or interface between SUD and stress responding. More than 25

years ago, Cummings, Gordon, and Marlett (1980) found that the most common types of stimuli predictive of relapse were intra-personal (negative emotional states), inter-personal (stressful interactions), or external cues (e.g., job stress, legal problems). The concept of a hybrid treatment program not only includes attempts at minimizing such stressors and providing individuals with more varied and effective coping strategies, but it also includes identifying and modifying linking factors such as tension-reduction alcohol outcome expectancies (Kushner et al., 2000) and identifying stress as a cue for drinking (Scott, Gilvarry, and Farrell, 1998).

A behavioral analysis of an individual's drug or alcohol use pattern in relationship to stress and anxiety is an important component of a hybrid treatment approach. For example, what are the external and internal events that relate to drug or alcohol use? What is the individuals coping or response repertoire in response to stressful experiences (Kadden, 1994)? Identifying these factors allows for the targeting of techniques such as stress management, relaxation training and systematic desensitization to feared situations via cue-exposure exercise, and cognitive strategies aimed at modifying misperceptions of events (Stockwell and Town, 1989).

Figure 15-1 provides an illustration of the interactive effects between anxiety and alcohol and the progression to disordered drinking. There are relatively equal proportions of individuals who begin the cycle with a SUD or begin with the anxiety disorder contributing to a feed-forward cycle of dual diagnosis. Drinking is maintained by the immediate reinforcement of anxiety reduction, contributing to an overall worsening of anxiety that, in turn, promotes more drinking, and so on (Kushner et al., 2000). The potential "buffering effects" of treating both the anxiety disorder and the SUD are also illustrated in the dual diagnosis model. If the anxiety disorder is effectively treated, there is still the likelihood of individuals experiencing a strong urge to use substances based on per-

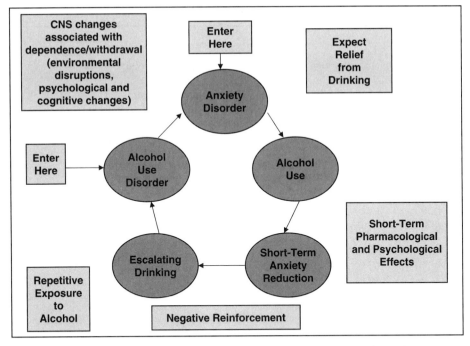

FIGURE 15-1   A working model of dual diagnosis (Kushner et al., 2000).

sisting alcohol and/or drug tension-reduction expectancies. Based on this model, it would be important to address both alcohol use and anxiety symptoms to minimize the risk that the vicious cycle would re-start (i.e., relapse).

VII. ANXIETY AND SUD TREATMENT OUTCOMES

The gist of this review so far has been that efforts at effectively treating both stress and SUD for comorbid individuals would improve outcomes over and above SUD treatment alone. Although a compelling idea, studies to date have reported mixed findings. In our discussion of treatment outcome studies, we will make an effort to categorize programs as sequential (serial) or parallel anxiety disorder and SUD treatment programs and will conclude with a review of so-called hybrid programs that consider anxiety

disorders and SR-SUD as a single problem with treatment needs that are unique to those of either condition alone. One must also keep in mind that treatment outcome must consider both the SUD and the stress/anxiety disorder. For example, the hypothesis that treating anxiety disorder improves the response to SUD treatment is only tested if the intervention actually improves the anxiety condition.

VIII. TREATMENT STUDIES REVIEWED

A. Parallel Treatment

The parallel treatment programs shown in Table 15-1 report mixed findings. Positive SUD treatment outcomes have been reported when comorbid mood and affective disorders are effectively treated (Fals-Stewart and Schafer, 1992; Kranzler et al., 1994). Fals-Stewart and Schafer (1992) noted

TABLE 15-1   SUD Treatment Outcome Studies

Program Type	Study	Population	Design	Follow-up	Outcome Mood/ Anxiety	Outcome SUD
Parallel	Fals-Stewart and Schafer (1992)	OCD/SUD N = 60	Three Conditions: SUD-TAU, SUD-TAU + CBT-OCD, Relaxation	1 year	+	+
	Kranzler et al. (1994)	Depressed + nondepressed subjects/ Alcohol N = 101	Two Conditions: SUD-TAU, Fluoxetine + CBT for SUD	9 months	+ (Depressed group only)	+
	Randall et al. (2001)	Social Phobia/ Alcohol N = 93	Two Conditions: CBT-SUD, CBT-SUD + CBT-Social Phobia	3 months	–	–
	Bowen et al. (2000) (Canada)	Alcohol/Panic N = 231	Two Conditions: TAU-SUD, CBT-Panic + TAU-SUD	1 year	=	=
Sequential	Toneatto (2005) (Canada)	Panic Disorder/ Alcohol (Community sample) N = 14	Within Group: CBT-SUD + Behavioral Therapy (BT)-Panic	1 year	+ within group change	+ within group change
Hybrid	Toneatto (2005) (Canada)	Panic Disorder/ Alcohol (Community sample) N = 14	Within Group: Hybrid Cognitive Therapy (CT) (Panic/SUD)	1 year	+ within group change	+ within group change
	Schade et al. (2005) (Amsterdam)	Social Phobia, Agoraphobia/ Alcohol N = 96	Two Conditions: TAU-SUD (Non-12 Step), TAU SUD + Hybrid CBT	1 year	+	–
	Kushner (2005)	Panic Disorder/ Alcohol N = 31	Two Condition: TAU-SUD, TAU-SUD + Hybrid CBT	4 months	+	+

Note: TAU = Treatment as usual for SUD, including 12-Step programs; SUD = Substance Use Disorder; CBT = Cognitive Behavioral Therapy, manual-driven treatments for SUD or anxiety disorder; Parallel = SUD and anxiety treatments provided concurrently; Sequential = SUD and anxiety treatments provided in sequential order; Hybrid = Integrated SUD and anxiety treatment; (+) = significant research outcomes; (–) = non-significant research outcomes; (=) = equivalent research outcomes.

superior outcomes at 1-year follow-up for individuals participating in parallel OCD and alcohol treatment as usual (TAU) on several treatment outcome indices, as compared to subjects who received TAU alone (Fals-Stewart and Schafer, 1994). Kranzler and colleagues (1994) reported fluoxetine to have limited efficacy in reducing relapse frequency or severity at follow-up, though medication along with CBT for SUD was helpful in reducing relapse risk during and post treatment, and significantly decreased symptoms of depression in individuals who met criteria for major depressive disorder.

Additional parallel treatment programs have reported nonsignificant as well as negative outcomes for alcohol and anxiety. Bowen, D'Arcy, Keegan, and Senthilselvan (2000) found nonsignificant differences in abstinence rates and anxiety severity ratings when comparing CBT for panic disorder and parallel TAU to TAU alone (in-patient). Important limitations to this study included limited support on the part of the chemical dependency treatment program for the separate anxiety treatment program and a lack of integration of the comorbid concerns in the CBT treatment program. Randall, Thomas, and Thevos (2001) utilized parallel CBT treatment programs for social phobia and SUD, as compared to CBT for SUD alone. An unexpected finding in the parallel CBT for social phobia group at follow-up was greater frequency of drinking episodes, more total drinks, and more frequent heavy drinking days. Also surprising was that both treatment and control groups improved equally on outcome measures of social anxiety. The subject population included a severe group of treatment (out-patient) seeking alcoholics attending from a program affiliated with a Veterans Affairs Medical Center and local county services. Randall et al. (2001) questioned the use of an individual CBT approach as used in this study, versus group CBT for social phobia. This study did not have a comparison with individuals going through standard 12-Step Alcoholism treatment, versus the individually administered CBT program for alcoholism.

In order to make sense of the parallel studies reviewed, we look to specific differences in the study populations, treatment approach employed, and treatment settings. Individuals who received parallel obsessive compulsive disorder (OCD) and SUD treatment demonstrated improvements in both anxiety and SUD (Fals-Stewart and Shafer, 1992), whereas, parallel treatment for social phobia and SUD actually resulted in worsening of SUD, with equivalent but nonsignificant changes in anxiety (Randall et al., 2001). The alcoholics with OCD studied by Fals-Stewart and Shafer consisted of mixed SUD (cocaine, alcohol, heroin, other). The social phobia group in Randall's study consisted of individuals with alcohol dependence. Randall et al. (2001) CBT for SUD program with social phobia group reported negative finding, while Kranzler and colleagues (1994) CBT for SUD and depression program found better alcoholism treatment outcomes.

One aspect of the parallel programs that may further explain differences in outcomes is the extent to which the anxiety treatment was integrated within the SUD program. Programs that did not have the support of the chemical dependency program (e.g., did not promote patients participation in parallel CBT for anxiety) (Bowen et al., 2000) reported poor outcomes, while other programs with positive outcomes appeared to have had institutional support. There are also significant differences in the treatment settings, with a drug-free therapeutic community (Fals-Stewart and Shafer, 1992), in-patient clinic (Bowen et al., 2000), and outpatient programs (Randall et al., 2001). The differences in study designs make it challenging to compare across parallel studies, with further research needed to determine if parallel treatment of anxiety disorders can consistently impact relapse rates in SUD treatment. We will further explore the evidence to determine impact of treating anxiety on SR-SUD.

B. Sequential Treatment

We defined sequential treatment as SUD and anxiety treatment programs provided in serial order. Toneatto (2005) compared sequential (behavioral therapy) and hybrid treatment (cognitive therapy) programs, obtaining equivalent results for anxiety and SUD. It was noted that anxiety diminished prior to exposure to the anxiety treatment components in the behavioral condition, leading to the conclusion that anxiety decreased relative to decreases in alcohol use. This study reported significant limitations with regard to group size, a lack of validation for self-reported alcohol and anxiety behaviors, and a lack of control for order effects. In addition, there was no control condition for individuals that participated in TAU only. Finally, within group improvements were emphasized as compared to between group changes. In light of this being a pilot study, the finding must be considered exploratory, requiring replication using improved methodological control (Toneatto, 2005). We will discuss the hybrid programs in this final section and the preliminary findings of this novel approach to treating comorbid anxiety and SUD.

C. Hybrid Treatment

Hybrid treatment is defined as a single integrated program to treat both SUD and anxiety. Kushner and colleagues (In press) suggested that it couldn't be assumed that anxiety treatments developed in psychiatric patients will work equally well in comorbid SUD treatment patients. In this regard, the effectiveness of hybrid treatment programs may depend on the integration of TAU for SUD and anxiety treatment programs (Kushner et al., 2000; Scott et al., 1998).

Schade and colleagues (2005) used a hybrid CBT program for anxiety disorders and found diminished anxiety symptoms but nonsignificant group differences with regard to relapse rates. The subject population was mixed, though 87 of 96 (91%) of the subjects reported social phobia as primary to alcoholism. The hybrid CBT and TAU treatment groups reported equivalent reductions in number of days of heavy drinking assessed 30 days prior to follow-up assessment (Schade et al., 2005). The findings from this study are limited by the use of self-report measures by phone interview for follow-up. This hybrid program provided evidence of successfully treating the anxiety disorder, yet there were nonsignificant group differences in relapse variables at the follow-up.

These findings are explicitly counter to the hypothesis that anxiety/stress contributes to SUD maintenance. For example, finding that neither the anxiety disorder nor the SUD is impacted by an anxiety intervention (e.g., Randall et al., 2001) could be a failure of the anxiety intervention rather than a disconfirmation of the hypothesis per se. However, finding that stress/anxiety disorder is effectively treated but SUD outcome is unaffected goes directly to disconfirming the core hypothesis functionally linking these disorders. However, additional research will be required due to the differences in treatment approaches and methods.

Kushner and colleagues (In press) developed a hybrid CBT treatment program. Subjects participating in the hybrid CBT also received parallel TAU for SUD and were compared to TAU for SUD alone. Approximately 78% of the eligible subjects completed the hybrid CBT treatment (31 of 40 subjects). In the analysis of baseline (30 days prior to treatment) and follow-up findings (30 days prior to 4-month follow-up period), Kushner and colleagues reported positive outcomes, with 16% of the treatment group still meeting criteria for panic disorder at follow-up, compared to 41% of the control group. Panic frequency diminished from 9 panic attacks per week to 1.5 (83% reduction) for the hybrid CBT group compared to a change of 11 to 9 panic attacks (18% reduction) in the control group over the same time. This effect change was found to be statistically significant. So far, these findings parallel those of Schade et al (2005).

However, unlike findings in the Schade study, Kushner and colleagues reported that alcohol relapse was significantly less severe among those receiving the hybrid CBT treatment. Subjects in the treatment group were significantly less likely than controls to meet criteria for alcohol dependence at follow-up, significantly less likely to have had any alcohol 30 days prior to follow-up, fewer total drinks and drinking days, and fewer heavy drinking days. Kushner and colleagues concluded that a hybrid-CBT treatment program for panic and alcohol dependence appeared to significantly decrease the severity of relapse on comorbid alcoholism treatment patients at 4-month follow-up. However, they caution that their control group was not randomly assigned and did not receive a sham or placebo treatment.

In comparing the different hybrid treatment programs, we are limited by the differences in treatment populations, treatment approaches, and methodological controls. Two of the three hybrid studies were conducted outside the United States (Amsterdam, Canada), and one study did not demonstrate adequate methodological control. Studies conducted in different countries have used different models for SUD treatment other than the 12-step model used predominantly in the United States. These differences present challenges in comparing across treatment approaches. The populations differed slightly, with Schade and colleagues treating primarily social phobia, while Kushner and colleagues (In press) treated individuals with primary panic disorder. Schade and colleagues (2005) offered a non-12-step program parallel to the hybrid program, which complicates comparison to treatment outcomes in other countries. Kushner and colleagues were able to demonstrate that treatment of comorbid panic disorder effected significant reductions in problem alcohol use. While Schade and

colleagues found that successfully treating symptoms of social phobia had no significant change over alcohol use rates, compared to the TAU for SUD program in Amsterdam. Kushner and colleagues reported a significant reduction in number of heavy drinking days, while Schade and colleagues found equivalent reductions in heavy drinking days between the hybrid and TAU programs. Additional studies of the hybrid approach using comparable TAU programs within the United States and abroad are needed to further evaluate the effectiveness of this approach to treating SUD and stress/anxiety disorders.

IX. CONCLUSIONS

Our discussion has focused on abnormal or a pathological response to stressors, including anxiety syndromes, as a risk for SUD with unique treatment features. The argument was made that individuals experiencing anxiety syndromes with comorbid SUD are at a significant disadvantage in their efforts to successfully abstain from alcohol and drug use given SUD treatment as usual. While SUD may develop as a short-term strategy for managing symptoms of anxiety, as supported in laboratory studies (stress-response dampening), the long-term effect is likely to be elevated anxiety, leading to a vicious cycle of continued and chronic drug and alcohol use to avoid heightened levels of stress, anxiety, and withdrawal. The treatment programs reviewed (parallel, sequential, hybrid) for individuals with comorbid anxiety disorders and SR-SUD were mixed, with some reporting positive, equivalent, and negative outcomes when treating the comorbid anxiety disorder. Our discussion also focused on the essential components of a successful comorbid treatment program and integrating SUD and anxiety disorder programs into one unique treatment approach. In order to further validate the efficacy of hybrid programs, additional randomized, controlled studies are needed.

As noted, one goal of the hybrid treatment approach is to ensure that individuals gain information into how their anxiety problems relate to alcohol and SUD. Individuals also need to develop the requisite coping skills in order to more appropriately contend with daily stressors, in order to limit the potential for relapse (anxiety and SUD). Further, the reduction of symptoms of anxiety would reduce relapse risk to the extent that such symptoms cue alcohol use. Individuals who did benefit from hybrid and other treatment approaches reviewed were taught (and presumably learned) to cope with high-risk situations (coping with internal and external triggers), received support in modifying alcohol expectancies, developed healthy social supports, and reported enhanced self-efficacy (i.e., ability to manage symptoms of anxiety and drinking urges). Based on the ongoing work of which we are aware (ours and others), we expect that clear-cut clinical recommendations and approaches for those with both SUD and stress/anxiety disorders will be in place within the current decade. Until then, it continues to make sense to screen for and, where found, treat stress-related problems among those with SUD. Prevention of SUD may also be aided by early intervention in stress-related problems.

ACKNOWLEDGMENTS

This research was supported, in part, by a grant from the National Institute on Alcoholism and Alcohol Abuse (AA015069) awarded to the second author.

REFERENCES

Abrams, K., Kushner, M. G., Lisdahl-Medina, K., and Voight, A. (2001). The expectancy and pharmacologic effects of alcohol on social anxiety in individuals with social phobia. *Drug and Alcohol Dependence, 64*, 219–231.

Abrams, K., Kushner, M. G., Lisdahl-Medina, K., and Voight, A. (2002). Self-administration of alcohol before and after a public speaking challenge by individuals with social phobia. *Psychology of Addictive Behaviors, 16*(2), 121–128.

American Psychiatric Association. (2000). *Diagnostic and statistical manual of mental disorders* (4th ed., text rev.). Washington, D.C.: Author.

Anisman, H., and Merali, Z. (1999). Understanding stress: Characteristics and caveats. *Alcohol Research and Health, 23*(4), 241–249.

Berkson, J. (1949). Limitations of the application of four-fold tables to hospital data. *Biological Bulletin, 2*, 47–53.

Bowen, R. C., D'Arcy, C., Keegan, D., and Senthilselvan, A. (2000). A controlled trial of cognitive behavioral treatment of panic in alcoholic inpatients with comorbid panic disorder. *Addictive Behavior, 4*, 593–597.

Brady, K. T., and Sonne, S. C. (1999). The role of stress in alcohol use, alcoholism, treatment, and relapse. *Alcohol Research and Health, 23*(4), 263–271.

Brown, S. A., Irwin, M., and Schuckit, M. A. (1991). Changes in anxiety among abstinent male alcoholics. *Journal of Studies on Alcohol, 52*, 55–61.

Brown, S. A., Vik, P.W., Patterson, T. L., Grant, I., and Schuckit, M. A. (1995). Stress, vulnerability, and adult alcohol relapse. *Journal of Studies on Alcohol, 56*, 538–545.

Chrousos, G., and Gold, P. W. (1992). The concepts of stress system disorders: Overview of behavioral and physical homeostasis. *Journal of the American Medical Association, 267*, 1244–1252.

Cooper, M. L., Russell, M., Skinner, J. B., Frone, M. R., and Mudar, P. (1992). Stress and alcohol use: Moderating effects of gender, coping, and alcohol expectancies. *Journal of Abnormal Psychology, 101*(1), 139–152.

Cummings, C., Gordon, J. R., and Marlatt, G. A. (1980). Relapse strategies of prevention and prediction. In W. R. Miller (Ed.), *The addictive behaviors: Treatment of alcoholism, drug abuse, smoking, and obesity* (pp. 291–321). Oxford: Pergamon Press.

Driessen, M., Meier, S., Hill, A., Wetterling, T., Lange, W., and Junghanns, K. (2001). The course of anxiety, depression, and drinking behaviors after completed detoxification in alcoholics with and without comorbid anxiety and depressive disorders. *Alcohol and Alcoholism, 36*(3), 249–255.

Fals-Stewart, W., and Schafer, J. (1992). The treatment of substance abusers diagnosed with obsessive-compulsive disorder: An outcome study. *Journal of Substance Abuse Treatment, 9*, 365–370.

Frone, M. R. (1999). Work stress and alcohol use. *Alcohol Research and Health, 23*(4), 284–291.

Frone, M. R., and Windle, M. (1997). Job dissatisfaction and substance use among employed high school students: The moderating influence of active and avoidant coping styles. *Substance Use and Misuse, 32*, 571–585.

Frone, M. R., Yardley, J. K., and Markel, K. (1997). Developing and testing and integrative model of the work-family interface. *Journal of Vocational Behavior, 50*, 145–167.

Kadden, R. M. (1994). Cognitive-behavioral approaches to alcoholism treatment. *Alcohol Health and Research World, 19*(4), 279–286.

Kessler, R. C., Crum, R. M., Warner, L. A., Nelson, C. B., Schulenberg, J., and Anthony, J. C. (1997). Lifetime co-occurrence of DSM-III alcohol abuse and dependence with other psychiatric disorders in the National Comorbidity Survey. *Archives of General Psychiatry, 54*, 313–321.

Kranzler, H. R., Burleson, J. A., DelBoca, F. K., Babor, T. F., Korner, P., Brown, J., and Bohn, M. J. (1994). Buspirone treatment of anxious alcoholics. *Archives of General Psychiatry, 51*, 720–731.

Kushner, M. G. (2005). Alcohol and anxiety treatment study. Unpublished manuscript, University of Minnesota, Minneapolis, MN.

Kushner, M. G., Abrahms, K., and Borchardt, C. (2000). The relationship between anxiety disorders and alcohol use disorders: A review of major prospectives and findings. *Clinical Psychology Review, 20*(2), 149–171.

Kushner, M. G., Abrams, K., Thunas, P., Hanson, K. L., Brekke, M., and Sletter, S. (2005). Follow up study of anxiety disorder and alcohol dependence in comorbid alcoholism treatment patients. Alcoholism Clinical and Experimental Research, 29(8), 1432–1443.

Kushner, M. G., Donahue, C., Sletten, S., Thunes, P., Abrams, K., Peterson, J., and Frye, B. (In Press: Cognitive behavioral treatment of comorbid anxiety disorder in alcoholism treatment patients: Presentation of a prototype program and future directions. Journal of Mental Health

Kushner, M. G., Mackenzie, T. B., Fiszdon, J., Valentiner, D. P., Foa, E., Anderson, N., and Wagensteen, D. (1996). The effects of alcohol consumption on laboratory-induced panic and state anxiety. *Archives of General Psychiatry, 53*, 264–270.

Kushner, M. G., Sher, K. J., and Beitman, B. D. (1990). The relation between alcohol problems and the anxiety disorders. *The American Journal of Psychiatry, 147*(6), 685–695.

Kushner, M. G., Sher, K. J., Wood, M. D., and Wood, K. W. (1994). Anxiety and drinking behavior: Moderating effects of tension reduction alcohol outcome expectancies. *Alcoholism: Clinical and Experimental Research, 18*, 852–860.

Lazarus, R. S., and Folkman, S. (1984). *Stress, appraisal, and coping*. New York, NY: Springer.

Levenson, R. W., Sher, K. J., Grossman, L. M., Neman, J., and Newlin, D. B. (1980). Alcohol and stress response dampening: Pharmacological effects, expectancy, and tension reduction. *Journal of Abnormal Psychology, 89*, 528–538.

Liu, X., and Weiss, F. (2002). Addictive effects of stress and drug cues on reinstatement of ethanol seeking: Exacerbation by history of dependence and role of concurrent activation of corticotropin-releasing factor and opioid mechanisms. *Journal of Neuroscience, 22*, 7856–7861.

Martin, J. K., Roman, P. M., and Blum, T. C. (1996). Job stress, drinking networks, and social support at work: A comprehensive model of employees, problem drinking. *Sociological Quarterly, 37*, 579–599.

McNally, M., and Noel, N. (1996). Effects of anticipatory versus impact stress on alcohol consumption. Paper presented at 30th annual convention of the Association for the Advancement of Behavior Therapy, New York.

Merikangas, K. R., Mehta, R. L., Molnar, B. E., Walters, E. E., Swendsen, J. D., Aguilar-Gaziola, S., Bijl, R., Borges, G., Caraveo-Anduaga, J. J., Dewit, D. J., Kolody, B., Vega, W. A., Wittchen, H. U., and Kessler, R. C. (1998). Comorbidity of substance use disorders with mood and anxiety disorders: Results of the International Consortium in Psychiatry Epidemiology. *Addictive Behaviors, 23*(6), 893–907.

Montoya, I. D., Covarrubias, L. D., Patek, J. A., and Graves, J. A. (2003). Posttraumatic stress disorder among Hispanic and African-American drug users. *The American Journal of Drug and Alcohol Abuse, 29*(4), 729–741.

Piazza, P. V., and Le Moal, M. (1998). Stress is a factor in addiction. In A. W. Graham and T. K. Schultz (Eds.). *Principles of addiction medicine* (pp. 83–93). Chevy Chase, MD: American Society of Addiction Medicine.

Randall, C. L., Thomas, S., and Thevos, A. K. (2001). Concurrent alcoholism and social anxiety disorder: A first step toward developing effective treatments. *Alcoholism: Clinical and Experimental Research, 25*(2), 210–220.

Regier, D. A., Farmer, M. E., Rae, D. S., Locke, B. Z., Keith, S. J., Judd, L. L., and Goodwin, F. K. (1990). Comorbidity of mental disorders with alcohol and other drug abuse: Results from the Epidemiologic Catchment Area (ECA) Study. *Journal of the American Medical Association, 264*, 2511–2518.

Schade, A., Marquenie, L. A., van Balkom, A. J. L. M., Koeter, M. W. J., de Beurs, E., van den Brink, W., and van Dyck, R. (2005). The effectiveness of anxiety treatment on alcohol dependent patients with a comorbid phobic disorder: A randomized controlled trial. *Alcoholism: Clinical and Experimental Research, 29*(5), 794–800.

Schuckit, M. A., and Hesselbrock, V. (1994). Alcohol dependence and anxiety disorders: What is the relationship? *American Journal of Psychiatry, 151*, 1723–1734.

Scott, J., Gilvarry, E., and Farrell, M. (1998). Managing anxiety and depression in alcohol and drug dependence. *Addictive Behaviors, 23*(6), 919–931.

Sher, K. G. (1987). Stress response dampening. In H. T. Blane and K. E. Leonard (Eds.), *Psychological theories of drinking and alcoholism* (pp. 227–271). New York: Guilford Press.

Sher, K. G., and Levenson, R. W. (1982). Risk for alcoholism and individual differences in the stress-response dampening effect of alcohol. *Journal of Abnormal Psychology, 91*, 350–368.

Sher, K. G., and Walitzer, K. S. (1986). Individual differences in the stress response dampening effect of alcohol: A dose response study. *Journal of Abnormal Psychology, 95*, 159–167.

Sinha, R., Catapano, D., and O'Malley, S. (1999). Stress induced craving and stress response in cocaine dependent individuals. *Psychopharmacology, 142*, 343–351.

Stockwell, T., and Town, C. (1989). Anxiety and stress management. In R. K. Hester and W. R. Miller (Eds.), *Handbook of alcoholism treatment approaches: Effective alternatives* (pp. 222–230). New York: Pergamon Press.

Toneatto, T. (2005). Cognitive versus behavioral treatment of concurrent alcohol dependence and ago-raphobia: A pilot study. *Addictive Behaviors, 30*, 115–125.

Tsigos, C., and Chrousos, G. (2002). Hypothalamic-adrenal-pituitary-axis: Neuroendocrine factors and stress. *Journal of Psychosomatic Research, 53*, 865–871.

Vasse, R. M., Nijhuis, F. J. N., and Kok, G. (1998). Associations between work stress, alcohol consumption, and sickness absence. *Addiction, 93*, 231–241.

Volpicelli, J. R., Balaraman, G., Hahn, J., Wallace, H., and Bux, D. (1999). The role of uncontrollable trauma in the development of PTSD and alcohol addiction. *Alcohol Research and Health, 23(4)*, 256–262.

Volpicelli, J. R., and Ulm, R. R. (1990). The influence of control over appetitive and aversive events on alcohol preference in rats. *Alcohol, 7*, 133–136.

Wilson, G. T., Abrams, D., and Lipscomb, T. (1980). Effects of increasing levels of intoxication and drinking pattern on social anxiety. *Journal of Studies on Alcohol, 41*, 250–264.

Young, R. McD., and Longmore, B. E. (1987 August). Alcohol-related beliefs and treatment success. Paper presented to the International Symposium of Alcohol and the Brain. Brisbane, Australia.

16

Post-traumatic Stress Disorder and Substance Use Disorders

MIGUEL E. ROBERTS, SCOTT D. MOORE, AND JEAN C. BECKHAM

The purpose of this chapter is to summarize current literature on the shared epidemiology, course, genetic, and neurobiological basis of post-traumatic stress disorder (PTSD) and substance use disorders (SUDs), as well as provide guidance on current treatment approaches. While the U.S. prevalence rates of PTSD are 7% to 9%, studies of at-risk populations yield substantially higher rates of PTSD with greater chronicity. A uniformly strong association between PTSD and SUDs has been reported (e.g., alcohol use disorders are found in approximately half of men and a fourth of women with PTSD). This association has a number of clinically important implications regarding the course, severity, additional comorbidity, daily functioning, and treatment outcomes for both PTSD and SUDs. Various theories regarding the nature of the causal relationship are reviewed including hypotheses that SUDs predispose to PTSD, SUDs are used to self-medicate PTSD, and that the co-occurrence is due to a shared genetic vulnerability. Relevant neurobiological literature on stress and substance use in both human and laboratory animal

research is reviewed, focusing on the role of norepinephrine, corticotropin-releasing factor (CRF), and dopamine. Finally, a functional relationship between PTSD symptomatology and substance cues and cravings are discussed as intricately related. The interplay between these two disorders is highlighted as they impact the form and nature of clinical treatment.

I. EPIDEMIOLOGY AND COURSE

There is a high incidence of exposure to traumatic experiences in the U.S. general population. The majority of the population at some time in their lives experiences a distressing and traumatic event (Gross et al., 2006; Kessler et al., 1995). Two common psychiatric conditions that occur post-trauma include post-traumatic stress disorder and substance use, abuse, or dependence. PTSD symptoms resolve for the large majority of individuals who experience a traumatic event. Two weeks after a traumatic event, 90% of individuals display PTSD symptoms, although only 7–9% of those exposed to a traumatic event will develop PTSD symptoms lasting at least 1 month or greater at some point in their life (Kessler et al., 1995). However, once present, post-traumatic reactions may be long lasting. For example, Kilpatrick and colleagues found that 16.5% of cases continue to meet diagnostic criteria for PTSD 17 years later (Kilpatrick et al., 1987). Similarly, other studies have found that 15% of combat veterans continue to meet diagnostic criteria 19 years post-trauma (Kulka et al., 1990), with chronicity being directly related to the degree of combat exposure (Roy-Byrne, 2004). Therefore, a subset of those individuals who experience a traumatic stressor will have a chronic course of PTSD.

National epidemiological studies reveal lifetime PTSD in 7–9% of the U.S. population (Kessler et al., 1995). Lifetime prevalence rates within at-risk populations, such as those serving in graves registration or rape survivors, are substantially higher, up to 70% (Foa, 1997; Resnick et al., 1993; Sutker et al., 1994). Epidemiological studies of substance disorders, such as O'Farrell (1994), have found 17% lifetime prevalence rates in the general population for abuse or dependence of any substance, although much higher lifetime prevalence rates have been observed depending on the methodology (Giaconia et al., 2000). Thus PTSD and SUDs are both highly prevalent conditions and can occur concurrently.

The relationship between post-traumatic stress disorder (PTSD) and the use, abuse, and dependence of a broad range of psychoactive substances has long been established, as can be seen in the extensive literature reviews of this relationship (Brady and Sinha, 2005; Jacobsen et al., 2001). Following the Civil War, veterans addicted to opioids, such as opium and morphine, were referred to as suffering from the "army disease" (Milby et al., 1997). More recent investigations of the co-occurrence of PTSD and SUDs have established a strong association between the two disorders (see Table

16-1 for a summary of the following studies; Kessler et al., 1995). Individuals with PTSD are at an increased risk for using a variety of substances and are at risk for substance use and dependence. A twofold increase in the risk of marijuana or illegal drug abuse or dependence in the past year was observed in one study (Kilpatrick et al., 2000). Complementary national epidemiological data have reported the prevalence of drug use disorders in individuals with PTSD to be 34.5% for men and 26.9% for women (Kessler et al., 1995). In this same sample, lifetime rates of alcohol use disorders for individuals with PTSD is approximately half of men and approximately one fourth of women were reported (Kessler et al., 1995). Epidemiologic data indicate a fourfold risk for adults (Breslau et al., 2003) and adolescents (Acierno et al., 2000) with PTSD to start smoking. Rates of cigarette smoking and nicotine dependence have been shown to be two to three times higher in help-seeking samples of individuals with PTSD than in the general population (Beckham et al., 1995; Beckham et al., 1997; Hourani et al., 1999). Conversely, in those seeking treatment for SUDs, an increased co-occurrence of PTSD and SUDs is also frequently reported. For instance, among individuals seeking treatment for SUDs, lifetime prevalence rates for PTSD have been observed as high as 45.3% for females and 24.3% for males, while current PTSD was seen in 40.0% of females and 12.2% of males (Deykin and Buka, 1997). In sum, a uniformly strong association between PTSD and SUDs has been observed in studies employing a broad range of methodologies and samples.

The co-occurrence of PTSD and SUDs has a number of important clinical implications relative to the occurrence of either disorder alone. First, those with comorbid PTSD and SUDs have a more chronic and severe course. For instance, Back and colleagues (2000) found that among treatment-seeking cocaine-dependent individuals, those with comorbid PTSD used larger amounts of drugs more frequently than

TABLE 16-1   Strength of Association between PTSD and Substance Use, Abuse, or Dependence

Substance Disorder or Use	Study Sample	PTSD and Substance	References Relationship
Drug abuse/ dependence	5,877 15–54-year-olds from the NCS; 4,023 boys and girls 12–17 years old from NSA; 899 men and women 21–30 years old; 1,007 21–30-year-old men and women	Lifetime prevalence rates men = 34.5%, women = 26.9% (PTSD) vs. men = 15.1%, women = 7.6% (No-PTSD); OR = 2.86; OR = 2.41; OR = 4.34 (CI = 1.63–11.53) OR = 3.0 (2.0–4.7)	Kessler et al., 1995; Kilpatrick et al., 2000; Breslau et al., 2003; Chilcoat and Breslau, 1998
Alcohol abuse/ dependence	NCS; NSA; 899 men and women 21–30 years old	Lifetime prevalence rates men = 51.9%, women = 27.9% (PTSD) vs. men = 34.4%, women = 13.5% (no-PTSD); OR = 1.56; OR = 1.45 (CI = 0.67–3.17)	Kessler et al., 1995; Kilpatrick et al., 2000; Breslau et al., 2003
Current cigarette smoking	NSA; 4,075 German men and women 18–64 years old; NCS; NCS; 124 help-seeking veterans; 98 combat veterans	Boys' OR = 2.10 Girls' OR = 4.22; OR = 2.76 (CI = 1.60–4.77) OR = 2.1 (CI = 1.6–2.9); Prevalence (current PTSD = 44.6% vs. 22.5% (no mental illness) Prevalence in combat veterans = 60%; 66% (PTSD)	Acierno et al., 2000; Hapke et al., 2005; Breslau et al., 2004a; Lasser et al., 2000; Beckham et al., 1995; Shalev et al., 1990
Nicotine dependence	899 men and women 21–30 years old; 4,075 German men and women 18–64 years old; NCS	OR = 4.03 (CI = 2.10–7.72); OR = 2.70 (CI = 1.57–4.65); OR = 1.7 (CI = 1.2–2.5)	Breslau et al., 2003; Hapke et al., 2005; Breslau et al., 2004a
Heavy cigarette smoking	445 help-seeking combat veterans	Prevalence = 48% (PTSD) vs. 28% (no-PTSD)	Beckham et al., 1997
PTSD in SUD help-seeking sample	297 adolescents 15–19 years old seeking SUDs treatment; NCS	OR of PTSD = 3.7 (CI = 2.0–6.8) OR of PTSD = 1.3 (CI = 0.6–2.9)	Deykin and Buka, 1997; Breslau et al., 2004b

Note: Information in columns for "Study Sample" and "PTSD and Substance Relationship" are presented in order of references. PTSD: Post-traumatic stress disorder; OR: Odds Ratio with 95% confidence interval in parentheses; NCS: National Comorbidity Survey; NSA: National Survey of Adolescents.

cocaine-dependent individuals without PTSD. The severity effect is also reflected in the higher number of additional comorbid Axis I and Axis II conditions (Back et al., 2000). Comorbid PTSD and SUDs are also associated with more severe avoidance and arousal PTSD symptoms (Saladin et al., 1995). Studies in men and women have reported that comorbid samples of PTSD and SUDs typically meet criteria for two additional Axis I disorders (Beckham et al., 2005b; Breslau et al., 1997; Labbate et al., 2004). Individuals with comorbid PTSD and SUDs are rated as more difficult to treat by providers (Najavits, 2002), and have poorer treatment outcomes than those with either disorder alone (Ouimette et al., 1998b). This is illustrated by higher rates of treatment attrition (Back et al., 2000), briefer abstinence periods following substance abuse treatment, and higher rates of relapse (Brown et al., 1996). Further, the outcomes following treatment worsen over time (e.g., at both 1 and 2 years post-treatment) for comorbid PTSD and SUDs individuals, relative to those with SUDs alone and those with SUDs and comorbid disorders apart from PTSD (Ouimette et al., 1998a; Ouimette et al., 1999). Finally, relative to individuals with either disorder alone, individuals with PTSD and SUDs have greater impairment in functioning across a number of important life domains. For example, individuals with comorbid PTSD and SUDs report worse physical health problems that more significantly interfere with daily functioning (Dobie et al., 2004; Larson et al., 2005), and are less likely to be employed 2 years following treatment (Ouimette et al., 1999). Compared to adolescents with either PTSD or SUDs, those with comorbid PTSD and SUDs have been observed to possess the poorest functioning in academic, interpersonal, and emotional functioning (Giaconia et al., 2000). Taken together, the data consistently suggest that individuals with comorbid PTSD and SUDs differ from those with either condition alone in clinically meaningful ways.

The complex relationship between PTSD and SUD is highlighted by the evidence that PTSD symptoms are differentially associated with the use of different substances (Bremner et al., 1996; McFall et al., 1992; Piasecki and Baker, 2000; Saladin et al., 1995). For example, McFall and colleagues (1992) found that re-experiencing and avoidance symptoms were associated with drug abuse more strongly than alcohol abuse, while hyperarousal symptoms were associated with alcohol abuse more strongly than drug abuse. This relationship between hyperarousal symptoms and drug (but not alcohol) use was also reported in first Gulf War veterans with PTSD (Shipherd et al., 2005).

Despite the well-documented relationship between PTSD and SUDs, the causal nature of this relationship is not completely settled. Several somewhat discrepant models and lines of evidence have emerged; however, the data are not wholly uniform with regards to the development, maintenance, and relapse of SUDs and PTSD. One model suggests that SUDs predispose individuals to PTSD via the increased risk of exposure to traumatic events that occur as a result of substance use. In partial support of this theory, several studies reported users of hard drugs, marijuana, and alcohol were at an increased risk of being physically or sexually assaulted relative to non-users (Breslau et al., 1991; Burnam et al., 1988; Cottler et al., 1992; Kessler et al., 1995) and that a majority of sexual assaults occur during the use of a psychoactive substance by at least one of the individuals involved (Gross et al., 2006). Further, a number of studies have demonstrated that SUDs predated PTSD (Cottler et al., 1992; Deykin and Buka, 1997; Giaconia et al., 2000; North et al., 2002).

A second model generated to investigate the casual relationship between PTSD and SUDs, often referred to as the self-medication model, posits that PTSD precedes or is concomitant with the development of SUDs and that the use of substances is a maladaptive coping strategy for management of the PTSD symptoms (Brown and Wolfe, 1994; Deykin and Buka, 1997; Giaconia et al., 2000; Jacobsen et al., 2001; Keane et al., 1988). A third model suggests that PTSD and SUDs commonly co-occur due to shared environmental, personality, neurobiological, or genetic factors.

The current weight of the evidence indicates that trauma exposure and PTSD are usually reported to have occurred first followed by the development of SUDs (Acierno et al., 2000; Brady et al., 1998; Bremner et al., 1996; Breslau et al., 1998; Chilcoat and Breslau, 1998; Kilpatrick et al., 2000; McFall et al., 1992). However, further prospective research is needed to address the multifactorial determination of comorbid PTSD and SUDs.

II. GENETICS OF PTSD AND ADDICTION

Early theories about PTSD conceptualized it as the direct result of exposure to a traumatic event. According to this view, the primary predictor of PTSD is trauma exposure, including parameters of the exposure severity, duration, and frequency. Despite empirical evidence supporting the presence of a dose-response relationship between the severity of trauma exposure and PTSD, the majority of individuals with trauma exposure do not develop the disorder (Breslau et al., 1998; Yehuda, 1999). In addition, Yehuda and McFarlane (1995) found that trauma exposure variables explained only a small proportion of the variance in PTSD symptoms. Furthermore, PTSD is not the only negative mental health outcome resulting from trauma exposure. Higher rates of major depression, panic, and substance abuse have all been documented among individuals with trauma exposure (Shalev et al., 1990; Yehuda et al., 1998a).

More recently, researchers have proposed that PTSD might be more fully explained by a diathesis-stress model in which trauma features and individual risk factors interact as determinants of PTSD. A large number of individual risk factors may be predictive of the development of PTSD including environmental, personality, and demographic factors; psychiatric history; dissociative symptoms; cognitive and biological systems; and genetic or familial predisposition (Yehuda, 1999).

Empirical evidence exists supporting the transmission of PTSD within families. Davidson and colleagues (1985) found that individuals who survived trauma but developed PTSD were more likely than those who did not develop PTSD to have parents and first-degree relatives with mood, anxiety, and substance abuse disorders. A study of Holocaust survivors and their families demonstrated that survivors with PTSD were more likely to have children with PTSD than were survivors without PTSD (Yehuda et al., 1998b; Yehuda et al., 1998c). More recently, a study by Davidson and colleagues (1998) showed that relatives of PTSD probands had higher rates of mental disorder; however, this finding was limited to only PTSD probands with a history of lifetime major depression. The family method of studying PTSD among biological relatives of the proband allows for comparing the frequency of PTSD between different degrees of relatives and is one basic methodology for studying the genetic influence on PTSD. It also allows for the evaluation of the rates of PTSD relative to the general population; however, this methodology has several limitations (Torgersen, 1997). First, higher morbidity risk among relatives does not prove genetic etiology of PTSD as a number of other causal factors can not be ruled out, such as common environment or imitation (Torgersen, 1997). Second, the disorder cannot be assessed in family members without trauma exposure, thus limiting the usefulness of family studies (Koenen, 2003; Segman and Shalev, 2003). Another limitation of this methodology is that the study design cannot separate the effects of genetic and environmental factors on concordance rates. As a result, the extent to which study findings support purely genetic explanations cannot be determined with this methodology.

In studying PTSD risk factors, twin studies have been used to estimate the heritability of certain traits or disorders, since they address the limitations of family genetic studies. Further, twin studies have been used to delineate the different roles of genetics and shared or family-wide environmental variables. The most basic twin method compares the concordance rates within identical or monozygotic (MZ) twins with those within fraternal or dizygotic (DZ) twins. MZ and DZ twins share 100% of their family environment; however, MZ twins have 100% of their genes in common, while DZ twins share an average of only 50% of their genes. According to the twin study methodology, relative to DZ twins, if MZ twins yield a higher concordance rate or similarity for a particular characteristic, such as PTSD, then that characteristic is considered to be influenced by genetics.

To date, twin studies generate the most compelling support for the influence of genetics on trauma exposure and PTSD risk. Despite being limiting to male veterans with combat exposure, most of the twin studies have utilized data from the Vietnam Era Twin (VET) Registry. This registry, created from military records, contains pairs of male twins with military service during the Vietnam era. For instance, True and colleagues (1993) studied PTSD prevalence rates among pairs of monozygotic and dizygotic twins. Their research showed that there appears to be a genetic component of up to 30% of PTSD symptoms and that, after controlling for differences in combat exposure, there is considerable genetic influence on all symptoms of PTSD. Similarly, genetic factors were found to explain 47% of the variance in combat exposure among VET Registry twin pairs (Lyons et al., 1993). Other studies using data from the VET Registry have demonstrated common genetic influences of a number of mental disorders including the following: alcohol and drug

dependence (McLeod et al., 2001; Xian et al., 2000); generalized anxiety and panic disorder symptoms (Chantarujikapong et al., 2001); and major depression (Koenen et al., 2003). Likewise, a study of a nonveteran volunteer community sample containing male and female twins obtained similar results (Stein et al., 2002). They found moderate heritability for exposure to physical violence (e.g., rape, combat, physical assault) and for PTSD symptoms.

In studies evaluating the degree to which genetic and environmental contribution overlap among PTSD and SUD, common genetic influences were identified, lending support for the shared vulnerability hypothesis. In Xian and colleagues' genetic model analysis (2000), the liability for PTSD was partially due to a 15.3% genetic contribution common to alcohol disorder (AD) and drug disorder (DD) and 20.0% genetic contribution specific to PTSD. Risk for AD was partially due to a 55.7% genetic contribution common to PTSD and DD. Genetic influences common to PTSD and AD accounted for 25.2% of the total risk for DD. Specific family environmental influence accounted for 33.9% of the total variance in risk for DD. Remaining variance for all three disorders was due to unique environmental factors both common and specific to each phenotype. No common family environmental influences on PTSD, AD, and DD were identified. In McLeod and colleagues' study (2001), unique environmental factors were more important than genetic factors for PTSD symptoms, whereas the occurrence of PTSD and alcohol use were associated through genetic contribution to personality. The influence of common environment was small. Environmental influences specific to PTSD symptoms were not associated with alcohol use. Thus, the covariation between PTSD symptoms and alcohol use was better explained by common genetic influences.

A more recent analysis of this data by Koenen and colleagues (2003) examined the effect of combat exposure and combat-related PTSD on the occurrence of SUD and other mental disorders. The purpose of the analyses was to evaluate whether the association between combat-related PTSD (C-PTSD) and other mental disorders is an artifact of shared familial vulnerability or whether the effect of combat-related PTSD comorbidity persists after controlling for shared vulnerability. Results indicated that combat exposure (adjusted for C-PTSD) was significantly associated with increased risk for alcohol and cannabis dependence, and that C-PTSD mediated the association between combat exposure and both major depression and tobacco dependence. These results suggested that combat exposure uniquely increased risk for substance dependence, while C-PTSD uniquely increased risk for major depression and tobacco dependence. Taken together, these studies suggest that genetic studies in the area of PTSD and SUD are useful, and future studies should combine genetically informative samples with longitudinal designs in order to specify the temporal relationship and comorbidity mechanisms among trauma exposure, SUD, and PTSD.

III. NEUROBIOLOGY OF STRESS AND SUBSTANCE ABUSE DISORDERS

Previous work addressing the intersection of PTSD and substance abuse in humans suggests a role for norepinephrine based on several parallel findings. Urinary excretion of norepinephrine metabolites is increased in PTSD (Southwick et al., 1999) and in withdrawal states (Hawley et al., 1985). In addition, the alpha-adrenergic agonist clonidine has been used to treat symptoms of both PTSD and drug withdrawal (Gowing et al., 2002; Southwick et al., 1999). However, since neurobiological studies of stress and substance abuse disorders in humans are limited to noninvasive techniques, researchers have since turned to well-characterized animal models and theoretical constructs.

Preclinical animal models of PTSD are currently not adequately developed, though the vast literature on neurobiological substrates of the response to stress facilitates understanding of the neurobiology of PTSD (McEwen, 2002). The emerging literature on neurobiological substrates of stress and substance abuse suggests several potential areas of convergence. These studies have been based on well-characterized animal models, including physical (foot shock, food deprivation), or psychological (predator threat, isolation, or social competition) stressors. Advantages of animal studies include the ability to control for genetics and prior history, intensity and frequency of stressors, and access to the drugs of interest (Piazza and Le Moal, 1998).

Generally, rodents exposed to stressors increase self-administration of drugs of abuse (alcohol, opiates, and stimulants; Piazza and Le Moal, 1998). Rats subjected to various types of stressors have a lower threshold for self-administering drugs, show greater motivation for continuing to self-administer, and are more likely to reinstate operant responding for drugs following extinction (Piazza and Le Moal, 1998).

Many neurotransmitter systems are involved in the interactions between stress and drug reinforcement. However, in addition to norephinephrine, two other systems appear to be highly relevant to both areas: corticotropin-releasing factor (CRF) and dopamine. Combat veterans with PTSD have increased concentrations of CRF in the cerebrospinal fluid (CSF), presumably reflecting increased central CRF-mediated neurotransmission (Bremner et al., 1997). Altered central CRF activity has also been suggested to occur in substance abusers in the absence of other psychiatric conditions (Contoreggi et al., 2003). These observations are paralleled in animal studies. In rats, acute restraint stress causes increased release of CRF in the amygdala (Pich et al., 1995). During acute withdrawal from virtually all drugs of abuse, release of CRF is enhanced in the central nucleus of the amygdala (Koob, 1999; Sarnyai et al., 2001). This acute withdrawal is associated with a behavioral syndrome suggestive of heightened anxiety; during alcohol withdrawal, these anxiety-like behaviors are reduced by local injection of CRF blockers into the central amygdala nucleus. However, acute alcohol-induced enhancement of GABAergic activity in the central nucleus is also dependent on local CRF actions (Nie et al., 2004). CRF also mediates the stress-induced reinstatement of previously extinguished conditioned responding for drugs, but is not involved in cue-induced reinstatement (Liu and Weiss, 2002).

Transgenic mice lacking the CRF receptor subtype CRF1 (CRF1 "knockout" mice) exhibit impaired responses to stress (Timpl et al., 1998). The CRF1 knockout mice do not differ from wild-type controls in the amount of ethanol voluntarily consumed; however, following a forced swim stressor, the CRF1 knockout mice exhibited a delayed enhancement in ethanol drinking (Sillaber et al., 2002), supporting the role of CRF in the stress responses.

Local administration of exogenous CRF into the amygdala elicits a fear response, and repeated injections of even small amounts of CRF result in a persistent state of elevated anxiety (Rainnie et al., 2004). This action of CRF results in persistent electrical hyperexcitability, although the mechanism is distinct from kindling. The demonstration of a prolonged increase in anxiety-like behaviors following a relatively brief exposure to CRF has been suggested to underlie the etiology and/or maintenance of anxiety disorders such as PTSD (Rainnie et al., 2004).

Dopamine has a well-established role in the reinforcing effects of drugs of abuse in animals; for a review, see Kreek and Koob (1998). In addition, dopamine may directly modulate activity of CRF in the amygdala (Eliava et al., 2003), and may underlie chronic changes in CRF activity in response to repeated drug administration (Goeders et al., 1990). Both acute stress and administration of drugs of abuse

result in dopamine release in the nucleus accumbens, while stress also potentiates the drug-induced dopamine release (Kalivas and Stewart, 1991). Social stress in socially housed cynomolgus monkeys alters both dopamine activity and propensity to self-administer drugs. Dominant monkeys showed increased central dopamine receptor binding compared to subordinate monkeys, yet only the subordinate monkeys were reinforced by cocaine (Morgan et al., 2002). Thus, there is a wealth of data showing that dopamine has a significant role in the reinforcing effects of drugs of abuse.

Future neurobiological animal research will likely aim to refine animal models of PTSD, possibly enabling comparisons of specific stress models on drug self-administration. In addition, although drugs of abuse clearly share actions on particular brain systems (Koob and Le Moal, 1997), the diversity of these agents implies multiple sites of interactions with stress pathways. Elucidation of these interactions may ultimately allow for more effective pharmacotherapeutics in the clinical treatment of substance abuse in the context of PTSD.

IV. TREATMENT IMPLICATIONS

Irrespective of the causal factors that lead to the comorbid relationship between PTSD and SUDs, a large number of those in a clinical population present with a densely intertwined symptomatic relationship that has deleterious effects for treatment of either condition. For instance, Read and colleagues (2004) found that those with unremitted PTSD had poorer SUD outcomes than those with remitted PTSD at 6 months following an inpatient SUD treatment. PTSD and SUD patients have posited that their comorbid conditions are functionally related (Brown et al., 1998). This supposition has now grown increasing support by a body of laboratory and clinical research demonstrating that mood states and trauma-related symptoms lead to increased urges and drug cravings in both current and abstinent substance users (Childress et al., 1994; Coffey and Lombardo, 1998; Saladin et al., 2003). For instance, negative affect, interpersonal conflict, and physical discomfort are all associated with increased urges to use drugs, alcohol, or nicotine Beckham et al., 1996; (Beckham et al., 2005b; Childress et al., 1994; Coffey and Lombardo, 1998; Sharkansky et al., 1999). Likewise, following the use of substances, significant reductions in negative affect are seen, thereby reinforcing both drug cravings and use (Bradizza et al., 1994; Coffey and Lombardo, 1998; Stasiewicz and Maisto, 1993). Substance cravings have recently been shown, via fMRI, to activate a set of neuroanatomical substrates (i.e., the ventral anterior cingulate gyrus, superior frontal gyrus, and ventral striatum) associated with attention, emotion, and the reward system (McClernon et al., 2005).

Experimental and ambulatory monitoring data have supported the relationship between smoking craving and negative affect in PTSD smokers (Beckham et al., 2005a; Beckham et al., 2005b). In an experimental study of 129 smokers evaluating the effect of trauma-related context and nicotinized versus denicotinized cigarettes, PTSD smokers demonstrated higher levels of craving, negative affect, and PTSD symptoms compared to trauma-exposed smokers without PTSD. Smoking either cigarette type results in decreased craving, negative affect, and PTSD symptoms. The results suggest that context and the nonpharmacologic effects of smoking are important variables in smoking craving and mood, particularly in smokers with PTSD. In an ambulatory study of PTSD and non-PTSD smokers, smoking was strongly related to craving, positive and negative affect, PTSD symptoms, restlessness, and several situational variables among PTSD smokers. However, for non-PTSD smokers, the only significant antecedent variables for smoking were craving, drinking coffee, being alone, not being with family, not working, and being

around others who were smoking. Further, in smokers unassessed for PTSD, lapses to smoking were significantly associated with high levels of negative affect, and a substantial subset of lapses took place under conditions of extreme negative affect (Shiffman et al., 1996), although this work needs to be completed in smokers with PTSD.

Other studies have found associations between types of PTSD symptom clusters and preferred substance, necessitating an ideographic examination of emotional states and urges in order for these to serve appropriate targets of treatment intervention (Ouimette et al., 1998b; Read et al., 2004; Saladin et al., 1995; Steindl et al., 2003). Further, Jacobsen and colleagues (2001) described a cycle of physiological withdrawal symptoms of CNS depressants mirroring the hyperarousal symptoms of PTSD, thus serving to increase trauma memories, and leading to further attempts to manage traumatic memories via substance use. Thus, following repeated pairings of use and attempts to manage such internal mood states, results suggest that these mood states and trauma symptoms become conditioned stimuli capable of triggering substance urges. A behaviorally oriented treatment of SUDs focused on such individualized trauma-related cues and the subsequent substance cravings are consistent with the relapse prevention efforts examining "high-risk situations" as seen in several efficacious substance treatment programs (Coffey et al., 2002; Marlatt, 1996). Figure 16-1 presents a conceptual model of the above-described relationship between PTSD and SUDs.

Given the established functional relationship between PTSD and SUDs, there is a treatment approach question of whether these conditions be treated separately or conjointly. Historically, comorbid PTSD and SUDs have been treated separately within clinical settings. While not without controversy (cf. Triffleman et al., 1999), a number of clinical researchers emphasize the need for concurrent treatment as a means of improving treatment efficacy and preventing relapse

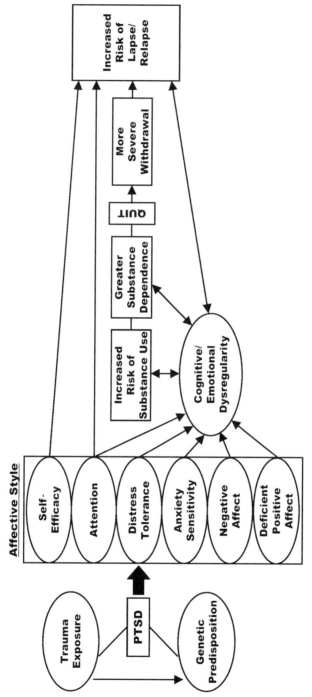

FIGURE 16-1   Conceptual model of the relationship between PTSD, affective style, and substance use or disorders.

(Back et al., 2000; Coffey et al., 2005). There are several detailed current clinical descriptions that provide guidance regarding the components and sequencing of concurrent rather than sequential treatment (Brady et al., 2001; Najavits et al., 1998).

The use of exposure-based treatments for PTSD has strong theoretical rationale, empirical support, and is recommended for the treatment of PTSD by the International Consensus Group on Depression and Anxiety and the Expert Consensus Guidelines (Ballenger et al., 2000; Foa et al., 1999). However, exposure appears to be underutilized in treating PTSD as seen in relatively low rates of use in "real world" settings (Becker et al., 2004). This may be due to the high rates of treatment noncompliance, high treatment dropout rates, and patients finding the treatment aversive (Brady et al., 2001; Foa et al., 1991; Scott and Stradling, 1997). Furthermore, the use of exposure therapy in those with comorbid PTSD and SUDs has been further complicated by limited data to guide treatment in comorbid populations (Cook et al., 2004) and concerns by clinicians that exposure would be too emotionally distressing for SUDs patients (Pitman et al., 1991; cf. Abueg and Fairbank, 1992), all with the connotation that separate treatment will lead to more effective treatment outcomes. However, the above noted relationship between PTSD and cravings indicates that failure to effectively treat PTSD may increase the likelihood of relapse. Therefore, there is a need to further develop effective concurrent treatments (reducing both PTSD and SUDs) that can be tolerated by most patients. Given the chronicity of both of the disorders, further investigation of long-term follow-up and retreatment is also needed.

The past decade has seen an increasing number of treatments developed for the purpose of treating PTSD and SUDs conjointly, each with efficacy data. In general, these approaches include cognitive behavioral methods for addressing PTSD symptoms with exposure-based treatment and

SUD symptoms with relapse prevention. Brady and colleagues developed a manualized "Concurrent Treatment of PTSD and Cocaine Dependence (CTPCD)" manualized treatment consisting of 16 individual 90-minute sessions over an 8-week period involving cognitive-behavioral components for cocaine dependence, exposure for PTSD, and psychoeducation (Back et al., 2001; Brady et al., 2001). Najavits and colleagues (1996) developed a manualized group treatment for PTSD and SUD, titled "safety seeking." This treatment approach consists of 24 sessions focusing on cognitive, behavioral, and interpersonal coping skills, and is novel in allowing patients to select the type of treatment session on any given visit (e.g., trauma focused or problem solving, relapse prevention focused). Similarly, Triffleman and colleagues developed an individual cognitive-behavioral treatment for PTSD and SUDs involving *in vivo* exposure (Trifffleman et al., 1999).

Acceptance and Commitment Therapy (ACT), a third generation cognitive behavioral treatment, is based on inclusion of personally chosen values, acceptance as formal treatment components, and focus on the functional relation of the relationship between PTSD and SUDs (Blackledge, 2004; Hayes et al., 1999; Mulick et al., 2005). In large part, ACT treatment is guided by the clinical conceptualization that many problems across the range of psychopathology are related to efforts to avoid or escape emotions, thoughts, memories, and other private experiences (Hayes et al., 1996). ACT has initial efficacy data supporting its use for SUDS alone (Batten and Hayes, 2005) and PTSD alone (Orsillo and Batten, 2005; Roberts and Wilson, 2002) and in concurrent treatment of PTSD and SUDs (Batten and Hayes, 2005).

In common across all the above-described treatments is the use of exposure as a core intervention component. For example, ACT treatment of PTSD and SUDs might include imaginal exposure to trauma memories, bodily sensation (e.g., drug cravings), or interoceptive cues (e.g., "butterflies in the stomach"). This use of exposure-based interventions may necessitate both a basic level of knowledge of learning theories and experience in the utilization of exposure on the part of the clinician (Coffey et al., 2005). In addition, these treatments also include a variety of skills components intended to not only initiate and maintain abstinence, but also to manage negative affect generated by the treatment (Back et al., 2001). For instance, Back and colleagues' CTPCD includes cognitive-behavioral techniques such as relaxation, thought-stopping, and identification of substance and trauma-related triggers.

While many of these treatments are in the early stages of development, the results thus far appear promising. Longitudinal clinical research indicates improved treatment efficacy when PTSD and SUDs are treated conjointly (Hien et al., 2004; Prochaska et al., 2004; Read et al., 2004; Zlotnick et al., 2003). Despite the above noted concerns that concurrent treatment involving exposure-based treatment for PTSD symptoms may impede SUD recovery, it has been shown to safely and more effectively lead to long-term abstinence without worsening psychiatric symptomatology relative to separate treatment for SUDs (McFall et al., 2005). Likewise, drug use has not been found to increase during or after the exposure phase of concurrent treatment via CTPCD, arguing against the notion that treating PTSD and SUD concurrently via exposure increases the chance of relapse (Brady et al., 2001). In other cases, significant reductions in substance use, current PTSD symptoms, and psychiatric symptomatology were seen post-treatment and at 3-month follow-up (Najavits et al., 1998; Zlotnick et al., 2003). Safety seeking has demonstrated improvements over treatment-as-usual and equivalence to relapse prevention in short- and long-term outcomes for both SUDs and PTSD (Hien et al., 2004). The data on these as well as other concurrent treatment programs are not without caveats, however, largely due to the early stage of the trials. Taken together, the available clinical research

on the concurrent treatment of PTSD and SUDs suggests that successful and effective treatment can occur concurrently via exposure-based therapy. Furthermore, contrary to reservations, those patients who are able to participate in concurrent treatment may increase the probability of their long-term substance use recovery.

V. SUMMARY AND FUTURE DIRECTIONS

The purpose of this chapter was to summarize the current research on PTSD and SUDs, focusing on the shared epidemiology, course, genetic, and neurobiological basis of PTSD and SUDs as well as the current available treatment approaches. The comorbidity of PTSD and SUDs is high. These disorders not only tend to co-occur, but the symptoms of each disorder are intricately related to the occurrence and course of the other. Available genetic and neurobiological information supports that these disorders are related but distinct.

REFERENCES

Abueg, F., and Fairbank, J. A. (1992). Behavioral treatment of posttraumatic stress disorder and co-occurring substance abuse. In P. A. Saigh, Ed. *Posttraumatic stress disorder. A behavioral approach to assessment and treatment*. Boston, MA: Allyn and Bacon.

Acierno, R., Kilpatrick, D. G., Resnick, H., Saunders, B., De Arellano, M., and Best, C. (2000). Assault, PTSD, family substance use, and depression as risk factors for cigarette use in youth: Findings from the national survey of adolescents. *Journal of Traumatic Stress, 13*(3), 381–396.

Back, S., Dansky, B. S., Coffey, S. F., Saladin, M. E., Sonne, S., and Brady, K. T. (2000). Cocaine dependence with and without post-traumatic stress disorder: A comparison of substance use, trauma history and psychiatric comorbidity. *American Journal on Addictions, 9*(1), 51–62.

Back, S. E., Dansky, B. S., Carrol, K. M., Foa, E. B., and Brady, K. T. (2001). Exposure therapy in the treatment of PTSD among cocaine-dependent individuals: Description of procedures. *Journal of Substance Abuse Treatment, 21*(1), 35–45.

Ballenger, J. C., Davidson, J. R. T., Lecrubier, Y., Nutt, D. J., Foa, E. B., Kessler, R. C., et al. (2000). Consensus statement on posttraumatic stress disorder from the international consensus group on depression and anxiety. *Journal of Clinical Psychiatry, 61*(Supplement 5), 60–66.

Batten, S. V., and Hayes, S. C. (2005). Acceptance and commitment therapy in the treatment of comorbid substance abuse and posttraumatic stress disorder: A case study. *Clinical Case Studies, 4*(3), 246–262.

Becker, C. B., Zayfert, C., and Anderson, E. (2004). A survey of psychologists' attitudes towards and utilization of exposure therapy for PTSD. *Behavior Research and Therapy, 42*(3), 277–292.

Beckham, J. C., Feldman, M. E., McClernon, F. J., and Vrana, S. R. (2005a). Cigarette smoking and script-driven imagery in smokers with and without posttraumatic stress disorder. *Manuscript submitted for publication.*

Beckham, J. C., Feldman, M. E., Vrana, S. R., Mozley, S. L., Erkanli, A., Clancy, C. P., et al. (2005b). Immediate antecedents of cigarette smoking in smokers with and without posttraumatic stress disorder: A preliminary study. *Experimental and Clinical Psychopharmacology, 13*(3), 218–228.

Beckham, J. C., Kirby, A. C., Feldman, M. E., Hertzberg, M. A., Moore, S. D., Crawford, A. L., et al. (1997). Prevalence and correlates of heavy smoking in Vietnam veterans with chronic posttraumatic stress disorder. *Addictive Behaviors, 22*, 637–647.

Beckham, J. C., Lytle, B. L., Vrana, S. R., Hertzberg, M. A., Feldman, M. E., and Shipley, R. H. (1996). Smoking withdrawal symptoms in response to a trauma-related stressor among Vietnam combat veterans with PTSD. *Addictive Behaviors, 21*, 93–101.

Beckham, J. C., Roodman, A. A., Shipley, R. H., Hertzberg, M. A., Cunha, G. H., Kudler, H. S., et al. (1995). Smoking in Vietnam combat veterans with posttraumatic stress disorder. *Journal of Traumatic Stress, 8*, 461–472.

Blackledge, J. T. (2004). Functional contextual processes in posttraumatic stress. *International Journal of Psychology and Psychological Therapy, 4*(3), 443–467.

Bradizza, C. M., Stasiewicz, P. R., and Maisto, S. A. (1994). A conditioning reinterpretation of cognitive events in alcohol and drug cue exposure. *Journal of Behavior Therapy and Experimental Psychiatry, 25*(1), 15–22.

Brady, K., Dansky, B. S., Sonne, S. C., and Saladin, M. E. (1998). Posttraumatic stress disorder and cocaine dependence: Order of onset. *American Journal on Addictions, 7*, 128–135.

Brady, K. T., Dansky, B. S., Back, S. E., Foa, E. B., and Carroll, K. M. (2001). Exposure therapy in the treatment of PTSD among cocaine-dependent individuals: Preliminary findings. *Journal of Substance Abuse Treatment, 21*(1), 47–54.

Brady, K. T., and Sinha, R. (2005). Co-occurring mental and substance use disorders: The neurobiological effects of chronic stress. *American Journal of Psychiatry, 162*(8), 1483–1493.

Bremner, J. D., Licinio, J., Darnell, A., Krystal, J. H., Owens, M. J., Southwick, S., et al. (1997). Elevated csf corticotropin-releasing factor concentrations in posttraumatic stress disorder. *American Journal of Psychiatry, 154*, 624–629.

Bremner, J. D., Southwick, S. M., Carnell, A., and Charney, D. S. (1996). Chronic PTSD in Vietnam combat veterans: Course of illness and substance abuse. *American Journal of Psychiatry, 153*, 369–375.

Breslau, N., Davis, G. C., Andreski, P., and Peterson, E. (1991). Traumatic events and posttraumatic stress disorder in an urban population of young adults. *Archives of General Psychiatry, 48*, 216–222.

Breslau, N., Davis, G. C., Peterson, E. G., and Schultz, L. (1997). Psychiatric sequelae of posttraumatic stress disorder in women. *Archives of General Psychiatry, 54*, 81–87.

Breslau, N., Davis, G. C., and Schultz, L. R. (2003). Posttraumatic stress disorder and the incidence of nicotine, alcohol, and other drug disorders in persons who have experienced trauma. *Archives of General Psychiatry, 60*, 289–294.

Breslau, N., Kessler, R., Chilcoat, H., Schultz, L., Davis, G., and Andreski, P. (1998). Trauma and posttraumatic stress disorder in the community: The 1996 Detroit area survey of trauma. *Archives of General Psychiatry, 55*, 627–632.

Breslau, N., Novak, S., and Kessler, R. (2004a). Psychiatric disorders and stages of smoking. *Biological Psychiatry, 55*, 69–76.

Breslau, N., Novak, S., and Kessler, R. (2004b). Daily smoking and the subsequent onset of psychiatric disorders. *Psychological Medicine, 34*, 323–333.

Brown, P. J., Stout, R. L., and Gannon-Rowley, J. (1998). Substance use disorder-PTSD comorbidity: Patients' perceptions of symptom interplay and treatment issues. *Journal of Substance Abuse Treatment, 14*, 1–4.

Brown, P. J., Stout, R. L., and Mueller, T. (1996). Posttraumatic stress disorder and substance abuse relapse among women: A pilot study. *Psychology of Addictive Behaviors, 10*, 124–128.

Brown, P. J., and Wolfe, J. (1994). Substance abuse and post-traumatic stress comorbidity. *Drug and Alcohol Dependence, 35*, 51–59.

Burnam, M. A., Stein, J. A., Golding, J. M., Siegel, J. M., Sorenson, S. B., Forsythe, A. B., et al. (1988). Sexual assault and mental disorders in the community population. *Journal of Consulting and Clinical Psychology, 56*(6), 843–850.

Chantarujikapong, S. I., Scherrer, J. F., Xian, H., Eisen, S., Lyons, M. J., Goldberg, J., et al. (2001). A twin study of generalized anxiety disorder symptoms, panic disorder symptoms and posttraumatic stress disorder in men. *Psychiatry Research, 103*, 133–146.

Chilcoat, H., and Breslau, N. (1998). Posttraumatic stress disorder and drug disorders: Testing causal pathways. *Archives of General Psychiatry, 46,* 913–917.

Childress, A. R., Ehrman, R. N., McLellan, A. T., MacRae, J., Natale, M., and O'Brien, C. P. (1994). Can induced moods trigger drug-related responses in opiate abuse patients? *Journal of Substance Abuse Treatment, 11,* 17–23.

Coffey, S. F., Dansky, B. S., and Brady, K. (2002). Exposure-based, trauma-focused therapy for substance abusers with PTSD. In P. Ouimette and P. J. Brown, Eds. Trauma and substance abuse: Causes, consequences, and treatment of comorbid disorders, (pp. 127–146). Washington, DC: American Psychological Association.

Coffey, S. F., and Lombardo, T. W. (1998). Effects of smokeless tobacco-related sensory and behavioral cues on urge, affect, and stress. *Experimental and Clinical Psychopharmacology, 6*(4), 406–418.

Coffey, S. F., Schumacher, J. A., Brimo, M. L., and Brady, K. T. (2005). Exposure therapy for substance abusers with PTSD: Translating research to practice. *Behavior Modification, 29*(1), 10–38.

Contoreggi, C., Herning, R. I., Na, P., Gold, P. W., Chrousos, G. P., Negro, P. J., et al. (2003). Stress hormone response to corticotropin-releasing hormone in substance abusers without severe comorbid psychiatric disease. *Biological Psychiatry, 54,* 873–878.

Cook, J. M., Schurr, P. P., and Foa, E. B. (2004). Bridging the gap between posttraumatic stress disorder research and clinical practice: The example of exposure therapy. *Psychotherapy: Theory, Research, Practice, Training, 41*(4), 374–387.

Cottler, L. B., Compton, W. M., Mager, D., Spitznagel, E. L., and Janca, A. (1992). Posttraumatic stress disorder among substance users from the general population. *American Journal of Psychiatry, 149,* 664–670.

Davidson, J. R. T., Swartz, M., Storck, M., Krishnan, R. R., and Hammett, E. (1985). A diagnostic and family study of posttraumatic stress disorder. *American Journal of Psychiatry, 142,* 90–93.

Davidson, J. R. T., Tupler, L. A., Wilson, W. H., and Connor, K. M. (1998). A family study of chronic posttraumatic stress disorder following rape trauma. *Journal of Psychiatric Research, 32,* 301–309.

Deykin, E. Y., and Buka, S. L. (1997). Prevalence and risk factors for posttraumatic stress disorder among chemically dependent adolescents. *American Journal of Psychiatry, 154*(6), 752–757.

Dobie, D. J., Kivlahan, D. R., Maynard, C., Bush, K. R., Davis, T. M., and Bradley, K. A. (2004). Posttraumatic stress disorder in female veterans: Association with self-reported health problems and functional impairment. *Archives of Internal Medicine, 164*(4), 394–400.

Eliava, M., Yilmazer-Hanke, D., and Asan, E. (2003). Interrelations between monoaminergic afferents and corticotropin-releasing factor-immunoreactive neurons in the rat central amygdaloid nucleus: Ultrastructural evidence for dopaminergic control of amygdaloid stress systems. *Histochemistry and Cell Biology, 120*(3), 183–197.

Foa, E. B. (1997). Trauma and women: Course, predictors, and treatment. *Journal of Clinical Psychiatry, 58*(Supplement 9), 25–28.

Foa, E. B., Davidson, J. R. T., Frances, A., Culpepper, L., Ross, R., and Ross, D. (Eds.). (1999). The expert consensus guideline series: Treatment of posttraumatic stress disorder. *Journal of Clinical Psychiatry, 60*(Supplement 16), 4–76.

Foa, E. B., Rothbaum, B. O., Riggs, D. S., and Murdock, T. B. (1991). Treatment of posttraumatic stress disorder in rape victims: A comparison between cognitive behavioral proceedings and counseling. *Journal of Consulting and Clinical Psychology, 59,* 715–723.

Giaconia, R. M., Reinherz, H. Z., Hauf, A. C., Paradis, A. D., Wasserman, M. S., and Langhammer, D. M. (2000). Comorbidity of substance use and posttraumatic stress disorders in a community sample of adolescents. *American Journal of Orthopsychiatry, 70*(2), 253–262.

Goeders, N. E., Bienvenu, O. J., and De Souza, E. B. (1990). Chronic cocaine administration alters corticotropin-releasing factor receptors in the rat brain. *Brain Research, 531,* 322–328.

Gowing, L. R., Farrell, M., Ali, R. L., and White, J. M. (2002). Alpha2-adrenergic agonist in opioid withdrawal. *Addiction, 97,* 49–58.

Gross, A. M., Winslett, A., Roberts, M. E., and Gohm, C. (2006). An examination of sexual violence against college women. *Violence Against Women, 12,* 288–300.

Hapke, U., Schumann, A., Rumpf, H., John, U., Konerding, U., and Meyer, C. (2005). Association of smoking and nicotine dependence with trauma and posttraumatic stress disorder in a general population sample. *Journal of Nervous and Mental Diseases, 193*(12), 843–846.

Hawley, R. J., Major, L. F., Schulman, E. A., and Linnoila, M. (1985). Cerebrospinal fluid 3-methoxy-4-hydroxyphenylglycol and norepinephrine levels in alcohol withdrawal: Correlations with clinical signs. *Archives of General Psychiatry, 42,* 1056–1062.

Hayes, S. C., Strosahl, K., and Wilson, K. G. (1999). *Acceptance and commitment therapy: An experiential approach to behavior change.* New York: Guilford.

Hayes, S. C., Wilson, K. G., Gilford, E. V., Follette, V. M., and Stosahl, K. (1996). Experiential avoidance and behavioral disorders: A functional dimensional approach to diagnosis and treatment. *Journal of Consulting and Clinical Psychology, 64,* 1152–1168.

Hien, D. A., Cohen, L. R., Miele, G. M., Litt, L. C., and Capstick, C. (2004). Promising treatments for women with comorbid PTSD and substance use disorders. *American Journal of Psychiatry, 161*(8), 1426–1432.

Hourani, L. L., Yuan, H., Bray, R. M., and Vincus, A. A. (1999). Psychosocial correlates of nicotine dependence among men and women in the U.S. Naval service. *Addictive Behaviors, 24*(4), 521–536.

Jacobsen, L. K., Southwick, S., and Kosten, T. B. (2001). Substance use disorders in patients with posttraumatic stress disorder: A review of the literature. *American Journal of Psychiatry, 158*(8), 1184–1190.

Kalivas, P. W., and Stewart, S. (1991). Dopamine transmission in the initiation and expression of drug- and stress-induced sensitization of motor activity. *Brain Research Reviews, 16*, 223–244.

Keane, T. M., Gerardi, R. J., Lyons, J. A., and Wolfe, J. (1988). The interrelationship of substance abuse and posttraumatic stress disorder: Epidemiological and clinical considerations. In M. Galanter, Ed. *Recent developments in alcoholism* (Vol. 6, pp. 27–48). New York: Plenum.

Kessler, R. C., Sonnega, A., Bromet, E., Hughes, M., and Nelson, C. B. (1995). Posttraumatic stress disorder in the national comorbidity survey. *Archives of General Psychiatry, 52*, 1048–1060.

Kilpatrick, D. B., Saunders, B. E., Veronen, L. J., and Best, C. L. (1987). Criminal victimization: Lifetime prevalence, reporting to police, and psychological impact. *Crime Delinquency, 33*, 479–489.

Kilpatrick, D. G., Acierno, R., Saunders, B., Resnick, H. S., Best, C. L., and Schnurr, P. P. (2000). Risk factors for adolescent substance abuse and dependence: Data from a national sample. *Journal of Consulting and Clinical Psychology, 68*(1), 19–30.

Koenen, K. C. (2003). A brief introduction to genetics research in PTSD. *PTSD Research Quarterly, 14*(3), 1–3.

Koenen, K. C., Lyons, M. J., Goldberg, J., Simpson, J., Williams, W. M., Toomey, R., et al. (2003). Co-twin control study of relationships among combat exposure, combat-related PTSD, and other mental disorder. *Journal of Traumatic Stress, 16*, 433–438.

Koob, G. F. (1999). Stress, corticotropin-releasing factor, and drug addiction. *Annals of the New York Academy of Sciences, 897*, 27–45.

Koob, G. F., and Le Moal, M. (1997). Drug abuse: Hedonic homeostatic dysregulation. *Science, 278*, 52–58.

Kreek, M. J., and Koob, G. F. (1998). Drug dependence: Stress and dysregulation of brain reward pathways. *Drug and Alcohol Dependence, 51*, 23–47.

Kulka, R. A., Schlenger, W. E., Fairbank, J. A., Hough, R. L., Jordon, B. K., Marmar, C. R., et al. (1990). *Trauma and the Vietnam War generation: Report of findings from the National Vietnam Veterans Readjustment Study*. New York: Brunner/Mazel.

Labbate, L. A., Sonne, S. C., Randal, C. L., Anton, R. F., and Brady, K. T. (2004). Does comorbid anxiety or depression affect clinical outcomes in patients with posttraumatic stress disorder and alcohol use disorders? *Comprehensive Psychiatry, 45*(4), 304–310.

Larson, M. J., Miller, L., Becker, M., Richardson, E., Kammerer, N., Thom, J., et al. (2005). Physical health burdens of women with trauma histories and co-occurring substance abuse and mental disorders. *Journal of Behavioral Health Services and Research, 32*(2), 128–140.

Lasser, K., Boyd, J. W., Woolhandler, S., Himmelstein, D., McCormick, D., and Bor, D. (2000). Smoking and mental illness: A population-based prevalence study. *JAMA, 284*(20), 2606–2610.

Liu, X., and Weiss, F. (2002). Additive effect of stress and drug cues on reinstatement of ethanol seeking: Exacerbation by history of dependence and role of concurrent activation of corticotropin-releasing factor and opioid mechanisms. *Journal of Neuroscience, 22*, 7856–7861.

Lyons, M. J., Goldberg, J., Eisen, S., True, W., Tsuang, M., Meyer, J. M., et al. (1993). Do genes influence exposure to trauma? A twin study of combat. *American Journal of Medical Genetics, 48*, 22–27.

Marlatt, G. A. (1996). Taxonomy of high-risk situations for alcohol relapse: Evolution and development of a cognitive-behavioral model. *Addiction, 91*(Supplement), S37–S49.

McClernon, F. J., Hiott, F. B., Huettel, S. A., and Rose, J. E. (2005). Abstinence-induced changes in self-reported craving correlate with event-related fMRI responses to smoking cues. *Neuropsychopharmacology, 30*, 1940–1947.

McEwen, B. S. (2002). The neurobiology and neuroendocrinology of stress: Implications for post-traumatic stress disorder from a basic science perspective. *Psychiatric Clinics of North America, 25*, 469–494.

McFall, M., Saxon, A. J., Thompson, C. E., Yoshimoto, D., Malte, C., Straits-Troster, K., et al. (2005). Improving the rates of quitting smoking for veterans with posttraumatic stress disorder. *American Journal of Psychiatry, 162*(7), 1311–1319.

McFall, M. E., Mackay, P. W., and Donovan, D. M. (1992). Combat-related posttraumatic stress disorder and severity of substance abuse in Vietnam veterans. *Journal of Studies on Alcohol, 53*(4), 357–363.

McLeod, D. S., Koenen, K. C., Meyer, J. M., Lyons, M. J., Eisen, S. A., True, W. R., et al. (2001). Genetic and environmental influences on the relationship among combat exposure, posttraumatic stress disorder symptoms, and alcohol use. *Journal of Traumatic Stress, 14*, 259–275.

Milby, J. B., Schumacher, J. E., and Stainback, R. D. (1997). Psychoactive substance use disorder: Drugs. In S. M. Turner and M. Hersen, Eds. Adult psychopathology and diagnosis (3rd ed., pp. 159–202). New York: John Wiley and Sons.

Morgan, D., Grant, K. A., Gage, H. D., Mach, R. H., Kaplan, J. R., Pioleau, O., et al. (2002). Social dominance in monkeys: Dopamine d2 receptors and cocaine self-administration. *Neuroscience, 5*, 169–174.

Mulick, P. S., Landes, S. J., and Kanter, J. W. (2005). Contextual behavior therapies in the treatment of

PTSD: A review. *International Journal of Behavioral Consulation and Therapy, 1*(3), 220–235.

Najavits, L. M. (2002). Clinicians' views on treating posttraumatic stress disorder and substance use disorder. *Journal of Substance Abuse Treatment, 22*(2), 79–85.

Najavits, L. M., Weiss, R. D., and Liese, B. S. (1996). Group cognitive behavioral therapy for women with PTSD and substance use disorder. *Journal of Substance Abuse Treatment, 13*(1), 13–22.

Najavits, L. M., Weiss, R. D., Shaw, S. R., and Muenz, L. R. (1998). "Seeking safety": Outcome of a new cognitive-behavioral psychotherapy for women with posttraumatic stress disorder and substance dependence. *Journal of Traumatic Stress, 11*(3), 437–456.

Nie, Z., Schweitzer, P., Roberts, A. J., Madamba, S. G., Moore, S. D., and Siggins, G. R. (2004). Ethanol augments gabaergic transmission in the central amygdala via crf1 receptors. *Science, 303*, 1512–1514.

North, C. S., Tivis, L., McMillen, J. C., Pfefferbaum, B., Spitznagel, E. L., Cox, J., et al. (2002). Psychiatric disorders in rescue workers after the Oklahoma City bombing. *American Journal of Psychiatry, 159*(5), 857–859.

O'Farrell, T. J. (1994). Substance abuse disorders. In V. B. Van Hasselt and M. Hersen, Eds. *Advanced abnormal psychology* (pp. 335–358). New York: Plenum.

Orsillo, S. M., and Batten, S. V. (2005). Acceptance and commitment therapy in the treatment of posttraumatic stress disorder. *Behavior Modification, 29*(1), 95–129.

Ouimette, P., Ahrens, C., Moos, R. H., and Finney, J. W. (1998a). During treatment changes in substance abuse patients with posttraumatic stress disorder: The influence of specific interventions and program environments. *Journal of Substance Abuse Treatment, 15*, 555–564.

Ouimette, P., Brown, P. J., and Najavits, L. M. (1998b). Course and treatment of patients with both substance use and posttraumatic stress disorders. *Addictive Behaviors, 6*, 785–795.

Ouimette, P., Finney, J. W., and Moos, R. H. (1999). Two-year posttreatment functioning and coping of substance abuse patients with posttraumatic stress disorder. *Psychology of Addictive Behaviors, 13*(2), 105–114.

Piasecki, T. M., and Baker, T. B. (2000). Does smoking amortize negative affect? *American Psychologist, 55*, 1156–1157.

Piazza, P. V., and Le Moal, M. (1998). The role of stress in drug self-administration. *Trends in Pharmacological Sciences, 19*, 67–74.

Pich, E. M., Lorang, M., Yeganeh, M., Rodriguez de Fonseca, F., Raber, J., Koob, G. F., et al. (1995). Increasing of extracellular corticotropin-releasing factor-like immunoreactivity levels in the amygdala of awake rats during restraint stress and ethanol

withdrawal as measured by microdialysis. *Journal of Neuroscience, 15*, 5439–5447.

Pitman, R. K., Altman, B., Greenwald, E., Longpre, R. E., Macklin, M. L., Poire, E., et al. (1991). Psychiatric complications during flooding therapy for posttraumatic stress disorder. *Journal of Clinical Psychiatry, 52*, 17–20.

Prochaska, J. J., Delucchi, K. L., and Hall, S. M. (2004). A meta-analysis of smoking cessation interventions with individuals in substance abuse treatment or recovery. *Journal of Consulting and Clinical Psychology, 72*(6), 1144–1156.

Rainnie, D. G., Bergeron, R., Sajdyk, T. J., Patil, M., Gehlert, D. R., and Shekhar, A. (2004). Corticotropin releasing factor-induced synaptic plasticity in the amygdala translates stress into emotional disorders. *Journal of Neuroscience, 24*, 3471–3479.

Read, J. P., Brown, P. J., and Kahler, C. W. (2004). Substance use and posttraumatic stress disorders: Symptom interplay and effects on outcome. *Addictive Behaviors, 29*(8), 1665–1672.

Resnick, H. S., Kilpatrick, D. G., Dansky, B. S., Saunders, B. E., and Best, C. L. (1993). Prevalence of civilian trauma and posttraumatic stress disorder in a representative sample of women. *Journal of Consulting and Clinical Psychology, 61*, 984–991.

Roberts, S. T., and Wilson, K. G. (2002, November). Acceptance and commitment therapy for PTSD: Single case study. *Association for the Advancement of Behavior Therapy*. Reno, NV.

Roy-Byrne, P., Arguelles, L., Vitek, M. E., Goldberg, J., Keane, T. M., True, W., Pitman, R. (2004). Persistence and change of PTSD symptomatology: A longitudinal co-twin control analysis of the Vietnam Era Twin Registry. *Social Psychiatry and Psychiatric Epidemiology, 39*, 681–685.

Saladin, M. E., Brady, K., Dansky, B. S., and Kilpatrick, D. (1995). Understanding comorbidity between PTSD and substance use disorder: Two preliminary investigations. *Addictive Behaviors, 20*, 643–655.

Saladin, M. E., Drobes, D. J., Coffey, S. F., Dansky, B. S., Brady, K. T., and Kilpatrick, D. G. (2003). PTSD symptom severity as a predictor of cue-elicited drug craving in victims of violent crime. *Addictive Behaviors, 28*(9), 1611–1629.

Sarnyai, Z., Shaham, Y., and Heinrichs, S. C. (2001). The role of corticotropin-releasing factor in drug addiction. *Pharmacological Review, 53*, 209–243.

Scott, M. J., and Stradling, S. G. (1997). Client compliance with exposure treatments for posttraumatic stress disorder. *Journal of Traumatic Stress, 10*(3), 523–526.

Segman, R. H., and Shalev, A. Y. (2003). Genetics of posttraumatic stress disorder. *CNS Spectrums, 8*(9), 693–698.

Shalev, A., Bleich, A., and Ursano, R. J. (1990). Posttraumatic stress disorder: Somatic comorbidity and effort tolerance. *Psychosomatics, 31*, 197–203.

Sharkansky, E. J., Brief, D. J., Peirce, J. M., Meehan, J. C., and Mannix, L. M. (1999). Substance abuse patients with posttraumatic stress disorder (PTSD): Identifying specific triggers of substance use and their associations with PTSD symptoms. *Psychology of Addictive Behaviors, 13*(2), 89–97.

Shiffman, S., Gnys, M., Richards, T. J., Paty, J. A., Hickcox, M., and Kassel, J. D. (1996). Temptations to smoke after quitting: A comparison of lapsers and maintainers. *Health Psychology, 15*, 455–461.

Shipherd, J. C., Stafford, J., and Tanner, L. R. (2005). Predicting alcohol and drug abuse in Persian Gulf War veterans: What role do PTSD symptoms play? *Addictive Behaviors, 30*(3), 595–599.

Sillaber, I., Rammes, G., Zimmermann, S., Mahal, B., Zieglgansberger, W., Wurst, W., et al. (2002). Enhanced and delayed stress-induced alcohol drinking in mice lacking functional crh1 receptors. *Science, 296*, 931–933.

Southwick, S., Bremner, J. D., Rasmusson, A., Morgan, C. A., Arnsten, A., and Charney, D. S. (1999). Role of norepinephrine in the pathophysiology and treatment of posttraumatic stress disorder. *Biological Psychiatry, 46*, 1192–1204.

Stasiewicz, P. R., and Maisto, S. A. (1993). Two-factor avoidance theory: The role of negative affect in the maintenance of substance use and substance use disorders. *Behavior Therapy, 24*, 337–356.

Stein, M. B., Jang, K. L., Taylor, S., Vernon, P. A., and Livesley, W. J. (2002). Genetic and environmental influences on trauma exposure and posttraumatic stress disorder symptoms: A twin study. *The American Journal of Psychiatry, 159*, 1675–1681.

Steindl, S. R., Young, R. M., Creamer, M., and Crompton, D. (2003). Hazardous alcohol use and treatment outcome in male combat veterans with posttraumatic stress disorder. *Journal of Traumatic Stress, 16*(1), 27–34.

Sutker, P. B., Uddo, M., Brailey, K., Allain, A. N., and Errera, P. (1994). Psychological symptoms and psychiatric diagnoses in Operation Desert Storm troops serving graves registration duty. *Journal of Traumatic Stress, 7*(2), 159–171.

Timpl, P., Spanagel, R., Sillaber, I., Kresse, A., Reul, J. M., Stalla, G. K., et al. (1998). Impaired stress response and reduced anxiety in mice lacking a functional corticotropin-releasing hormone receptor 1. *Nature Genetics, 19*, 162–166.

Torgersen, S. (1997). Genetic basis and psychopathology. In S. M. Turner and M. Hersen, Eds. *Adult psychopathology and diagnosis* (3rd ed., pp. 58–85). New York: John Wiley and Sons.

Triffleman, E., Carroll, K., and Kellogg, S. (1999). Substance dependence posttraumatic stress disorder therapy: An integrated cognitive-behavioral approach. *Journal of Substance Abuse Treatment, 17*(1–2), 3–14.

True, W. R., Rice, J., Eisen, S. A., and Heath, A. C. (1993). A twin study of genetic and environmental contributions to liability for posttraumatic stress symptoms. *Archives of General Psychiatry, 50*, 257–265.

Xian, H., Chantarujikapong, S. I., Scherrer, J. F., Eisen, S. A., Lyons, M. J., Goldberg, J., et al. (2000). Genetic and environmental influences on posttraumatic stress disorder, alcohol and drug dependence in twin pairs. *Drug and Alcohol Dependence, 61*(1), 95–102.

Yehuda, R. (1999). Biological factors associated with susceptibility to posttraumatic stress disorder. *Canadian Journal of Psychiatry, 44*, 34–39.

Yehuda, R., and McFarlane, A. C. (1995). Conflict between current knowledge about posttraumatic stress disorder and its original conceptual basis. *American Journal of Psychiatry, 152*, 1705–1713.

Yehuda, R., McFarlane, A., and Shalev, A. (1998a). Predicting the development of posttraumatic stress disorder from the acute response to a traumatic event. *Biological Psychiatry, 44*, 1305–1313.

Yehuda, R., Schmeidler, J., Giller, E., Binder-Brynes, K., and Siever, L. J. (1998b). Relationship between PTSD characteristics of Holocaust survivors and their adult offspring. *American Journal of Psychiatry, 155*, 841–843.

Yehuda, R., Shmeidler, J., Wainberg, M., Binder-Brynes, K., and Duvdevani, T. (1998c). Increased vulnerability to posttraumatic stress disorder in adult offspring of Holocaust survivors. *American Journal of Psychiatry, 155*, 1163–1171.

Zlotnick, C., Najavits, L. M., Rohsenow, D. J., and Johnson, D. M. (2003). A cognitive-behavioral treatment for incarcerated women with substance abuse disorder and posttraumatic stress disorder: Findings from a pilot study. *Journal of Substance Abuse Treatment, 25*(2), 99–105.

17

Novel Pharmacologic Treatment of Stress and Addiction: The Role of CRF and Glucocorticoid Antagonists

DANIEL SAAL AND CHARLES B. NEMEROFF

Historically, addiction has been among the most intractable psychiatric conditions. Standard therapies, both behavioral and pharmacological, are moderately effective in the short term and even less so for the long term. The serious medical and psychosocial effects of addiction are well documented. Despite this frustrating track record, new advances in understanding the basic neurobiological mechanisms that underlie addiction have served as an impetus for considerably intense research efforts in this field. A prominent issue in the treatment of addiction is the propensity for stress to induce relapse of addictive behaviors. This has prompted an interest in treatments that focus on stress response mechanisms in the context of addiction. This chapter reviews some of the promising directions in the development of such novel treatments. We will describe the basic mechanisms that serve as the rationale for each of these treatment modalities.

I. GENERAL MECHANISMS OF ADDICTION

An abundance of data points to a relatively circumscribed set of brain structures as central to addiction. The ventral tegmental area (VTA) is a midbrain nucleus composed of dopamine and GABA-producing cells. A burgeoning database, reviewed below, suggests that the initiation of addictive processes occur in the VTA. The VTA projects DA efferents broadly, but the targets important for stress and addiction are primarily the nucleus accumbens (NAc), prefrontal cortex (PFC), and certain amygdaloid nuclei. Other critical structures include the hippocampus and pedunculopontine nucleus (PPN). The nucleus accumbens projects GABA-ergic efferents to the VTA and PFC. The PFC projects excitatory, glutamatergic efferents to the NAc and VTA. The balance of the synaptic and neuromodulatory outputs of each of these nuclei is critical for acquisition and

Stress and Addiction: Biological and Psychological Mechanisms
Edited by **Mustafa al'Absi, Ph.D.**

maintenance of addiction. In this chapter we will scrutinize these pathways and their modulation by the stress response. It is important to note that although the various addictive substances act via distinct initial receptors, they all appear to similarly activate this circuit (Koob et al., 1998; Nestler and Malenka, 2004; Thomas and Malenka, 2003).

A critical shift in understanding the mechanisms of addiction follow the recognition that these circuits are modulated in response to both rewards such as juice (Schultz, 2005; Tobler et al., 2003; Tobler et al., 2005), cocaine, amphetamine, and nicotine, as well as distress. Interestingly, this reward circuit is active in the human response to monetary gain and even laughter (Berns, 2004; Montague and Berns, 2002). This convergence of reward and stress at the circuit and cellular level has been demonstrated repeatedly and, as will be discussed below, has now been extended to the molecular and synaptic levels. In fact this convergence has resulted in the modification of the view that the addiction process is one of reward seeking to a misappropriation of salience mechanisms (Nestler, 1993). This explains why a painful experience, such as a divorce, might act in the same way for an addict as a pleasurable one, such as a dose of morphine: Both are experienced by the brain as highly important and salient. As such, it becomes easier to understand why just as a drink can send an abstinent alcoholic onto a drinking binge, a stressful experience can trigger a relapse as well.

II. BEHAVIORAL PARADIGMS

In order to review the literature on addiction and stress, we will first describe the basic behavioral paradigms used to explore these phenomena. The behavioral paradigms upon which we will focus are behavioral sensitization, operant conditioning, and conditioned place preference.

We will briefly review these paradigns here to allow a better understanding of the treatments presented in the monograph.

A. Sensitization

Sensitization is both the simplest addiction behavioral paradigm and the most difficult to conceptualize. In this paradigm, rodents are given repeated doses of cocaine, amphetamine, or morphine and placed in a device that measures their ambulation. This is termed the *induction phase*. Animals demonstrate "reverse tolerance" to the substance in that their activity increases with each subsequent injection. The truly interesting aspect of this is that after the induction phase animals can be withdrawn and after as much as 1 year, when, given a test dose of drug, will resume the enhanced activity pattern in response to the drug (Berridge and Robinson, 2003; Robinson and Berridge, 2000). In this respect the paradigm is similar to the long-term craving that addicts experience long after withdrawal. This technique has been used to map the anatomical (Bjijou et al., 1996; Deroche et al., 1995; Li et al., 1999), pharmacologic (Bjijou et al., 1996; David et al., 2002; W. Lu et al., 1997), molecular (Nestler, 1993), and synaptic (Carlezon and Nestler, 2002; Kalivas and Stewart, 1991; J. A. Kim et al., 2003; W. Lu and Wolf, 1999; Szumlinski et al., 2000; Thomas et al., 2001) events that may underlie addiction. The same paradigm can be performed by injecting cocaine into the VTA for the training phase and into the NAc for the expression of sensitization (Wolf, 1998). This is historically how the hypothesis was developed that the VTA is the gatekeeper for addiction, whereas the NAc is the site of long-term storage of the addicted state. It is a somewhat difficult paradigm to apply because a core aspect of human drug addiction is the decrease in efficacy of the substance to trigger reward responses (tolerance). However, the reliability, ease, and robust nature of the technique have made it invaluable (Berridge and Robinson, 2003;

Robinson and Becker, 1986). Interestingly, Miczek and colleagues demonstrated that stress alone can act to induce sensitization that is expressed in response to amphetamine. Rats were exposed to repeated brief social defeat stress, in which a male animal is introduced into a dominant male's cage, four times over the course of 10 days. This treatment produces a significant and reproducible stress response in the nondominant animal. Animals were then tested for their locomotor response to amphetamine and found to be sensitized relative to control animals. This motor effect persisted for at least 70 days (Covington and Miczek, 2001; Nikulina et al., 2004). This effect appears to involve the same CNS structures described above. Indeed, Fos–like immunoreactive proteins were upregulated in the VTA and NAc in this paradigm (Nikulina et al., 2004) in very much the same way as they are following repeated cocaine (J. Chen et al., 1995; Nikulina et al., 2004; Nye et al., 1995), amphetamine (Dalia and Wallace, 1995), morphine (J. Liu et al., 1994; Sharp et al., 1995), ethanol (in the NAc) (Yoshimoto et al., 2000), and nicotine (Schilstrom et al., 2000) (for review, see Nestler, 1993). Thus sensitization is a useful tool for exploring the neurobiological underpinnings of stress and addiction.

B. Operant Conditioning

Operant conditioning is a paradigm in which animals (rodents and primates) press a lever or poke their nose in a hole to obtain a drug reward. There are a number of variations of this paradigm. The simplest is that an animal receives a reward each time the lever is pressed. However, experiments can be designed in which the animal must perform the task with increasing repetition for each subsequent reward, the so-called progressive ratio paradigm. The value of the latter modality is that one can measure the point at which the animal stops performing the task because it is no longer sufficiently motivated. This is termed a *breaking point* and is a relevant measure for certain experimental manipulations discussed below. In many ways, operant conditioning is most like human addiction, in that it requires active participation of the subject. It is a good measure of motivation for the drug in question. Furthermore, as in human addiction, if the reward is removed the animal will eventually stop performing the task, a phenomenon known as extinction. In a manner strikingly similar to human behavior, once an animal demonstrates extinction, a subsequent dose of the addictive substance will promote a return of the extinguished behavior. An important aspect of this paradigm is that animals will also return to the active behavior following a stressor. Interestingly, this applies to opiates (L. Lu et al., 2003b; Shalev et al., 2000), cocaine (Shaham et al., 2003), nicotine (Buczek et al., 1999), ethanol (Le and Shaham, 2002; Little et al., 2005), and amphetamine (Shepard et al., 2004) (for review, see Bossert et al., 2005; Shaham et al., 2003).

C. Conditioned Place Preference (CPP)

This paradigm is generally performed with rodents. Animals are placed in a behavioral apparatus that measures their time spent in one of two chambers of a box.[1] Initially, the chambers of the box are accessible to the animal. Animals are tested for initial preference and then assigned to one of two groups. At this time the door between the chambers is closed such that the animal cannot move between them. One group receives a drug injection and is placed in a given chamber of the box. This injection is alternated with saline injections paired with the other chamber. The control group receives only saline injections paired with both chambers. After the training phase the door between the chambers

---

[1] In fact there are usually three chambers in CPP. There are the saline paired, drug paired, and a central vestibule that is neutral. However, for simplicity and clarity, only the two-chamber approach is discussed here.

is opened and animals are allowed to explore both chambers. The time spent in the drug-paired side is compared to pre-training values. An increase in time spent on the drug-paired side indicates drug-seeking or reward-seeking behavior. This place preference diminishes with time and can be reinstated after re-exposure to drug even when the drug is administered out of context. As we will see below, stress can affect both the training and reinstatement of CPP. Also relevant to this technique is the related paradigm, conditioned place aversion, in which animals are trained to avoid the chamber paired with an aversive stimulus (Bardo, 1998; L. Lu et al., 2003b; Tzschentke, 1998). This paradigm has been informative in elucidating the neuroanatomy of addiction. For example, injection of NMDA receptor antagonists directly into the VTA blocks synaptic adaptation required for acquisition of CPP (J. A. Kim et al., 2004).

III. GENERAL MECHANISMS OF STRESS RESPONSE

As discussed in other chapters in this publication, corticotropin-releasing factor (CRF) plays a preeminent role in the organization of the response to stress. Classically, this peptide has been viewed primarily in its role as a hypothalamic releasing factor in promotion of ACTH release. However, more recently, CRF has been recognized as an important extrahypothalamic neuromodulator (Koob and Heinrichs, 1999) where it integrates the effects of stress including autonomic and immune responses. A number of preclinical studies have demonstrated that CRF directly affects key CNS structures involved in addiction (Ungless et al., 2003; Wang et al., 2005). These structures include the amygdala, a likely source of CRF neurons that are involved in stress responsiveness (Dunn et al., 2004) and the VTA (Ungless et al., 2003).

IV. CORTICOTROPIN-RELEASING FACTOR

Corticotropin-releasing factor (CRF) is a 41 amino acid peptide that is the secretory product of a 196 amino acid precursor. It is conserved across species (about 40% identity) (Dautzenberg and Hauger, 2002; Vale et al., 1981). It is found in neurons heterogeneously distributed throughout the CNS with a particularly high density in the medial parvocellular division of the hypothalamic paraventricular nucleus (PVN). This particular cell group is the primary source of CRF secreted into the hypothalamic hypophyseal portal circulation (Sawchenko et al., 1993). CRF in turn acts on corticotrophs of the anterior pituitary to release adrenocorticotropin (ACTH), which circulates through the body and stimulates release of glucocorticoids from the adrenal cortex. Cortisol is the main glucocorticoid in man and serves as an integral component of the sympatho-adrenal response. It also provides a signal for feedback inhibition at the level of the PVN, anterior pituitary, and extrahypothalamic sites such as the hippocampus. In addition to its role in the hypothalamic-pituitary-adrenal (HPA) axis regulation of the stress response, considerable interest has recently been focused on the extra-endocrine role of CRF in neuromodulation of other brain systems. CRF-containing neural circuits in the amygdala, cortex, hippocampus, and brain stem also contribute to the stress response, as well as modulate a variety of other physiologic and behavioral processes (Koob and Heinrichs, 1999; Nemeroff, 2002; Sawchenko et al., 1993).

A functionally related peptide, urocortin I, shares 43% sequence identity with CRF and is highly conserved across species. To date, two other related peptides, urocortin II (in humans, termed *stresscopin-related peptide*) and III (termed *stresscopin*) have been identified (Hsu and Hsueh, 2001). Urocortin I is primarily expressed in the Edinger-Westfall nucleus, the forebrain, and hypothalamus. Functionally, urocortins interact with CRF receptors as discussed below. Urocortin II is expressed in the paraventricular, supraoptic, and arcuate nuclei of the hypothalamus, the locus coeruleus, and motor nuclei of the brain stem and spinal cord (Dautzenberg and Hauger, 2002), and urocortin III is found in the bed nucleus of the stria terminalis as well as the lateral septum and medial amygdaloid nucleus. Unlike CRF and urocortin I, urocortin II and III do not stimulate the release of ACTH (Bale and Vale, 2004; Hsu and Hsueh, 2001).

V. GLUCOCORTICOIDS

Peripherally, corticosteroids exert a vast array of effects ranging from regulation of metabolism and the immune system to blood pressure. In humans, activation of the HPA axis results in release of cortisol from the adrenal cortex, whereas in rats the predominant stress steroid is corticosterone. Remarkably, there is relatively little information on the use of glucocorticoid receptor antagonists on modulation of addiction behaviors in spite of the fact that these agents may block stress-induced addiction behaviors. However, whether corticosteroids may play a role in addiction behaviors in the absence of stress remains unclear (Piazza and Le Moal, 1998). We review the evidence that supports such an approach (Saal et al., 2003).

VI. CRF RECEPTORS

CRF receptors are divided into CRFr1 and CRFr2 subtypes. There is 70% identity between CRFr1 and CRFr2 receptors (Lovenberg et al., 1995). The specifics of CRF receptor subtype localization are still evolving. For example, Ungless et al. (2003) performed RT-PCR and demonstrated CRFr2 expression in the VTA, where it had not been previously described. Both urocortin I and CRF bind both to the CRFr1 and CRFr2, whereas urocortin II and III bind only to CRFr2. There is an associated, membrane-bound protein distinct from the receptor that is required for the association of CRF receptors (Bale and Vale, 2004; Ungless et al., 2003). Urocortins do not bind this secondary protein (Bale and Vale, 2004). Both CRFr1 and CRFr2 are G-protein coupled receptors. Here again, there is growing complexity. Early data indicated that Gs and the cyclic-AMP system were the primary downstream mediators of receptor CRF binding. However, in the VTA, CRFr2 appears to mediate its actions via phospholipase C and not cyclic-AMP (Ungless et al., 2003).

VII. CRF PHARMACOLOGY

A number of antagonists of the CRF receptors are now available. Because CRF is a peptide, structurally related compounds are not useful for *in vivo* studies or subsequent clinical studies because of their inability to cross the blood-brain barrier. These peptide-based compounds have been of use only in preclinical studies of stress and addiction. In addition to those enumerated below, a number of lipophilic CRF receptor antagonists have not yet been studied in models of addiction and in the interest of brevity will not be comprehensively described.

Antalarmin: (N-Butyl-N-ethyl-[2,5,6-trimethyl-7-(2,4,6-trimethylphenyl)-7H-pyrrolo[2,3-d]pyrimidin-4-yl]amine) is an antagonist of the CRFr1 with a K_i of 1.3 to 1.9 nM depending on the brain region studied. It is bioavailable to CNS sites following IP injection in rats (Webster et al., 1996). Antalarmin significantly reduced ethanol seeking in a modified operant conditioning model in which mice were trained to press a lever for a 10% ethanol solution and then exposed to ethanol vapors to maintain dependence. Animals were withdrawn for 14 days and then treated with either saline or Antalarmin IP. Antalarmin-treated animals demonstrated decreased lever pressing compared to saline animals (Breese et al., 2005).

CP-154,526: This Pfizer compound is a centrally bioavailable CRFr1 antagonist following an IP injection. This compound has been shown to mitigate anxiety and depression symptoms in rodent models (Seymour et al., 2003). A recent and unexpected finding is that CP-154,526 administered systemically enhances dopamine release in the PFC but not in the nucleus accumbens in response to cocaine. The authors of this study suggest that this effect may underlie the observed blunting of cocaine seeking by CRF antagonists (Gurkovskaya et al., 2005). Shaham et al. (1998) used this compound to demonstrate that inhibition of CRFr1 reduces stress-induced reinstatement for both cocaine and heroin.

R121919: This compound, 5-dimethyl-3-(6-dimethyl-4-methylpyridin-3-yl)-7-dipropylaminopyrazolo[1,5-a]pyrimidine, is a CRFr1 antagonist synthesized by Neurocrine Biosciences and studied in depression (Kunzel et al., 2003; Zobel et al., 2000) in a partnership with Janssen and is now the property of GlaxoSmithKline. It has a K_i of 3.5 nM and an IC 50 of 50 nM in culture. It is bioavailable to the CNS after oral administration (C. Chen et al., 2004).

Other lipophilic CRFr1 antagonists include NBI 27914, NBI 30775, and SSR125543A (Bale and Vale, 2004).

Peptide antagonists of CRF receptors: As noted above, there are a number of peptide analogs of CRF, but these compounds must be administered directly into the CNS. α-helical $CRF_{(9-41)}$ and Astressin are antagonists of both CRFr1 and r2. The former has a greater affinity for CRFr2 than CRFr1 (Spina et al., 2000). Astressin 2B is CRFr2 selective as is anti-sauvagine-30. These compounds are truncated versions of CRF in which individual amino acids are substituted with D isoforms (Spina et al., 2000).

VIII. CRF IN ADDICTION AND STRESS

There are several rationales for CRF antagonists as potential therapeutic agents in addiction treatment. The first is the well-established connection between stress and addiction behaviors. The second is that CRF expression is affected by treatment with various drugs of abuse (Bruijnzeel and Gold, 2005; S. Lee and Rivier, 1997; Maj et al., 2003; Rivier and Lee, 1996). Third, as noted earlier, CRF has been recently shown to modulate synaptic events in the VTA (Ungless et al., 2003). A number of groups have obtained preclinical data that collectively support CRF antagonists as promising treatments for stress-induced relapse of drug abuse behaviors. Some of these treatments were noted in the "CRF Pharmacology" section. In this section we provide examples of the use of CRF receptor antagonists in each class of addictive substance. Early studies largely focused on peripheral measures of the HPA axis, such as plasma glucocorticoids and made inferences about CNS mechanisms. A valid question to ask is whether extra-hypothalamic CRF circuits, independent of the HPA axis, are most relevant to addiction neurophysiology. As such, corticosterone levels may be irrelevant to these circuits.

A. Ethanol

Acute administration of ethanol increases CRF-dependent release of ACTH (Rivier and Lee, 1996) and alters the expression of CRFr1 mRNA in the PVN (S. Lee and Rivier, 1997). Thus ethanol apparently directly activates the hypothalamic CRF system (S. Lee and Rivier, 1997; Rivier and Lee, 1996). Chronic ethanol use results in long-standing disregulation of the HPA axis (Adinoff et al., 1990; Adinoff et al., 1991). Alcoholics' plasma cortisol levels are elevated during withdrawal and after 3 weeks of abstinence ACTH responses to CRF are blunted (Adinoff et al., 1990). One difference between addiction and drug use is that, in abstinence, the addict is in a state of withdrawal. Withdrawal is a stressed state and relief of that stress by further substance use may be the reward being sought. In rodent models, acute withdrawal is associated with elevated levels of CRF in the rat extended amygdala (Koob, 1999; Merlo Pich et al., 1995). In the acute ethanol withdrawal phase, CSF CRF levels are elevated in human subjects (Adinoff et al., 1996; Hawley et al., 1994). Furthermore, in abstinent ethanol-addicted human subjects, stress increased ethanol craving (Brown et al., 1990; Cooney et al., 1997; Litt et al., 2000). As such, relieving withdrawal stress may be a key aspect of minimizing addiction behaviors in the newly sober addict (Cooney et al., 1997). This is modeled closely by rodent studies of stress-induced increases in ethanol consumption (Breese et al., 2005) and stress-induced reinstatement of operant conditioning for ethanol (Le and Shaham, 2002; X. Liu and Weiss, 2002). CP154,526 (CRFr1 antagonist) and CRA1000 (CRFr1 antagonist) blocked the anxiogenic effects of early withdrawal (Breese et al., 2005; Knapp et al., 2004). Nonspecific CRF receptor antagonists block reinstatement to ethanol (X. Liu and Weiss, 2002). These studies strongly argue that moderating CRF availability may be a fruitful approach to moderating withdrawal stress-induced relapse to ethanol use.

B. Cocaine

Cocaine-addicted humans subjectively report increased cocaine craving to both stress and images of cocaine and drug paraphernalia. Sinha et al. demonstrated that both of these stimuli induce increases in plasma ACTH concentrations. By inference, these conditions have been posited to induce an increase in central CRF neuronal activity (Sinha et al., 2003). In the rat, chronic cocaine exposure increases levels of CRF and its mRNA in the central nucleus of the amygdala. This effect is transient and resolves 48 hours after the last cocaine dose (Maj et al., 2003). Additionally, anterior pituitary CRFr1 binding is elevated by repeated cocaine exposure (Zhou et al., 2003). This increased CRFergic activity may mediate some of the behavioral effects of cocaine. CP-154,526 (a CRFr1 antagonist) or α heli-

cal CRF_{9-41} (a CRFr1 antagonist), given ICV, diminished cocaine-induced dopamine increases in the NAc and motor activation. In contrast anti-sauvagine-30 (a CRFr2 antagonist) did not affect the motor response to cocaine. Of particular interest is the observation that CRFr1 antagonists block the induction of CPP for cocaine (L. Lu et al., 2003a). Others have shown that expression of sensitization is blocked by CP-154,526. CP-154,526 did not block lever pressing for cocaine or the ability of a rat to distinguish the cocaine and saline levers. However, the CRFr1 antagonist right shifted the dose response curve of cocaine required to promote reinstatement following a 10-day extinction (Przegalinski et al., 2005). This suggests that CRF mediates the cocaine-induced increase in dopamine required for the rewarding and perhaps the addictive aspects of the drug but did not impair basic cognitive or motor properties of the animal.

There are also discordant findings. Lee et al. found that in squirrel monkeys CRF, ACTH, or cortisol were incapable of inducing cocaine reinstatement. Furthermore, in their animals, CP-154,526 had no effect on reinstatement of lever pressing despite demonstrable effects on salivary cortisol (B. Lee et al., 2003). These authors noted that prior work in rats demonstrated corticosterone-induced reinstatement (Deroche et al., 1997). However, their data and a number of other studies argue for a limited role of cortisol or CRF in cocaine addiction. Of note, they administered all drugs IV, including peptides that cannot cross the blood-brain barrier. Though this may explain the lack of CRF effect, it does not explain the failure of CP-154,526, which presumably can cross the blood-brain barrier, to block reinstatement. It should, however, be noted that our studies using this compound to develop a PET ligand revealed limited brain permeability (Martarello et al., 2001). One hopes future work with more potent and membrane-permeant CRF antagonists will clarify this issue.

C. Opiates

A well-established link exists between stress and opiate abuse (Piazza and Le Moal, 1998). Acute and chronic morphine exposure increase expression of CRF mRNA in the rat central nucleus of the amygdala (Maj et al., 2003; McNally and Akil, 2002), whereas chronic morphine treatment decreased hypothalamic CRF mRNA expression (Laorden et al., 2003). Acute, naloxone-induced withdrawal caused an increase of CRF mRNA expression in the paraventricular nucleus of the hypothalamus (McNally and Akil, 2002). Mice that are chronically exposed to morphine were less likely to show signs of acute naloxone-induced withdrawal if pretreated with CRA1000, a CRFr1 antagonist. Similarly, ICV α-helical CRF$_{9-14}$ blunted the physiologic signs of withdrawal in rats (McNally and Akil, 2002), suggested to be mediated by changes in the turnover of noradrenaline (Funada et al., 2001). Our group similarly has shown that R121919 (CRFr1 antagonist) attenuates the physical signs of opiate withdrawal, as well as the elevated expression of CRF hnRNA in the paraventricular nucleus of the hypothalamus (K. Skelton et al., 2006). Beyond the physical effects of withdrawal, others have shown that CP-154,526 (IP) or α-helical CRF$_{9-14}$ (ICV) blocks foot shock or morphine-induced reinstatement of place preference, whereas anti-sauvagine-30 (a CRFr2 antagonist) did not (L. Lu et al., 2000a; L. Lu et al., 2000b). Thus there may be a role for CRFr1 receptor antagonists in both mitigating the symptoms of withdrawal and opiate-induced relapse.

D. Benzodiazepines

There is a substantial literature on the use of CRF antagonists to blunt anxiety symptoms in animals and a limited literature in humans. On its face, one might expect that benzodiazepines, which are potent anti-anxiety agents, would interact with the

CRF system. Both chronic and acute alprazolam reduced CRF concentrations in the locus coeruleus, CRFr1 mRNA, and CRF ligand binding in the basolateral amygdala. In addition, CRF mRNA expression in the central nucleus of the amygdala was decreased. In contrast, mRNA and CRFr2a protein were increased (K. H. Skelton et al., 2000). Withdrawal from benzodiazepines causes an acute increase in activity of the HPA axis (Owens and Nemeroff, 1991). We have recently shown that in animals chronically exposed to lorazepam and acutely withdrawn with flumazenil, a benzodiazepine receptor antagonist, the CRFr1 antagonist R121919 blunted the plasma ACTH, corticosterone increases, and withdrawal behaviors (K. Skelton et al., 2006).

E. Nicotine

Acute nicotine exposure stimulates the HPA axis via activation of brain stem nuclei that activate the PVN (Matta et al., 1998). The literature describing the effects of chronic nicotine exposure is quite contradictory. Semba et al. found that chronic nicotine treatment resulted in decreased corticosterone responses to stress, implying blunting of the CRF system. However, the animals in this study did not exhibit abnormal dexamethasone suppression test results, nor were changes in CRF mRNA in the PVN detected (Semba et al., 2004). They did not measure CRF mRNA expression in the amygdala and therefore may have missed the source of the altered stress response (Bruijnzeel and Gold, 2005). These studies are complicated by the very short active phase of nicotine and relatively rapid onset of withdrawal due to receptor desensitization by the drug. As such this activation may be due to either the physiologic consequences of the drug or the stress of withdrawal. There is limited data as to whether nicotine withdrawal alters CRF systems. Foot shock can evoke reinstatement for nicotine self-administration (Buczek et al., 1999).

There are no published reports of the use of CRF receptor antagonists to blunt nicotine withdrawal or stress-induced reinstatement.

IX. CORTICOSTEROIDS AND ADDICTION

Studies in which the glucocorticoid receptor was manipulated both genetically and pharmacologically demonstrate that this receptor is involved in cocaine-relevant behaviors. Mice in which the central nervous system glucocorticoid receptor are specifically knocked out[2] are able to learn to self-administer high dose cocaine (2 mg/kg). However, at lower doses knockout animals are less sensitive to cocaine than control animals. In addition, though the acute response to cocaine was unchanged by this genetic manipulation, sensitization was abolished when tested both 3 and 30 days following the induction of sensitization. These results were consistent with the finding that mifepristone decreases the breaking point for cocaine self-administration (Deroche et al., 1995). Stress potentiates behavioral sensitization to both amphetamine and morphine. Deroche et al. (1995) used food deprivation as a stressor in adrenalectomized animals to demonstrate that this stress-induced potentiation is mediated by adrenal glucocorticoids. Furthermore, the same group showed that corticosterone replacement is required in adrenalectomized rats for both induction and reinstatement of cocaine self-administration (Deroche et al., 1997).

X. STRESS AND ADDICTION: MECHANISTIC OVERVIEW

As noted above, the VTA is often conceptualized as the gatekeeper for addiction behaviors. We and a number of other groups have looked at modulation of synaptic and intrinsic membrane properties in the context of stress and addiction. This is one of the rare examples of an *in vivo* manipulation of an animal that results in a measurable physiologic change at the synaptic level. The VTA dopamine cells are, in part, driven by excitatory inputs from the prefrontal cortex and the PPN. A series of publications examined the excitatory inputs to dopamine cells in the VTA following *in vivo* exposures. These papers demonstrated that a single exposure to cocaine, amphetamine, nicotine, morphine, or alcohol increases the strength of these synapses (Borgland et al., 2004; Dong et al., 2004; Saal et al., 2003; Ungless et al., 2001). The most direct interpretation of these data is that a single exposure to addictive substances results in an increase in the gain of the dopamine release circuit. Thus VTA cells in animals that have been exposed to psychostimulants are more likely to fire upon excitatory stimulation and thereby release more dopamine for any given excitatory input to these cells (Overton and Clark, 1997; Overton et al., 1999; Zhang et al., 1997). The critical connection of this finding to stress-induced addiction behaviors is that a single exposure to a cold-water forced swim stress results in a similar synaptic enhancement. This stress-induced enhancement of synaptic strength occludes further enhancement by cocaine indicating that there is some mechanistic overlap between the two processes. However, the stress-induced synaptic changes are blocked by mifepristone, whereas the cocaine-induced changes are not (Dong et al., 2004; Saal et al., 2003). Unfortunately, it has not yet been shown that the synaptic changes are causal in either relapse or acquisition of addiction. What has been shown is that GluR1 knockout mice, which

***

[2] The general method to create this mouse is to generate a mouse with so-called loxP flanked glucocorticoid receptor gene and cross that animal with a mouse expressing the CRE recombinase on a CNS-specific promoter. The cells in which the CRE recombinase is expressed will excise the GR gene. The value of this approach, as opposed to a global knockout, is that the peripheral glucocorticoid system remains intact.

lack a particular class of glutamate receptors, do not demonstrate the VTA synaptic enhancement to either stress or cocaine and have impaired acquisition of conditioned place preference to cocaine (Dong et al., 2004). These results suggest a mechanistic nexus for stress and addiction that involves the HPA axis. A critical aspect of this literature is that it suggests that mifepristone and other glucocorticoid antagonists should affect some aspect of addiction. Conversely, corticosteroids should facilitate acquisition or relapse. In fact there is evidence for both of these phenomena, as noted previously.

Ungless et al. used whole cell slice recordings to demonstrate that CRF, applied acutely to midbrain dopamine cells, increases the postsynaptic responsiveness to NMDA. This was mediated by both the CRFr2 and required the CRF binding protein. The implication of these findings is that stress may render cells more sensitive to the modulatory effects of NMDA receptor activation. In particular, this NMDA receptor potentiation may be upstream of the increase in synaptic strength described above, or due to other cellular changes (Ungless et al., 2003). In addition to the synaptic changes, simultaneous activation of CRFr1 and CRFr2 receptors results in increased firing of midbrain dopamine cells (Wanat and Bonci, 2005). A different mechanism that may act in concert with the postsynaptic effects of CRF was recently described by Wang et al. They observed that in rats exposed to cocaine, but not drug naïve animals, CRF in the VTA is required for reinstatement of lever pressing by foot shock; moreover, CRF in the drug-experienced, but not the naïve, animals causes enhanced release of presynaptic glutamate (Wang et al., 2005). This is yet another form of priming, in which cocaine alters the synaptic properties such that stress can act as an initiator of drug-related behaviors. The implication is that a presynaptic modulation promotes the enhanced activity of DA cells following stress exposure. These data are consistent with the finding that animals exposed to seven daily cocaine doses and then allowed to withdraw for 28 days are psychomotor activated in response to ICV injection over a range of doses of CRF (Erb et al., 2003).

XI. CLINICAL TRIALS WITH CRF COMPOUNDS

To date there have been no human trials using CRF receptor antagonists to target addiction. There has been one published early clinical trial of a CRF receptor antagonist, R121919, for depression. Zobel et al. found no endocrine alteration with respect to thyroid, gonadal, and renin-angiotensin systems. Initially they found no change in liver enzymes, EEG, or ECG (Kunzel et al., 2003). There was also no change in body weight or leptin levels (Kunzel et al., 2005). They did find that, in this open label trial, with doses up to 80 mg, there were improvements in depression and anxiety symptom severity (Zobel et al., 2000). This trial was not placebo controlled or blinded and as such is of limited predictive value. Unfortunately, this compound is no longer under investigation in clinical trials due to concerns over hepatotoxicity (Nemeroff and Vale, 2005). Several other CRF antagonists are currently being studied in randomized controlled clinical trials in patients with major depression. However these results are not yet available (Nemeroff and Vale, 2005).

XII. CONCLUSIONS

A number of new systems are being examined for their putative role in addiction. We have reviewed the role of various components of the stress. As further advances occur in the biochemistry, physiology, molecular biology, pharmacology, and clinical medicine of this system, one hopes additional advances will follow. Beyond the core actors in this system, we cannot lose sight of the complex relationship of stress, anxiety and other neuromodulators and neurotransmitters such as the monoamines, glutamate, or GABA. There is already a growing interest in glutamate for depression and addiction. Notably, the metabotropic glutamate receptors have been implicated in the addiction process and are likely to be a target in the near future (Rauhut et al., 2003). In all likelihood, no one modality will act as a "silver bullet" to undo the synaptic and behavioral changes incurred in the addiction process. Furthermore, some of the mechanisms that underlie the stress and addiction processes are critical for learning, memory, physiologic stress responses, and regulation of an array of nonpathologic biological processes. As such, manipulation of these systems may not be specific to addiction and may impair other forms of learning and memory.

DISCLOSURE

Dr. Nemeroff consults to, serves on the Speakers' Bureau and/or Board of Directors of, and has been a grant recipient and/or owns equity in one or more of the following: Abbott Laboratories, Acadia Pharmaceuticals, AFSP, APIRE, Astra Zeneca, BMC-JR LLC, Bristol-Myers-Squibb, CeNeRx, Corcept, Cypress Biosciences, Cyberonics, Eli Lilly, Entrepreneur's Fund, Forest Laboratories, George West Mental Health Foundation, GlaxoSmithKline, i3 DLN, Janssen Pharmaceutica, Lundbeck, NARSAD, NIMH, NFMH, NovaDel Pharma, Otsuka, Pfizer Pharmaceuticals, Quintiles, Reevax, UCB Pharma, Wyeth-Ayerst. Dr. Saal serves on the Scientific Advisory Board of Intellihealth Corp.

ACKNOWLEDGMENTS

The authors are supported by NIH MH-42088 (CBN), MH-39415 (CBN), MH-58299 (CBN), DA-17872 (DBS), NARSAD Young Investigators Award (DBS).

REFERENCES

Adinoff, B., Anton, R., Linnoila, M., Guidotti, A., Nemeroff, C. B., and Bissette, G. (1996). Cerebrospinal fluid concentrations of corticotropin-releasing hormone (CRH) and diazepam-binding inhibitor (DBI) during alcohol withdrawal and abstinence. *Neuropsychopharmacology, 15*(3), 288–295.

Adinoff, B., Martin, P. R., Bone, G. H., Eckardt, M. J., Roehrich, L., George, D. T., et al. (1990). Hypothalamic-pituitary-adrenal axis functioning and cerebrospinal fluid corticotropin releasing hormone and corticotropin levels in alcoholics after recent and long-term abstinence. *Arch Gen Psychiatry, 47*(4), 325–330.

Adinoff, B., Risher-Flowers, D., De Jong, J., Ravitz, B., Bone, G. H., Nutt, D. J., et al. (1991). Disturbances of hypothalamic-pituitary-adrenal axis functioning during ethanol withdrawal in six men. *Am J Psychiatry, 148*(8), 1023–1025.

Bale, T. L., and Vale, W. W. (2004). CRF and CRF receptors: Role in stress responsivity and other behaviors. *Annu Rev Pharmacol Toxicol, 44*, 525–557.

Bardo, M. T. (1998). Neuropharmacological mechanisms of drug reward: Beyond dopamine in the nucleus accumbens. *Crit Rev Neurobiol, 12*(1–2), 37–67.

Berns, G. S. (2004). Something funny happened to reward. *Trends Cogn Sci, 8*(5), 193–194.

Berridge, K. C., and Robinson, T. E. (2003). Parsing reward. *Trends Neurosci, 26*(9), 507–513.

Bjijou, Y., Stinus, L., Le Moal, M., and Cador, M. (1996). Evidence for selective involvement of dopamine d1 receptors of the ventral tegmental area in the behavioral sensitization induced by intra-ventral tegmental area injections of d-amphetamine. *J Pharmacol Exp Ther, 277*(2), 1177–1187.

Borgland, S. L., Malenka, R. C., and Bonci, A. (2004). Acute and chronic cocaine-induced potentiation of synaptic strength in the ventral tegmental area: Electrophysiological and behavioral correlates in individual rats. *J Neurosci, 24*(34), 7482–7490.

Bossert, J. M., Ghitza, U. E., Lu, L., Epstein, D. H., and Shaham, Y. (2005). Neurobiology of relapse to heroin and cocaine seeking: An update and clinical implications. *Eur J Pharmacol.*

Breese, G. R., Chu, K., Dayas, C. V., Funk, D., Knapp, D. J., Koob, G. F., et al. (2005). Stress enhancement of craving during sobriety: A risk for relapse. *Alcohol Clin Exp Res, 29*(2), 185–195.

Brown, S. A., Vik, P. W., McQuaid, J. R., Patterson, T. L., Irwin, M. R., and Grant, I. (1990). Severity of psychosocial stress and outcome of alcoholism treatment. *J Abnorm Psychol, 99*(4), 344–348.

Bruijnzeel, A. W., and Gold, M. S. (2005). The role of corticotropin-releasing factor-like peptides in cannabis, nicotine, and alcohol dependence. *Brain Res Brain Res Rev, 49*(3), 505–528.

Buczek, Y., Le, A. D., Wang, A., Stewart, J., and Shaham, Y. (1999). Stress reinstates nicotine seeking but not sucrose solution seeking in rats. *Psychopharmacology (Berl), 144*(2), 183–188.

Carlezon, W. A., Jr., and Nestler, E. J. (2002). Elevated levels of glur1 in the midbrain: A trigger for sensitization to drugs of abuse? *Trends Neurosci, 25*(12), 610–615.

Chen, C., Wilcoxen, K. M., Huang, C. Q., Xie, Y. F., McCarthy, J. R., Webb, T. R., et al. (2004). Design of 2,5-dimethyl-3-(6-dimethyl-4-methylpyridin-3-yl)-7-dipropylaminopyrazolo[1,5-a]pyrimidine (nbi 30775/r121919) and structure—activity relationships of a series of potent and orally active corticotropin-releasing factor receptor antagonists. *J Med Chem, 47*(19), 4787–4798.

Chen, J., Nye, H. E., Kelz, M. B., Hiroi, N., Nakabeppu, Y., Hope, B. T., et al. (1995). Regulation of delta Fosb and Fosb-like proteins by electroconvulsive seizure and cocaine treatments. *Mol Pharmacol, 48*(5), 880–889.

Cooney, N. L., Litt, M. D., Morse, P. A., Bauer, L. O., and Gaupp, L. (1997). Alcohol cue reactivity, negative-mood reactivity, and relapse in treated alcoholic men. *J Abnorm Psychol, 106*(2), 243–250.

Covington, H. E., 3rd, and Miczek, K. A. (2001). Repeated social-defeat stress, cocaine or morphine. Effects on behavioral sensitization and intravenous cocaine self-administration "binges." *Psychopharmacology (Berl), 158*(4), 388–398.

Dalia, A., and Wallace, L. J. (1995). Amphetamine induction of c-Fos in the nucleus accumbens is not inhibited by glutamate antagonists. *Brain Res, 694*(1–2), 299–307.

Dautzenberg, F. M., and Hauger, R. L. (2002). The CRF peptide family and their receptors: Yet more partners discovered. *Trends Pharmacol Sci, 23*(2), 71–77.

David, V., Durkin, T. P., and Cazala, P. (2002). Differential effects of the dopamine d2/d3 receptor antagonist sulpiride on self-administration of morphine into the ventral tegmental area or the nucleus accumbens. *Psychopharmacology (Berl), 160*(3), 307–317.

Deroche, V., Marinelli, M., Le Moal, M., and Piazza, P. V. (1997). Glucocorticoids and behavioral effects of psychostimulants. II: Cocaine intravenous self-administration and reinstatement depend on glucocorticoid levels. *J Pharmacol Exp Ther, 281*(3), 1401–1407.

Deroche, V., Marinelli, M., Maccari, S., Le Moal, M., Simon, H., and Piazza, P. V. (1995). Stress-induced sensitization and glucocorticoids. I. Sensitization of dopamine-dependent locomotor effects of amphetamine and morphine depends on stress-induced corticosterone secretion. *J Neurosci, 15*(11), 7181–7188.

Dong, Y., Saal, D., Thomas, M., Faust, R., Bonci, A., Robinson, T., et al. (2004). Cocaine-induced potentiation of synaptic strength in dopamine neurons: Behavioral correlates in glura(-/-) mice. *Proc Natl Acad Sci U S A, 101*(39), 14282–14287.

Dunn, A. J., Swiergiel, A. H., and Palamarchouk, V. (2004). Brain circuits involved in corticotropin-releasing factor-norepinephrine interactions during stress. *Ann N Y Acad Sci, 1018*, 25–34.

Erb, S., Funk, D., and Le, A. D. (2003). Prior, repeated exposure to cocaine potentiates locomotor responsivity to central injections of corticotropin-releasing factor (CRF) in rats. *Psychopharmacology (Berl), 170*(4), 383–389.

Funada, M., Hara, C., and Wada, K. (2001). Involvement of corticotropin-releasing factor receptor subtype 1 in morphine withdrawal regulation of the brain noradrenergic system. *Eur J Pharmacol, 430*(2–3), 277–281.

Gurkovskaya, O. V., Palamarchouk, V., Smagin, G., and Goeders, N. E. (2005). Effects of corticotropin-releasing hormone receptor antagonists on cocaine-induced dopamine overflow in the medial prefrontal cortex and nucleus accumbens of rats. *Synapse, 57*(4), 202–212.

Hawley, R. J., Nemeroff, C. B., Bissette, G., Guidotti, A., Rawlings, R., and Linnoila, M. (1994). Neurochemical correlates of sympathetic activation during severe alcohol withdrawal. *Alcohol Clin Exp Res, 18*(6), 1312–1316.

Hsu, S. Y., and Hsueh, A. J. (2001). Human stresscopin and stresscopin-related peptide are selective ligands for the type 2 corticotropin-releasing hormone receptor. *Nat Med, 7*(5), 605–611.

Kalivas, P. W., and Stewart, J. (1991). Dopamine transmission in the initiation and expression of drug- and stress-induced sensitization of motor activity. *Brain Res Brain Res Rev, 16*(3), 223–244.

Kim, J. A., Pollak, K., Hjelmstad, G. O., and Fields, H. L. (2003). Single dose cocaine sensitization of both a morphine place-preference and a u69593 place aversion: Reversal by intra-vta mk-801. Paper presented at the Society for Neuroscience, New Orleans.

Kim, J. A., Pollak, K. A., Hjelmstad, G. O., and Fields, H. L. (2004). A single cocaine exposure enhances both opioid reward and aversion through a ventral tegmental area-dependent mechanism. *Proc Natl Acad Sci U S A, 101*(15), 5664–5669.

Knapp, D. J., Overstreet, D. H., Moy, S. S., and Breese, G. R. (2004). Sb242084, flumazenil, and cra1000 block ethanol withdrawal-induced anxiety in rats. *Alcohol, 32*(2), 101–111.

Koob, G. F. (1999). Stress, corticotropin-releasing factor, and drug addiction. *Ann N Y Acad Sci, 897*, 27–45.

Koob, G. F., and Heinrichs, S. C. (1999). A role for corticotropin releasing factor and urocortin in behavioral responses to stressors. *Brain Res, 848*(1–2), 141–152.

Koob, G. F., Sanna, P. P., and Bloom, F. E. (1998). Neuroscience of addiction. *Neuron, 21*(3), 467–476.

Kunzel, H. E., Ising, M., Zobel, A. W., Nickel, T., Ackl, N., Sonntag, A., et al. (2005). Treatment with a CRH-1-receptor antagonist (R121919) does not affect weight or plasma leptin concentration in patients with major depression. *J Psychiatr Res, 39*(2), 173–177.

Kunzel, H. E., Zobel, A. W., Nickel, T., Ackl, N., Uhr, M., Sonntag, A., et al. (2003). Treatment of depression with the CRH-1-receptor antagonist R121919: Endocrine changes and side effects. *J Psychiatr Res, 37*(6), 525–533.

Laorden, M. L., Milanes, M. V., Angel, E., Tankosic, P., and Burlet, A. (2003). Quantitative analysis of corticotropin-releasing factor and arginine vasopressin mRNA in the hypothalamus during chronic morphine treatment in rats: An in situ hybridization study. *J Neuroendocrinol, 15*(6), 586–591.

Le, A., and Shaham, Y. (2002). Neurobiology of relapse to alcohol in rats. *Pharmacol Ther, 94*(1–2), 137–156.

Lee, B., Tiefenbacher, S., Platt, D. M., and Spealman, R. D. (2003). Role of the hypothalamic-pituitary-adrenal axis in reinstatement of cocaine-seeking behavior in squirrel monkeys. *Psychopharmacology (Berl), 168*(1–2), 177–183.

Lee, S., and Rivier, C. (1997). Alcohol increases the expression of type 1, but not type 2 alpha corticotropin-releasing factor (CRF) receptor messenger ribonucleic acid in the rat hypothalamus. *Brain Res Mol Brain Res, 52*(1), 78–89.

Li, Y., Hu, X. T., Berney, T. G., Vartanian, A. J., Stine, C. D., Wolf, M. E., et al. (1999). Both glutamate receptor antagonists and prefrontal cortex lesions prevent induction of cocaine sensitization and associated neuroadaptations. *Synapse, 34*(3), 169–180.

Litt, M. D., Cooney, N. L., and Morse, P. (2000). Reactivity to alcohol-related stimuli in the laboratory and in the field: Predictors of craving in treated alcoholics. *Addiction, 95*(6), 889–900.

Little, H. J., Stephens, D. N., Ripley, T. L., Borlikova, G., Duka, T., Schubert, M., et al. (2005). Alcohol withdrawal and conditioning. *Alcohol Clin Exp Res, 29*(3), 453–464.

Liu, J., Nickolenko, J., and Sharp, F. R. (1994). Morphine induces c-Fos and Junb in striatum and nucleus accumbens via d1 and n-methyl-d-aspartate receptors. *Proc Natl Acad Sci U S A, 91*(18), 8537–8541.

Liu, X., and Weiss, F. (2002). Additive effect of stress and drug cues on reinstatement of ethanol seeking: Exacerbation by history of dependence and role of concurrent activation of corticotropin-releasing factor and opioid mechanisms. *J Neurosci, 22*(18), 7856–7861.

Lovenberg, T. W., Liaw, C. W., Grigoriadis, D. E., Clevenger, W., Chalmers, D. T., De Souza, E. B., et al. (1995). Cloning and characterization of a functionally distinct corticotropin-releasing factor receptor subtype from rat brain. *Proc Natl Acad Sci U S A, 92*(3), 836–840.

Lu, L., Ceng, X., and Huang, M. (2000a). Corticotropin-releasing factor receptor type I mediates stress-induced relapse to opiate dependence in rats. *Neuroreport, 11*(11), 2373–2378.

Lu, L., Liu, D., Ceng, X., and Ma, L. (2000b). Differential roles of corticotropin-releasing factor receptor subtypes 1 and 2 in opiate withdrawal and in relapse to opiate dependence. *Eur J Neurosci, 12*(12), 4398–4404.

Lu, L., Liu, Z., Huang, M., and Zhang, Z. (2003a). Dopamine-dependent responses to cocaine depend on corticotropin-releasing factor receptor subtypes. *J Neurochem, 84*(6), 1378–1386.

Lu, L., Shepard, J. D., Scott Hall, F., and Shaham, Y. (2003b). Effect of environmental stressors on opiate and psychostimulant reinforcement, reinstatement and discrimination in rats: A review. *Neurosci Biobehav Rev, 27*(5), 457–491.

Lu, W., Chen, H., Xue, C. J., and Wolf, M. E. (1997). Repeated amphetamine administration alters the expression of mRNA for ampa receptor subunits in rat nucleus accumbens and prefrontal cortex. *Synapse, 26*(3), 269–280.

Lu, W., and Wolf, M. E. (1999). Repeated amphetamine administration alters ampa receptor subunit expression in rat nucleus accumbens and medial prefrontal cortex. *Synapse, 32*(2), 119–131.

Maj, M., Turchan, J., Smialowska, M., and Przewlocka, B. (2003). Morphine and cocaine influence on CRF biosynthesis in the rat central nucleus of amygdala. *Neuropeptides, 37*(2), 105–110.

Martarello, L., Kilts, C. D., Ely, T., Owens, M. J., Nemeroff, C. B., Camp, M., et al. (2001). Synthesis and characterization of fluorinated and iodinated pyrrolopyrimidines as pet/spect ligands for the CRF1 receptor. *Nucl Med Biol, 28*(2), 187–195.

Matta, S. G., Fu, Y., Valentine, J. D., and Sharp, B. M. (1998). Response of the hypothalamo-pituitary-adrenal axis to nicotine. *Psychoneuroendocrinology, 23*(2), 103–113.

McNally, G. P., and Akil, H. (2002). Role of corticotropin-releasing hormone in the amygdala and bed nucleus of the stria terminalis in the behavioral, pain modulatory, and endocrine consequences of opiate withdrawal. *Neuroscience, 112*(3), 605–617.

Merlo Pich, E., Lorang, M., Yeganeh, M., Rodriguez de Fonseca, F., Raber, J., Koob, G. F., et al. (1995). Increase of extracellular corticotropin-releasing factor-like immunoreactivity levels in the amygdala of awake rats during restraint stress and ethanol withdrawal as measured by microdialysis. *J Neurosci, 15*(8), 5439–5447.

Montague, P. R., and Berns, G. S. (2002). Neural economics and the biological substrates of valuation. *Neuron, 36*(2), 265–284.

Nemeroff, C. B. (2002). New directions in the development of antidepressants: The interface of neurobiology and psychiatry. *Hum Psychopharmacol, 17* (Suppl 1), S13–16.

Nemeroff, C. B., and Vale, W. W. (2005). The neurobiology of depression: Inroads to treatment and new drug discovery. *J Clin Psychiatry, 66*(Suppl 7), 5–13.

Nestler, E. J. (1993). Cellular responses to chronic treatment with drugs of abuse. *Crit Rev Neurobiol, 7*(1), 23–39.

Nestler, E. J., and Malenka, R. C. (2004). The addicted brain. *Sci Am, 290*(3), 78–85.

Nikulina, E. M., Covington, H. E., 3rd, Ganschow, L., Hammer, R. P., Jr., and Miczek, K. A. (2004). Long-term behavioral and neuronal cross-sensitization to amphetamine induced by repeated brief social defeat stress: Fos in the ventral tegmental area and amygdala. *Neuroscience, 123*(4), 857–865.

Nye, H. E., Hope, B. T., Kelz, M. B., Iadarola, M., and Nestler, E. J. (1995). Pharmacological studies of the regulation of chronic Fos-related antigen induction by cocaine in the striatum and nucleus accumbens. *J Pharmacol Exp Ther, 275*(3), 1671–1680.

Overton, P. G., and Clark, D. (1997). Burst firing in midbrain dopaminergic neurons. *Brain Res Brain Res Rev, 25*(3), 312–334.

Overton, P. G., Richards, C. D., Berry, M. S., and Clark, D. (1999). Long-term potentiation at excitatory amino acid synapses on midbrain dopamine neurons. *Neuroreport, 10*(2), 221–226.

Owens, M. J., and Nemeroff, C. B. (1991). Physiology and pharmacology of corticotropin-releasing factor. *Pharmacol Rev, 43*(4), 425–473.

Piazza, P. V., and Le Moal, M. (1998). The role of stress in drug self-administration. *Trends Pharmacol Sci, 19*(2), 67–74.

Przegalinski, E., Filip, M., Frankowska, M., Zaniewska, M., and Papla, I. (2005). Effects of CP 154,526, a CRF1 receptor antagonist, on behavioral responses to cocaine in rats. *Neuropeptides, 39*(5), 525–533.

Rauhut, A. S., Neugebauer, N., Dwoskin, L. P., and Bardo, M. T. (2003). Effect of bupropion on nicotine self-administration in rats. *Psychopharmacology (Berl), 169*(1), 1–9.

Rivier, C., and Lee, S. (1996). Acute alcohol administration stimulates the activity of hypothalamic neurons that express corticotropin-releasing factor and vasopressin. *Brain Res, 726*(1–2), 1–10.

Robinson, T. E., and Becker, J. B. (1986). Enduring changes in brain and behavior produced by chronic amphetamine administration: A review and evaluation of animal models of amphetamine psychosis. *Brain Res, 396*(2), 157–198.

Robinson, T. E., and Berridge, K. C. (2000). The psychology and neurobiology of addiction: An incentive-sensitization view. *Addiction, 95*(Suppl 2), S91–117.

Saal, D., Dong, Y., Bonci, A., and Malenka, R. C. (2003). Drugs of abuse and stress trigger a common synaptic adaptation in dopamine neurons. *Neuron, 37*(4), 577–582.

Sawchenko, P. E., Imaki, T., Potter, E., Kovacs, K., Imaki, J., and Vale, W. (1993). The functional neuroanatomy of corticotropin-releasing factor. *Ciba Found Symp, 172*, 5–21; discussion 21–29.

Schilstrom, B., De Villiers, S., Malmerfelt, A., Svensson, T. H., and Nomikos, G. G. (2000). Nicotine-induced Fos expression in the nucleus accumbens and the medial prefrontal cortex of the rat: Role of nicotinic and NMDA receptors in the ventral tegmental area. *Synapse, 36*(4), 314–321.

Schultz, W. (2005). Behavioral theories and the neurophysiology of reward. *Annu Rev Psychol.*

Semba, J., Wakuta, M., Maeda, J., and Suhara, T. (2004). Nicotine withdrawal induces subsensitivity of hypothalamic-pituitary-adrenal axis to stress in rats: Implications for precipitation of depression during smoking cessation. *Psychoneuroendocrinology, 29*(2), 215–226.

Seymour, P. A., Schmidt, A. W., and Schulz, D. W. (2003). The pharmacology of CP-154,526, a non-peptide antagonist of the CRH1 receptor: A review. *CNS Drug Rev, 9*(1), 57–96.

Shaham, Y., Erb, S., Leung, S., Buczek, Y., and Stewart, J. (1998). CP-154,526, a selective, non-peptide antagonist of the corticotropin-releasing factor-1 receptor attenuates stress-induced relapse to drug seeking in cocaine- and heroin-trained rats. *Psychopharmacology (Berl), 137*(2), 184–190.

Shaham, Y., Shalev, U., Lu, L., De Wit, H., and Stewart, J. (2003). The reinstatement model of drug relapse: History, methodology and major findings. *Psychopharmacology (Berl), 168*(1–2), 3–20.

Shalev, U., Highfield, D., Yap, J., and Shaham, Y. (2000). Stress and relapse to drug seeking in rats: Studies on the generality of the effect. *Psychopharmacology (Berl), 150*(3), 337–346.

Sharp, F. R., Liu, J., Nickolenko, J., and Bontempi, B. (1995). NMDA and d1 receptors mediate induction of c-Fos and Junb genes in striatum following morphine administration: Implications for studies of memory. *Behav Brain Res, 66*(1–2), 225–230.

Shepard, J. D., Bossert, J. M., Liu, S. Y., and Shaham, Y. (2004). The anxiogenic drug yohimbine reinstates methamphetamine seeking in a rat model of drug relapse. *Biol Psychiatry, 55*(11), 1082–1089.

Sinha, R., Talih, M., Malison, R., Cooney, N., Anderson, G. M., and Kreek, M. J. (2003). Hypothalamic-pituitary-adrenal axis and sympatho-adreno-medullary responses during stress-induced and drug cue-induced cocaine craving states. *Psychopharmacology (Berl), 170*(1), 62–72.

Skelton, K., Oren, D., Gutman, D. A., O'Brien, D., Easterling, K., Holtzman, S. G., et al. (2006). The CRF1 receptor antagonist, R121919, attenuates the effects of drug withdrawal. *J Pharmacol Exp Ther.*

Skelton, K. H., Nemeroff, C. B., Knight, D. L., and Owens, M. J. (2000). Chronic administration of the triazolobenzodiazepine alprazolam produces opposite effects on corticotropin-releasing factor and urocortin neuronal systems. *J Neurosci, 20*(3), 1240–1248.

Spina, M. G., Basso, A. M., Zorrilla, E. P., Heyser, C. J., Rivier, J., Vale, W., et al. (2000). Behavioral effects of central administration of the novel CRF antagonist astressin in rats. *Neuropsychopharmacology, 22*(3), 230–239.

Szumlinski, K. K., Herrick-Davis, K., Teitler, M., Maisonneuve, I. M., and Glick, S. D. (2000). Behavioural sensitization to cocaine is dissociated from changes in striatal NMDA receptor levels. *Neuroreport, 11*(12), 2785–2788.

Thomas, M. J., Beurrier, C., Bonci, A., and Malenka, R. C. (2001). Long-term depression in the nucleus accumbens: A neural correlate of behavioral sensitization to cocaine. *Nat Neurosci, 4*(12), 1217–1223.

Thomas, M. J., and Malenka, R. C. (2003). Synaptic plasticity in the mesolimbic dopamine system. *Philos Trans R Soc Lond B Biol Sci, 358*(1432), 815–819.

Tobler, P. N., Dickinson, A., and Schultz, W. (2003). Coding of predicted reward omission by dopamine neurons in a conditioned inhibition paradigm. *J Neurosci, 23*(32), 10402–10410.

Tobler, P. N., Fiorillo, C. D., and Schultz, W. (2005). Adaptive coding of reward value by dopamine neurons. *Science, 307*(5715), 1642–1645.

Tzschentke, T. M. (1998). Measuring reward with the conditioned place preference paradigm: A comprehensive review of drug effects, recent progress and new issues. *Prog Neurobiol, 56*(6), 613–672.

Ungless, M. A., Singh, V., Crowder, T. L., Yaka, R., Ron, D., and Bonci, A. (2003). Corticotropin-releasing factor requires CRF binding protein to potentiate NMDA receptors via CRF receptor 2 in dopamine neurons. *Neuron, 39*(3), 401–407.

Ungless, M. A., Whistler, J. L., Malenka, R. C., and Bonci, A. (2001). Single cocaine exposure in vivo induces long-term potentiation in dopamine neurons. *Nature, 411*(6837), 583–587.

Vale, W., Spiess, J., Rivier, C., and Rivier, J. (1981). Characterization of a 41-residue ovine hypothalamic peptide that stimulates secretion of corticotropin and beta-endorphin. *Science, 213*(4514), 1394–1397.

Wanat, M. J., and Bonci, A. (2005). Corticotropin-releasing factor (CRF) increases the firing rate of dopamine neurons in the ventral tegmental area (VTA). [Abstract]. Society for Neuroscience.

Wang, B., Shaham, Y., Zitzman, D., Azari, S., Wise, R. A., and You, Z. B. (2005). Cocaine experience establishes control of midbrain glutamate and dopamine by corticotropin-releasing factor: A role in stress-induced relapse to drug seeking. *J Neurosci, 25*(22), 5389–5396.

Webster, E. L., Lewis, D. B., Torpy, D. J., Zachman, E. K., Rice, K. C., and Chrousos, G. P. (1996). In vivo and in vitro characterization of antalarmin, a nonpeptide corticotropin-releasing hormone (CRH) receptor antagonist: Suppression of pituitary ACTH release and peripheral inflammation. *Endocrinology, 137*(12), 5747–5750.

Wolf, M. E. (1998). The role of excitatory amino acids in behavioral sensitization to psychomotor stimulants. *Prog Neurobiol, 54*(6), 679–720.

Yoshimoto, K., Ueda, S., Nishi, M., Yang, Y., Matsushita, H., Takeuchi, Y., et al. (2000). Changes in dopamine transporter and c-Fos expression in the nucleus accumbens of alcohol-tolerant rats. *Alcohol Clin Exp Res, 24*(3), 361–365.

Zhang, X. F., Hu, X. T., White, F. J., and Wolf, M. E. (1997). Increased responsiveness of ventral tegmental area dopamine neurons to glutamate after repeated administration of cocaine or amphetamine is transient and selectively involves AMPA receptors. *J Pharmacol Exp Ther, 281*(2), 699–706.

Zhou, Y., Spangler, R., Schlussman, S. D., Ho, A., and Kreek, M. J. (2003). Alterations in hypothalamic-pituitary-adrenal axis activity and in levels of proopiomelanocortin and corticotropin-releasing hormone-receptor 1 mRNAs in the pituitary and hypothalamus of the rat during chronic 'binge' cocaine and withdrawal. *Brain Res, 964*(2), 187–199.

Zobel, A. W., Nickel, T., Kunzel, H. E., Ackl, N., Sonntag, A., Ising, M., et al. (2000). Effects of the high-affinity corticotropin-releasing hormone receptor 1 antagonist R121919 in major depression: The first 20 patients treated. *J Psychiatr Res, 34*(3), 171–181.

Current and Future Directions of Research on Stress and Addictive Behaviors

MUSTAFA AL'ABSI

I. INTRODUCTION

This book includes the latest discoveries on the interactions of stress neurobiology and addiction. It addresses the role of stress in addiction vulnerability, maintenance, and relapse from basic and clinical perspectives. Special attention is given to new and promising lines of inquiry that have implications in the development of novel treatment strategies. While there is recognition among scientists and practitioners about the role it plays in addiction, stress has received relatively less empirical attention in the context of addiction etiology and treatment compared with depression and anxiety. Nevertheless, the chapters included in this book provide compelling evidence of the importance of considering stress when addressing addiction vulnerability and tackling issues related to treatment and recovery. It is evident throughout this book that major advances have been accomplished in the understanding of addiction neurobiology and the interactions with different

systems involved in the stress response. The multidisciplinary approach that has been used in addressing these interactions reflects a high level of sophistication and provides a strong promise for the long-term impact of the work accomplished to date.

In this chapter we highlight some of these discoveries and relate them to conceptual framework linking stress and addiction processes. In subsequent sections of this chapter we discuss in more detail components of this model, focusing first on the role of stress in addiction vulnerability and the physiological mechanisms mediating this risk. We then highlight the role of stress in maintaining addiction and in precipitating relapse. Next, we highlight issues that moderate the interaction of stress and addiction, including genetics, sex, and coping style. We briefly discuss how impulsivity and cognitive deficits may mediate the effects of stress on addiction processes. Finally, we outline a research agenda for the future that builds on the current state of knowledge and advances it toward more discoveries to improve diagnosis and treatment of addictions.

II. WORKING MODEL

The model takes a multivariate approach to defining risk factors for addiction vulnerability, maintenance, and relapse. It includes three categories of variables: dispositional, situational, and interactive variables. Dispositional factors include biological, genetic, and trait variables, while situational factors include early life experiences as well as psychological and environmental stressors. The interaction of these factors influences how an individual responds both behaviorally and physiologically, and includes variables such as the intensity and manner by which the individual responds to stress.

As shown in Figure 18-1, prenatal and postnatal experiences as well as childhood exposure to adverse experiences during childhood may lead to an overall hypersensitivity to environmental and psychosocial stressors. This enhanced sensitivity may contribute to chronic or frequent experiences of negative affective states, thus increasing vulnerability and subsequent reinforcement of drug use. Exaggerated affective states are also associated with prolonged perturbations of the stress response systems (e.g., hormonal and sympathetic responses), eventually leading to an altered stress response as well as cognitive and behavioral consequences, including deficits in response inhibition. These altered responses may play a role in increasing the risk for drug use. This is supported by evidence suggesting that increased vulnerability to addiction in individuals with early childhood stress exposure may be mediated by stress-induced alterations in the hypothalamic-pituitary-adrenocortical (HPA) and mesolimbic dopamine functions (as discussed later).

These stress effects contribute directly and indirectly to all addiction phases (i.e., initiation, maintenance, and relapse). While we include these processes in a sequential manner and include all addiction processes as the outcome, we note that certain elements of the model may have greater influence during one phase of addiction than the others. For example, prenatal-postnatal experience may be most relevant to the initiation of an addictive behavioral cascade, starting with engaging in experimental behaviors and leading to a period of habitual behaviors that facilitate the entry into the addiction cycle. Similarly, altered neurobiological stress response may be more relevant to addiction maintenance and relapse than to initiation.

In addition to these interactions, other dispositional and trait factors as well as social, cultural, and environmental factors may have influences on multiple levels of risk. Genetic and sex-related factors may influence the impact of prenatal and postnatal exposure to stress and may also influence different parameters of the stress response and the extent to which these predisposing factors translate into addictive behaviors. Similarly, parental use and psychosocial factors could directly and indirectly influence the impact of early stress and its influence on the stress response later in life and may also influence the expression of risk. Personality traits, congnitive styles, and learning history may influence perception of stress and directly influence addiction risk. Peer pressure and expectancy of benefits from drug use may have its effect most on the addictive behavior itself. On the other hand, coping resources and social support reinforcing self-efficacy and ability to avoid drug use may have a buffering effect promoting a healthy response to stress as well as reducing risk for drug use and/or strengthening the individual's ability to abstain from drug use.

We note the bidirectional relationships between addictive processes and altered stress response and between the altered

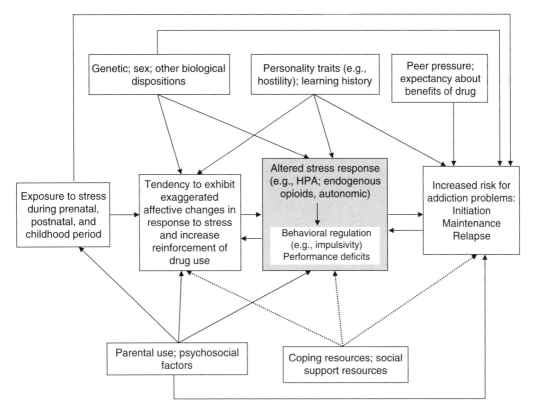

FIGURE 18-1 A diagram illustrating the relationship between stress and addictive processes. The model indicates that childhood exposure to adverse experiences may cause hypersensitivity to stress and contribute to experiences of negative affective states when confronting stress later in life. This hypersensitivity may increase vulnerability for drug use and contribute to the maintenance of drug-taking behavior. Influence of stress on these addictive behaviors is mediated by exaggerated affective changes and perturbations of the stress response systems.

responses and stress-related affective changes. There may also be other facets of interactions that were not specifically depicted in the model (e.g., the influence of ongoing addictions on various affective and behavioral regulatory processes discussed below). We have limited elements of the model in order to maintain clarity in an already complicated figure. We note that this working model is presented as a framework for organizing and stimulating future research rather than to provide definitive answers to the challenging questions at hand. Next, we discuss the role of stress in addiction vulnerability and review work on physiological mechanisms that may mediate effects of early stress on addiction.

III. STRESS AND VULNERABILITY TO ADDICTION

Both animal and human research provides ample evidence that prenatal and postnatal stress increases vulnerability to use and abuse of drugs. Kosten and Kehoe (2007) have reviewed growing literature demonstrating the influence of various stress paradigms used to investigate stress, including neonatal isolation, on vulnerability to drug use. Manipulations that involve social separation or isolation, in contrast to group housing, were found to increase self-administration of different drugs of abuse (e.g., Alexander et al., 1978; Schenk et al., 1987). Experiments using rhesus monkeys found that monkeys that were reared by their peers during the first 6 months of their life consumed more alcohol than monkeys reared by their mothers (Higley et al., 1993). Interestingly, social separation in adult monkeys that were reared by their mothers led to increases in alcohol consumption to a level comparable to that seen in the peer-reared monkeys. This suggests that exposure to stress, whether during childhood or later in life, leads to increased drug self-administration.

Research with humans has demonstrated that adverse childhood experiences such as emotional, physical, and sexual abuse are associated with increased risk for addiction and with initiation of substance abuse at an early age (Bensley et al., 1999; Dembo et al., 1988; Harrison et al., 1997; Widom et al., 1999). Consistent with this literature, studies have shown that exposure to physical or sexual abuse increases likelihood to continue drug use (e.g., Harrison et al., 1997), and high levels of social and environmental stress predict a rapid progression in tobacco, marijuana, and alcohol use (Kaplan and Johnson, 1992; Wills et al., 1996). Studies have also demonstrated increased frequency of history of trauma among drug-dependent individuals, especially women, than non-drug users (Najavits et al., 1998).

Mechanisms mediating effects of early childhood adversity are likely to include biological, social, and behavioral processes reflecting the long-term consequences of childhood stress. These effects may also resemble those produced by chronic stress. To this end, there is evidence demonstrating that chronic stress and exposure to hardship in early life contribute to significant alterations in the stress response systems. For example, research has shown that animals that were reared under various stressful conditions exhibited significant alterations in the HPA stress response throughout development and adult life (Plotsky and Meaney, 1993). Increased levels of corticotropic-releasing factor (CRF) in the cerebrospinal fluid were found in chronically stressed infant monkeys, reflecting enhanced output of the CRF-HPA system similar to that found in mood disorders (Arborelius et al., 1999; Coplan et al., 1996). Research in wild baboons has shown enhanced adrenocortical production associated with chronic social stress produced by social subordination in these animals (Sapolsky et al., 1997). This is similar to enhanced HPA activation frequently found in depression, where greater adrenocorticotropic hormone (ACTH) and cortisol secretion (Rubin et al., 1987), greater free cortisol in urine (Carroll et al., 1976), increased cortisol and CRF level in cerebrospinal fluid (Nemeroff et al., 1984), and a greater incidence of escape from the Dexamethasone Suppression Test (Carroll et al., 1981) are usually found.

Altered HPA responses are also related to the risk for addiction. Primates that exhibited enhanced cortisol responses to stress early in life showed increased alcohol consumption during adulthood (Fahlke et al., 2000). Furthermore, experiments in rats have shown that increased reactivity, as evidenced by greater or longer corticosterone response to a stress (Kabbaj et al., 2000; Piazza et al., 1991), was associated with increased self-administration of psychostimulants (Grimm and See, 1997; Piazza et al., 1990). Extensive basic research also suggests the possibility that stress-related effects on dopaminergic activity may be one mechanism through which stress increases the risk for drug addiction. Animal experiments show that various acute stressors increase the dopamine release (Imperato et al., 1992; Kalivas and Duffy, 1995). As reviewed by Marinelli (2007), animals with higher reactivity to mild stress exhibit enhanced dopaminergic activity relative to animals with lower reactivity. Increased reactivity was defined in terms of greater or longer corticosterone or greater or longer locomotor response to a stressful situation, such as the exposure to a novel setting or to restraint stress (Kabbaj et al., 2000; Marinelli, 2007; Piazza et al., 1991).

Evidence is currently available in humans indicating that stress-related vulnerability may be due to a dysregulated or blunted stress response by the HPA axis. Blunted HPA stress response has been documented in abstinent alcoholics (Adinoff et al., 2005) and smokers (al'Absi et al., 2003), and is thought to be a result of allostatic adjustment that contributes to increased feelings of discomfort, possibly leading to maintained drug use. Another line of research, however, indicates that this attenuated activity represents a risk factor associated with vulnerability to drug dependence. This is supported by results showing that nonalcoholics with a family history of alcoholism exhibit blunted responses to stress (Dai et al., 2005). Research has also shown lower levels of plasma β-endorphin in individuals with positive family history for alcoholism than in those without a positive family history (Gianoulakis et al., 2005). Furthermore, alcohol consumption was associated with increased plasma β-endorphin levels in the high-risk but not in the low-risk group (Gianoulakis, 1996), and consumption of alcohol was associated with smaller attenuation of plasma β-endorphin responses to stress in individuals with positive family history for alcoholism (Dai et al., 2002). A similar pattern of reactivity was also found in individuals at high risk for addictive problems, including boys with persistent antisocial behaviors (Snoek et al., 2004) and women with increased trait anxiety (Oswald et al., 2006).

It is possible that these alterations are linked to reduced central opioid tone (Wand et al., 1998). This has been directly evaluated by assessing HPA response to opioid receptor blockade, a protocol that is believed to be a useful functional assessment of hypothalamic opioid activity (Wand et al., 1998). The prediction was that the stronger the opioidergic inhibition of CRF neurons, the higher the dose of opioid antagonist needed for disinhibition. Compared to individuals with a negative family history for alcoholism, individuals with a positive family history require lower concentrations of naloxone to remove the opioid inhibitory control of the CRF neurons (Wand et al., 1998). They also exhibit higher ACTH and cortisol responses to administration of similar doses of naloxone and naltrexone, demonstrating an altered HPA axis response to opioid receptor blockade in individuals at high risk for alcoholism (Hernandez-Avila et al., 2002; Wand et al., 2001). For more details on this literature, the reader is referred to Chapter 4, by Chong (2007). There may be multiple sources that contribute to diminished opioid activity, including reduced opioid receptor density, decreased synaptic opioid content, and differences in the types of opioid receptors or their binding affinities. These changes may in turn contribute to attenuated basal levels of dopaminergic activity and concentrations, increasing vulnerability to drug use, as a compensatory means to stimulate the opioid-mesolimbic dopaminergic activity.

Accumulating literature indicates the close interactions between the HPA activity and mesolimbic dopamine (DA) and how these interactions influence drug-seeking behaviors (Piazza and Le, 1998). Mesolimbic DA is activated by many drugs of abuse (Epping-Jordan et al., 1998; Salamone, 1994), and is directly involved in the reinforcing and mood-regulating effects of drug use. This system is stimulated by aversive conditions (Salamone, 1994) and may facilitate coping with these conditions (Salamone, 1994). The nucleus accumbens appears to play an important role in these adaptive processes. The dopaminergic-mesolimbic system also interacts with various limbic structures, such as the amygdala and hippocampus. These systems are modulated by glucocorticoids. Experiments have shown that stress-induced increases in DA synaptic transmission are blocked by glucocorticoid receptor antagonist (Saal et al., 2003), and that administering corticotropin-releasing hormone potentiates N-methyl-D-aspartate (NMDA) receptor-mediated synaptic transmission in DA neurons (Ungless et al., 2003). On the other hand, adrenalectomy reduces extracellular concentrations of DA in the nucleus accumbens (Barrot et al., 2000; Piazza et al., 1996), and this effect seems to be due to corticosterone, as administration of this hormone reverses that effect. Glucocorticoid receptors rather than mineralocorticoid receptors mediate these effects. Administration of a glucocorticoid receptor antagonist decreases DA levels in a dose-dependent manner, with no change in response to mineralocorticoid antagonist (Marinelli et al., 1998). A relevant line of research shows that administration of corticosterone produces an increase in DA in the nucleus accumbens (Imperato et al., 1991; Mittleman et al., 1992). Mechanisms of DA-glucocorticoid interaction may include glucocorticoid facilitatory effects on glutamate-induced activity (Cho and Little, 1999; Overton et al., 1996), leading to increased DA neuron activity and release. Glucocorticoids may also increase DA neurotransmitter synthesis through their facilitatory action on tyrosine hydroxylase (Dunn et al., 1978; Iuvone et al., 1977; Ortiz et al., 1995) and may also reduce DA metabolism and clearance from the synaptic region by decreasing the activity of metabolizing enzymes, such as monoamine oxidase (Parvez and Parvez, 1973; Veals et al., 1977).

In summary, exposure to stressful events early in life or to chronic stress may increase vulnerability to addiction. Mechanisms of this risk may include altered HPA and endogenous opioid stress response. Stress-related effects on dopaminergic activity may also be a mechanism, although results have not been systematically confirmed in humans. For example, while animal experiments suggest that stress-related hyper-responsiveness predicts risk for drug self-administration, human studies suggest that it is the hypoactivation of the stress response systems that seem to relate to risk for drug addiction. Systematic research examining this question in a prospective fashion and across multiple addiction stages

may provide clarity on this set of associations and their significance in the etiology and treatment of addiction. Next, we highlight the role of stress in maintaining addiction and in relapse. We also briefly review recent research on potential mechanisms of the stress effects.

IV. STRESS AND ONGOING ADDICTION AND RELAPSE

Drug use is known to escalate under conditions of high stress and negative affect, especially when there are expectations that drug use will alleviate these discomforting feelings (Copeland et al., 1995; Kassel et al., 2007; Sinha, 2001). Subsequently, through repeated associations of stress with drug use, external and internal stimuli associated with the stress response may become conditioned stimuli that trigger increased craving (Childress et al., 1993; Stewart et al., 1984). In addition, abstinence from drug use is usually associated with several aversive affective states, including anxiety, depression, restlessness, irritability, physical symptoms, and detriment in cognitive performance (American Psychiatric Association, 1994; Cooney et al., 1997). These symptoms may be intensified under conditions of stress (al'Absi et al., 2002a), leading to increased craving. The reduction of these negative affective states then reinforces drug use, increasing the likelihood in the future of experiencing craving for drugs in the presence of stress-related cues and negative affective states.

As shown in Figure 18-2, while initial drug use may be associated with euphoria, positively reinforcing drug use, continued use leads to the development of tolerance. During periods of abstinence and/or under conditions of high stress, negative affect, and craving increase, leading to further drug use. This in turn leads to subsequent relief of these symptoms, further reinforcing drug-taking behaviors. Abstinence may also occur in the context of a cessation attempt and may be maintained over an extended period. Exposure to acute stress or to drug-related cues may increase craving and negative affect, possibly contributing to relapse to drug use. This drug use is reinforced by the reduction of craving and negative affect, increasing risk for reinstatement of regular drug-using behavior (see Figure 18-2).

In addition to the stress-related affect regulation, drug use may also be maintained through a complex set of cognitive-affective interactions. Chronic drug use contributes to neuropsychological and physiological changes that may themselves contribute to maintaining drug-taking behavior. Performance deficits in attention, concentration, working memory, and other intellectual impairments have been frequently cited among various groups of drug dependents (e.g., al'Absi et al., 2002b; Simon et al., 2000) and are thought to exacerbate abstinence effects. Functional as well as structural brain changes have also been documented (Thompson et al., 2004; Volkow et al., 2001). There are also indications of significant deficits in response inhibition and impulsivity (Monterosso et al., 2005; Salo et al., 2005). In combination, these deficits may play a role in maintaining drug-using behavior (Fillmore and Rush, 2002; Jentsch and Taylor, 1999). Furthermore, evidence suggests that response inhibition may be impaired under conditions of high stress and withdrawal-related negative affect, leading to drug use, rapid progress from initiation to dependence, and relapse (Gonzalez Castro et al., 2000).

There is also evidence to suggest a role for stress in relapse. Both correlational and laboratory-based studies have demonstrated the role of stress as a trigger for relapse (Fox et al., 2005; McFall et al., 1992; McKay et al., 1995). Animal experiments have noted a role for exposure to aversive experiences in reinstatement and relapse (Kreek and Koob, 1998). Human studies frequently show that stress is a widely cited reason for relapse (Bradley et al., 1989;

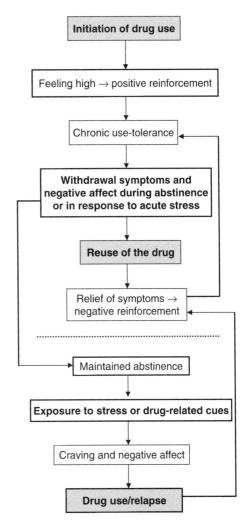

FIGURE 18-2 Illustration of how stress and negative affect contribute to maintenance of drug use and to relapse. Initial drug use may be associated with euphoric effects, but with continued use tolerance develops. During abstinence or under conditions of high stress, negative affect and craving increase leading to drug use and to subsequent relief of these symptoms. Exposure to acute stress or to drug-related cues may also increase craving, contributing to relapse in individuals who are abstinent.

Cohen and Lichtenstein, 1990; Wallace, 1989. For example, Cohen and Lichtenstein (1990) found that smokers who failed to quit cigarette smoking or relapsed after a short period reported higher levels of stress prior to initial abstinence or at 1, 3, and 6 months after cessation. Decreased reported stress was associated with changes in status from smoking to abstinence, and increased reported stress was associated with changes from abstinence to smoking (Cohen and Lichtenstein, 1990). Participants whose lapses were precipitated by stress moved faster to a full relapse than those whose lapses were triggered by eating or drinking (Shiffman et al., 1996). Since abstinence from drug use may lead to increases in perceived stress (Parrott, 1999), it is possible that those who experience heightened negative affect after initial abstinence are at high risk for early relapse (al'Absi et al., 2004a; Burgess et al., 2002; Kenford, et al. 2002).

Risk for relapse has also been studied in laboratory settings owing to the methodological advances in the assessment of stress and the development of refined methodology to simulate stress in the laboratory that facilitated the assessment of various biological, behavioral, and psychological indices of reactivity (Kudielka and Kirschbaum, 2007). Our own research with smokers has demonstrated the utility of several laboratory stressors, such as public speaking, extended mental arithmetic, and pain-induction procedures. We have used these probes to examine various biological and psychophysiological functions in dependent tobacco users (al'Absi et al., 2002a; 2003). We have also used similar laboratory-based procedures to identify predictors of smoking relapse (al'Absi et al., 2005). In one study we found that smokers who relapsed within 4 weeks of a quit attempt showed attenuated hormonal and cardiovascular responses to stress, exaggerated withdrawal symptoms, and mood deterioration after quitting. When analyzing the data using regression analyses, we found that attenuated responses to stress predicted a shorter time to relapse (al'Absi et al., 2005), supporting the utility of this paradigm to assess the integrity of the stress response among drug users and the use of the results to identify those at high risk for early relapse. In addition to using circumscribed challenges in laboratory settings, other studies using recall and imaginary

experiences have also been useful. Studies using guided imagery involving recall of personal stressful experiences were found to increase craving for cocaine and alcohol in abstinent cocaine-dependent participants (Fox et al., 2005; Sinha et al., 1999), and these reports predicted the incidence of relapse following treatment (Fox et al., 2005).

Our understanding of how stress triggers relapse is still evolving, although there are several neurobiological and behavioral mechanisms that have been identified based on basic research in animals. One stress model that has been used to investigate these mechanisms is foot-shock–induced relapse. Experiments using pharmacological, neurochemical, and behavioral methods have demonstrated the role of CRF in stress-induced relapse. As reviewed by Erb (2007), CRF within the extended amygdala circuitry seems to play a primary role in foot-shock–induced reinstatement (Erb et al., 2001). Other mechanisms include DA and glutamatergic systems. The DA projections terminate at the prefrontal cortex (PFC), while glutamatergic projections originate from the PFC to the nucleus accumbens, in addition to other projections involving multiple brain structures (McFarland et al., 2004). These structures are also involved in emotion regulation and affective response to stress, providing a likely pathway through which stress and addiction relapse interface.

In summary, there is growing evidence demonstrating that stress and negative affect contribute to addiction maintenance and relapse. The reduction of negative affective states by drug use negatively reinforces this behavior, increasing the likelihood of experiencing craving for drugs in the presence of stress-related cues in the future. Advances in the scientific study of stress and addiction suggest a role for multiple neurobiological systems including CRF and DA. In the next sections we highlight factors that are known to moderate the effects of stress on addiction, including sex differences, genetic factors, coping resources, and behavioral traits. We note that our discussion is rather brief and meant to emphasize certain findings. More comprehensive sections are found in other chapters of this book.

V. FACTORS AFFECTING STRESS AND ADDICTION INTERACTIONS

Sex Differences

Sex differences have significant implications in the understanding of stress-related addiction vulnerability and relapse. Several indications in both human and animal studies suggest that sex mßoderates effects of stress on drug administration. Animal experiments using foot shock have shown enhanced HPA responses as well as other behavioral and neuronal activity in female compared with male rats (Beatty and Beatty, 1970; Kosten et al., 2005). Early life stress has greater effects on cocaine self-administration in female rats than control (Kosten and Kehoe, 2007). On the other hand, certain drugs, such as cocaine, produce greater behavioral and hormonal responses in female than in male rats, and these effects seem to be independent of ovarian hormones (Bowman et al., 1999; Kuhn and Francis, 1997). Consistent with these results are findings indicating that neonatal isolation facilitated acquisition and maintenance of food intake in female but not in male rats (Kosten et al., 2000; Zhang et al., 2005). Effects of stress on drug administration may also be mediated by different neurophysiological changes in males and females. For example, experiments found that NMDA receptor binding in dorsal striatum was upregulated in isolated males but downregulated in isolated females (Sircar et al., 2001). Similar sex differences were found showing that neonatal isolation was associated with increased corticosterone levels in female but not in male pups (Knuth and Etgen, 2005).

In humans, clinical and epidemiological reports indicate that stress is more frequently reported by women than men with addiction problems, and that stress is more frequently cited as a reason for drug use, maintenance, and relapse in women than in men (e.g., Najavits et al., 1998; Wechsberg et al., 1998). Women who experienced childhood sexual abuse exhibited a four-fold increase in risk for lifetime prevalence of both alcoholism and other drug abuse relative to women who did not experience such abuse (Wilsnack et al., 1997; Winfield et al., 1990). They are also more likely to produce symptoms of post-traumatic stress disorder (PTSD) and comorbid substance abuse problems than men (Newton-Taylor et al., 1998). On the other hand, 70% of female drug users report childhood sexual abuse (NIDA, 1994). Research suggests that environmental context plays a greater role in determining perception of drug effects in women than in men (Perkins, 1999). Women who smoke are more likely to use smoking to cope with negative affect than men (Dicken, 1978). They report more urges to smoke (Abrams et al., 1987) and more distress after exposure to acutely stressful situations and to smoking-specific stimuli than male smokers (Abrams et al., 1987; Swan et al., 1993), and they are less likely to maintain long-term smoking abstinence than men (D'Angelo et al., 2001; Wetter et al., 1999).

Stress-related effects on addiction may work through different mechanisms in men and women. Differences in the patterns, intensity, and frequency of the stress response may contribute to these differences in patterns and severity of addiction (Grunberg et al., 1991; Staley et al., 2001). For example, in one study that used responses to stress as potential predictors of relapse, we found different patterns of relapse predictors in men and women. Attenuated cortisol and ACTH responses to stress were associated with early relapse in men. Intensity of withdrawal symptoms after exposure to acute stress predicted time to relapse in women (al'Absi, 2006).

We recently compared tobacco-dependent men and women and found another facet of regulatory changes that indicate a possible source of differences between men and women. In that study we found that sex differences in pain measures were consistently diminished among smokers relative to nonsmokers (see Figure 18-3). The literature in nondrug users has consistently demonstrated marked sex differences in pain perception, with women exhibiting greater sensitivity to pain than men (al'Absi et al., 1999; Feine et al., 1991; Jensen et al., 1992; Maixner and Humphrey, 1993). In a recent study, we found that women who were dependent smokers exhibited comparable pain sensitivity to that of men. Since the endogenous opioid system interacts with the hypothalamic-pituitary-gonadal axis and indirectly influences estrogen production from the ovaries (al'Absi et al., 2002c; Ferin, 1989), it is conceivable that female smokers exhibit reduced production of estradiol that contributes to reduced pain sensitivity in this group. This possibility is supported by recent research showing that female smokers have reduced estradiol production relative to nonsmoking women (Girdler et al., 2005). Animal experiments have demonstrated that reduced estrogen production leads to increased sensitivity to pain (Frye et al., 1993; Ratka and Simpkins, 1991), and one study in humans showed that higher estrogen concentrations were associated with increased thermal pain sensitivity (Fillingim et al., 1997).

Previous research has also shown a differential effect of the endogenous opioid system on pain and blood pressure regulation (al'Absi et al., 2004b). We found that opioid blockade, using 50 mg of naltrexone, was associated with analgesia and with attenuated systolic and diastolic blood pressure responses to acute stressors in women but not in men. These effects

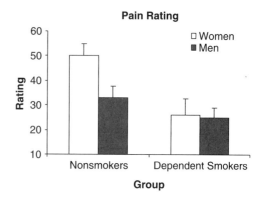

Pain Rating

FIGURE 18-3   Mean pain ratings after exposure to the cold pressor test. The hand cold pressor test (temperature range: 0–4 °C) lasted for 90 seconds. Line bars indicate standard error of the mean. During the test, nonsmoking women reported greater pain than nonsmoking men ($p < 0.01$), but no such difference was found among smoking men and women.

were the opposite of the expected increase in pain sensitivity and blood pressure after opioid blockade. These sex differences may be in part due to effects of steroids on opiate receptors in several areas of the brain and to differences in the role of the opioid system in the stress response (Cicero et al., 2002; Hammer et al., 1994; Zubieta et al., 1999). It is possible that sex differences exist in the sensitivity, quantity, and ratio of the different classes of opioid receptors (Hammer, 1985; Sershen et al., 1998). For example, a recent study demonstrated sex differences in the mu-opioid receptors' responses to sustained pain (Zubieta et al., 2002), and higher mu-opioid binding was previously found in women (Zubieta et al., 1999). It is intriguing to speculate that these sex differences in endogenous opioids play a role in the observed sex differences in behavioral and pharmacological responses to drugs, severity of substance abuse, and outcome of treatment efforts (Clemmey et al., 1997; Dudish and Hatsukami, 1996; Etter et al., 2002; Kandel et al., 1997).

In summary, there are clear sex differences in the patterns of addiction vulnerability, motivators for drug use, and risk factors for relapse. The influence of stress also seems to vary. Clinical and epidemiological studies indicate that stress may be a more potent risk factor for drug initiation, maintenance, and relapse in women than in men. There are also indications that effects of stress may be mediated by different effectors in men and women. While no specific mechanisms have been identified to account for these sex differences, it is likely that multiple systems are involved, including systems involved in the stress and reinforcement regulation as well as sex-specific hormonal characteristics. Finally, it is critical to recognize that these sex differences have implications in terms of approach to the assessment and treatment of stress-related problems and addiction in men and women.

Genetic Factors

Research into the role of genetic factors in addiction has witnessed significant growth in recent years as evidenced in multiple chapters of this book (e.g., Enoch, 2007; Lovallo, 2007). We highlight here findings that bear directly on systems involved in stress and addiction, the HPA, and the endogenous opioid systems. There is evidence indicating that variability in cortisol responses to stress is determined in part by genetic factors. Twin studies have shown high heritability of more than 97% for sustained cortisol response to stress (Federenko et al., 2004). Cortisol responses to awakening have also been found to have heritability of 40–60% (Bartels et al., 2003; Wust et al., 2000). Genetic factors may influence functionality of glucocorticoid receptor activity, especially related to negative feedback (Bartels et al., 2003). Previous research has described multiple glucocorticoid receptor polymorphisms, including the Asn363Ser exon 2 variant and BclI variant (DeRijk and de Kloet, 2005). These polymorphisms seem to be associated with variance in HPA stress response, with Asn363Ser variant associated with increased cortisol response to acute psychosocial stress and a BclI variant associated with diminished cortisol response (Wust et al., 2004).

In addition to the role of genetic variations related to the HPA system, genetic factors related to the endogenous opioid functions are also important in the understanding of the stress response. Research to identify polymorphisms associated with the opioid system functions has demonstrated that the functional polymorphism Asn40Asp (+118A/G) in the mu opioid receptor gene (OPRM1) is closely involved in regulating the functions of this system. This poly-mporphism is associated with a threefold increase in mu-endorphin binding affinity and potency. Thus, it is likely that this polymorphism is also associated with increased inhibition of the CRF neurons (Bond et al., 1998). Studies have shown that relative to Asn40 allele, OPRM1 Asp40 variant was associated with lower cortisol responses to psychological stressors in healthy men (Chong et al., 2007). Consistent with these results, OPRM1 Asp40 was associated with enhanced HPA activation, as evidenced by larger cortisol responses to opioid receptor blockade (Hernandez-Avila et al., 2003, Wand et al., 2002). Research in rhesus monkeys provides consistent information demonstrating that a similar polymorphism was associated with reduced ACTH-stimulated plasma cortisol levels (Miller et al., 2004), although the association of this polymorphism with drug dependence has not been established (Arias et al., 2005).

In summary, there are promising lines of research to identify specific functional polymorphisms implicated in regulating the stress response and reinforcement-related neurobiological functions. Future research should determine the extent to which these polymorphisms may inform the development of new intervention strategies. For example, there is interesting evidence to suggest that naltrexone, an opioid receptor antagonist acting primarily at the mu-opioid receptor, is helpful in the treatment of alcoholism, and recent results suggest that its effects on the HPA axis may predict intensity of alcohol craving (O'Malley et al., 2002). If Asp40 variant is associated with enhanced endogenous opioid tone and with enhanced inhibitory effects on HPA functions, it would be reasonable to predict that individuals with this variant would benefit from opiate blockade treatment. Recent research findings lend support to this prediction. Alcoholics with one or two copies of the Asp40 allele who were treated with naltrexone had significantly lower relapse rates and moderated their drinking for a longer period of time compared with Asn40 homozygotes alcoholics (Oslin et al., 2003). Asp40 variant was also associated with enhanced benefits from nicotine replacement therapy in smoking cessation treatment (Lerman et al., 2004).

VI. STRESS, POOR BEHAVIORAL REGULATION, AND ADDICTION

Poor behavioral regulation, impulsivity, and other cognitive deficits are considered important behavioral mechanisms that increase risk for addiction and contribute to its maintenance. Research has shown that impulsivity in children is a risk factor for substance abuse during adulthood (Dawes et al., 2000; White et al., 1994). Impulsivity is higher among various drug dependent groups relative to respective control groups (Kirby and Petry, 2004; Mitchell, 1999). Impulsivity is associated with greater severity of drug use (Reynolds, 2004; Semple et al., 2005). Donahue and Grant (2007) discussed the possibility that stress may contribute to different facets of impulse control problems, and this may be mediated by deficits in regulating emotion. In this case, stress may lead to maladaptive behavioral responses and sensation- or reward-seeking behaviors, likely leading to decreased self-control and increased impulsive behaviors (Muraven and Baumeister, 2000). These behavioral deficits may contribute to drug use behavior and may increase difficulties in maintaining abstinence when confronted with situational demands. Consistent with this prediction, studies have found a relationship between impulsivity and treatment outcome in cocaine abusers (Patkar et al., 2004), tobacco smokers (Doran et al., 2004), and poly-substance abusers (McCown, 1990).

Impulsive control problems may also be related to cognitive functions. Growing evidence indicates that cognitive and executive functioning may influence risk for initiation and maintenance of addiction (Hyman and Malenka, 2001; Kalivas et al., 2005; Robinson and Berridge, 2003). One of these functions is response inhibition. Deficits in this function may predispose the individual to take risks leading to drug-taking behavior with rapid progression to dependence (Gonzalez Castro et al., 2000). On the other hand, effects of stress on cognitive functions (such as attention, working memory, and response inhibition) have been established (al'Absi, et al., 2002a; Cohen, 1980; Glass et al., 1971; Hockey, 1970). Direct evidence in primates has shown that uncontrollable stress (exposure to noise) produced significant impairments in prefrontal cognitive function in monkeys (Arnsten and Goldman-Rakic, 1998). These functions are modulated by dopaminergic activity, which itself is altered by chronic drug use (Kalivas et al., 1998). It is possible that these changes contribute to deficits in stress-related cognitive and affective regulation (Jentsch and Taylor, 1999; Robbins and Everitt, 1996), leading to difficulties in mounting an adaptive response to stress, increasing the risk for maintaining drug use.

In summary, stress may impact risk of addiction initiation and maintenance through increasing impulsive behaviors and increasing risk for other cognitive deficits. Chronic drug use itself may contribute to these effects, perpetuating a positive feedback cycle that leads to maintained drug use, escalation, and relapse.

substance use and stress or negative affect is reinforced.

VII. COPING RESOURCES

There is some support to suggest that individuals with adequate coping and social support resources are able to buffer effects of stress on addiction vulnerability and relapse. This has led to the notion that teaching individuals who have addiction problems coping skills and cognitive behavioral strategies to address stress may help them in their recovery (Carroll et al., 1994; Monti et al., 1989). The issue of addressing stress in the context of addictive problems, however, remains challenging and relatively less developed. High impact of exposure to ongoing or childhood stress when combined with addictive problems may present a set of complex challenges to researchers and clinicians that require more sophisticated approaches than have been utilized to date.

Research on comorbidity illustrates that individuals with substance use problems and who suffer from psychological problems may face significant hurdles in their efforts to overcome their addictions (Donahue and Kushner, 2007; Roberts et al., 2007). This may be a result of a history of using substances to cope with negative affective states. The negative reinforcement of this drug-using behavior increases chances of using the drug to deal with stress or negative affect in the future, including those caused by temporary abstinence (Ahmed and Koob, 2005; Childress et al., 1994). This leads to a vicious cycle of substance use to regulate affect. This cycle occurs during active drug use as well as in relapse. In this context, it is important to recognize and account for the role of expectancy in the interaction between stress and addiction. As discussed by Kassel et al. (2007), there are reasons to believe that expectancy is one mechanism through which the link between

VIII. DISCUSSION AND FUTURE DIRECTIONS

In this section we outline specific themes that require further discussion and warrant more attention in future research.

1. While evidence demonstrates the influence of childhood adversity on stress vulnerability, various environmental and biological factors moderate this long-lasting effect of early adversity. For example, there is evidence that low levels of expression of the monoamine-oxidase A gene is associated with increased risk for conduct and antisocial behavior, factors that in turn are associated with addiction (Caspi et al., 2002; Foley et al., 2004). Evidence also suggests that many psychosocial factors directly influence the degree to which stress impacts the individual. As discussed in this book (Steptoe and Hamer, 2007), factors such as social, demographic, and economic status, in addition to recent and early life adversity and patterns of coping, determine the intensity and manner by which an individual responds to stress. The manners by which individuals are affected by various social and environment factors should also be considered when examining the impact of stress in individuals who have addiction problems. Such research must have both laboratory and population-based focus and must take into account the complexity of psychosocial factors that affect propensity to respond to stress in an unhealthy manner.

2. As discussed earlier (e.g., Tate et al., 2007), stress is widely cited as being one reason for drug use among adolescents. It is not clear when and how stress promotes transitions to ongoing drug

use and dependence. As an example, of the approximately 75% of adolescents who have tried cigarettes or used alcohol, only a minority continue to use and become dependent on these substances (Johnston et al., 2004; Wills and Stoolmiller, 2002). An important item on the research agenda addressing the interaction of stress and addiction should be to develop methods to identify individuals and situational characteristics that are associated with increased risk for dependence in adolescents. Related to this question is identifying those who may be at risk for other behavioral or mood problems and who may initiate drug use as a method to manage increased sensitivity to stress and negative affect. This information is critical for developing appropriate prevention and intervention strategies.

3. We have noted that various cognitive and behavioral deficits are associated with the stress response among drug-dependent individuals, and there are indications that these deficits lead to maintained drug use and relapse. It is, however, not yet clear the extent to which these deficits result from chronic exposure to the drug or represent a risk factor that precedes drug use. This is an important issue that requires further research, taking into account developmental issues and stages of progression of the addiction process. In addition, the growing recognition of the role of impulsive behaviors in addiction and the role of stress in this behavioral regulation provide an important area for intervention. As noted in this book, the current literature on the assessment and intervention of impulse control problems is rather limited (Donahue and Grant, 2007). A new approach to address the role of stress across multiple addictive problems would benefit from directly addressing impulsive behaviors and the propensity to engage in drug-taking behaviors under conditions of high stress.

4. There is a need to determine the extent to which certain behavioral or neurochemical manifestations of the relationship between stress and addiction liability are common across multiple drugs of abuse or other addictive behaviors. There are indications that certain neural and biological processes (e.g., dopamine activation) are common across multiple addictive behaviors. There may be unique interactions and drug-specific idiosyncrasies of the effects of stress in each type of addiction. Addressing these issues should directly assist in guiding efforts to develop effective prevention and treatment strategies to buffer effects of stress and directly combat addiction problems.

5. Treatment strategies to address addiction remain crude and largely ineffective. Efforts that address specific risk factors for addiction and relapse are sorely needed. These treatments should integrate multiple biobehavioral approaches and focus on helping patients at multiple levels, including gaining insight on the role of stress and negative affect in their addictions and learning coping skills to deal with ongoing or daily stressors (Donahue and Kushner, 2007). These methods should take into consideration the role played by expectations that drug use may lead to the reduction of negative affect. Other approaches may also include developing an abstinence-focused social support network, promoting self-efficacy about the ability to manage stress, in addition to taking advantage of available pharmacological treatments. This hybrid approach should help reduce stress-triggered drug use and relapse. Specific scientific investigation to guide this treatment is still needed.

6. Future research should also provide specific information on who may benefit more from this type of stress-focused approach. For example, it is

conceivable that patients with stress-related problems (e.g., individuals who have been exposed to trauma) would benefit from such interventions, in light of the fact that they are usually overrepresented among patients with addictive disorders. Furthermore, a proactive approach to care for this high-risk group may be needed in order to prevent escalation of their problems. This in turn would require means to screen for these problems early and tailor management of addiction liability in conjunction with approaches to address stress-related complications.

7. There are indications that multimodal intervention programs incorporating psychosocial and pharmacological interventions could be useful in addressing risk factors for addiction, such as impulsive behaviors, but there is very little research to identify specific components of these interventions and efficiently integrate them into prevention and treatment efforts. For example, it would be important to identify the therapeutic strategies most effective in addressing impulsive behaviors in individuals who have high levels of stress or other comorbidities, such as anxiety and depression. In that context it would be important to develop interventions that provide effective means of coping with stress in individuals who are predisposed to impulsive behaviors. These may include skills that help in managing tension and regulating affective state, and may also include ongoing help and support to prevent relapse to dysfunctional behaviors when experiencing negative affect and stress. Research is needed to develop and evaluate the extent to which such strategies reduce impulsive decision making when exposed to stressful events. The impact of such efforts may expand across all addictive stages:

initiation, maintenance, abstinence, and relapse.

8. Evidence reviewed in this book confirms that trauma and other stress-related problems are associated with increased risk for addiction initiation, maintenance, and relapse. The causal direction, however, remains unclear. For example, it is not clear if PTSD leads to drug addiction or if addiction increases chances to witness or be victimized by a traumatic event and subsequently develop this disorder. Although there is significant overlap in the two disorders (i.e., addiction and PTSD), there is still a critical gap in our knowledge about who develops PTSD and addiction problems and how to identify risk for either disorder. Such knowledge can prove helpful in the treatment approaches used with both disorders.

9. Research has provided evidence demonstrating the role of CRF as an extra-hypothalamic neuromodulator (Koob and Heinrichs, 1999) directly involved in integrating different facets of the stress response, including autonomic, hormonal, and immune responses. More relevant to this book is the direct CRF interactions with several key structures, such as the amygdala, ventral tegmental area, cortex, and hippocampus, that are involved in addictive processes and in orchestrating the stress response (Dunn et al., 2004; Ungless et al., 2003; Wang et al., 2005). These interactions have stimulated efforts to explore pharmacological agents that interact with this system. Animal studies show that systemic injections of CRF receptor antagonists or alpha-2 adrenoceptor agonists prevent stress-induced reinstatement. Specifically, there is evidence (see Goeders, 2007) from animal experiments demonstrating effectiveness of CRF receptor antagonists in treating ongoing addiction and reducing risk for relapse

in response to stress and drug-related cues. Research is still needed to identify potential therapeutic effects of CRF-probing agents. The nature of how the CRF system interacts with the endogenous opioid and dopaminergic systems in the context of stress and addiction is still in need of further study. Translational extension of this work to human laboratory studies is critical in guiding future discoveries for treatment of stress-related problems and addiction.

10. Finally there are still unanswered questions related to the effects of abstinence on stress biological and behavioral function and the extent to which stress exacerbates withdrawal syndrome. The interactive effects of stress and abstinence may be critical in determining risk for relapse. Identifying neurobiological mechanisms of this interaction is an important step toward identifying specific circuitry that link stress with maintained drug use and relapse. Answering these questions should also inform future efforts toward developing new treatment procedures to prevent stress-triggered relapse.

IX. CONCLUSIONS

There has been a great deal of scientific progress over the recent decade delineating the neurobiological circuitry underlying effects of stress on addiction. In addition, some progress has been made addressing how stress in early life alters the regulation of the stress response, influences motivated behavior, and increases risk for addiction. Research has also progressed to explore how genetic risk for addiction may relate to different patterns of stress response, how these differences manifest in terms of biological and behavioral responses, the role and characteris-

tics of the stress response in the context of risk for addiction, as well as alterations after chronic drug use. Complementary to this progress, there have been efforts to improve tools to assess addiction and stress, and to develop or refine existing treatment strategies.

Notwithstanding these advances, much remains to be accomplished to translate the wealth of basic knowledge into clinical practice. To that end, there are encouraging results (Goeders, 2007; Saal and Nemeroff, 2007) pointing toward the potential of HPA-related pharmacological interventions in the treatment of addictions in humans, although more work is still needed to understand the specific nature of how stress and the subsequent activation of the HPA axis impact addiction. Until new medications targeting stress-related systems are added to existing treatment methods, strategies such as learning means to reduce and cope with stress should be integrated into addiction treatments as tools to manage triggers that may promote drug use and relapse. Eventually a combination of pharmacotherapies targeting stress response systems such as HPA and other cognitive behavioral stress management techniques may prove effective in managing withdrawal symptoms and craving and leading to improved outcomes of addiction treatment.

REFERENCES

Abrams, D. B., Monti, P. M., Pinto, R. P., Elder, J. P., Brown, R. A., and Jacobus, S. I. (1987). Psychosocial stress and coping in smokers who relapse or quit. *Health Psychology, 6,* 289–303.

Ahmed, S. H., and Koob, G. F. (2005). Transition to drug addiction: A negative reinforcement model based on an allostatic decrease in reward function. *Psychopharmacology (Berl), 180,* 473–490.

al'Absi, M., (2006). Altered psychoendocrine responses to psychological stress and smoking relapse. *International Journal of Psychophysiology, 59,* 218–227.

al'Absi, M., Amunrud, T., and Wittmers, L. E. (2002a). Psychophysiological effects of nicotine abstinence and behavioral challenges in habitual smokers. *Pharmacol Biochem Behav, 72,* 707–716.

al'Absi, M., Buchanan, T. W., Marrero, A., and Lovallo W. R. (1999). Sex differences in pain perception and cardiovascular responses in persons with parental history for hypertension. *Pain, 83*, 331–338.

al'Absi, M., Hatsukami, D., and Davis, G. (2005). Attenuated adrenocorticotropic responses to stress predict early relapse. *Psychopharmacology, 181*, 107–117.

al'Absi, M., Hatsukami, D., Davis, G. L., and Wittmers, L. (2004a) Prospective examination of effects of smoking abstinence on cortisol and withdrawal symptoms as predictors of early smoking relapse. *Drug and Alcohol Dependence, 73*, 267–278.

al'Absi, M., Hugdahl, K., and Lovallo, W. R. (2002b). Adrenocortical responses and cognitive performance. *Psychophysiology, 39*, 95–99.

al'Absi, M., Petersen, K. L., and Wittmers, L. E. (2002c). Adrenocortical and hemodynamic predictors of pain perception in men and women. *Pain, 92*, 197–205.

al'Absi, M., Wittmers, L., Ellestad, D., Nordehn, G., Kim, S. W., Kirschbaum, C., and Grant, J. E. (2004b). Sex differences in pain and hypothalamic-pituitary-adrenocortical responses to opioid blockade. *Psychosomatic Medicine, 166*, 198–206.

al'Absi, M., Wittmers, L. E., Erickson, J., Hatsukami, D., and Crouse, B. (2003). Attenuated adrenocortical and blood pressure responses to psychological stress in ad libitum and abstinent smokers. *Pharmacol Biochem Behav, 74*, 401–410.

Alexander, B. K., Coambs, R. B., and Hadaway, F. F. (1978). The effect of housing and gender on morphine self-administration in rats. *Psychopharmacology, 58*, 175–179.

American Psychiatric Association. (1994). Diagnostic and statistical manual (4th ed.). Washington D.C., Author.

Arborelius, L., Owens, M. J., Plotsky, P. M., and Nemeroff, C. B. (1999). The role of corticotrophin-releasing factor in depression and anxiety disorders. *J Endocrinol, 160*, 1–12.

Arias, A., Fein, R., Kranzler, H. R. (2006). Association of an Asn40Asp (A118G) polymorphism in the mu-opioid receptor gene with substance dependence: a meta-analysis. Drug Alcohol Depend. *83*: 262–268.

Arnsten, A.F.T and Goldman-Rakic, P. S. (1998). Noise stress impairs prefrontal cortical cognitive function in monkeys. *Arch Gen Psychiatry, 55*, 362–368.

Barrot, M., Marinell, M., Abrous, D. N., Rouge-Pont, Le Moal, M., and Piazza, P. V. (2000). The dopaminergic hyper-responsiveness of the shell of the nucleus accumbens is hormone-dependent. *Eur J Neurosci, 12*, 973–979.

Bartels, M., de Geus, E. J., Kirschbaum, C., and Sluyter, F. (2003). Heritability of daytime cortisol levels in children. *Behav Genet, 33*, 421–433.

Beatty, W. W., and Beatty, P. A. (1970). Hormonal determinants of sex differences in avoidance behavior and reactivity to electric shock in the rat. *Journal of Comparative and Physiological Psychology, 73*, 446–455.

Bond, C., LaForg, K. S., Tian, M., Melia, D., Zhang, S., Borg, L., Gong, J., Schluger, J., Strong, J. A., Leal, S. M., Tischfield, J. A., Kreek, M. J., and Yu, L. (1998). Single-nucleotide polymorphism in the human mu opioid receptor gene alters beta-endorphin binding and activity: Possible implications for opiate addictiction. *Proc Natl Acad Sci USA, 95*, 9608–9613.

Bowman, B. P., Vaughan, S. R., Walker, Q. D., Davis, S. L., Little, P. J., Scheffler, N. M., Thomas, B. F., and Kuhn, C. M. (1999). Effects of sex and gonadectomy on cocaine metabolism in the rat. *Journal of Pharmacology and Experimental Therapeutics, 290*, 1316–1323.

Bradley, B. P., Phillips, G., Green, and Gossop, M. (1989). Circumstances surrounding the initial lapse to opiate use following detoxification. *Br J Psychiatry, 154*, 354–359.

Burgess, E. S., Brown, R. A., Kahler, C. W., Niaura, R., Abrams, D. B., Goldstein, M. G., and Miller, I. W. (2002). Patterns of change in depressive symptoms during smoking cessation: Who's at risk for relapse? *J Consult Clin Psychol, 70*, 356–361.

Carroll, B. J., Curtis, G. C., Davies, B. M., Mendels, J., and Sugerman, A. A. (1976). Urinary free cortisol excretion in depression. *Psychol Med, 6*, 43–50.

Carroll, B. J., Feinberg, M., Greden, J. F., Tarika, J. Albala, A. A., Haskett, R. F., et al. (1981). A specific laboratory test for the diagnosis of melancholia. Standardization, validation, and clinical utility. *Arch Gen Psychiatr, 38*, 15–22.

Carroll, K., Rounsaville, B., Gordon, L., Nich, C., Jatlo, Bisighini, R., and Gawin, F. (1994). Psychotherapy and pharmacotherapy for ambulatory cocaine abusers. *Arch Gen Psychiatry, 51*, 177–187

Caspi, A., McClay, J., Moffitt, T. E., Mill, J., Martin, J., Craig, I. W., Taylor, A., and Poulton, R. (2002). Role of genotype in the cycle of violence in maltreated children. *Science, 297*, 851–853.

Childress, A. R., Ehrman, R., McLellan, A. T., MacRae, J., Natale, M., and O'Brien, C. P. (1994). Can induced moods trigger drug-related responses in opiate abuse patients? *J Subst Abuse Treat, 11*, 17–23.

Childress, A., Hole, A., Ehrman, R., Robbins, S., McLellan, A., and O'Brien, C. (1993). Cue reactivity and cue reactivity interventions in drug dependence. *NIDA Res Monogr, 137*, 73–95.

Cho, K., and Little, H. J. (1999). Effects of corticosterone on excitatory amino acid responses in dopamine-sensitive neurons in the ventral tegmental area. *Neuroscience, 88*, 837–845.

Chong, R. Y., Uhart, M., and Wand, G. S. (2007). Endogenous opiates, addiction, and the stress response. In al'Absi, M. (ed), Stress and addiction: Biological and psychological mechanisms. London, UK: Elsevier, Ltd.

Cicero, T. J., Nock, B., O'Connor, L., and Meyer, E. R. (2002). Role of steroids in sex differences in morphine-induced analgesia: Activational and organizational effects. *J Pharmacol Exp Ther, 300*, 695–701.

Clemmey, P., Brooner, R., Chutuape, M. A., Kidorf, M., and Stitzer, M. (1997). Smoking habits and attitudes in a methadone maintenance treatment population. *Drug Alcohol Depend, 44*, 123–132.

Cohen, S. (1980). Aftereffects of stress on human performance and social behavior: A review of research and theory. *Psychol Bull, 88*, 82–108.

Cohen, S., and Lichtenstein, E. (1990). Perceived stress, quitting smoking and smoking relapse. *Health Psychol, 9*, 466–478.

Cooney, N., Litt, M., Morse, P., and Bauer, L. (1997). Alcohol cue reactivity, negative mood reactivity and relapse in treated alcoholics. *J Abnorm Psychol, 106*, 243–250.

Copeland, A. L., Brandon, T. H., and Quinn, E. P. (1995). The Smoking Consequences Questionnaire—Adult: Measurement of smoking outcome expectancies of experienced smokers. *Psychological Assessment, 7*, 484–494.

Coplan, J. D., Andrews, M. W., Rosenblum, L. A., Owens, M. J., Friedman, S., Gorman, J. M., and Nemeroff, C. B. (1996). Persistent elevations of cerebrospinal fluid concentrations of corticotrophin-releasing factor in adult non-human primates exposed to early-life stressors: Implications for the pathophysiology of mood and anxiety disorders. *Proc Natl Acad Sci, 93*, 1619–1623.

Dai, X., Thavundayil, J., and Gianoulakis, C. (2002). Differences in the responses of the pituitary beta-endorphin and cardiovascular system to ethanol and stress as a function of family history. *Alcohol Clin. Exp. Res., 26*, 1171–1180.

Dai, X., Thavundayil, J., and Gianoulakis, C. (2005). Differences in the peripheral levels of beta-endorphin in response to alcohol and stress as a function of alcohol dependence and family history of alcoholism. *Alcohol Clin. Exp. Res., 29*, 1965–1975.

D'Angelo, M. E., Reid, R. D., Brown, K. S., and Pipe, A. L. (2001). Gender differences in predictors for long-term smoking cessation following physician advice and nicotine replacement therapy. *Can J Public Health, 92*, 418–422.

Dawes, M. A., Antelman, S. M., Vanyukov, M. M., Giancola, P., Tarter, R. E., Susman, E. J., et al. (2000). Developmental sources of variation in liability to adolescent substance use disorders. *Drug and Alcohol Dependence, 61*, 3–14.

Dembo, R., Dertke, M., Borders, S., Washburn, M., and Schmeidler, J. (1988). The relationship between physical and sexual abuse and tobacco, alcohol, and illicit drug use among youths in a juvenile detention center. *Int J Addict, 23*, 351–378.

DeRijk, R., and de Kloet, E. R. (2005). Corticosteroid receptor genetic polymorphisms and stress responsivity. *Endocrine, 28*, 263–270.

Dicken, C. (1978). Sex roles, smoking, and smoking cessation. *J Health Soc Behav, 19*, 324–334.

Donahue, C. B., and Grant, J. E. (2007). Stress and impulsive behaviors. In al'Absi, M. (ed), *Stress and addiction: Biological and psychological mechanisms.* London, UK: Elsevier, Ltd.

Donahue, C. B., and Kushner, M. G. (2007). Stress, anxiety and addiction: Intervention strategies. In al'Absi, M. (ed), *Stress and addiction: Biological and psychological mechanisms.* London, UK: Elsevier, Ltd.

Doran, N., Spring, B., McChargue, D., Pergadia, M., and Richmond, M. (2004). Impulsivity and smoking relapse. *Nicotine and Tobacco Research, 6*, 641–647.

Dudish, S. A., and Hatsukami, D. K. (1996). Gender differences in crack users who are research volunteers. *Drug Alcohol Depend, 42(1)*, 55–63.

Dunn, A. J., Gildersleeve, N. B., and Gray, H. E. (1978). Mouse brain tyrosine hydroxylase and glutamic acid decarboxylase following treatment with adrenocorticotropic hormone, vasopressin or corticosterone. *J. Neurochem., 31*, 977–982.

Dunn, A. J., Swiergiel, A. H., and Palamarchouk, V. (2004). Brain circuits involved in corticotropin-releasing factor-norepinephrine interactions during stress. *Ann N Y Acad Sci, 1018*, 25–34.

Enoch, M. A. (2007). Genetics, stress, and risk for addiction. In al'Absi, M. (ed), *Stress and addiction: Biological and psychological mechanisms.* London, UK: Elsevier, Ltd.

Epping-Jordan, M. P., Watkins, S. S., Koob, G. F., and Markou, A. (1998). Dramatic decreases in brain reward function during nicotine withdrawal. *Nature, 393*, 76–79.

Erb, S. (2007). Neurobiology of stress and risk for relapse. In al'Absi, M. (ed), *Stress and addiction: Biological and psychological mechanisms.* London, UK: Elsevier, Ltd.

Erb, S., Shaham Y., and Stewart, J. (2001). Stress-induced relapse to drug seeking in the rat: Role of the bed nucleus of the stria terminalis and amygdala. *Stress, 4*, 289–303.

Etter, J. F., Prokhorov, A. V., and Perneger, T. V. (2002). Gender differences in the psychological determinants of cigarette smoking. *Addiction, 97(6)*, 733–743.

Federenko, I. S., Nagamine, M., Hellhammer, D. H., Wadha, P. D., and Wust, S. (2004). The heritability of hypothalamus pituitary adrenal axis responses to psychosocial stress is context dependent. *J Clin Endocrinol Metab, 89*, 6244–6250.

Feine, J., Bushnell, M., and Miron, D. (1991). Sex differences in the perception of noxious heat stimuli. *Pain, 44*, 255–262.

Ferin, M. (1989). The role of endogenous opioid peptides in the regulation of the menstrual cycle. *J Steroid Biochem, 33*, 683–685.

Fillingim, R. B., Maixner, W., Girdler, S. S., Light, K. C., Harris, M. B., Sheps, D. S., and Mason, G. A. (1997). Ischemic but not thermal pain sensitivity varies across the menstrual cycle. *Psychosom Med, 59*, 512–520.

Fillmore, M. T., and Rush, C. R. (2002). Impaired inhibitory control of behavior in chronic cocaine users. *Drug Alcohol Depend, 66*, 265–273.

Foley, D. L., Eaves, L. J., Wormley, B., Silberg, J. L., Maes, H. H., Kuhn, J., and Riley, B. (2004). Childhood adversity, monoamine oxidase a genotype, and risk for conduct disorder. *Arch Gen Psychiatry, 61,* 738–744.

Fox, H. C., Talih, M., Malison, R., Anderson, G. M., Kreek, M. J., and Sinha, R. (2005). Frequency of recent cocaine and alcohol use affects drug craving and associated responses to stress and drug-related cues. *Psychoneuroendocrinology, 30,* 880–891.

Frye, C. A., Cuevas, C. A., and Kanarek, R. B. (1993). Diet and estrous cycle influence pain sensitivity in rats. *Pharmacol Biochem Behav, 45,* 255–260.

Gianoulakis, C. (1996). Implications of endogenous opioids and dopamine in alcoholism: Human and basic science studies. *Alcohol Alcohol Suppl, 1,* 33–42.

Gianoulakis, C., Dai, X., Thavundayil, J., and Brown, T. (2005). Levels and circadian rhythmicity of plasma ACTH, cortisol, and beta-endorphin as a function of family history of alcoholism. *Psychopharmacology (Berl), 181,* 437–444.

Girdler, S. S., Maixner, W., Naftel, H. A., Stewart, P. W., Moretz, R. L., and Light, K. C. (2005). Cigarette smoking, stress-induced analgesia and pain perception in men and women. *Pain, 114,* 372–385.

Glass, D. C., Reim, B., and Singer, J. E. (1971). Behavioral consequences of adaptation to controllable and uncontrollable noise. *J Exp Soc Psychol, 7,* 244–257.

Goeders, N. E. (2007). The hypothalamic-pituitary-adrenal axis and addiction. In al'Absi, M. (ed), *Stress and addiction: Biological and psychological mechanisms.* London, UK: Elsevier, Ltd.

Gonzalez Castro, F., Barrington, E. H., Walton, M. A., and Rawson, R. A. (2000). Cocaine and methamphetamine: Differential addiction rates. *Psychol Addict Behav, 14,* 390–396.

Grimm, J. W., and See, R. E. (1997). Cocaine self-administration in ovariectomized rats is predicted by response to novelty, attenuated by 17-beta estradiol, and associated with abnormal vaginal cytology. *Physiol Behav, 61,* 755–761.

Grunberg, N. E., Winders, S. E., and Wewers, M. E. (1991). Gender differences in tobacco use. *Health Psychol, 10,* 143–153.

Hammer, R. P., Jr. (1985). The sex hormone-dependent development of opiate receptors in the rat medial preoptic area. *Brain Res, 360(1–2),* 65–74.

Hammer, R. P., Jr, Zhou, L., and Cheung, S. (1994). Gonadal steroid hormones and hypothalamic opioid circuitry. *Horm Behav, 28(4),* 431–437.

Harrison, P. A., Fulkerson, J. A., and Beebe, T. J. (1997). Multiple substance use among adolescent physical and sexual abuse victims. *Child Abuse Neglect, 21,* 529–539.

Hernandez-Avila, C. A., Oncken, C., Van, K. J., Wand, G, and Kranzler, H. R. (2002). Adrenocorticotropin and cortisol responses to a naloxone challenge and risk of alcoholism. *Biol. Psychiatry, 51,* 652–658.

Hernandez-Avila, C. A., Wand, G., Luo, X., Gelernter, J., and Kranzler, H. R. (2003). Association between the cortisol response to opioid blockade and the Asn40Asp polymorphism at the mu-opioid receptor locus (OPRM1). *Am J. Med Genet B Neuropsychiatr Genet, 118,* 60–65.

Higley, J. D., Thompson, W. N., Champoux, M., Goldman, D., Hasert, M. F., Kraemer, G. W., Scanlon, J. M., Suomi, S. J., and Linnoila, M. (1993). Paternal and maternal genetic and environmental contributions to cerebrospinal fluid monoamine metabolites in rhesus monkeys (Macaca mulatta). *Arch Gen Psychiatry, 50,* 615–623.

Hockey, G. R. J. (1970). Effect of loud noise on attentional selectivity. *Q J Exp Psychol, 22,* 28–36.

Hyman, S. E., and Malenka, R. C. (2001). Addiction and the brain: The neurobiology of compulsion and its persistence. *Nat Rev Neurosci, 2,* 695–703.

Imperato, A., Angelucci, L., Casolini, P., Zocchi, A., and Puglisi-Allegra, S. (1992). Repeated stressful experiences differently affect limbic dopamine release during and following stress. *Brain Res, 577,* 194–199.

Imperato, A., Puglisi-Allegra, S., Casolini, P., and Angelucci, L. (1991). Changes in brain dopamine and acetylcholine release during and following stress are independent of the pituitary-adrenocortical axis. *Brain Res., 538,* 111–117.

Iuvone, P. M., Morasco, J., and Dunn, A. J. (1977). Effect of corticosterone on the synthesis of [3H]catecholamines in the brains of CD-1 mice. *Brain Res., 120,* 571–576.

Jensen, R., Rasmussen, B., and Pedersen, B. (1992). Cephalic muscle tenderness and pressure pain threshold in a general population. *Pain, 48,* 197–203.

Jentsch, J. D., and Taylor, J. R. (1999). Impulsivity resulting from frontostriatal dysfunction in drug abuse: Implications for the control of behavior by reward-related stimuli. *Psychopharmacology, 146,* 373–390.

Johnston, L. D., O'Malley, P. M., Bachman, J. G., and Schulenberg, J. E. (2004). *Monitoring the future national results on adolescent drug use: Overview of key findings, 2004.* Bethesda, MD: National Institute on Drug Abuse.

Kabbaj, M., Devine, D. P., Savage, V. R., and Akil, H. (2000). Neurobiological correlates of individual differences in novelty-seeking behavior in the rat: Differential expression of stress-related molecules. *J Neurosci., 20,* 6983–6988.

Kalivas, P. W., and Duffy, P. (1995). Selective activation of dopamine transmission in the shell of the nucleus accumbens by stress. *Brain Res, 675,* 325–328.

Kalivas, P. W., Pierce, R. C., Cornish, J., and Sorg, B. A. (1998). A role for sensitization in craving and relapse in cocaine addiction. *J Psychopharmacol, 12,* 49–53.

Kandel, D., Chen, K., Warner, L. A., Kessler, R. C., and Grant, B. (1997). Prevalence and demographic correlates of symptoms of last year dependence on alcohol, nicotine, marijuana and cocaine in the U.S. population. *Drug Alcohol Depend, 44,* 11–29.

Kaplan, H. B., and Johnson, R. J. (1992). Relationships between circumstances surrounding initial illicit drug use and escalation of use: Moderating effects of gender and early adolescent experiences. In Glantz M., Pickens R. (eds), *Vulnerability to drug abuse.* pp. 299–358. Washington, D.C. American Psychological Association.

Kassel, J. D., Veilleux, J. C., Wardle, M. C., Yates, M. C., Greenstein, J. E., Evatt, D. P., and Roesch, L. L. (2007). Negative affect and addiction. In al'Absi, M. (ed), *Stress and addiction: Biological and psychological mechanisms.* London, UK: Elsevier, Ltd.

Kenford, S. L., Smith, S. S., Wetter, D. W., Jorenby, D. E., Fiore, M. C., and Baker, T. B. (2002). Predicting relapse back to smoking: Contrasting affective and physical models of dependence. *J Consult Clin Psychol, 70,* 216–227.

Kirby, K. N., and Petry, N. M. (2004). Heroin and cocaine abusers have higher discount rates for delayed rewards than alcoholics or non-drug-using controls. *Addiction, 99,* 461–471.

Knuth, E. D., and Etgen, A. M. (2005). Corticosterone secretion induced by chronic isolation in neonatal rats is sexually dimorphic and accompanied by elevated ACTh. *Hormones and Behavior, 47,* 65–75.

Koob, G. F., and Heinrichs, S. C. (1999). A role for corticotropin releasing factor and urocortin in behavioral responses to stressors. *Brain Res, 848(1–2),* 141–152.

Kosten, T. A., and Kehoe, P. (2007). Early life stress and vulnerability to addiction. In al'Absi, M. (ed), *Stress and addiction: Biological and psychological mechanisms.* London, UK: Elsevier, Ltd.

Kosten, T. A., Miserendino, M. J. D., Bombace, J. C., Lee H. J., and Kim, J. J. (2005). Sex-selective effects of neonatal isolation on fear conditioning and foot shock sensitivity. *Behavioural Brain Research, 157,* 235–244.

Kosten, T. A., Miserendino, M. J. D., and Kehoe, P. (2000). Enhanced acquisition of cocaine self-administration in adult rats with neonatal isolation stress experience. *Brain Research, 875,* 44–50.

Kreek, M. J., and Koob, G. F. (1998). Drug dependence: Stress and dysregulation of brain reward pathways. *Drug Alcohol Depend, 51,* 23–47.

Kudielka, B. M., and Kirschbaum, C. (2007). Biological bases of the stress response. In al'Absi, M. (ed), *Stress and addiction: Biological and psychological mechanisms.* London, UK: Elsevier, Ltd.

Kuhn, C., and Francis, R. (1997). Gender differences in cocaine-induced HPA axis activation. *Neuropsychopharmacology, 16,* 399–407.

Lerman, C., Wileyto, E. P., Patterson, F., Rukstalis, M., Audrain-McGovern, J., Restine, S., Shields, P. G., Kaufmann, V., Redden, D., Benowitz, N., and Berrettini, WH. (2004). The functional mu opioid receptor (OPRM1) Asn40Asp variant predicts short-term response to nicotine replacement therapy in a clinical trial. *Pharmacogenomics J, 4,* 184–192.

Lovallo, W. R. (2007). Individual differences in response to stress and risk for addiction. In al'Absi, M. (ed),

Stress and addiction: Biological and psychological mechanisms. London, UK: Elsevier, Ltd.

Maixner, W., and Humphrey, C. (1993). Gender differences in pain and cardiovascular responses to forearm ischemia. *The Clinical Journal of Pain, 2,* 16–25.

Marinelli, M. (2007). Dopaminergic reward pathways and effects of stress. In al'Absi, M. (ed), *Stress and addiction: Biological and psychological mechanisms.* London, UK: Elsevier, Ltd.

Marinelli, M., Aouizerate, B., Barrot, M., Le Moal, M., and Piazza P. V. (1998). Dopamine-dependent responses to morphine depend on glucocorticoid receptors. *Proc Natl Acad Sci U. S. A., 95,* 7742–7747.

McCown, W. (1990). The effect of impulsivity and empathy on abstinence of poly-substance abusers: A prospective study. *British Journal of Addictions, 85,* 635–637.

McFall, M. E., Mackay, P. W., and Donovan, D. M. (1992). Combat-related posttraumatic stress disorder and severity of substance abuse in Vietnam veterans. *J. Stud. Alcohol., 53,* 357–363.

McFarland, K., Davidge, S. B., Lapish, C. C., and Kalivas, P. W. (2004). Limbic and motor circuitry underlying footshock-induced reinstatement of cocaine seeking behavior. *Journal of Neuroscience, 24,* 1551–1560.

McKay, J. R., Rutherford, M. J., Alterman, A. I., Cacciola, J. S., and Kaplan, M. R. (1995). An examination of the cocaine relapse process. *Drug and Alcohol Dependence, 38,* 35–43.

Miller, G. M., Bendor, J., Tiefenbacher, S., Yang, H., Novak, M. A., and Madras, B. K. (2004). A mu-opioid receptor single nucleotide polymorphism in rhesus monkey: Association with stress response and aggression. *Mol Psychiatry, 9,* 99–108.

Mitchell, S. H. (1999). Measures of impulsivity in cigarette smokers and non-smokers. *Psychopharmacology, 146,* 455–464.

Mittleman, G., Blaha, C. D., and Phillips, A. G. (1992). Pituitary-adrenal and dopaminergic modulation of schedule-induced polydipsia: Behavioral and neurochemical evidence. *Behav. Neurosci., 106,* 408–420.

Monterosso, J. R., Aron, A. R., Cordova, X., Xu, J., and London, ED. (2005). Deficits in response inhibition associated with chronic methamphetamine abuse. *Drug Alcohol Depend, 79,* 273–277.

Monti, P. M., Abrams, D. B., Kadden, R. M., and Cooney, N. L. (1989). *Treating alcohol dependence: A coping skills training guide.* New York: Guilford Press.

Muraven, M., and Baumeister, R. F. (2000). Self-regulation and depletion of limited resources: Does self-control resemble a muscle? *Psychol Bull, 126,* 247–259.

Najavits, L. M., Gastfriend, D. R., Barber, J. P., Reif, S., Muenz, L. R., Blaine, J., Frank, A., Crits-Christoph, Z., Thase, M., and Weiss, R. D. (1998). Cocaine dependence with and without PTSD among subjects in the National Institute on Drug Abuse Collaborative

Cocaine Treatment Study. *American Journal of Psychiatry, 155*, 214–219.

National Institute on Drug Abuse. (1994). *Capsules, women and drug abuse*, 6, 2.

Nemeroff, C. B., Widerlov, E., Bissette, G., Walleus, H., Karlsson, I., Eklund, K., Kilts, C. D., Loosen, P. T., and Vale, W. (1984). Elevated concentations of CSF corticotropin-releasing factor-like immunoreactivity in depressed patients. *Science, 226*, 1342–1344.

Newton-Taylor, B., DeWit, D., and Gliksman, L. (1998). Prevalence and factors associated with physical and sexual assault of female university students in Ontario. *Health Care Women Int., 19*, 155–164.

O'Malley, S. S., Krishnan-Sarin, S., Farren, C., Sinha, R., and Kreek, M. J. (2002). Naltrexone decreases craving and alcohol self-administration in alcohol-dependent subjects and activates the hypothalamo-pituitary-adrenocortical axis. *Psychopharmacology (Berl), 160*, 19–29.

Ortiz, J., DeCaprio, J. L., Kosten, T. A., and Nestler, E. J. (1995). Strain-selective effects of corticosterone on locomotor sensitization to cocaine and on levels of tyrosine hydroxylase and glucocorticoid receptor in the ventral tegmental area. *Neuroscience, 67*, 383–397.

Oslin, D. W., Berrettini, W., Kranzler, H. R., Pettinati, H., Gelernter, J., Volpicelli, J. R., and O'Brien, C. P. (2003). A functional polymorphism of the mu-opioid receptor gene is associated with naltrexone response in alcohol-dependent patients. *Neuropsychopharmacology, 28*, 1546–1552.

Oswald, L. M., Zandi, P., Nestadt, G., Potash, J. B., Kalaydjian, A. E., and Wand, G. S. (2006). Relationship between cortisol responses to stress and personality. *Neuropsychopharmacology* [Epub ahead of print].

Overton, P. G., Tong, Z. Y., Brain, P. F., and Clark, D. (1996). Preferential occupation of mineralocorticoid receptors by corticosterone enhances glutamate-induced burst firing in rat midbrain dopaminergic neurons. *Brain Res., 737*, 146–154.

Parrott, A. (1999). Does cigarette smoking cause stress? *American Psychologist, 54*, 817–820.

Parvez, H., and Parvez, S. (1973). The regulation of monoamine oxidase activity by adrenal cortical steroids. *Acta Endocrinol (Copenh), 73*, 509–517.

Patkar, A. A., Murray, H. W., Mannelli, P., Gottheil, E., Weinstein, S. P., and Vergare, M. J. (2004). Pre-treatment measures of impulsivity, aggression and sensation seeking are associated with treatment outcome for African-American cocaine-dependent patients. *Journal of Addictive Disorders, 23*, 109–122.

Perkins, K. A. (1999). Nicotine discrimination in men and women [In Process Citation]. *Pharmacol Biochem Behav, 64*, 295–299.

Piaza, P. V., Barrot, M., Rouge-Pont, F., Marinelli, M., Maccari, S., Abrou, D. N., Simon, H., and Le Moal, M. (1996). Suppression of glucocorticoid secretion and antipsychotic drugs have similar effects on the mesolimbic dopaminergic transmission. *Proc Natl Acad Sci U.S.A., 93*, 15445-15450.

Piazza, P. V., Deminiere, J. M., Maccari, S., Mormede, P., Le Moal, M., and Simon, H. (1990). Individual reactivity to novelty predicts probability of amphetamine self-administration. *Behav. Pharmacol., 1*, 339–345.

Piazza, P. V., and Le, M. M. (1998). The role of stress in drug self-administration. *Trends Pharmacol. Sci., 19*, 67–74.

Piazza, P. V., Maccari, S, Deminiere, J. M., Le Moal, M., Mormede, P., and Simon, H. (1991). Corticosterone levels determine individual vulnerability to amphetamine self-administration. *Proc. Natl. Acad. Sci. U. S. A., 88*, 2088–2092.

Plotsky, P. M., and Meaney, M. J. (1993). Early postnatal experience alters hypothalamic corticotropin-releasing factor (CRF) mRNA, median eminence CRF content, and stress induced release in adult rats. *Mol Brain Res, 18*, 195–200.

Ratka, A., and Simpkins, J. W. (1991). Effects of estradiol and progesterone on the sensitivity to pain and on morphine-induced antinociception in female rats. *Horm Behav, 25*, 217–228.

Reynolds, B. (2004). Do high rates of cigarette consumption increase delay discounting? A cross-sectional comparison of adolescent smokers and young-adult smokers and nonsmokers. *Behavioral Processes, 67*, 545–549.

Robbins, T. W., and Everitt, B. J. (1996). Neurobehavioral mechanisms of reward and motivation. *Curr Opin Neurobiol, 6*, 228–236.

Roberts, M. E., Moore, S. D., and Beckham, J. C. (2007). PTSD and substance use disorders. In al'Absi, M. (ed), *Stress and addiction: Biological and psychological mechanisms*. London, UK: Elsevier, Ltd.

Robinson, T. E., and Berridge, K. C. (2003). Addiction. *Annu Rev Psychol, 54*, 25–53.

Rubin, R. T., Poland, R. E., Lesser, I. M., Winston, R. A., and Blodgett, N. (1987). Neuroendocrine aspects of primary endogenous depression I. Cortisol secretory dynamics in patients and matched controls. *Arch Gen Psychiatry, 44*, 328–336.

Saal, D., Dong, Y., Bonci, A., and Malenka, R. C. (2003). Drugs of abuse and stress trigger a common synaptic adaptation in dopamine neurons. *Neuron, 37*, 577–582.

Saal, D., and Nemeroff, C. B. (2007). Novel pharmacologic treatment of stress and addiction: The role of CRF and glucocorticoid antagonists. In al'Absi, M. (ed), *Stress and addiction: Biological and psychological mechanisms*. London, UK: Elsevier, Ltd.

Salamone, J. D. (1994). The involvement of nucleus accumbens dopamine in appetitive and aversive motivation. *Behav. Brain Res., 61*, 117–133.

Salo, R., Nordahl, T. E., Moore, C., Waters, C., Natsuaki, Y., Galloway, G. P., Kile, S., and Sullivan, E. V. (2005). A dissociation in attentional control: Evidence from methamphetamine dependence. *Biol Psychiatry, 57*, 310–313.

Sapolsky, R. M., Alberts, S. C., and Altman, J. (1997). Hypercortisolism associated with social subordinance or social isolation among wild baboons. *Arch Gen Psychiatry, 54,* 1137–1143.

Schenk, S., Lacelle, G., Gorman, K., and Amit, Z. (1987). Cocaine selfadministration in rats influenced by environmental conditions: Implications for the etiology of drug abuse. *Neurosci Lett, 81,* 227–231.

Semple, S. J., Zians, J., Grant, L., and Patterson, T. L. (2005). Impulsivity and methamphetamine use. *Journal of Substance Abuse Treatment, 29,* 85–93.

Sershen, H., Hashim, A., and Lajtha, A. (1998). Gender differences in kappa-opioid modulation of cocaine-induced behavior and NMDA-evoked dopamine release. *Brain Res, 801(1–2),* 67–71.

Shiffman, S, Hickcox, M., Paty, J. A., Gnys, M., Kassel, J. D., and Richards, T. J. (1996). Progression from a smoking lapse to relapse: Prediction from abstinence violation effects, nicotine dependence, lapse characteristics. *J Consult Clin Psychol, 64,* 993–1002.

Simon, S. L., Domier, C., Carnell, J., Brethen, P., Rawson, R., and Ling, W. (2000). Cognitive impairment in individuals currently using methamphetamine. *Am J Addict, 9,* 222–231.

Sinha, R. (2001). How does stress increase risk of drug abuse and relapse? *Psychopharmacology, 158,* 343–359.

Sinha, R., Catapano, D., and O'Malley, S. (1999). Stress-induced craving and stress response in cocaine dependent individuals. *Psychopharmacology, 142,* 343–351.

Sircar, R., Mallinson, K., Goldbloom, L. M., and Kehoe, P. (2001). Postnatal stress selectively upregulates striatal N-methyl-D-aspartate receptors in male rats. *Brain Research, 904,* 145–148.

Snoek, H., Van Goozen, S. H., Matthys, W., Buitelaar, J. K., and van Engeland, H. (2004). Stress responsivity in children with externalizing behavior disorders. *Dev Psychopathol, 16,* 389–406.

Staley, J. K., Krishnan-Sarin, S., Zoghbi, S., Tamagnan, G., Fujita, M., Seibyl, J. P., Maciejewski, P. K., O'Malley, S., and Innis, R. B. (2001). Sex differences in [123I]beta-CIT SPECT measures of dopamine and serotonin transporter availability in healthy smokers and nonsmokers. *Synapse, 41,* 275–284.

Steptoe, A., and Hamer, M. (2007). Psychosocial determinants of the stress response. In al'Absi, M. (ed), Stress and addiction: Biological and psychological mechanisms. London, UK: Elsevier, Ltd.

Stewart, J., de Wit, H., and Eikelboom, R. (1984). The role of unconditioned and conditioned drug effects in the self-administration of opiates and stimulants. *Psychol Rev, 91,* 251–268.

Swan, G. E., Ward, M. M., Jack, L. M., and Javitz, H. S. (1993). Cardiovascular reactivity as a predictor of relapse in male and female smokers. *Health Psychol, 12,* 451–458.

Tate, S. R., Patterson, K. A., Nagel, B. J., Anderson, K. G. and Brown, S. A. (2007). Addiction and stress in adolescents. In al'Absi, M. (ed), *Stress and addiction: Biological and psychological mechanisms.* London, UK: Elsevier, Ltd.

Thompson, P. M., Hayashi, K. M., Simon, S. L., Geaga, J. A., Hong, M. S., Sui, Y, Lee, J. Y., Toga, A. W., Ling, W., and London E. D. (2004). Structural abnormalities in the brains of human subjects who use methamphetamine. *J Neurosci, 24,* 6028–6036.

Ungless, M. A., Singh, V., Crowder, T. L., Yaka, R., Ron, D., and Bonci, A. (2003). Corticotropin-releasing factor requires CRF binding protein to potentiate NMDA receptors via CRF receptor 2 in dopamine neurons. *Neuron, 39,* 401–407.

Veals, J. W., Korduba, C. A., and Symchowicz, S. (1977). Effect of dexamethasone on monoamine oxidase inhibiton by iproniazid in rat brain. *Eur J Pharmacol., 41,* 291–299.

Volkow, N. D., Chang, L., Wang, G. J., Fowler, J. S., Franceschi, D., Sedler, M. J., Gatley, S. J., Hitzemann, R, Ding, Y. S., Wong, C, and Logan, J. (2001) Higher cortical and lower subcortical metabolism in detoxified methamphetamine abusers. *Am J Psychiatry, 158,* 383–389.

Wallace, B. C (1989). Psychological and environmental determinants of relapse in crack cocaine smokers. *J Subst Abuse Treat, 6,* 95–106.

Wand, G. S., Mangold, D., El, D. S., McCaul, M. E., and Hoover, D. (1998). Family history of alcoholism and hypothalamic opioidergic activity. *Arch Gen Psychiatry, 55,* 1114–1119.

Wand, G. S., McCaul, M., Yang, X., Reynolds, J., Gotjen, D, Lee, S, and Ali, A. (2002). The mu-opioid receptor gene polymorphism (A118G) alters HPA axis activation induced by opioid receptor blockade. *Neuropsychopharmacology, 26,* 106–114.

Wand, G. S., McCaul, M. E., Gotjen, D., Reynolds, J., and Lee, S. (2001). Confirmation that offspring from families with alcohol-dependent individuals have greater hypothalamic-pituitary-adrenal axis activation induced by naloxone compared with offspring without a family history of alcohol dependence. *Alcohol Clin. Exp. Res., 25,* 1134–1139.

Wang, B., Shaham, Y., Zitzman, D., Azari, S, Wise, R. A., and You, Z.B. (2005). Cocaine experience establishes control of midbrain glutamate and dopamine by corticotropin-releasing factor: A role in stress-induced relapse to drug seeking. *J Neurosci, 25(22),* 5389–5396.

Wechsberg, W. M., Craddock, S. G., and Hubbard, R. L. (1998). How are women who enter substance abuse treatment different than men? A gender comparison from the Drug Abuse Treatment Outcome Study (DATOS). *Drugs and Society, 13,* 97–115.

Wetter, D. W., Kenford, S. L., Smith, S. S., Fiore, M. C., Jorenby, D. E., and Baker, T. B. (1999). Gender differences in smoking cessation. *J Consult Clin Psychol, 67,* 555–562

White, J. L., Moffitt, T. E., Caspi, A., Bartusch, D. J., Needles, D. J., and Stouthamer-Loeber, M. (1994).

Measuring impulsivity and examining its relationship to delinquency. *Journal of Abnormal Psychology, 103*, 192–205.

Widom, C. S., Weiler, B. L., and Cottler, L. B. (1999). Childhood victimization and drug abuse: A comparison of prospective and retrospective findings. *J Consult Clin Psychol, 67*, 867–880.

Wills, T. A., McNamara, G, Vaccaro, D., and Hirky, A. E. (1996). Escalated substance use: A longitudinal grouping analysis from early to middle adolescence. *J Abnorm Psychol, 105*, 166–180.

Wills, T. A., and Stoolmiller, M. (2002). The role of self-control in early escalation of substance use: A time-varying analysis. *Journal of Consulting & Clinical Psychology, 70*, 986–997.

Wilsnack, S. C., Vogeltanz, N. D., Klassen, A. D., and Harris, T. R. (1997). Childhood sexual abuse and women's substance abuse: National survey findings. *J Stud Alcohol, 58*, 264–271.

Winfield I, George, L. K., Swartz, M., and Blazer, D. G. (1990). Sexual assault and psychiatric disorders among a community sample of women. *Am J Psychiatry, 147*, 335–341.

Wust, S., Federenko, I., Hellhammer, D. H., and Kirschbaum, C. (2000). Genetic factors, perceived chronic stress, the free cortisol response to awakening. *Psychoneuroendocrinology, 25*, 707–720.

Wust, S., van Rossum, E. F., Federenko, I. S., Koper, J. W., Kumsta, R., and Hellhammer, D.H. (2004). Common polymorphisms in the glucocorticoid receptor gene are associated with adrenocortical responses to psychosocial stress. *J Clin Endocrinol Metab, 89*, 565–573.

Zhang, X. Y., Sanchez, H., Kehoe, P., and Kosten, T. A. (2005). Neonatal isolation enhances maintenance but not reinstatement of cocaine self-administration in adult male rats. *Psychopharmacology, 177*, 391–399.

Zubieta, J. K., Dannals, R. F., and Frost, J. J. (1999). Gender and age influences on human brain mu-opioid receptor binding measured by PET. *Am J Psychiatry, 156(6)*, 842–848.

Zubieta, J. K., Smith, Y. R., Bueller, J. A., Xu, Y., Kilbourn, M. R., Jewett, D. M et al. (2002). Mu-opioid receptor-mediated antinociceptive responses differ in men and women. *J Neurosci, 22(12)*, 5100–5107.

Subject Index

Author Index

Aarons, G.A., 129, 187, 252, 259, 262, 296, 299
Abdullah, L., 102, 103, 145
Abela, J.R., 186
Abelson, J.A., 146
Abelson, M.L., 100
Abercrombie, E.D., 44, 54, 67, 72, 75
Abrahms, K., 303, 304, 313
Abrams, D., 187, 303, 314
Abrams, D.B., 357, 365, 369
Abrams, K., 312
Abrams, M., 270, 272, 282
Abrantes, A., 261
Abrantes, A.M., 232, 248
Abrous, 369
Abrous, D., 165
Abrous, D.N., 68, 78, 365
Abrous, N., 36
Abueg, F., 325, 326
Acierno, R., 261, 316, 317, 319, 326, 329
Ackl, N., 344, 347
Acquas, E., 71
Adam, A., 142
Adams, C.E., 80
Adams, D., 144
Adams, M.L., 88, 97
Adams, R.N., 69, 79, 83
Adell, A., 43, 67
Ader, R., 111, 120, 281
Adinoff, B., 22, 23, 48, 35, 67, 130, 139, 195,
    209, 230, 231, 242, 244, 338, 339, 343, 353
Adkins, A., 205, 209
Adlaf, E.M., 259
Adson, D.E., 208
Advis, J.P., 98

Aghajanian, G.K., 47, 51, 61, 67, 69, 73, 74
Agnati, L.F., 73, 121
Agrawal, A., 174, 184
Aguilar-Gaziola, S., 144, 313
Aharoni, S., 142
Ahmed, S.H., 28, 35, 108, 120, 148, 151, 162, 166,
    181, 182, 184, 230, 242, 244, 361, 365
Ahrens, C., 330
Ainette, M.G., 262
Aitken, D.H., 124
Akana, S.F., 70
Akerstedt, T., 276, 280, 281
Akil, H., 16, 74, 79, 86, 97, 100, 101, 162, 163, 340,
    345, 368
Akirav, I., 42, 67
al'Absi, M., 16, 234, 238, 244, 274, 353, 355, 356,
    358, 360, 365, 367, 368, 370
Alarcon, M., 98
Albala, A.A., 365
Albaugh, B., 140, 141
Alberts, S.C., 370
Albrecht, S., 99
Alcaro, A., 146
Alexander, B.K., 352, 365
Alexander, D.M., 38
Alheid, G.F., 152, 160, 162
Ali, A., 146, 370
Ali, M., 103
Ali, R.L., 328
Alikaridis, F., 124
Allain, A.N., 331
Allan, C.A., 268, 280
Allen, A., 197, 208
Allen, B.A., 286, 291, 300

Beckman, J.C., 327
Beebe, T.J., 122, 367
Begleiter, H., 140, 141
Beites, F.J., 193, 209
Beitman, B.D., 313
Belfer, I., 138, 140
Beliveau, D., 99
Belknap, J.K., 100
Bell, G.I., 86, 102
Bell, H., 287, 298
Bell, V., 37
Beltramino, C.A., 162
Belzung, C., 108, 120
Bencherif, B., 90, 98, 99
Bendor, J., 144, 368
Benes, F.M., 42, 68
Bengel, D., 143
Bengoechea, T.G., 76
Beninger, R.J., 102
Benjamin, D., 88, 98
Benjamin, J., 143
Benke, D., 143
Benkelfat, C., 75, 101
Bennet, A., 142
Bennete, M.C., 71
Bennett, B., 141
Bennett, J.A., 80
Bennett, J.P., Jr., 79
Benowitz, N., 143, 368
Ben-Shahar, O., 40, 82
Ben-Shlomo, Y., 144
Bensley, 352
Bensley, L.S., 119, 120
Benson, J.A., 143
Bentgen, K.M., 80
Benwell, M.E., 44, 68
Berendse, H.W., 73
Berga, S.L., 11, 15
Bergen, A.W., 95, 97, 98, 134, 140
Berger, S., 18
Bergeron, R., 330
Bergerson, R., 247
Bergman, J., 107, 120
Bergstrom, B.P., 72
Berke, J.D., 120, 162
Berkson, J., 305, 312
Berlin, J., 141
Berlinguet, L., 74
Berman, S.M., 185
Bernardi, G., 68, 72, 77
Bernardini, R., 14, 15, 19
Bernardy, N.C., 231, 233, 245
Berney, T.G., 345

Berns, G.S., 334, 343, 345
Bernston, G., 224
Berntson, G.G., 175, 185
Berrendero, F., 134, 140
Berrettini, W., 102, 144, 369
Berrettini, W.H., 72, 98, 100, 143, 368
Berridge, C.W., 68, 106, 121
Berridge, K.C., 48, 79, 116, 125, 177, 187, 334, 343, 346, 360, 369
Berry, M.S., 345
Berry, R., 166
Bertolucci-D'Angio, M., 54, 55, 68
Berton, O., 140
Besedovsky, H.O., 14, 15
Bespalov, A.Y., 68
Besser, G.M., 92, 100
Best, C., 326
Best, C.L., 261, 329, 330
Betito, K., 18
Bettschen, D., 124
Beurrier, C., 346
Beuten, J., 241, 245
Beyer, A., 95, 98
Beyer, C.E., 81
Bhatnagar, S., 18, 123
bi-Dargham, A., 101
Bienvenu, O.J., 37, 328
Bierut, L.J., 129, 140
Bigelow, G.E., 149, 162, 165
Bijl, R., 144, 313
Bilkei-Gorzo, A., 145
Bilsky, E.J., 102
Binder-Brynes, K., 331
Bingham, C.R., 260
Binnekade, R., 163
Biondi, M., 5, 11, 12, 15
Birch, C.D., 295, 298
Bird, C., 99
Birmaher, B., 283
Birman, S., 66, 68
Bíró, É., 39, 125, 165
Biron, C.A., 17
Bisighini, R., 365
Bissette, G., 142, 343, 344, 369
Bjijou, Y., 334, 343
Bjorklund, A., 70
Black, C.A., 67, 120
Blackledge, J.T., 325, 327
Blackson, T., 189
Blaha, C.D., 77, 121, 369
Blaine, J., 124, 369
Blakely, R.D., 141
Blanc, G., 53, 68, 73, 75, 81

Datla, K., 74
Daunais, J.B., 91, 99
Dautzenberg, F.M., 336, 337, 344
Davey Smith, G., 213, 223
David, V., 334, 344
Davidge, S.B., 124, 164, 368
Davidson, D., 91, 99
Davidson, J.R.T., 319, 327, 328
Davidson, R.J., 205, 207
Davies, B.M., 365
Davies, J.B., 252, 261, 267, 282
Davies, M., 300
Davila, V., 61, 70
Davis, C.G., 142
Davis, C.S., 286, 298
Davis, G., 327, 365
Davis, G.C., 36, 327
Davis, G.L., 365
Davis, H., 224, 248
Davis, J.M., 37
Davis, M., 154, 160, 162, 164, 228, 245
Davis, S.L., 120, 365
Davis, T.M., 328
Davis, W.M., 28, 36
Dawes, M., 189
Dawes, M.A., 234, 245, 255, 260, 360, 366
Dawson, D.A., 141, 145, 181, 185
Day, R., 267, 280
Dayan, P., 80
Dayas, C.V., 245, 343
Dayton, M.A., 72
De Arellano, M., 326
de Beurs, E., 195, 208
de Geus, E.J., 140, 225, 365
de Jong, I.E., 59, 70, 231, 245
De Jong, J., 343
de Kloet, E.R., 8, 16, 23, 38, 41, 59, 70, 125, 126,
    131, 141, 229, 231, 245, 247, 359, 366
de la Garza, R., 181, 185
De Luca, M.A., 71
De Montis, M.G., 72, 75, 76
de Olmos, J.S., 154, 162, 163
de Sliva Lobo, D.S., 196, 208
De Souza, E., 162
De Souza, E.B., 37, 159, 163, 328, 345
De Villiers, S., 346
De Vries, J., 273, 281
de Vries, J.B., 72
De Vries, T., 149, 163
De Waele, J.P., 87, 89, 99
de Wit, H., 28, 36, 39, 80, 91, 99, 141, 148, 149,
    163, 166, 177, 188, 346, 370
De, V.J., 103

Deadwyler, S.A., 107, 120
deBeurs, E., 313
DeCaprio, J.L., 77, 123, 369
Decker, P.A., 259
DeDourin, C., 126
Deffenbacher, J.L., 205, 207
Degenhardt, L., 173, 185
Deicke, J., 246
deJong, J., 124
Del Boca, F., 294, 299
Del Boca, F.K., 178, 186, 244, 313
del Rey, A., 15
Delconte, J.D., 102
Delcore, R., Jr., 83
Delfino, R.J., 184, 185
Delfs, J., 166
Delfs, J.M., 65, 70, 154, 160, 162, 163
Delitala, G., 11, 12, 16
Dellu, F., 41, 70
DeLuca, J.W., 179, 186
Delucchi, K.L., 330
Delville, Y., 203, 207
Demaria, P.A., Jr., 98
Dembo, R., 352, 366
DeMichele, A., 141
Deminière, J.M., 23, 36, 38, 39, 71, 78, 108, 113,
    121, 124, 165, 369
Demura, H., 104
Denenberg, V.H., 122
Denollet, J., 270, 273, 281
Denver, R.J.M., 165
Der-Avakian, A., 68
Derevensky, J.L., 196, 208
DeRijk, R., 131, 141, 359, 366
Deroche, V., 42, 57, 65, 70, 71, 78, 80, 165, 334,
    339, 341, 344
Deroche-Gamonet, V., 82
Dertke, M., 366
DeUrrutia, J., 36
Deutch, A.Y., 44, 53, 54, 71, 80, 106, 121
Devine, D.P., 8, 74, 87, 99, 368
DeVries, A.C., 28, 36, 106, 121
DeVries, G.J., 107, 121
deVries, M., 187
DeVry, J., 91, 99
DeWit, D., 39, 369
DeWit, D.J., 144, 313
DeWitte, P., 75
Deykin, E.Y., 316, 317, 319, 328
Dhabhar, F.S., 12, 14, 16, 17
Dhar, V., 37, 38
Di Chiara, G., 43, 48, 50, 56, 69, 71, 73, 79, 162
Di, S., 135, 141

Tischfield, J.A., 98, 140, 365
Tivis, L., 330
Tobe, S.W., 217, 224
Tobler, P.N., 72, 229, 248, 334, 346
Todd, M., 184
Toga, A.W., 40, 370
Tokola, R., 203, 210
Toland, A.M., 287, 300
Tolin, D.F., 198, 200, 201, 207
Tollison, R.D., 188
Tomasi, P., 16
Tomboly, C., 98
Tominaga, T., 18
Tomlinson, K., 179, 187, 261
Tomori, N., 104
Toneatto, T., 308, 310, 314
Toner, B.B., 200, 207
Tong, Z.Y., 77, 369
Tonigan, J.S., 287, 296, 297, 299
Tontoni, A., 142
Toomey, R., 126, 145, 329
Torgersen, S., 319, 320, 331
Torpy, D.J., 26, 40, 347
Torres, E.M., 83
Toru, M., 239, 246
Tosi, H., 282
Toth, G., 98
Toth, Z.E., 145
Totterdell, S., 81
Town, C., 314
Town, T., 95, 102, 103, 145
Townsley-Stemberger, R.M., 199, 209
Tracy, K.A., 205, 208
Tran-Nguyen, L.T., 49, 82, 124
Travis, E.R., 69
Treasure, J., 282
Treiber, F.A., 224
Trell, E., 287, 299
Tremblay, L., 250, 262
Triano, L., 122
Triffleman, E., 325, 331
Trimmel, M., 180, 189
Tronche, F., 76, 82
Troughton, E., 243, 245
Troughton, E.P., 232, 246
Troxel, W.M., 215, 224
True, W., 126, 145, 329, 330
True, W.R., 129, 145, 320, 329, 331
Trujols, J., 100
Trulson, M.E., 57, 80, 82
Tsai, G., 133, 145
Tsai, J., 260
Tsai, T.H., 123

Tsigos, C., 8, 19, 302, 314
Tsigoulis, M., 224
Tsuang, M., 145, 329
Tsuang, M.T., 105, 126, 129, 145
Tsuchiya, K., 74
Tsuda, A., 75
Tsutsumi, A., 220, 224
Tu, W., 189
Tulevski, I.G., 287, 300
Tuomainen, T.P., 142
Tupala, E., 87, 103
Tupler, L.A., 328
Turchan, J., 345
Turiault, M., 60, 76, 82
Turner, L., 180, 189
Turner, N.E., 286, 294, 300
Turner, S.M., 331
Turrina, C., 268, 283
Tutek, D.A., 205, 208
Twining, C., 68
Tyrer, P., 184
Tzschentke, T.M., 336, 346

Uchino, B.N., 220, 224
Uddo, M., 331
Udry, J.R., 261
Ueda, S., 347
Ueki, S., 175, 186
Uhart, M., 94, 98, 103, 140, 234, 248, 366
Uhde, T.W., 124
Uhl, G.R., 100, 145, 146, 241, 248
Uhlenhuth, E., 124
Uhlenhuth, E.H., 36, 40
Uhr, M., 77, 104, 248, 344
Ujike, H., 100
Ulibarri, C., 68, 79, 165
Ullsperger, M., 228, 238, 247
Ulm, R.R., 304, 314
Ungerstedt, U., 44, 74, 77, 81, 83
Ungless, M.A., 47, 58, 59, 62, 82, 155, 166, 336, 337, 338, 341, 342, 347, 354, 364, 370
Unis, A.S., 105, 126
United States Department of Health and Human Services (USDHHS), 176, 189
Unrod, M., 183, 186
Unterwald, E.M., 91, 97, 103
Urn, J.B., 118, 120
Ursano, R.J., 331
Ursin, H., 4, 5, 17
Urwyler, S., 100, 103
Ushiyama, T., 104
Ussher, M., 22, 23, 39
Uusitupa, M.I., 142